AF687519

Dendritic Spines: Modeling, Function and Properties

Dendritic Spines: Modeling, Function and Properties

Editor: Latosha Anderson

AMERICAN
MEDICAL PUBLISHERS
www.americanmedicalpublishers.com

AMERICAN
MEDICAL PUBLISHERS
www.americanmedicalpublishers.com

Cataloging-in-Publication Data

Dendritic spines : modeling, function and properties / edited by Latosha Anderson.
p. cm.
Includes bibliographical references and index.
ISBN 979-8-88740-042-6
1. Dendrites. 2. Neurons. 3. Synapses. 4. Nervous system. 5. Neurology. I. Anderson, Latosha.
QP363 .D46 2023
591.188--dc23

© American Medical Publishers, 2023

American Medical Publishers,
41 Flatbush Avenue,
1st Floor, New York,
NY 11217, USA

ISBN 979-8-88740-042-6 (Hardback)

This book contains information obtained from authentic and highly regarded sources. Copyright for all individual chapters remain with the respective authors as indicated. All chapters are published with permission under the Creative Commons Attribution License or equivalent. A wide variety of references are listed. Permission and sources are indicated; for detailed attributions, please refer to the permissions page and list of contributors. Reasonable efforts have been made to publish reliable data and information, but the authors, editors and publisher cannot assume any responsibility for the validity of all materials or the consequences of their use.

Trademark Notice: Registered trademark of products or corporate names are used only for explanation and identification without intent to infringe.

Contents

Preface

Dendritic spine is a small membranous protrusion from the dendrite of a neuron that takes input from a single axon at the synapse. It serves as a storage site for synaptic strength and it aids in the transmission of electrical signals to the neuron's cell body. In addition to providing an anatomical substrate for synaptic transmission and memory storage, dendritic spines can also increase the number of probable contacts between neurons. Dendritic spines are also hypothesized to have electrical properties, which are studied through the development of modeling techniques. A few of such models are Baer and Rinzel's continuum model, and spike-diffuse-spike model. Abnormalities within the spines can result in cognitive disorders such as ADHD, Alzheimer's disease, autism and intellectual disability. This book is compiled in such a manner, that it will provide in-depth knowledge about the modeling, function and properties of dendritic spines. It is appropriate for students seeking detailed information in this area as well as for experts.

The researches compiled throughout the book are authentic and of high quality, combining several disciplines and from very diverse regions from around the world. Drawing on the contributions of many researchers from diverse countries, the book's objective is to provide the readers with the latest achievements in the area of research. This book will surely be a source of knowledge to all interested and researching the field.

In the end, I would like to express my deep sense of gratitude to all the authors for meeting the set deadlines in completing and submitting their research chapters. I would also like to thank the publisher for the support offered to us throughout the course of the book. Finally, I extend my sincere thanks to my family for being a constant source of inspiration and encouragement.

Editor

1

Endoplasmic reticulum calcium stores in dendritic spines

Menahem Segal * and Eduard Korkotian

Department of Neurobiology, The Weizman Institute, Rehovot, Israel

*Correspondence:
Menahem Segal, Department of Neurobiology, The Weizmann Institute, Rehovot 76100, Israel e-mail: Menahem.segal@weizmann.ac.il

Despite decades of research, the role of calcium stores in dendritic spines structure, function and plasticity is still debated. The reasons for this may have to do with the multitude of overlapping calcium handling machineries in the neuron, including stores, voltage and ligand gated channels, pumps and transporters. Also, different cells in the brain are endowed with calcium stores that are activated by different receptor types, and their differential compartmentalization in dendrites, spines and presynaptic terminals complicates their analysis. In the present review we address several key issues, including the role of calcium stores in synaptic plasticity, their role during development, in stress and in neurodegenerative diseases. Apparently, there is increasing evidence for a crucial role of calcium stores, especially of the ryanodine species, in synaptic plasticity and neuronal survival.

Keywords: dendritic spines, ryanodine receptors, IP3 receptors, STIM, Orai

INTRODUCTION

Dendritic spines are the locus of most excitatory synapses in the forebrain, and are subject to extensive modifications in the process of growth, maturation and aging (Sala and Segal, 2014). The main route for modifying the structure and functions of dendritic spines is through influx of calcium from the extra synaptic space into the dendritic spine, where an excess calcium concentration triggers cascades of molecular events leading to these changes. While the concentration of free intracellular calcium concentration $[Ca^{2+}]_i$ in neurons is very low (in the range of 10–100 nM), about four order of magnitude below the ambient extracellular $[Ca^{2+}]$, some intracellular organelles contain fairly high $[Ca^{2+}]_i$, similar to that of $[Ca^{2+}]$o, and are considered to be "calcium stores". Under certain conditions, the nucleus can contain high concentrations of calcium (Korkotian and Segal, 1996). A more ubiquitous organelle is the mitochondrion, where $[Ca^{2+}]$ can reach 100 μM by pumping it in using a specialized uniporter (Rizzuto et al., 2012). Mitochondrial calcium plays an important role in energy metabolism and cell survival, but will not be dealt with herein. The other organelle containing a high $[Ca^{2+}]_i$ which is considered to be a "calcium store" is the endoplasmic reticulum (ER), which is ubiquitous in dendrites, and is assumed to extend into spines. The first suggestion for a possible calcium store in dendritic spines, and more specifically in the spine apparatus (SA) is that of Fifková et al. (1983) who conducted one of the earliest electron microscopic (EM) studies to find apparent calcium deposits in the dendritic spines, in close association with the SA. They suggested that the SA is a calcium sequestering organelle, which regulates intraspinal calcium concentration during synaptic activity. A later study using three-dimensional reconstruction of dendritic spines (Spacek and Harris, 1997) revealed a continuum of the smooth ER into the SA, where it forms the typical lamellar structure, which may occasionally reach the postsynaptic density (PSD) at the synapse. Thus, there is a putative structure within the dendritic spine, which may serve a role as a calcium store. The identity and putative functions of this store in dendritic spines is currently subject to extensive analysis.

THE IP3 RECEPTOR

The ER calcium stores are activated by two types of receptors, the inositol 1,4,5 trisphosphate receptor (IP3R), and the ryanodine receptor (RyR). The IP3R is of three isoforms, 1–3, and the predominant neuronal one is the IP3R1, whereas the other two are found primarily in non neuronal tissue (Fujino et al., 1995). The RyR, which is activated by low concentrations of ryanodine also has three isoform, RyR1–3, which are found primarily in muscle cells, and are responsible for contraction, but are also found throughout the brain (Galeotti et al., 2008; Kushnir et al., 2010). Both IP3R1 and RyR are distributed across the entire nervous system, with differential distribution in different neuron type and neuronal compartment. EM analysis of the hippocampus indicated that IP3R are present at high concentrations in dendritic shafts and cell bodies, whereas RyR are present primarily in dendritic spines and axons (Sharp et al., 1993). In contrast, GABAergic neurons of the cerebellum contain high concentrations of IP3R, also in dendritic spines. Consequently, IP3Rs were studied extensively in cerebellar purkinje cells (Goto and Mikoshiba, 2011). IP3 stores are important for maintenance of dendritic spine morphology of purkinje cells in the cerebellum (Sugawara et al., 2013). A slow $[Ca^{2+}]_i$ surge, resulting from activation of the IP3-receptors has been described in dendritic spines of cerebellar purkinje cells which may have some functional significance in these dendritic spines (Rose and Konnerth, 2001).

Even though the IP3 receptor is not localized in dendritic spines of hippocampal neurons, its involvement in plastic processes in this structure is well documented. IP3Rs are assumed to mediate the action of acetylcholine (ACh) and other neuromodulators, to cause release of calcium from stores and a subsequent change in AMPA and NMDA receptor functions (Raymond and Redman, 2006; Fernández de Sevilla et al., 2008; Fernández de Sevilla and Buño, 2010). IP3Rs probably mediate the effects of brain derived neurotrophic factor (BDNF) on neuronal plasticity in cultured cortical neurons (Nakata and Nakamura, 2007). One possible mode of involvement of ER in calcium release from IP3 stores has been proposed recently (Holbro et al., 2009); synaptic activation of glutamate receptors could evoke a delayed calcium surge in large spines that was blocked by metabotropic glutamate receptor (mGluR) antagonists and heparin (an antagonist of calcium release from IP3 stores). The role of these delayed calcium surges in synaptic plasticity is not entirely clear. A more direct role of IP3Rs in synaptic functions is indicated by Sala et al. (2005), suggesting that activation of mGluR which are located in dendritic spines, recruits IP3Rs to release calcium from stores, so as to activate calcium-gated K currents, which will modulate the efficacy of the transfer of synaptic currents from the synapse on the spine head to the dendritic shaft.

THE RYANODINE RECEPTOR

The more controversial store is the one associated with the brain RyR (Verkhratsky, 2005; Zalk et al., 2007). There are three isoforms of ryanodine receptors (RyR1–3) that are differentially localized in dendrites and spines of central neurons. Several RyR gene knockdown express specific behavioral phenotypes including an antidepressant effect (Galeotti et al., 2008; Kushnir et al., 2010). Its main attribute is that it is activated by calcium influx into the cell, such that the influx of calcium ions through the plasma membrane is amplified by release of calcium from RyR-associated calcium stores. Caffeine, and low concentration of ryanodine (0.5–1 μM) are agonists for this receptor, and high concentration of ryanodine (100 μM) or cyclopiazonic acid (CPA) are antagonists of the RyR. Initial studies (Mainen et al., 1999; Kovalchuk et al., 2000) were unable to detect an effect of CPA on subthreshold synaptically evoked rise of $[Ca^{2+}]i$ in CA1 neurons of the hippocampus, a response that was shown to be primarily mediated by activation of the NMDA receptor. In contrast, Emptage et al. (1999) demonstrated that release from stores is responsible for the rise of $[Ca^{2+}]i$ that is seen following synaptic activation of CA1 neurons of cultured hippocampal slices in that this rise is completely blocked by CPA or ryanodine, an antagonist of the RyR. Interestingly, they did confirm that blockade of calcium-induced release of calcium from stores prolongs the decay of the calcium rise following back propagating action potential, as seen by Mainen et al. (1999) and Sabatini et al. (2002). All three groups found that the size of the calcium transient associated with an action potential is not affected by CPA. The reasons for the difference in the assumed store involvement in the synaptic calcium rise between the Sabatini/Mainen and the Emptage groups is not entirely clear, and it may have to do with the type of preparation, acute slices vs. cultured slice or the intracellular concentration and affinity of calcium sensor used by the three groups (Fluo-4, low concentration, high affinity dye, vs. high concentration, low affinity Oregon Green dye, in the Sabatini/Mainen and Emptage groups, respectively), as well as the sensitivity of the method of recording/imaging.

The issue remained controversial when Brünig et al. (2004) reported that they could not detect any effect of caffeine on spine motility, unlike the effects of NMDA or AMPA receptor activation. Furthermore, Harvey and Svoboda (2007) could not confirm an involvement of RyR in tetanic stimulation-induced spine head expansion, although Harvey and Collingridge (1992) reported that thapsigargin blocks LTP in hippocampal slices. These observations contrast with the effects of caffeine on $[Ca^{2+}]i$ and spine morphology reported before (Korkotian and Segal, 1999), and the description of the presence of calcium stores in dendritic spines (Harris, 1999). A more recent study supported the link between stores and spines by proposing that the RyR 2 and 3 isoforms mediate the action of BDNF on dendritic spines and on cognitive tasks associated with the hippocampus (Adasme et al., 2011).

A possible molecular and structural substrate associated with the RyR is the SA, which is enriched with synaptopodin (SP), an actin binding protein that was originally detected in the kidney, and later in the brain (Mundel et al., 1997; Deller et al., 2003; Asanuma et al., 2005). Several studies contributed to the initial association of SP with synaptic plasticity. In one, SP expression was found to be enhanced following tetanic stimulation, an effect that is assumed to underlie a transition from short to long-term potentiation (Yamazaki et al., 2001; Fukazawa et al., 2003). It was also demonstrated recently that rats exposed to an acute swim stress expressed a rapid increase in SP-density specifically in the dorsal hippocampus (Vlachos et al., 2008). Thus, dynamic changes in SP accompany plasticity-related stimulation, and are expected to play a role in enhanced memory formation in the behaving animal. It has been proposed that SP is co-localized with the RyR in dendritic spines of rat hippocampus (Vlachos et al., 2009; Segal et al., 2010). Furthermore, a reduction in SP in cultured hippocampal neurons by transfection with RNAi construct led to a marked reduction in plasticity of dendritic spines following several procedures commonly known to generate spine plasticity (ibid). The association of SP with RyR may resolve the inconsistencies among reports on the involvement of RyR in synaptic plasticity, as only about a third of the spines contain the spine apparatus and SP, while the others may not be affected by activators of the RyR (Segal et al., 2010).

A more direct indication for a role of RyR in dendritic spine $[Ca^{2+}]_i$ variations has been proposed recently by the use of flash photolysis of caged calcium inside dendritic spines (Korkotian and Segal, 2011; **Figure 1**). A momentary increase in $[Ca^{2+}]_i$ in dendritic spines by photolysis of caged calcium is followed by an exponential decay back to baseline level. However, in spines that are endowed with a SP puncta, an additional slow non-exponential component of elevated $[Ca^{2+}]_i$ was seen, and this was abrogated by RyR antagonists, indicating that a rise in free $[Ca^{2+}]_i$ is followed by a further increase, caused by its release from local stores.

CALCIUM STORES AND PLASTICITY

The involvement of calcium stores in generation and maintenance of long term potentiation has been studied extensively over the past two decades (Meldolesi, 2001; Shimuta et al., 2001; Fitzjohn and Collingridge, 2002; Bardo et al., 2006; Baker et al., 2013).

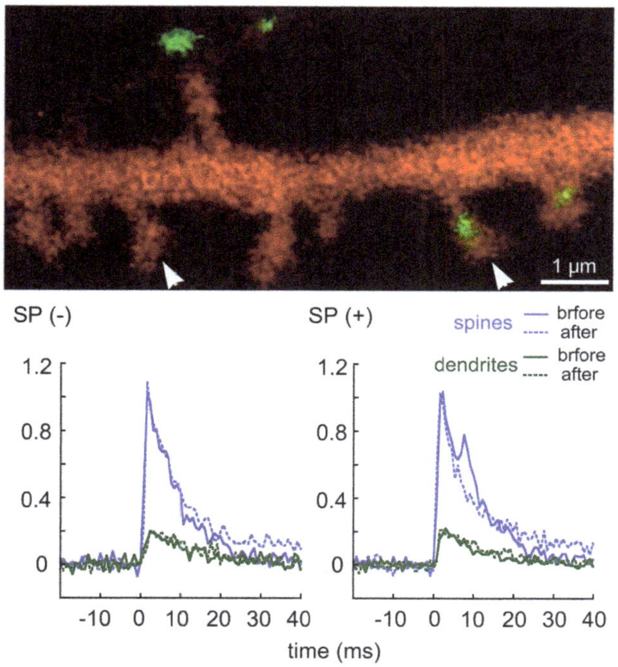

FIGURE 1 | Transient rise of $[Ca^{2+}]_i$ following flash photolysis of caged EGTA in dendritic spines of cultured hippocampal neurons. DsRed-transfected cells were loaded with a calcium indicator Fluo-4, and with the caged EGTA, the flash was focused on different dendritic spines in the field of view, and the transient elevation of $[Ca^{2+}]_i$ was recorded using line scan mode across the spine head and parent dendrite. The culture was then exposed to thapsigargin, and the same spines were imaged again. Following the experiment, cultures were fixed and immunostained for SP. Comparisons were made between SP-containing (right arrowhead) and SP-lacking spines (left arrowhead). For each sample ($n = 9$ spines), the transient rise of $[Ca^{2+}]_i$ in both the spine head (blue) and parent dendrite (green) were plotted, before (continuous line) and after thapsigargin (dotted line). A secondary "hump" in the transient rise of $[Ca^{2+}]i$ was seen only in the SP(+) spines but not in the SP(−) ones. This hump was erased in the presence of thapsigargin (after). Scale in image, 1 µm, ordinate is the averaged transients (df/f). (modified from Korkotian and Segal, 2011).

Several compounds, known to produce long term enhancement of synaptic reactivity, have been suggested to act by releasing of calcium from stores (Auerbach and Segal, 1994; Welsby et al., 2006). Furthermore, direct release of calcium from stores, using caffeine, produced a calcium store-dependent, NMDA-independent LTP (Martin and Buno, 2003). These authors suggest that the LTP is mediated presynaptically, to affect release of glutamate from terminals. Likewise, a brief exposure to caffeine, acting via a RyR, primed the conversion of short term to long term potentiation (Sajikumar et al., 2009). These and similar studies where tetanus-induced LTP could be blocked by drugs which interfere with the release of calcium from stores (Harvey and Collingridge, 1992) demonstrate the importance of calcium stores in the generation and maintenance of LTP. An interesting intra-hippocampal differential distribution of RyRs across the septo-temporal axis has been demonstrated (Grigoryan et al., 2012), which affects the ability of ryanodine and caffeine to enhance LTP in CA1 region of the hippocampal slice. This indicates that the activation of RyR in relation to neuronal plasticity is likely to be region-specific. Furthermore, the involvement of the stores can be exerted through the regulation of delivery of glutamate receptors to the synaptic site (Korkotian and Segal, 2006, 2007), or through regulation of one of several calcium-dependent processes in the dendrite, the spine or the synapse.

LOADING OF CALCIUM INTO STORES

RyRs are unique in that they are activated by an influx of calcium to induce release of calcium from the stores. That is, if calcium ions enter the cell via voltage or ligand gated channels, the RyR store cause further release of calcium ions, so as to amplify the action of the influxed ions. However, the influx of calcium through ion and ligand gated channels is only one of two main mechanisms that feed calcium into the stores. The other one is independent of the synapse-related ion channels, and is unique in that it senses a reduction in calcium concentrations in the store, to activate influx of calcium directly through the membrane, irrespective of afferent activity. This process is called store-operated calcium entry (SOCE) and has been studied extensively in non-neuronal tissue, with only few studies examining its role in central neurons. The reduction of $[Ca^{2+}]_i$ in the stores is sensed by stromal interacting protein (STIM), which is localized to the cytoplasm. Upon demand (i.e., low $[Ca^{2+}]_i$), STIM moves to the plasma membrane where it binds to Orai, a calcium channel that is voltage and extracellular ligand-independent. Both STIM and Orai are found in some dendritic spines (**Figure 2**). Following binding to STIM, Orai allows influx of calcium ions into the cytoplasm, where they are pumped into the ER stores. The malfunctioning of peripheral STIM/Orai complex has been associated with severe immunodeficiency syndrome (Feske et al., 2010). In the brain there are two species of STIM, STIM1, which has been shown recently to link to mGluRs and play a critical role in cerebellar neurons (Hartmann et al., 2014), and STIM2 (Sun et al., 2014) which appears to regulate influx of calcium in forebrain neurons, and be related to Alzheimer's disease (AD) (below). STIM and Orai have been identified in several neuronal compartments (Korkotian et al., 2014), and they are assumed to play an important role in the formation and maturation of dendritic spines.

There is a long standing issue concerning the development of spines; what is formed first, spines which grow in search for a presynaptic partner, or synapses that are made first on the dendritic shaft, followed by extension and formation of spines. If indeed Orai allows influx of calcium that is independent of synaptic activity, it can be considered to have a pivotal role in spine formation, and help form spines even in the absence of a synapse. Consequently, spines are not formed by an extrinsic factor, e.g., presynaptic activity, but by an intrinsic need to fill up stores, which allows a local rise of $[Ca^{2+}]_i$, sufficient to activate actin polymerization and formation of spines, which then hunt for a presynaptic partner, or collapse, in its absence. In any case, the presence of Orai in dendritic spines is an additional evidence for the important role of calcium stores in dendritic spine formation and plasticity.

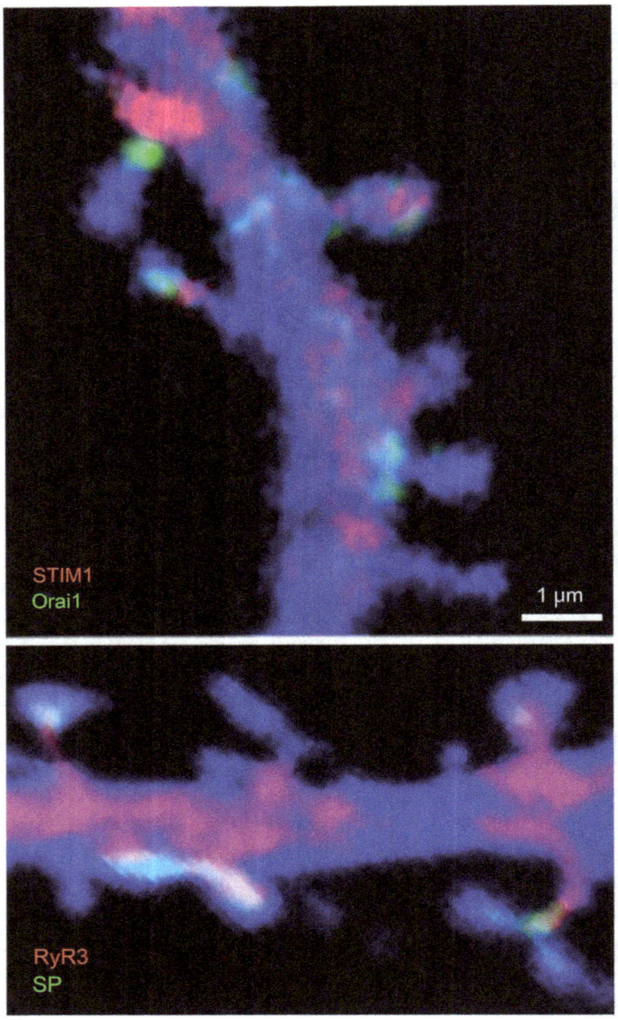

FIGURE 2 | Colocalization of STIM1 and Orai1 (top) and RyR3 and SP (bottom) in cultured hippocampal neurons. Cells were transfected with DsRed to image morphology (blue) and subsequently immunostained for STIM1 (red, top) and Orai1(green), or RyR (red) and SP (green, bottom). Scale 1 μm for both images. Colocalization of STIM and Orai are obvious in some but not all spines, such that either both or none were immunostained in the dendritic spines. Similarly, RyR and SP were colocalized in some but not all dendritic spines.

CALCIUM STORES AND STRESS

Exposure to stress can cause lasting effects in specific regions in the brain including the hippocampus. Following stressful experience, CA1 region of the dorsal hippocampus shows a lower ability to express LTP, and a larger long term depression (LTD) (Maggio and Segal, 2007). Surprisingly, CA1 of ventral hippocampus (VH) expresses larger LTP following the same stress. In previous studies we ascribed this metaplastic properties of VH to the recruitment of calcium stores (Grigoryan et al., 2012). In more recent studies, stress has been shown to cause an increase in beta adrenergic receptor activation of protein kinase A (PKA), which in turn regulates release of calcium from stores (Grigoryan and Segal, 2013). Dysregulation of RyR activation by the enhanced PKA results in release of calcium from stores, which perhaps can enhance ability to express LTP, but may also have long term detrimental consequences to cell function and survival (Stutzmann and Mattson, 2011; Liu et al., 2012). While these studies do not address directly the role of RyR in dendritic spines, there is accumulating evidence that chronic stress severely reduces dendritic spine density as well as ability to express LTP, which may be directly related to the deterioration of mechanisms for regulation of release of calcium from stores (Andres et al., 2013).

CALCIUM STORES IN NEURODEGENERATIVE DISEASES

Several studies suggest that synapse and dendritic spines dysfunctions are preceding and contributing to the eventual neuronal death and neurodegeneration in AD (Youn et al., 2007; Yu et al., 2012). Strikingly, recent work by Stutzmann and Mattson (2011) associates AD neuropathology with an over-expression of RyRs in dendrites and particularly in spines. Furthermore, caffeine caused a large facilitation of reactivity to tetanic stimulation in neurons from young 3xTg mouse hippocampus but not from controls (Grigoryan et al., 2014). This supersensitivity to activation of the RyR was noticed before the emergence of neuropathology in these mice, indicating that activation of RyR stores may lead rather than lag behind the pathology of AD. These results indicate that the association of RyR with dendritic spines, and their role in release of calcium from stores in relation to synaptic plasticity may be more important than originally suggested, especially in the development of AD.

This is also supported by post-mortem tissue sample analysis from patients with AD that consistently showed prominent synapse and dendritic spine loss in the hippocampus and throughout the cortex, the principal areas affected by AD-related pathology (DeKosky and Scheff, 1990; Knafo et al., 2009).

Indeed the number of synapses and spines elimination is often greater than the expected level for the amount of lost neurons and better correlates with the cognitive decline, suggesting that the primary synaptic failure is a prominent pathogenic cause of AD (Walsh and Selkoe, 2004; Verpelli and Sala, 2012).

The identification of specific genes associated with the pathogenesis of AD will lead to a better understanding of the molecular mechanisms underlying synapse and spine alterations. Mutations in three major genes implicated in beta amyloid (Aβ) metabolism, amyloid precursor protein (APP) and presenilin1 (PS1) have been associated to familial AD with an autosomal dominant form of inheritance and early onset of the disease (Bertram and Tanzi, 2008; Bertram et al., 2010). These mutations cause a well-documented increase in production of Aβ oligomers that at the end are responsible for inducing spine alterations, and reduce spine density (Shankar et al., 2007).

Mouse models of AD show behavioral deficits in reference and working memory but also dendritic and synaptic alterations, similar to what can be described in human patients. For example the human APP Tg2576 transgene mouse model shows a reduced spine density in hippocampal neurons from CA1 and dentate gyrus, even before the development of amyloid plaques, suggesting that soluble pathological Aβ oligomers initiate synapses alterations before neurodegeneration (Middei et al., 2008). Similarly, APP/PS1 transgenic mice showed alterations in spine density and morphology in dendrites in proximity of plaques but also a significant decrease in the frequency of large spines in neurons of plaque-free regions (Knafo et al., 2009).

Amyloid peptides have been shown to cause calcium rise, and neuronal degeneration. Paula-Lima et al. (2011) proposed that the amyloid oligomers stimulate RyR mediated calcium release, to induce mitochondrial fragmentation and loss of calcium regulation, ending in cell death. On the other hand, Zeiger et al. (2013) suggest that calcium influx through SOCE actually reduces formation of amyloid beta peptide, the evil molecule in AD. Thus, whether activation of SOCE is beneficial or detrimental to cell function in an AD environment remains to be elucidated. A more recent study, using Presenilin-mutant, familial AD-like mouse model, found that suppression of IP3Rs alleviates the AD symptoms. This study links calcium stores to AD, and proposes novel strategies for the treatment of the disease.

Many other genes have been identified as high risk factors to develop AD in the elderly. Among these genes apolipoprotein E (APOE) is the most important and studied risk factor. ApoE has three major isoforms, apoE2, E3 and E4 and apoE4 is associated with high risk of developing the disease, while the other ApoE seem to be neuroprotective. Transgenic mice for the human ApoE isoforms showed that indeed ApoE4 transgene has reduced spine density in the dentate gyrus and in the cortex in an age-dependent manner, while mice expressing human ApoE2 and ApoE3 have normal numbers of spines. One study also showed that in the human brain there is an inverse correlation between ApoE4 expression and spine density in dentate gyrus neurons (Dumanis et al., 2009). Interestingly the transgene expression of ApoE2 in two different mouse models of AD (Tg2576 and PDAPP mice) can rescue spine density to normal levels (Lanz et al., 2003). Thus all the mouse models of AD show alteration of spine morphology that correlates well with synaptic and behavioral dysfunctions. Consequently, measuring spine morphology is a good readout of the progression and severity of the pathology.

Which are the molecular mechanisms causing spine degeneration in AD? Recent results suggest that some signalling pathways regulating synaptic plasticity are involved. For example cofilin and drebrin, the actin-binding proteins with opposite effects on actin dynamics (see above), are both affected in AD. Cofilin phosphorylation and activity is up-regulated by Aβ 1–42 peptide in a concentration-dependent manner thus causing alteration in actin polymerization (Knobloch and Mansuy, 2008). In striking contrast, drebrin, the postsynaptic protein that binds and stabilizes actin in spines, is severely reduced in the brains of patients with AD and in transgenic animal models of the disease (Counts et al., 2012). Thus, a major initiating factor is probably associated with the malfunction of the RyR, causing a change in basal $[Ca^{2+}]_i$, and consequently changes in calcium associated processes responsible for the spine cytoskeleton. Current studies (Shilling et al., 2014; Sun et al., 2014) attempt to ameliorate the AD-associated morphological deterioration by addressing specifically calcium stores.

CONCLUSIONS

Recent accumulating evidence indicates that calcium stores of the RyR type have a pivotal role in dendritic spine development, plasticity and longevity. Disruption of this role of RyR in any stage of life will retard the functionality of the spine, the parent dendrite and the neuron of origin, leading to mental deterioration and AD. Recent attempts to ameliorate AD development focus on the RyR, and the regulation of $[Ca^{2+}]_i$ in the affected neurons.

AUTHOR CONTRIBUTIONS

Both Menahem Segal and Eduard Korkotian wrote the manuscript.

ACKNOWLEDGMENTS

Supported by grants from the Israel Science Foundation and The German Israel Foundation.

REFERENCES

Adasme, T., Haeger, P., Paula-Lima, A. C., Espinoza, I., Casas-Alarcón, M. M., Carrasco, M. A., et al. (2011). Involvement of ryanodine receptors in neurotrophin-induced hippocampal synaptic plasticity and spatial memory formation. *Proc. Natl. Acad. Sci. U S A* 108, 3029–3034. doi: 10.1073/pnas.1013580108

Andres, A. L., Regev, L., Phi, L., Seese, R. R., Chen, Y., Gall, C. M., et al. (2013). NMDA receptor activation and calpain contribute to disruption of dendritic spines by the stress neuropeptide CRH. *J. Neurosci.* 33, 16945–16960. doi: 10.1523/JNEUROSCI.1445-13.2013

Asanuma, K., Kim, K., Oh, J., Giardino, L., Chabanis, S., Faul, C., et al. (2005). Synaptopodin regulates the actin-bundling activity of alpha-actinin in an isoform-specific manner. *J. Clin. Invest.* 115, 1188–1198. doi: 10.1172/jci200523371

Auerbach, J. M., and Segal, M. (1994). A novel cholinergic induction of long-term potentiation in rat hippocampus. *J. Neurophysiol.* 72, 2034–2040.

Baker, K. D., Edwards, T. M., and Rickard, N. S. (2013). The role of intracellular calcium stores in synaptic plasticity and memory consolidation. *Neurosci. Biobehav. Rev.* 37, 1211–1239. doi: 10.1016/j.neubiorev.2013.04.011

Bardo, S., Cavazzini, M. G., and Emptage, N. (2006). The role of the endoplasmic reticulum Ca2+ store in the plasticity of central neurons. *Trends Pharmacol. Sci.* 27, 78–84. doi: 10.1016/j.tips.2005.12.008

Bertram, L., Lill, C. M., and Tanzi, R. E. (2010). The genetics of Alzheimer disease: back to the future. *Neuron* 68, 270–281. doi: 10.1016/j.neuron.2010.10.013

Bertram, L., and Tanzi, R. E. (2008). Thirty years of Alzheimer's disease genetics: the implications of systematic meta-analyses. *Nat. Rev. Neurosci.* 9, 768–778. doi: 10.1038/nrn2494

Brünig, I., Kaech, S., Brinkhaus, H., Oertner, T. G., and Matus, A. (2004). Influx of extracellular calcium regulates actin-dependent morphological plasticity in dendritic spines. *Neuropharmacology* 47, 669–676. doi: 10.1016/j.neuropharm.2004.07.038

Counts, S. E., He, B., Nadeem, M., Wuu, J., Scheff, S. W., and Mufson, E. J. (2012). Hippocampal drebrin loss in mild cognitive impairment. *Neurodegener. Dis.* 10, 216–219. doi: 10.1159/000333122

DeKosky, S. T., and Scheff, S. W. (1990). Synapse loss in frontal cortex biopsies in Alzheimer's disease: correlation with cognitive severity. *Ann. Neurol.* 27, 457–464. doi: 10.1002/ana.410270502

Deller, T., Korte, M., Chabanis, S., Drakew, A., Schwegler, H., Stefani, G. G., et al. (2003). Synaptopodin-deficient mice lack a spine apparatus and show deficits in synaptic plasticity. *Proc. Natl. Acad. Sci. U S A* 100, 10494–10499. doi: 10.1073/pnas.1832384100

Dumanis, S. B., Tesoriero, J. A., Babus, L. W., Nguyen, M. T., Trotter, J. H., Ladu, M. J., et al. (2009). ApoE4 decreases spine density and dendritic complexity in cortical neurons in vivo. *J Neurosci.* 29, 15317–15322. doi: 10.1523/JNEUROSCI.4026-09.2009

Emptage, N., Bliss, T. V., and Fine, A. (1999). Single synaptic events evoke NMDA receptor-mediated release of calcium from internal stores in hippocampal dendritic spines. *Neuron* 22, 115–124. doi: 10.1016/s0896-6273(00)80683-2

Fernández de Sevilla, D., and Buño, W. (2010). The muscarinic long-term enhancement of NMDA and AMPA receptor-mediated transmission at Schaffer collateral synapses develop through different intracellular mechanisms. *J. Neurosci.* 30, 11032–11042. doi: 10.1523/JNEUROSCI.1848-10.2010

Fernández de Sevilla, D., Núñez, A., Borde, M., Malinow, R., and Buño, W. (2008). Cholinergic-mediated IP3-receptor activation induces long-lasting synaptic enhancement in CA1 pyramidal neurons. *J. Neurosci.* 28, 1469–1478. doi: 10.1523/JNEUROSCI.2723-07.2008

Feske, S., Picard, C., and Fischer, A. (2010). Immunodeficiency due to mutations in ORAI1 and STIM1. *Clin. Immunol.* 135, 169–182. doi: 10.1016/j.clim.2010.01.011

Fifková, E., Markham, J. A., and Delay, R. J. (1983). Calcium in the spine apparatus of dendritic spines in the dentate molecular layer. *Brain Res.* 266, 163–168. doi: 10.1016/0006-8993(83)91322-7

Fitzjohn, S. M., and Collingridge, G. L. (2002). Calcium stores and synaptic plasticity. *Cell Calcium* 32, 405–411. doi: 10.1016/s0143416002001999

Fujino, I., Yamada, N., Miyawaki, A., Hasegawa, M., Furuichi, T., and Mikoshiba, K. (1995). Differential expression of type 2 and type 3 inositol 1,4,5-trisphosphate receptor mRNAs in various mouse tissues: in situ hybridization study. *Cell Tissue Res.* 280, 201–210. doi: 10.1007/bf00307790

Fukazawa, Y., Saitoh, Y., Ozawa, F., Ohta, Y., Mizuno, K., and Inokuchi, K. (2003). Hippocampal LTP is accompanied by enhanced F-actin content within the dendritic spine that is essential for late LTP maintenance in vivo. *Neuron* 38, 447–460. doi: 10.1016/s0896-6273(03)00206-x

Galeotti, N., Vivoli, E., Bartolini, A., and Ghelardini, C. (2008). A gene-specific cerebral types 1, 2 and 3 RyR protein knockdown induces an antidepressant-like effect in mice. *J. Neurochem.* 106, 2385–2394. doi: 10.1111/j.1471-4159.2008.05581.x

Goto, J., and Mikoshiba, K. (2011). Inositol 1,4,5-trisphosphate receptor-mediated calcium release in Purkinje cells: from molecular mechanism to behavior. *Cerebellum* 10, 820–833. doi: 10.1007/s12311-011-0270-5

Grigoryan, G., Biella, G., Albani, D., Forloni, G., and Segal, M. (2014). Stress impairs synaptic plasticity in triple-transgenic Alzheimer's disease mice: rescue by ryanodine. *Neurodegener. Dis.* 13, 135–138. doi: 10.1159/000354231

Grigoryan, G., Korkotian, E., and Segal, M. (2012). Selective facilitation of LTP in the ventral hippocampus by calcium stores. *Hippocampus* 22, 1635–1644. doi: 10.1002/hipo.22000

Grigoryan, G., and Segal, M. (2013). Prenatal stress alters noradrenergic modulation of LTP in hippocampal slices. *J. Neurophysiol.* 110, 279–285. doi: 10.1152/jn.00834.2012

Harris, K. M. (1999). Calcium from internal stores modifies dendritic spine shape. *Proc. Natl. Acad. Sci. U S A* 96, 12213–12215. doi: 10.1073/pnas.96.22.12213

Hartmann, J., Karl, R. M., Alexander, R. P., Adelsberger, H., Brill, M. S., Rühlmann, C., et al. (2014). STIM1 controls neuronal Ca(2+) signaling, mGluR1-dependent synaptic transmission and cerebellar motor behavior. *Neuron* 82, 635–644. doi: 10.1016/j.neuron.2014.03.027

Harvey, J., and Collingridge, G. L. (1992). Thapsigargin blocks the induction of long-term potentiation in rat hippocampal slices. *Neurosci. Lett.* 139, 197–200. doi: 10.1016/0304-3940(92)90551-h

Harvey, C. D., and Svoboda, K. (2007). Locally dynamic synaptic learning rules in pyramidal neuron dendrites. *Nature* 450, 1195–1200. doi: 10.1038/nature06416

Holbro, N., Grunditz, A., and Oertner, T. G. (2009). Differential distribution of endoplasmic reticulum controls metabotropic signaling and plasticity at hippocampal synapses. *Proc. Natl. Acad. Sci. U S A* 106, 15055–15060. doi: 10.1073/pnas.0905110106

Knafo, S., Alonso-Nanclares, L., Gonzalez-Soriano, J., Merino-Serrais, P., Fernaud-Espinosa, I., Ferrer, I., et al. (2009). Widespread changes in dendritic spines in a model of Alzheimer's disease. *Cereb. Cortex* 19, 586–592. doi: 10.1093/cercor/bhn111

Knobloch, M., and Mansuy, I. M. (2008). Dendritic spine loss and synaptic alterations in Alzheimer's disease. *Mol. Neurobiol.* 37, 73–82. doi: 10.1007/s12035-008-8018-z

Korkotian, E., and Segal, M. (1999). Release of calcium from stores alters the morphology of dendritic spines in cultured hippocampal neurons. *Proc. Nat. Acad. Sci. U S A* 96, 12068–12072. doi: 10.1073/pnas.96.21.12068

Korkotian, E., and Segal, M. (2007). Morphological constraints on calcium dependent glutamate receptor trafficking into individual dendritic spine. *Cell Calcium* 42, 41–57. doi: 10.1016/j.ceca.2006.11.006

Korkotian, E., and Segal, M. (2011). Synaptopodin regulates release of calcium from stores in dendritic spines of cultured hippocampal neurons. *J. Physiol.* 589, 5987–5995. doi: 10.1113/jphysiol.2011.217315

Korkotian, E., Frotscher, M., and Segal, M. (2014). Synaptopodin regulates spine plasticity: mediation by calcium stores. *J. Neurosci.* (in press).

Korkotian, E., and Segal, M. (1996). Lasting effects of glutamate on nuclear calcium concentration in cultured rat hippocampal neurons: regulation by calcium stores. *J. Physiol.* 496, 39–48.

Korkotian, E., and Segal, M. (2006). Spatially confined diffusion of calcium in dendrites of hippocampal neurons revealed by flash photolysis of caged calcium. *Cell Calcium* 40, 441–449. doi: 10.1016/j.ceca.2006.08.008

Kovalchuk, Y., Eilers, J., Lisman, J., and Konnerth, A. (2000). NMDA receptor-mediated subthreshold Ca(2+) signals in spines of hippocampal neurons. *J. Neurosci.* 20, 1791–1799.

Kushnir, A., Betzenhauser, M. J., and Marks, A. R. (2010). Ryanodine receptor studies using genetically engineered mice. *FEBS Lett.* 584, 1956–1965. doi: 10.1016/j.febslet.2010.03.005

Lanz, T. A., Carter, D. B., and Merchant, K. M. (2003). Dendritic spine loss in the hippocampus of young PDAPP and Tg2576 mice and its prevention by the ApoE2 genotype. *Neurobiol. Dis.* 13, 246–253. doi: 10.1016/s0969-9961(03)00079-2

Liu, X., Betzenhauser, M. J., Reiken, S., Meli, A. C., Xie, W., Chen, B. X., et al. (2012). Role of leaky neuronal ryanodine receptors in stress-induced cognitive dysfunction. *Cell* 150, 1055–1067. doi: 10.1016/j.cell.2012.06.052

Maggio, N., and Segal, M. (2007). Striking variations in corticosteroid modulation of long-term potentiation along the septotemporal axis of the hippocampus. *J. Neurosci.* 27, 5757–5765. doi: 10.1523/jneurosci.0155-07.2007

Mainen, Z. F., Malinow, R., and Svoboda, K. (1999). Synaptic calcium transients in single spines indicate that NMDA receptors are not saturated. *Nature* 399, 151–155. doi: 10.1038/20187

Martin, E. D., and Buno, W. (2003). Caffeine-mediated presynaptic long term potentiation in hippocampal CA1 pyramidal neurons. *J. Neurophysiol.* 89, 3029–3038. doi: 10.1152/jn.00601.2002

Meldolesi, J. (2001). Rapidly exchanging Ca2+ stores in neurons: molecular, structural and functional properties. *Prog. Neurobiol.* 65, 309–338. doi: 10.1016/s0301-0082(01)00004-1

Middei, S., Restivo, L., Caprioli, A., Aceti, M., and Ammassari-Teule, M. (2008). Region-specific changes in the microanatomy of single dendritic spines over time might account for selective memory alterations in ageing hAPPsweTg2576 mice, a mouse model for Alzheimer disease. *Neurobiol. Learn. Mem.* 90, 467–471. doi: 10.1016/j.nlm.2008.04.008

Mundel, P., Heid, H. W., Mundel, T. M., Kruger, M., Reiser, J., and Kriz, W. (1997). Synaptopodin: an actin-associated protein in telencephalic dendrites and renal podocytes. *J. Cell Biol.* 139, 193–204. doi: 10.1083/jcb.139.1.193

Nakata, H., and Nakamura, S. (2007). Brain-derived neurotrophic factor regulates AMPA receptor trafficking to post-synaptic densities via IP3R and TRPC calcium signaling. *FEBS Lett.* 581, 2047–2054. doi: 10.1016/j.febslet.2007.04.041

Paula-Lima, A. C., Adasme, T., SanMartín, C., Sebollela, A., Hetz, C., Carrasco, M. A., et al. (2011). Amyloid β-peptide oligomers stimulate RyR-mediated Ca2+ release inducing mitochondrial fragmentation in hippocampal neurons and prevent RyR-mediated dendritic spine remodeling produced by BDNF. *Antioxid. Redox Signal.* 14, 1209–1223. doi: 10.1089/ars.2010.3287

Raymond, C. R., and Redman, S. J. (2006). Spatial segregation of neuronal calcium signals encodes different forms of LTP in rat hippocampus. *J. Physiol.* 570, 97–111. doi: 10.1113/jphysiol.2005.098947

Rizzuto, R., De Stefani, D., Raffaello, A., and Mammucari, C. (2012). Mitochondria as sensors and regulators of calcium signaling. *Nat. Rev. Mol. Cell Biol.* 13, 566–578. doi: 10.1038/nrm3412

Rose, C. R., and Konnerth, A. (2001). Stores not just for storage. Intracellular calcium release and synaptic plasticity. *Neuron* 31, 519–522. doi: 10.1016/S0896-6273(01)00402-0

Sabatini, B. L., Oertner, T. G., and Svoboda, K. (2002). The life cycle of Ca(2+) ions in dendritic spines. *Neuron* 33, 439–452. doi: 10.1016/s0896-6273(02)00573-1

Sajikumar, S., Li, Q., Abraham, W. C., and Xiao, Z. C. (2009). Priming of short term potentiation and synaptic tagging/capture mechanisms by ryanodine receptor activation in rat hippocampal CA1. *Learn. Mem.* 16, 178–186. doi: 10.1101/lm.1255909

Sala, C., Roussignol, G., Meldolesi, J., and Fagni, L. (2005). Key role of the postsynaptic density scaffold proteins Shank and Homer in the functional architecture of Ca2+ homeostasis at dendritic spines in hippocampal neurons. *J. Neurosci.* 25, 4587–4592. doi: 10.1523/jneurosci.4822-04.2005

Sala, C., and Segal, M. (2014). Dendritic spines: the locus of structural and functional plasticity. *Physiol. Rev.* 94, 141–188. doi: 10.1152/physrev.00012.2013

Segal, M., Vlachos, A., and Korkotian, E. (2010). The spine apparatus, synaptopodin and dendritic spine plasticity. *Neuroscientist* 16, 125–131. doi: 10.1177/1073858409355829

Shankar, G. M., Bloodgood, B. L., Townsend, M., Walsh, D. M., Selkoe, D. J., and Sabatini, B. L. (2007). Natural oligomers of the Alzheimer amyloid-beta protein induce reversible synapse loss by modulating an NMDA-type glutamate receptor-dependent signaling pathway. *J. Neurosci.* 27, 2866–2875. doi: 10.1523/jneurosci.4970-06.2007

Sharp, A. H., McPherson, P. S., Dawson, T. M., Aoki, C., Campbell, K. P., and Snyder, S. H. (1993). Differential immunohistochemical localization of inositol 1,4,5-trisphosphate- and ryanodine-sensitive Ca2+ release channels in rat brain. *J. Neurosci.* 13, 3051–3063.

Shilling, D., Müller, M., Takano, H., Mak, D. O., Abel, T., Coulter, D. A., et al. (2014). Suppression of InsP3 receptor-mediated Ca2+ signaling alleviates mutant presenilin-linked familial Alzheimer's disease pathogenesis. *J. Neurosci.* 34, 6910–6923. doi: 10.1523/JNEUROSCI.5441-13.2014

Shimuta, M., Yoshikawa, M., Fukaya, M., Watanabe, M., Takeshima, H., and Manabe, T. (2001). Postsynaptic modulation of AMPA receptor mediated synaptic responses and LTP by the type 3 Ryanodine receptor. *Mol. Cell. Neurosci.* 17, 921–930. doi: 10.1006/mcne.2001.0981

Spacek, J., and Harris, K. M. (1997). Three-dimensional organization of smooth endoplasmic reticulum in hippocampal CA1 dendrites and dendritic spines of the immature and mature rat. *J. Neurosci.* 17, 190–203.

Stutzmann, G. E., and Mattson, M. P. (2011). Endoplasmic reticulum Ca(2+) handling in excitable cells in health and disease. *Pharmacol. Rev.* 63, 700–727. doi: 10.1124/pr.110.003814

Sugawara, T., Hisatsune, C., Le, T. D., Hashikawa, T., Hirono, M., Hattori, M., et al. (2013). Type 1 inositol trisphosphate receptor regulates cerebellar circuits by maintaining the spine morphology of purkinje cells in adult mice. *J. Neurosci.* 33, 12186–12196. doi: 10.1523/JNEUROSCI.0545-13.2013

Sun, S., Zhang, H., Liu, J., Popugaeva, E., Xu, N. J., Feske, S., et al. (2014). Reduced synaptic STIM2 expression and impaired store-operated calcium entry cause destabilization of mature spines in mutant presenilin mice. *Neuron* 82, 79–93. doi: 10.1016/j.neuron 2014.02.019

Verkhratsky, A. (2005). Physiology and pathophysiology of the calcium store in the endoplasmic reticulum of neurons. *Physiol. Rev.* 85, 201–279. doi: 10.1152/physrev.00004.2004

Verpelli, C., and Sala, C. (2012). Molecular and synaptic defects in intellectual disability syndromes. *Curr. Opin. Neurobiol.* 22, 530–536. doi: 10.1016/j.conb.2011.09.007

Vlachos, A., Korkotian, E., Schonfeld, E., Copanaki, E., Deller, T., and Segal, M. (2009). Synaptopodin regulates plasticity of dendritic spines in hippocampal neurons. *J. Neurosci.* 29, 1017–1033. doi: 10.1523/JNEUROSCI.5528-08.2009

Vlachos, A., Maggio, N., and Segal, M. (2008). Lack of correlation between synaptopodin expression and the ability to induce LTP in the rat dorsal and ventral hippocampus. *Hippocampus* 18, 1–4. doi: 10.1002/hipo.20373

Walsh, D. M., and Selkoe, D. J. (2004). Deciphering the molecular basis of memory failure in Alzheimer's disease. *Neuron* 44, 181–193. doi: 10.1016/j.neuron.2004.09.010

Welsby, P., Rowan, M., and Anwyl, R. (2006). Nicotinic receptor-mediated enhancement of long term potentiation involves activation of metabotropic glutamate receptors and ryanodine-sensitive calcium stores in the dentate gyrus. *Eur. J. Neurosci.* 24, 3109–3118. doi: 10.1111/j.1460-9568.2006.05187.x

Yamazaki, M., Matsuo, R., Fukazawa, Y., Ozawa, F., and Inokuchi, K. (2001). Regulated expression of an actin-associated protein, synaptopodin, during long-term potentiation. *J. Neurochem.* 79, 192–199. doi: 10.1046/j.1471-4159.2001.00552.x

Youn, H., Jeoung, M., Koo, Y., Ji, H., Markesbery, W. R., Ji, I., et al. (2007). Kalirin is under-expressed in Alzheimer's disease hippocampus. *J. Alzheimers Dis.* 11, 385–397.

Yu, W., Polepalli, J., Wagh, D., Rajadas, J., Malenka, R., and Lu, B. (2012). A critical role for the PAR-1/MARK-tau axis in mediating the toxic effects of Aβ on synapses and dendritic spines. *Hum. Mol. Genet.* 21, 1384–1390. doi: 10.1093/hmg/ddr576

Zalk, R., Lehnart, S. E., and Marks, A. R. (2007). Modulation of the ryanodine receptor and intracellular calcium. *Annu. Rev. Biochem.* 76, 367–385. doi: 10.1146/annurev.biochem.76.053105.094237

Zeiger, W., Vetrivel, K. S., Buggia-Prévot, V., Nguyen, P. D., Wagner, S. L., Villereal, M. L., et al. (2013). Ca2+ influx through store-operated Ca2+ channels reduces Alzheimer disease β-amyloid peptide secretion. *J. Biol. Chem.* 288, 26955–26966. doi: 10.1074/jbc.M113.473355

2

Matrix metalloproteinase-9 involvement in the structural plasticity of dendritic spines

Michal Stawarski[1†], Marzena Stefaniuk[2†] and Jakub Wlodarczyk[1*]

[1] Laboratory of Cell Biophysics, Department of Molecular and Cellular Neurobiology, Nencki Institute of Experimental Biology, Warsaw, Mazowieckie, Poland
[2] Laboratory of Neurobiology, Department of Molecular and Cellular Neurobiology, Nencki Institute of Experimental Biology, Warsaw, Mzowieckie, Poland

***Correspondence:**
Jakub Wlodarczyk, Laboratory of Cell Biophysics, Department of Molecular and Cellular Neurobiology, Nencki Institute of Experimental Biology, Ul. Ludwika Pasteura 3, Warszawa 02-093, Mazowieckie, Poland
e-mail: j.wlodarczyk@nencki.gov.pl

Dendritic spines are the locus for excitatory synaptic transmission in the brain and thus play a major role in neuronal plasticity. The ability to alter synaptic connections includes volumetric changes in dendritic spines that are driven by scaffolds created by the extracellular matrix (ECM). Here, we review the effects of the proteolytic activity of ECM proteases in physiological and pathological structural plasticity. We use matrix metalloproteinase-9 (MMP-9) as an example of an ECM modifier that has recently emerged as a key molecule in regulating the morphology and dysmorphology of dendritic spines that underlie synaptic plasticity and neurological disorders, respectively. We summarize the influence of MMP-9 on the dynamic remodeling of the ECM via the cleavage of extracellular substrates. We discuss its role in the formation, modification, and maintenance of dendritic spines in learning and memory. Finally, we review research that implicates MMP-9 in aberrant synaptic plasticity and spine dysmorphology in neurological disorders, with a focus on morphological abnormalities of dendritic protrusions that are associated with epilepsy.

Keywords: matrix metalloproteinase-9, dendritic spines, structural synaptic plasticity, extracellular matrix, epilepsy

INTRODUCTION

Structural plasticity is an active field in neuroscience, with pivotal implications for the understanding of many different levels of learning and memory and a wide range of neurological and cognitive disorders (Sala and Segal, 2014; Penzes et al., 2011). Dendritic spines are plastic structures that undergo morphological changes in response to stimuli that modulate neuronal activity. Such remodeling underlies the formation and long-term storage of information in the brain, and spine remodeling frequently accompanies neurodegenerative diseases, i.e., ischemia (Brown et al., 2008b) or spinal cord injury (Kim et al., 2006) lead to a reduction in spine density and elongation of the remaining spines; traumatic brain injury alters dendritic spines stability (Campbell et al., 2012). The extracellular matrix (ECM) of the brain mediates structural stability by creating a scaffold for dendritic spines (de Vivo et al., 2013). ECM components do not constitute only a passive environment. Some ECM components (e.g., matrix metalloproteinase-9 [MMP-9]) also actively participate in synaptic plasticity. Growing evidence indicates a particular role for MMP-9 in the mediation of structural plasticity in the brain.

In the present review, we discuss the concept of the tetrapartite synapse, with a particular emphasis on ECM proteins, and highlight both the beneficial and detrimental roles of MMP-9 in pathological structural brain plasticity. We focus on epileptogenesis as an example of a disease in which the role of MMP-9 in aberrant synaptic plasticity and permanent impairment is particularly significant (Wilczynski et al., 2008).

TETRAPARTITE SYNAPSE

The first high-resolution observations of neurons by Ramón y Cajal unveiled the existence of dendritic spines, small membranous protrusions on the surface of dendrites (Ramón y Cajal, 1888, 1899). Ramón y Cajal theorized that they could be involved in signal transmission within the brain (Ramón y Cajal, 1891, 1893), giving rise to the classical theory of a dipartite synapse as a basic unit of neuronal information processing. The dipartite synapse is formed by presynaptic and postsynaptic parts that are found on presynaptic boutons and dendritic spines, respectively, separated by the synaptic cleft. In the decades that followed, research showed that this model was overly simplified, and additional players were added to the picture. The concept of a tripartite synapse appeared, in which the astrocyte, once believed to be an inert, "neuron-feeding" cell, actively participates in synaptic transmission (Araque et al., 1999). Soon new components of the synapse were discovered, giving rise to the tetrapartite or even pentapartite concept of the synapse. In one conceptualization, microglia (reviewed in De Leo et al., 2006) join pre- and postsynaptic neurons and astrocytes to form the synapse. In another conceptualization, the ECM is added as a key component of the synapse (reviewed in Dityatev and Rusakov, 2011). The ECM is a complex protein network that fills the extracellular space and is secreted by neurons, glia, and non-neuronal cells. It was previously seen as an inert component of the synapse, a scaffold that maintains synaptic integrity, with no effect on synaptic transmission. The reality, however, turned out to be quite different. Recent research has shown that the ECM actively regulates a plethora of cellular functions, from the initial establishment of the synapse to the regulation of synaptic transmission and synaptic plasticity (reviewed in Dityatev et al., 2010). The ECM has begun to be recognized as a critical factor that affects synapses by enveloping them and forming a synaptic element. ECM components with known roles in the regulation of synaptic transmission include laminin, tenascins, thrombospondin, lectins, and MMPs, to name a few (comprehensively reviewed in Dansie and Ethell, 2011). Among the numerous ECM components that have been proposed to play roles in brain plasticity, MMP-9 has recently emerged as a key molecule involved in long-term memory and the underlying synaptic changes (Rivera et al., 2010; Huntley, 2012; Tsien, 2013). The focal point of synaptic changes within the brain are dendritic spines that harbor synaptic contacts. Their stability is correlated with their shape, in which mushroom-like spines are generally more stable than thin, long spines. The size of the spine head is well known to be correlated with the area of the postsynaptic density (PSD; Harris and Stevens, 1989; Meyer et al., 2014) and AMPA receptor number (Nusser et al., 1998; Kharazia and Weinberg, 1999; Takumi et al., 1999; Szepesi et al., 2014). Dendritic spine neck length on the other hand is correlated with postsynaptic potential (Araya et al., 2006; Tønnesen et al., 2014). Thus, dendritic spine morphology has been accepted to determine the strength of synaptic connections. The structural plasticity of dendritic spines is widely seen as the basis of the primary functions of the central nervous system, including learning and memory. The influence of MMP-9 on dendritic spine morphology makes it a perfect candidate molecule for synaptic remodeling.

MATRIX METALLOPROTEINASE-9

MMP-9 is a 92 kDa protein that belongs to a family of zinc- and calcium-dependent endopeptidases. Because of its ability to cleave gelatin, it is classified as a gelatinase. It is encoded in the human genome by a gene located on chromosome 20 (20q13.12). The molecular biology of MMP-9 was summarized in an excellent, exhaustive review by Vandooren et al. (2013).

MMP-9 has a complex domain structure, with a signal peptide at the N-terminus, followed by a propeptide, a catalytic domain with a zinc ion binding site, three fibronectin type II inserts, a proline-rich and heavily *O*-glycosylated linker, and a hemopexin domain located at the C-terminus of the protein (Stute et al., 2003). The propeptide contains an evolutionarily conserved PRCGVPDV domain that binds the zinc ion in the catalytic domain and blocks the activity of the enzyme until it is cleaved (Van Wart and Birkedal-Hansen, 1990; Becker et al., 1995). The overlapping substrate specificity of MMPs (to date, 25 MMPs have been identified in humans) is attributable to a zinc-binding motif, HExGHxxGxxH (where x signifies any amino acid), within the catalytic domain, which is shared by all MMPs. Tandemly repeated fibronectin type II inserts within the catalytic domain are responsible for gelatin binding. The linker allows for independent movement of the catalytic and hemopexin domains, which influence enzyme conformation (Rosenblum et al., 2007) and the substrate specificity of MMP-9. The hemopexin domain is able to bind an endogenous MMP-9 inhibitor called tissue inhibitor of matrix metalloproteinases-1 (TIMP-1) and several MMP-9 substrates. It is also responsible for the membrane docking of MMP-9 (Bode et al., 1999) and formation of homo- and heterodimers with neutrophil gelatinase-associated lipocalin (NGAL; Kjeldsen et al., 1993; Cha et al., 2002).

MMP-9 is ubiquitously expressed throughout the body. Within the resting brain, it is mostly synthesized by neurons but to some extent also by glia in such structures as the hippocampus, cerebral cortex, and cerebellum. It is extracellularly secreted, although recent studies have also revealed its presence in the nucleus of muscle cells (Yeghiazaryan et al., 2012), neurons (Yang et al., 2010; Hill et al., 2012), human glial cells (Pirici et al., 2012), and mitochondria of retinal capillary cells. MMP-9 may act as a negative regulator of mitochondrial function and may be involved in apoptosis (Kowluru et al., 2011).

The expression of MMP-9 is regulated on multiple levels: (1) transcription (for a comprehensive review of the transcriptional and epigenetic regulation of MMP-9 expression, including regulation through non-coding RNAs, see Labrie and St-Pierre, 2013; several studies also indicate that reactive oxygen species (ROS) activate MMP-9 expression through AP-1 transcription factors; Hasebe et al., 2007; Hsieh et al., 2014); (2) posttranslation (also involving non-proteolytic activation); (3) local translation (Dziembowska et al., 2012); (4) sequestration on the cell membrane (e.g., binding to cell adhesion molecules, such as hyaluronian receptor CD44 (Bourguignon et al., 1998), integrins (Wang et al., 2003), lipoprotein receptor-related protein-1 (LRP-1), and megalin/LRP-2 (Van den Steen et al., 2006)); (5) internalization (Hahn-Dantona et al., 2001); and (6) delayed activation that involves cleavage of the propeptide and co-secretion with TIMP-1, its endogenous inhibitor (Sbai et al., 2010). In the brain, the primary transcriptional regulators of MMP-9 expression are AP-1 and nuclear factor-κB (NF-κB). Yin Yang 1 (YY1) was identified as a strong repressor of MMP-9 transcription in the rat hippocampus *in vivo* and cultured neurons (Rylski et al., 2008).

MMP-9 activation usually occurs through the cleavage of a propeptide that disrupts its zinc ion binding properties. Cleavage may also be performed by other MMPs and the tissue plasminogen activator (tPA)-plasmin system (Bruno and Cuello, 2006). However, non-proteolytic activation/inactivation is also possible through posttranslational modification. The thiol modification of methionine and cysteine residues within the catalytic domain and nitration or oxidation of the propeptide cysteine that is responsible for zinc ion binding are also able to activate MMPs without propeptide removal. Finally, nitric oxide, a commonly occurring secondary messenger in the brain, is able to regulate the stability of MMP-9 mRNA (Akool et al., 2003).

MMP-9 and TIMP-1 are secreted by neurons in a Golgi-dependent manner in 160–200 nm vesicles. The vesicles move along microtubules and microfilaments. They are distributed in the somatodendritic compartment and can be found in dendritic spines (Sbai et al., 2008).

MMP-9 regulates numerous cell activities through its involvement in matrix remodeling and the liberation of macromolecules (e.g., growth factors) that are embedded within the ECM. MMP-9 is involved in various physiological functions, such as tissue remodeling, cellular differentiation (Zimowska et al., 2013), cell-cell contact and cell migration (Kim et al., 2012), the release of cytokines and regulation of growth factor activity (Schonbeck et al., 1998), survival and apoptosis (Kowluru et al., 2011), angiogenesis, inflammation, and signaling (for a comprehensive review of MMP-9 function, see Vandooren et al., 2013; Verslegers et al., 2013). Aside from maintaining tissue homeostasis, MMP-9 plays a role in a range of pathologies (comprehensively reviewed in Rivera et al., 2010; Kaczmarek, 2013).

Polymorphisms that have been identified in the MMP-9 gene promoter ([CA]n microsatellite at position -90 and SNP at -1562) that affect the binding of nuclear proteins and thus the expression levels of the protein were correlated with an increased incidence of several pathologies in human populations (Ye, 2000). Additionally, a functional polymorphism that might affect the binding of non-coding RNAs and thus mRNA transport and translation was identified within the 3' untranslated region of MMP-9 mRNA (Yuan et al., 2013).

The monitoring of MMP-9 activity originally took advantage of its gelatinolytic properties in the form of zymography, in which MMP-9 cleaves an FITC-tagged gelatin (DQ-gelatin). Under normal conditions, FITC fluorescence is almost completely quenched unless DQ-gelatin is cleaved by MMP-9. In such a case, fluorescence increases and can be readily monitored using confocal microscopy. However, DQ-gelatin does not enable the tracking of MMP-9 activity with high spatial and temporal resolution because it is freely diffusive. Moreover, DQ-gelatin is also cleaved by MMP-2, which generally has a much higher level of expression than MMP-9. Therefore, assays that utilize DQ-gelatin, with the exception of gel zymography, are highly nonspecific. In recent years, a number of new MMP-9 activity biosensors have been developed (Faust et al., 2008; Fudala et al., 2011; Akers et al., 2012; Gustafson et al., 2013) in response to the perceived shortcomings of classical zymographic approaches. The potential of MMP-9 as a prognostic marker of cancer led to considerable interest in developing diagnostic and analytical probes to detect the proteolytic activity of MMP-9 in cancer (for a survey of several MMP-9 activity probes used in cancer detection, see Roy et al., 2011; for a review of MMP-9 detection methods in cancer, see Scherer et al., 2008; for MMP-9 near-infrared fluorescence probes in *in vivo* imaging, see Wallis de Vries et al., 2009; Kaijzel et al., 2010; Akers et al., 2012; Lee et al., 2012). We recently developed a genetically encoded fluorescence resonance energy transfer (FRET)-based MMP-9 activity biosensor (Stawarski et al., 2014) that is compatible with live cell imaging approaches and can be used to study the effects of MMP-9 on structural plasticity with very high spatiotemporal resolution. It is membrane-anchored and utilizes the teal fluorescent protein (mTFP1) as a donor of energy and two tandemly repeated Venus proteins as energy donors to increase the resonant energy transfer level (**Figure 1**). The biosensor was engineered for the highest possible FRET efficiency and incorporates a synthetic MMP-9 cleavage site within an α-helical region, giving the biosensor high sensitivity to MMP-9 action and improved specificity. The biosensor can be used to study the action of MMP-9 at the level of single dendritic spines, providing an opportunity to unambiguously correlate endogenous MMP-9 activity with the plastic changes of dendritic spines. Furthermore, by combining the biosensor with one of several recently described brain optical clearing techniques (several optical clearing agents were recently reviewed in Zhu et al., 2013; see also Chung et al. (2013) for CLARITY, Hama et al. (2011) for Scale and Susaki et al. (2014) for CUBIC) bridging the gap between studies of the global anatomical changes that occur because of synaptic plasticity and locally regulated extremely low-level proteolytic activity around single neurons might be possible, thus providing insights into the basic mechanisms of brain plasticity.

MMP-9 IN PHYSIOLOGICAL STRUCTURAL PLASTICITY

Research on MMP-9 was originally concentrated on its role in the pathology of the central nervous system (e.g., post-injury and post-stroke damage to brain tissue) due to its ECM-cleavage properties. However, the first indication that MMP-9 may play a role beyond the pathology of the brain came from research on the kainate-induced epilepsy models in mice. Kainate-induced seizures lead to massive cell death in CA regions of the hippocampus, the limbic cortex, and the amygdala but a pronounced plasticity in the dentate gyrus (DG; Zagulska-Szymczak et al., 2001). Nedivi et al. (1993) demonstrated that TIMP-1 mRNA (i.e., an endogenous inhibitor of MMPs, including MMP-9) is upregulated following kainate-induced seizures. A follow-up study (Szklarczyk et al., 2002) revealed that MMP-9 mRNA, protein, and activity levels are also upregulated in the DG of the hippocampus under the same experimental conditions. Furthermore, Jaworski et al. (1999) observed that the expression of TIMP-1 is coupled to neuronal excitation and spatially and temporarily overlaps with c-Fos expression. Kuzniewska et al. (2013) and Ganguly et al. (2013) also demonstrated that MMP-9 expression depends on the c-Fos transcriptional regulation. C-Fos role in brain plasticity was postulated already by Kaczmarek et al. (2002). Nagy et al. (2006) and Bozdagi et al. (2007) demonstrated that MMP-9 is a necessary component of long-term potentiation (LTP; i.e., an experimental paradigm that mimics certain aspects of physiological plasticity) both in acute hippocampal slices and *in vivo* in urethane-anesthetized rats. They discovered that MMP-9 is required in the late phase of LTP in the CA1 field, and MMP-9 inhibition by whatever means (e.g., inhibitors and antisense RNA) leads to a rapid return of synaptic potentiation to baseline levels. Research on MMP-9 knockout mice revealed diminished LTP that could be rescued by exogenously applied recombinant MMP-9 (Nagy et al., 2006). Meighan et al. (2006) demonstrated that spatial learning leads to alterations in MMP-9 mRNA and protein levels. The injection of either the broad-spectrum MMP inhibitor FN-439 or antisense RNA led to markedly diminished learning in the Morris water maze. A similar effect was achieved with the *N*-methyl-D-aspartate (NMDA) receptor antagonist MK801. Finally, Meighan et al. (2006) demonstrated that the effect of MMPs on learning is facilitated through changes of the actin cytoskeleton. Recent studies also revealed that MMP-9 is required for cortical

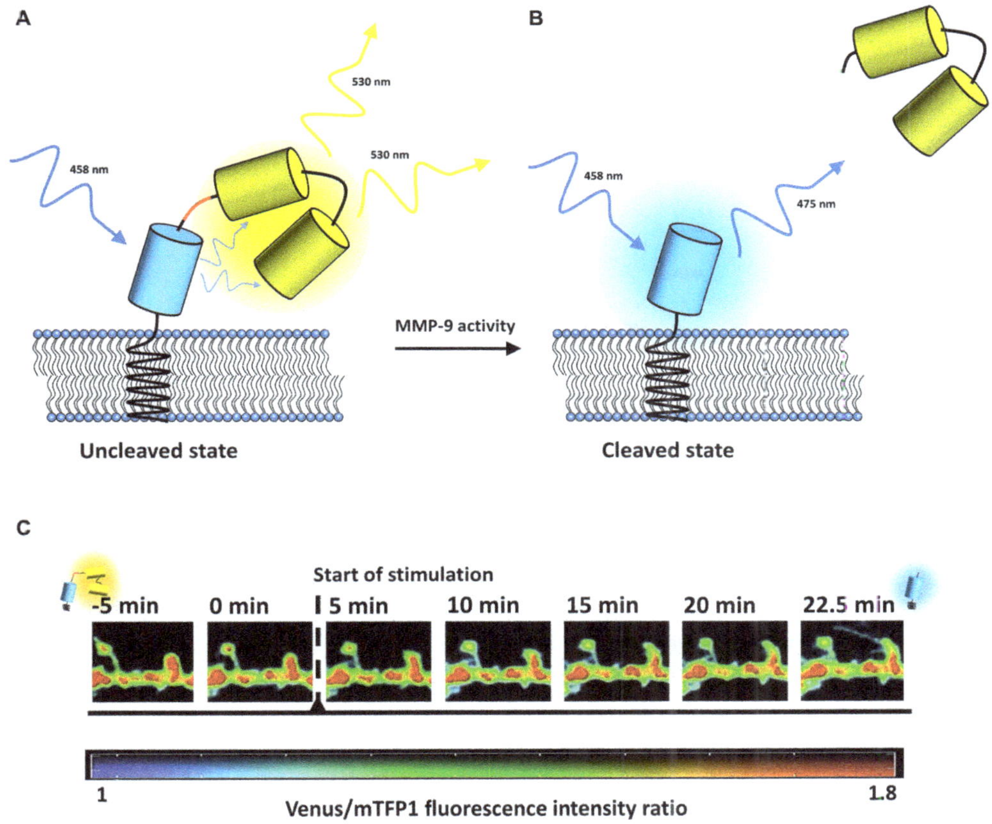

FIGURE 1 | MMP-9 activity detection mechanism of the biosensor. (A) In an uncleaved state, the excitation energy is transferred from mTFP1 (depicted in blue) to Venus (depicted in yellow), resulting in the fluorescence of the yellow fluorescent protein. **(B)** Once MMP-9 cleaves the biosensor (sequence recognized by MMP-9 is marked in red), the Venus proteins are released, the FRET phenomenon disappears, and the fluorescence of mTFP1 increases. **(C)** Time-lapse imaging of endogenous MMP-9 activity visualized with the MMP-9 activity biosensor expressed in a primary rat hippocampal culture. Colors indicate the value of Venus-to-mTFP1 fluorescence intensity ratio (reds—high values of the ratio/uncleaved biosensor; blues—low values of the ratio/cleaved biosensor; see the color bar below image insets). Stimulation was performed with the chemical long-term potentiation (LTP) protocol (see Stawarski et al., 2014). Biosensor pictures in the left and right of the diagram indicate visually the state of the biosensor (uncleaved/cleaved).

plasticity evoked by sensory deprivation (e.g., whisker plucking (Kaliszewska et al., 2012) and monocular deprivation (Spolidoro et al., 2012)) and LTP in the mossy fiber-CA3 pathway (Wiera et al., 2012, 2013). Physiological remodeling is also strongly influenced by experience-dependent mechanisms that imply an interaction between neural circuits and the external world. An enriched environment has been shown to influence brain plasticity by inducing MMP-9 activity (Foscarin et al., 2011; Cao et al., 2014). More information on the role of MMP-9 in physiological plasticity can be found in recently published reviews (Rivera et al., 2010; Wlodarczyk et al., 2011).

Matrix metalloproteinases are functionally involved in the regulation of synaptic plasticity (Nagy et al., 2006; Bozdagi et al., 2007; Okulski et al., 2007; Rivera et al., 2010; Huntley, 2012; Szepesi et al., 2013) and formation and maintenance of dendritic spines (Wang et al., 2008; Bilousova et al., 2009; Michaluk et al., 2011). Although details of MMP-9 action on dendritic spines are not fully elucidated, the research performed so far allowed to construct a model of MMP-9 activity around dendritic spines, which is presented in **Figure 2**. The model postulates that MMP-9 is released from dendritic spines following a stimulus. MMP-9 activity, possibly mediated through β1 integrin signaling causes the elongation of dendritic spines and increases the mobility of NMDA receptors. The time window in which MMP-9 is active is brief, as it is almost immediately inactivated by its endogenous inhibitor TIMP-1. MMP-9 inhibition allows the dendritic spines to mature, incorporate AMPA receptors and form active synapses. The model presented above is supported by numerous observations, which are briefly summarized in the next paragraph.

The presence of MMP-9-coding mRNA, protein, and enzymatic activity at the level of dendritic spines was confirmed by recent studies (Konopacki et al., 2007; Wilczynski et al., 2008; Gawlak et al., 2009; Dziembowska et al., 2012). The activity-dependent local translation of MMP-9 mRNA and protein release was recently demonstrated by Dziembowska et al. (2012), supporting the hypothesis that locally secreted MMP-9 and other dendritically synthesized proteins are involved in the structural

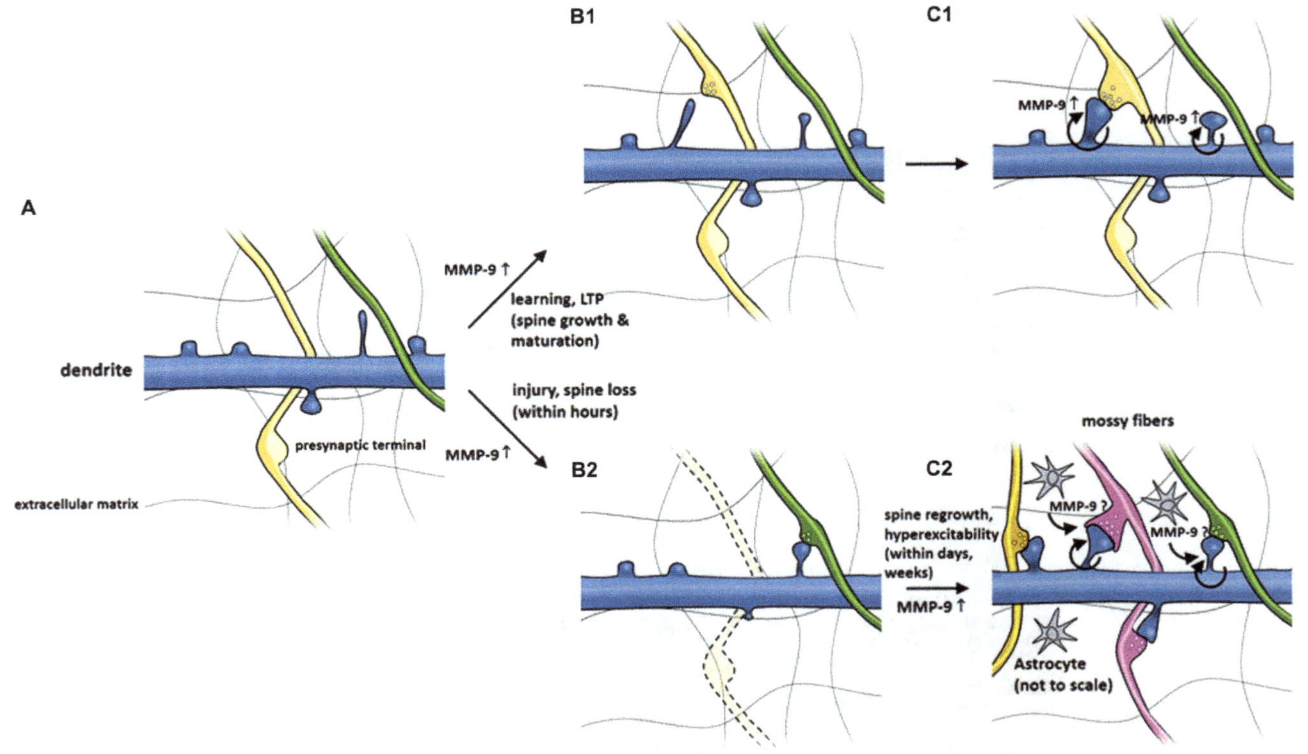

FIGURE 2 | MMP-9 involvement in morphological changes of dendritic spines in LTP and possible role in epileptogenesis-related spine pathology. (A) Dendritic spines extend as small protrusions from dendritic shaft. **(B1)** MMP-9 level is elevated upon stimulus which leads to spine elongation and **(C1)** maturation. **(B2)** Fast (within minutes) activation of MMP-9 by injury or seizures may induce spine loss. **(C2)** Continuous increase of MMP-9 (secondary to seizures, within days) may cause regrowth of dendritic spines and contribute to long-term circuitry remodeling underlying seizures.

and functional plasticity of activated synapses. MMP-9 also increases the lateral mobility of NMDARs (Michaluk et al., 2009). Michaluk et al. (2011) also demonstrated that elongation and spine thinning are regulated by integrin β1 signaling and are accompanied by changes in the decay time of miniature synaptic currents. The blockade of integrin β1 signaling with an integrin β1 antibody abolished both the MMP-9-dependent increase in NMDAR mobility and its ability to affect spine morphology. The ICAM-5 ectodomain produced by MMP-9 cleavage stimulates an increase in AMPA mini excitatory postsynaptic current (mEPSC) frequency and leads to recruitment of the AMPAR GluA1 subunit to the membrane (Lonskaya et al., 2013).

The activity of MMP-9 that was locally released in response to stimuli was also recently reported to modulate the morphology of dendritic spines (Wang et al., 2008; Bilousova et al., 2009). Admittedly, there is some confusion on how exactly MMP-9 affects the spine morphology, with different groups reporting markedly different effects, with some groups observing spine maturation following MMP-9 activity, while others report dendritic spine elongation. Wang observed that MMP-9 was required in spine enlargement associated with LTP in acute hippocampal slices. That observation indicates that MMP-9 may drive the establishment of persistent modification of both synapse structure and function (Wang et al., 2008). Intracellular adhesion molecule-5 (ICAM-5) cleavage by MMP-9 causes the elongation of dendritic filopodia in dissociated neuronal cultures (Tian et al., 2007) and influences AMPAR-dependent glutamatergic transmission. Our research indicates that the enzymatic activity of MMP-9 is able to cause an elongation and thinning of dendritic spines on hippocampal neurons in three experimental models: transgenic rats that overexpress auto-activating MMP-9, dissociated hippocampal cultures, and organotypic cultures (Michaluk et al., 2011). Bilousova observed that the incubation of dissociated neuronal cultures with recombinant MMP-9 led to the transformation of mushroom-shaped dendritic spines into filopodia-like protrusions (Bilousova et al., 2009). Minocycline, a drug whose pleiotropic effects include the inhibition of MMP-9 activity, reverses filopodia transformation toward mature spines in an animal model of fragile X syndrome (Fmr1 knockout mice). Apparently conflicting effects of MMP-9 on spine structure and dynamics can be explained by different research protocols, including enzyme concentration, treatment duration, and age and developmental stage of the neurons. The research discussed above also differs in the manner by which MMP-9 was applied (i.e., bath application *vs.* local application), the duration of MMP-9 activity influenced by the inhibitory effect of TIMP-1 (an endogenous MMP-9 inhibitor), and the maturity of neurons. Wang et al. (2008) observed that MMP-9 promotes the maturation of dendritic spines, whereas Tian et al. (2007) and Michaluk et al. (2011) reported something markedly different (i.e., MMP-9 or MMP-9-released products stimulated spine elongation). Wang et al. (2008) performed their studies using acute slices from postnatal day 14 (PD14) to PD21 rats, whereas Michaluk et al. (2011) chose an organotypic culture model from PD7 rats. Furthermore, Wang et al. (2008) applied MMP-9 locally with a stimulating electrode, which more closely resembles physiological conditions, in contrast to the study by Michaluk et al. (2011), who used bath application, which is closer to pathological conditions. MMP-9 activity is thus believed to be strictly regulated, local, and transient, and the inhibition of MMP-9 may be the final step in spine maturation, in which a filopodium-like protrusion matures into a mushroom-like dendritic spine (Tian et al., 2007; Bilousova et al., 2009). Studying the effect of TIMP-1 sequestration on spine morphology might be advantageous.

Spine head protrusions (SHPs) are small filopodia-like processes that extend from the dendritic spine head. They represent a new type of postsynaptic structural remodeling that follows neuronal activity. We recently reported the role of MMP-9 in the formation of SHPs (Szepesi et al., 2013). Chemically induced LTP (cLTP) leads to the upregulation of MMP-9 activity in dissociated hippocampal cultures and appears to control SHP formation. The growth of SHPs is abolished by inhibiting MMP activity or influencing microtubule dynamics. Recombinant auto-activating MMP-9 promotes the formation of SHPs in organotypic hippocampal slices. Spines with SHPs were also shown to recruit new postsynaptic AMPA receptors following cLTP, and AMPAR recruitment was MMP-dependent.

Research indicates that the effect of MMP-9 on spine morphology may be mediated not by a general disruption of ECM structure (Michaluk et al., 2009) but rather by the tightly regulated cleavage of specific ECM proteins that would then trigger the intracellular integrin signaling pathway (Wang et al., 2008; Michaluk et al., 2011). The modifications of spine morphology appear to involve MMP-9 cleavage of the following proteins: β-dystroglycan, ICAM-5, integrins (MMP-9 is known to cleave integrin β2; Vaisar et al. (2009), and β4 (Pal-Ghosh et al., 2011). Indirect evidence also suggests that MMP-9 may drive the cleavage of integrin β1 (Kim et al., 2009), neuroligin-1, and ephrin (Nagy et al., 2006; Michaluk et al., 2007, 2009; Tian et al., 2007; Conant et al., 2010; Peixoto et al., 2012). The MMP-9-driven cleavage of ICAM-5, a negative regulator of spine maturation, was observed following neuronal stimulation and led to spine maturation (Tian et al., 2007; Conant et al., 2010). Peixoto et al. (2012) observed that neuroligin-1 cleavage by MMP-9 at the postsynaptic site of glutamatergic synapses resulted in a destabilized presynaptic site and modification of synaptic transmission. The Ephrin/Eph receptor complex, cleaved by MMP-9 following hippocampal LTP, is involved in learning and memory (Klein, 2004; Murai and Pasquale, 2004). Therefore, MMP-9 is clearly an important player in the dynamic remodeling of dendritic spines, and its affinity for numerous proteins supports the concept of a tetrapartite synapse (Dityatev and Rusakov, 2011).

Matrix metalloproteinases also process various non-ECM proteins, such as growth factor precursors, cell-surface receptors, and adhesion molecules (Nagase and Woessner, 1999; Ethell and Ethell, 2007; Michaluk and Kaczmarek, 2007). Several MMP-9 substrates were identified only *in vitro* (e.g., the ECM and the basement membrane molecules brevican, laminin and aggrecan; Nakamura et al., 2000; Overall, 2002; Morrison et al., 2009) and not confirmed *in vivo*. β-dystroglycan (β-DG) was confirmed to be cleaved by MMP-9 *in vivo* in response to enhanced neuronal activity (Michaluk et al., 2007). β-DG is a transmembrane protein that serves as a cell-surface anchor for α-dystroglycan, which binds to the extracellular domains of β-DG and laminin, agrin, and perlecan (Ervasti and Campbell, 1993; Gee et al., 1993; Bowe et al., 1994; Campanelli et al., 1996; Peng et al., 1998; Henry et al., 2001) in non-neuronal cells and neurexins in the central nervous system (Sugita et al., 2001). Thus, MMP-9 activity may uncouple the cytoskeleton from the ECM. Other cell-surface receptors that were confirmed to be MMP-9 substrates include the interleukin-2 (IL-2) receptor α chain (CD25; Sheu et al., 2001; De Paiva et al., 2009), ephrin B (Lin et al., 2008), and NG2 proteoglycan in the spinal cord (Larsen et al., 2003).

Bajor et al. (2012) isolated two synaptic proteins that are cleaved *in vivo* by MMP-9: synaptic cell adhesion molecule-2 (synCAM-2) and collapsin response mediator protein-2 (CRMP-2). CRMP-2 is involved in axon guidance, neurite outgrowth, and the regulation of neuronal differentiation (Inagaki et al., 2001; Fukata et al., 2002; Yoshimura et al., 2005). It was suggested to play a role in numerous neurological diseases, such as Alzheimer's disease, epilepsy, and ischemia (Gu and Ihara, 2000; Czech et al., 2004; Uchida and Goshima, 2005). SynCAM-2 (also known as Necl-3, IgSF4D, and Cadm-2) is a Ca^{2+}-binding immunoglobulin-like transmembrane protein that is expressed by neurons in the developing and adult brain. It is localized to the synaptic cleft and contributes to synaptic organization and function (Fogel et al., 2007).

Growth factors and signaling molecules that were confirmed to be processed by MMP-9 *in vivo* include IL-8 (Van den Steen et al., 2000), pro brain-derived neurotrophic factor (BDNF; Hwang et al., 2005; Mizoguchi et al., 2011a), pro tumor necrosis factor α (TNF-α; Roghani et al., 1999), and pro transforming growth factor β (TGF-β; Yu and Stamenkovic, 2000). The ability of MMP-9 to cleave β-amyloid peptide is particularly interesting because an increase in MMP-9 expression was observed in Alzheimer's disease patients by several research groups (Backstrom et al., 1996; Yan et al., 2006; Mizoguchi et al., 2011a; Filippov and Dityatev, 2012).

MMP-9 IN ABERRANT STRUCTURAL PLASTICITY

Accumulating evidence suggests that MMP-9 may also play a relatively direct role in other forms of learning and memory, including those associated with addiction. Many drugs and alcohol induce neuroplastic changes in pathways that subserve emotion and cognition. Elevated MMP-9 activity has been implicated in the synaptic remodeling that is important for the reactivation of cocaine memory in rats (Brown et al., 2008a). In mice, methamphetamine treatment resulted in the rapid upregulation of MMP-9 (Liu et al., 2008; Conant et al., 2011). MMP-9 has also been implicated in the plastic changes induced by alcohol addiction (Samochowiec et al., 2010). Importantly, both drug and chronic alcohol exposure cause structural alterations of dendrites and their spines (Zhou et al., 2007; Shen et al., 2009).

The importance of MMP-9 in shaping dendritic spine architecture in disease is further supported by autism and mental retardation studies. Fragile X syndrome is a form of inherited intellectual disability (Hagerman et al., 2005; Bagni et al., 2012). Patients with fragile X syndrome have aberrant dendritic spine morphology (Rudelli et al., 1985). Long and thin immature dendritic spines are also observed in Fmr1 knockout mice, a model of fragile X syndrome (Comery et al., 1997). MMP-9 has been shown to be highly increased in the fragile X syndrome mouse model (Bilousova et al., 2009). The reduction of MMP-9 levels induced by minocycline promoted dendritic spine maturation and improved general behavioral performance. High MMP-9 activity levels are also lowered by minocycline in fragile X syndrome patients (Dziembowska et al., 2013). Notably, minocycline has been tested in clinical trials to treat fragile X syndrome and shown to provide significant functional benefits (Paribello et al., 2010; Utari et al., 2010; Leigh et al., 2013). Matrix metalloproteinases have also been implicated in other forms of autism (Abdallah and Michel, 2013). MMP-9 levels are elevated in patients with Autism Spectrum Disorder (Abdallah et al., 2012). MMP-9 levels are also increased in patients with schizophrenia (Rybakowski et al., 2013), and dendritic spine alterations have been identified in multiple brain regions in schizophrenia (Glausier and Lewis, 2013).

Aberrant structural plasticity is a major phenomenon associated with epilepsy (Scharfman, 2002). Epilepsy is a brain disorder characterized by an enduring predisposition to the generation of epileptic seizures, understood as sudden excessive neuronal discharges. In many cases, epilepsy develops as a result of brain damage caused by traumatic brain injury, stroke, or infection (Banerjee and Hauser, 2008). The primary insult is associated with an increased incidence of secondary injuries that can develop within hours to days or even weeks. Secondary brain injury is thought to be responsible for the development of many of the aforementioned sustained neurological deficits (Bolkvadze and Pitkanen, 2012; Rezaei et al., 2012; Mollayeva et al., 2013). Patients with epilepsy frequently suffer from memory impairment, behavioral problems, and psychiatric disorders (Dodrill, 2002; Helmstaedter, 2002; Williams, 2003; Elger et al., 2004; Berg, 2011). Dendritic spines receive a majority of excitatory synaptic inputs. Transmission and dendritic spine shape and function are strictly related, and such structural changes likely constitute hallmarks of pathology and the observed cognitive deficits.

Indeed, abnormalities in dendritic spines have been commonly associated with human epilepsy and animal models of epilepsy (Swann et al., 2000; Wong, 2005). A prominent decrease in dendritic spine density has been observed in pyramidal neurons in the hippocampus and neocortex and dentate granule cells in patients with temporal lobe epilepsy (Multani et al., 1994; Jiang et al., 1998; Blümcke et al., 1999; Freiman et al., 2011; Kitaura et al., 2011). Similar aberrations have been observed in animal models of epilepsy (Jiang et al., 1998; González-Burgos et al., 2004; Ampuero et al., 2007). Notably, other alterations, such as an increase in dendritic spine number or size, have also been reported (Represa et al., 1993; Suzuki et al., 1997; Isokawa, 2000). These common features of both human and animal studies indicate that dendritic spine abnormalities represent an important factor in the pathological mechanisms of posttraumatic epilepsy, but it is still unclear whether they are more related to the cause or consequence of seizures (Wong and Guo, 2013). Furthermore, dendritic spine pathology may be both the cause and consequence of seizures. Alterations in dendritic spine structure or function can affect the processing of synaptic inputs. Seizures are implicated in excessive neuronal excitability, and these changes may constitute a compensatory response in the form of a homeostatic mechanism. However, the loss of excitatory input eventually affects inhibitory networks, which in turn may cause increased excitability and an inclination toward seizures.

An important issue are the mechanisms that are involved in dendritic spine pathology in epilepsy. The ECM constitutes a natural milieu for dendritic spines, and ECM remodeling may potentially influence epileptogenesis on many different levels, predominantly related to structural reorganization. Extracellular structural networks stabilize cellular and synaptic components. When pathology occurs, however, these stable components break down, which may lead to abnormal structural reorganization (i.e., dendritic spine loss or axonal sprouting) that promotes circuitry reorganization and epileptogenesis. Seizures lead to striking remodeling of the ECM, which may be essentially engaged in different aspects of epileptogenesis (Dityatev, 2010; Lukasiuk et al., 2011). Metalloproteinases, enzymes that modulate the ECM, grow to be important players in these processes. Evidence for a role of MMP-9 in physiological and aberrant synaptic plasticity and posttraumatic epileptogenesis is especially strong, in contrast to other MMPs (Lukasiuk et al., 2011).

Some evidence also comes from human studies. The critical role of MMP-9 in pathology following trauma is supported by clinical studies, in which elevated levels of MMP-9 were detected in cerebrospinal fluid from patients with severe traumatic brain injury (Grossetete et al., 2009). Prolonged seizures are also related to high serum MMP-9 levels in patients (Suenaga et al., 2008). MMP-9 is also upregulated in the cortex in patients with focal cortical dysplasia, a disorder associated with intractable cortical epilepsy (Konopka et al., 2013). Notably, the prominent upregulation of MMP-9 was observed mainly at postsynaptic sites (i.e., at dendritic spines).

The involvement of the MMP-9 proteolytic system has been widely studied in animal models of epilepsy. After traumatic brain injury, the activation of MMP-9 in lesioned cortex occurred within 1 day following trauma and remained elevated for 7 days after the initial insult (Hadass et al., 2013). Moreover, treatment with an MMP-9 inhibitor effectively attenuated MMP-9 activity, reduced brain lesion volume, and prevented neuronal loss and dendritic degeneration (Hadass et al., 2013). Similarly, after brain trauma, MMP-9 protein levels are increased compared with the contralateral cortex, with a peak 24 h following injury and elevations that persist for up to 1 week. Moreover, MMP-9 knockout mice have smaller traumatic brain lesion volumes (Wang et al., 2000).

MMP-9 is also induced during status epilepticus after treatment with kainate (Zhang et al., 2000; Szklarczyk et al., 2002;

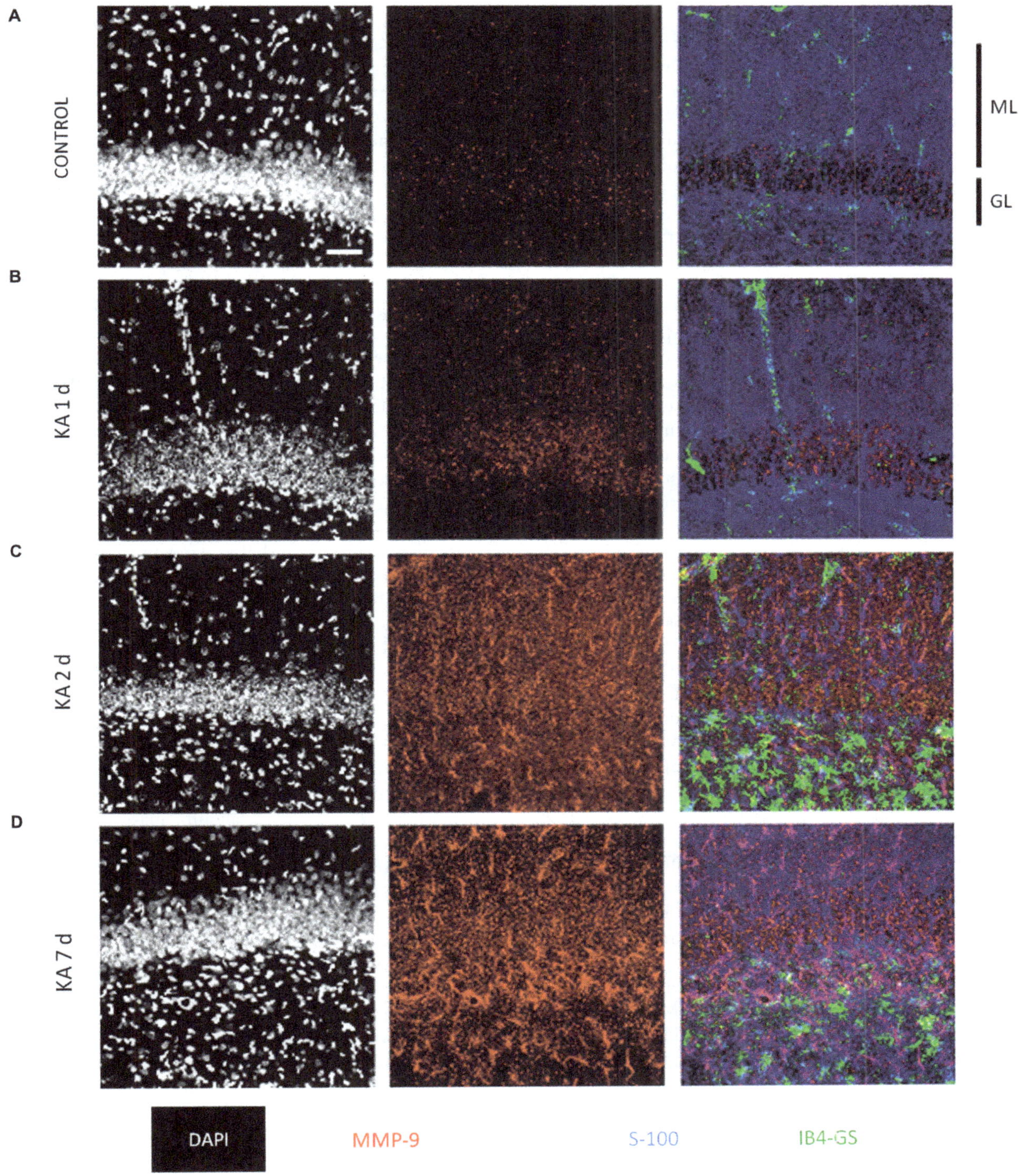

FIGURE 3 | MMP-9 immunoreactivity (IR) in the Dentate Gyrus (DG) of control animal and 1–7 days following intra-amygdalar kainic acid (KA) administration. (A) Immediately after KA administration MMP-9 IR is low and distributed equally across DG layers. **(B–D)** MMP-9 IR increases after KA injection. **(C–D)** Note increased IR of MMP-9 predominantly in molecular layer (ML). **(D)** Seven days post KA administration neuronal MMP-9 reservoir is enriched with astrocytic pool. Confocal images from brain tissue labeled with nuclear marker (DAPI—white), MMP-9 antibody (red), astrocyte marker anitbody (S-100, blue), microglia marker antibody (IB4-GS, green). GL—granular layer, ML—molecular layer. Scale bar 50 μm. The experiment was performed by dr Grzegorz Wilczynski. For further reference, see Wilczynski et al. (2008).

Jourquin et al., 2003; Konopacki et al., 2007) and pilocarpine (Kim et al., 2009). MMP-9 immunoreactivity (IR) is increased 24 h after kainic acid (KA) administration. IR is initially observed in neurons, and expression remains elevated for up to 7 days. Notably, MMP-9 IR is also observed in astrocytes (**Figure 3**). The increased expression and activity of MMP-9 has been shown to also occur with pentylenetetrazol (PTZ)-induced seizures (Michaluk et al., 2007; Rylski et al., 2009; Mizoguchi et al., 2011b). In these models, MMP-9 has been suggested to contribute to neuronal death (Jourquin et al., 2003; Kim et al., 2009), dendritic spine pruning (Szklarczyk et al., 2002), and the formation of aberrant synaptic contacts (Szklarczyk et al., 2002).

Strong evidence for a pivotal role of MMP-9 in epileptogenesis-related plasticity was provided by Mizoguchi and Wilczynski (Wilczynski et al., 2008; Mizoguchi et al., 2011a). Repeated treatment with PTZ produced kindled seizure, accompanied by enhanced MMP-9 activity and expression in the hippocampus (Mizoguchi et al., 2011a). The sensitivity to PTZ kindling was decreased in MMP-9 knockout mice (Wilczynski et al., 2008; Mizoguchi et al., 2011a). These mice also exhibited less severe seizures. In contrast, rats with constitutive neuronal MMP-9 overexpression that received PTZ treatment were more susceptible to seizures than wildtype animals. MMP-9 has been suggested to facilitate the development of seizures by affecting epilepsy-related synaptic plasticity. Seizure-induced MMP-9 expression was previously shown to be localized to dendrites and synapses and implicated in synaptic remodeling and mossy fiber sprouting, pathological structural phenomena associated with epilepsy (Szklarczyk et al., 2002; Michaluk and Kaczmarek, 2007; Gawlak et al., 2009). Indeed, MMP-9 protein levels and activity localized at synapses were strongly upregulated following intraperitoneal kainate treatment (Wilczynski et al., 2008). In the same study, unilateral kainate injections into the amygdala were used to induce status epilepticus. Twenty-four hours after seizure onset, spine density decreased in the DG on the injected side compared with the contralateral side in MMP-9 wildtype animals. In contrast, no difference in spine density was found between the injected and contralateral sides in MMP-9 knockout mice. Overall, status epilepticus-induced dendritic spine loss in the ML of the DG appears to be mediated by MMP-9 release from spines in response to seizures. In MMP-9 knockout animals the pruning of dendritic spines is abolished, despite the presence of stimulus. MMP-9 was also shown to be involved in mossy fiber sprouting and aberrant synaptogenesis in hippocampal epileptogenesis, in which neither of these phenomena develop in the absence of the enzyme. Interestingly, mossy fiber sprouting sites have been associated with the regrowth of dendritic spines in this region after status epilepticus (Isokawa, 2000).

MMP-9 activity was also considerably enhanced in other epilepsy models that do not involve neuronal cell loss (Baracskay et al., 2008; Gallyas et al., 2008; Sarkisova and van Luijtelaar, 2011). MMP-9 may be involved in generalized absence epilepsy, in which increased activity was found in WAG/Rij rats (Takacs et al., 2010). These rats spontaneously produce absence-like seizures caused by the hypersynchronic activity of thalamocortical and corticothalamic neurons and are commonly used as an animal model of human absence epilepsy (Coenen and Van Luijtelaar, 2003). Interestingly, the administration of doxycycline, an MMP inhibitor, aggravated epileptiform activity in WAG/Rij rats (Kovács et al., 2011). Matrix metalloproteinases were previously shown to act directly on NMDA and AMPA receptors (Michaluk et al., 2009; Gorkiewicz et al., 2010). This may, in turn, provide a sort of balanced homeostatic synaptic plasticity during seizures. NMDA and AMPA receptors are involved in the genesis of absence seizures (Coenen and Van Luijtelaar, 2003). Therefore, MMP-9 inhibition may increase the net level of excitability and increase absence-like epileptic activity in WAG/Rij rats (Takacs et al., 2010).

Considering the extant evidence, MMP-9 might play a dual role in epilepsy, with distinct roles in pathogenesis at various time-points after seizures (Michaluk and Kaczmarek, 2007). Aside from contributing to structural remodeling, MMP-9 may also be involved in maintaining homeostatic synaptic plasticity to counteract epileptic seizures. Fast activation of MMP-9 by seizures (i.e., within minutes) may induce spine loss (which is not observed in MMP-9 knockout mice) that initially alters neuronal excitability and reduces the effects of seizures. Sustained increases in MMP-9 levels (secondary to seizures, within days) may be hypothesized to push the balance toward the regrowth of dendritic spines and restore system balance but in effect contribute to long-term circuitry remodeling. Such aberrant plasticity may underlie epileptogenesis and lead to the formation of epileptic foci in the brain (**Figure 2**).

CONCLUSIONS

Brain plasticity relies on modifications in synaptic connectivity that are driven by molecular changes in neurons and the ECM. The ability to change synaptic connections comprises alterations of dendritic spines at the morphological level. We reviewed the role of ECM metalloproteinase activity in physiological and pathological structural plasticity. We summarized the contribution of MMP-9 in the dynamic remodeling of the ECM via the cleavage of numerous extracellular substrates and its role in the formation, modification, and maintenance of dendritic spines. Importantly, MMP-9 may serve as an example of a proteolytic modifier of the ECM, thus supporting the concept of a tetrapartite synapse. Finally, we examined the morphological abnormalities of dendritic protrusions that are well known to be associated with neuropsychiatric disorders, particularly those that involve cognitive deficits. We reviewed evidence that implicates MMP-9 in aberrant synaptic plasticity and spine dysmorphology in neuropsychiatric disorders.

ACKNOWLEDGMENTS

This work was supported by the Ministry of Science and Higher Education (grant no. IP2011 060671), the European Regional Development Fund (POIG 01.01.02-00-008/08), and an ERA-NET-NEURON/09/2013 grant to Marzena Stefaniuk.

We would like to thank prof. Leszek Kaczmarek for the critical review of the manuscript. We would like to thank prof. Wilczynski for kindly providing **Figure 3**.

Marzena Stefaniuk, Michal Stawarski and Jakub Wlodarczyk drafted and critically revised the manuscript. Jakub Wlodarczyk contributed to the general conception of the work and approved the final version of the manuscript.

REFERENCES

Abdallah, M. W., and Michel, T. M. (2013). Matrix metalloproteinases in autism spectrum disorders. *J. Mol. Psychiatry* 1:16. doi: 10.1186/2049-9256-1-16

Abdallah, M. W., Pearce, B. D., Larsen, N., Greaves-Lord, K., Nørgaard-Pedersen, B., Hougaard, D. M., et al. (2012). Amniotic fluid MMP-9 and neurotrophins in autism spectrum disorders: an exploratory study. *Autism Res.* 5, 428–433. doi: 10.1002/aur.1254

Akers, W. J., Xu, B., Lee, H., Sudlow, G. P., Fields, G. B., Achilefu, S., et al. (2012). Detection of MMP-2 and MMP-9 activity in vivo with a triple-helical peptide optical probe. *Bioconjug. Chem.* 23, 656–663. doi: 10.1021/bc300027y

Akool, E. S., Kleinert, H., Hamada, F. M., Abdelwahab, M. H., Forstermann, U., Pfeilschifter, J., et al. (2003). Nitric oxide increases the decay of matrix metalloproteinase 9 mRNA by inhibiting the expression of mRNA-stabilizing factor HuR. *Mol. Cell. Biol.* 23, 4901–4916. doi: 10.1128/mcb.23.14.4901-4916.2003

Ampuero, E., Dagnino-Subiabre, A., Sandoval, R., Zepeda-Carreno, R., Sandoval, S., Viedma, A., et al. (2007). Status epilepticus induces region-specific changes in dendritic spines, dendritic length and TrkB protein content of rat brain cortex. *Brain Res.* 1150, 225–238. doi: 10.1016/j.brainres.2007.02.089

Araque, A., Parpura, V., Sanzgiri, R. P., and Haydon, P. G. (1999). Tripartite synapses: glia, the unacknowledged partner. *Trends Neurosci.* 22, 208–215. doi: 10.1016/s0166-2236(98)01349-6

Araya, R., Jiang, J., Eisenthal, K. B., and Yuste, R. (2006). The spine neck filters membrane potentials. *Proc. Natl. Acad. Sci. U S A* 103, 17961–17966. doi: 10.1073/pnas.0608755103

Backstrom, J. R., Lim, G. P., Cullen, M. J., and Tokes, Z. A. (1996). Matrix metalloproteinase-9 (MMP-9) is synthesized in neurons of the human hippocampus and is capable of degrading the amyloid-β peptide (1–40). *J. Neurosci.* 16, 7910–7919.

Bagni, C., Tassone, F., Neri, G., and Hagerman, R. (2012). Fragile X syndrome: causes, diagnosis, mechanisms and therapeutics. *J. Clin. Invest.* 122, 4314–4322. doi: 10.1172/JCI63141

Bajor, M., Michaluk, P., Gulyassy, P., Kekesi, A. K., Juhasz, G., and Kaczmarek, L. (2012). Synaptic cell adhesion molecule-2 and collapsing response mediator protein-2 are novel members of the matrix metalloproteinase-9 degradome. *J. Neurochem.* 122, 775–788. doi: 10.1111/j.1471-4159.2012.07829.x

Banerjee, P. N., and Hauser, W. A. (2008). "Incidence and prevalence," in *Epilepsy. A Comprehensive Textbook*, eds J. Engel and T. A. Pedley (Philadelphia: Wolters Kluwer Health/Lippincott Williams and Wilkins), 45–56.

Baracskay, P., Szepesi, Z., Orban, G., Juhasz, G., and Czurko, A. (2008). Generalization of seizures parallels the formation of "dark" neurons in the hippocampus and pontine reticular formation after focal-cortical application of 4-aminopyridine (4-AP) in the rat. *Brain Res.* 1228, 217–228. doi: 10.1016/j.brainres.2008.06.044

Becker, J. W., Marcy, A. I., Rokosz, L. L., Axel, M. G., Burbaum, J. J., Fitzgerald, P. M., et al. (1995). Stromelysin-1: three-dimensional structure of the inhibited catalytic domain and of the C-truncated proenzyme. *Protein Sci.* 4, 1966–1976. doi: 10.1002/pro.5560041002

Berg, A. T. (2011). Epilepsy, cognition and behavior: the clinical picture. *Epilepsia* 52(Suppl. 1), 7–12. doi: 10.1111/j.1528-1167.2010.02905.x

Bilousova, T. V., Dansie, L., Ngo, M., Aye, J., Charles, J. R., Ethell, D. W., et al. (2009). Minocycline promotes dendritic spine maturation and improves behavioural performance in the fragile X mouse model. *J. Med. Genet.* 46, 94–102. doi: 10.1136/jmg.2008.061796

Blümcke, I., Zuschratter, W., Schewe, J. C., Suter, B., Lie, A. A., Riederer, B. M., et al. (1999). Cellular pathology of hilar neurons in Ammon's horn sclerosis. *J. Comp. Neurol.* 414, 437–453. doi: 10.1002/(sici)1096-9861(19991129)414:4<437::aid-cne2>3.0.co;2-3

Bode, W., Fernandez-Catalan, C., Nagase, H., and Maskos, K. (1999). Endoproteinase-protein inhibitor interactions. *APMIS* 107, 3–10. doi: 10.1111/j.1699-0463.1999.tb01520.x

Bolkvadze, T., and Pitkanen, A. (2012). Development of post-traumatic epilepsy after controlled cortical impact and lateral fluid-percussion-induced brain injury in the mouse. *J. Neurotrauma* 29, 789–812. doi: 10.1089/neu.2011.1954

Bourguignon, L. Y., Zhu, D., and Zhu, H. (1998). CD44 isoform-cytoskeleton interaction in oncogenic signaling and tumor progression. *Front. Biosci.* 3, d637–d649.

Bowe, M. A., Deyst, K. A., Leszyk, J. D., and Fallon, J. R. (1994). Identification and purification of an agrin receptor from Torpedo postsynaptic membranes: a heteromeric complex related to the dystroglycans. *Neuron* 12, 1173–1180. doi: 10.1016/0896-6273(94)90324-7

Bozdagi, O., Nagy, V., Kwei, K. T., and Huntley, G. W. (2007). In vivo roles for matrix metalloproteinase-9 in mature hippocampal synaptic physiology and plasticity. *J. Neurophysiol.* 98, 334–344. doi: 10.1152/jn.00202.2007

Brown, T. E., Forquer, M. R., Harding, J. W., Wright, J. W., and Sorg, B. A. (2008a). Increase in matrix metalloproteinase-9 levels in the rat medial prefrontal cortex after cocaine reinstatement of conditioned place preference. *Synapse* 62, 886–889. doi: 10.1002/syn.20562

Brown, C. E., Wong, C., and Murphy, T. H. (2008b). Rapid morphologic plasticity of peri-infarct dendritic spines after focal ischemic stroke. *Stroke* 39, 1286–1291. doi: 10.1161/STROKEAHA.107.498238

Bruno, M. A., and Cuello, A. C. (2006). Activity-dependent release of precursor nerve growth factor, conversion to mature nerve growth factor and its degradation by a protease cascade. *Proc. Natl. Acad. Sci. U S A* 103, 6735–6740. doi: 10.1073/pnas.0510645103

Campanelli, J. T., Gayer, G. G., and Scheller, R. H. (1996). Alternative RNA splicing that determines agrin activity regulates binding to heparin and α-dystroglycan. *Development* 122, 1663–1672.

Campbell, J. N., Low, B., Kurz, J. E., Patel, S. S., Young, M. T., and Churn, S. B. (2012). Mechanisms of dendritic spine remodeling in rat model of traumatic brain injury. *J. Neurotrauma* 29, 218–234. doi: 10.1089/neu.2011.1762

Cao, W., Duan, J., Wang, X., Zhong, X., Hu, Z., Huang, F., et al. (2014). Early enriched environment induces an increased conversion of proBDNF to BDNF in the adults rat's hippocampus. *Behav. Brain Res.* 265, 76–83. doi: 10.1016/j.bbr.2014.02.022

Cha, H., Kopetzki, E., Huber, R., Lanzendorfer, M., and Brandstetter, H. (2002). Structural basis of the adaptive molecular recognition by MMP9. *J. Mol. Biol.* 320, 1065–1079. doi: 10.1016/s0022-2836(02)00558-2

Chung, K., Wallace, J., Kim, S.-Y., Kalyanasundaram, S., Andalman, A. S., Davidson, T. J., et al. (2013). Structural and molecular interrogation of intact biological systems. *Nature* 497, 332–337. doi: 10 1038/nature12107

Coenen, A. M., and Van Luijtelaar, E. L. (2003). Genetic animal models for absence epilepsy: a review of the WAG/Rij strain of rats. *Behav. Genet.* 33, 635–655. doi: 10.1023/A:1026179013847

Comery, T. A., Harris, J. B., Willems, P. J., Oostra, B. A., Irwin, S. A., Weiler, I. J., et al. (1997). Abnormal dendritic spines in fragile X knockout mice: maturation and pruning deficits. *Proc. Natl. Acad. Sci. U S A* 94, 5401–5404. doi: 10.1073/pnas.94.10.5401

Conant, K., Lonskaya, I., Szklarczyk, A., Krall, C., Steiner, J., Maguire-Zeiss, K., et al. (2011). Methamphetamine-associated cleavage of the synaptic adhesion molecule intercellular adhesion molecule-5. *J. Neurochem.* 118, 521–532. doi: 10.1111/j.1471-4159.2010.07153.x

Conant, K., Wang, Y., Szklarczyk, A., Dudak, A., Mattson, M. P., and Lim, S. T. (2010). Matrix metalloproteinase-dependent shedding of intercellular adhesion molecule-5 occurs with long-term potentiation. *Neuroscience* 166, 508–521. doi: 10.1016/j.neuroscience.2009.12.061

Czech, T., Yang, J. W., Csaszar, E., Kappler, J., Baumgartner, C., and Lubec, G. (2004). Reduction of hippocampal collapsin response mediated protein-2 in patients with mesial temporal lobe epilepsy. *Neurochem. Res.* 29, 2189–2196. doi: 10.1007/s11064-004-7025-3

Dansie, L. E., and Ethell, I. M. (2011). Casting a net on dendritic spines: the extracellular matrix and its receptors. *Dev. Neurobiol.* 71, 956–981. doi: 10.1002/dneu.20963

De Leo, J. A., Tawfik, V. L., and Lacroix-Fralish, M. L. (2006). The tetrapartite synapse: path to CNS sensitization and chronic pain. *Pain* 122, 17–21. doi: 10.1016/j.pain.2006.02.034

De Paiva, C. S., Yoon, K. C., Pangelinan, S. B., Pham, S., Puthenparambil, L. M., Chuang, E. Y., et al. (2009). Cleavage of functional IL-2 receptor alpha chain (CD25) from murine corneal and conjunctival epithelia by MMP-9. *J. Inflamm. (Lond)* 6:31. doi: 10.1186/1476-9255-6-31 de Vivo, L., Landi, S., Panniello, M., Baroncelli, L., Chierzi, S., Mariotti, L., et al. (2013). Extracellular matrix inhibits structural and functional plasticity of dendritic spines in the adult visual cortex. *Nat. Commun.* 4:1484. doi: 10.1038/ncomms2491

Dityatev, A. (2010). Remodeling of extracellular matrix and epileptogenesis. *Epilepsia* 51(Suppl. 3), 61–65. doi: 10.1111/j.1528-1167.2010.02612.x

Dityatev, A., and Rusakov, D. A. (2011). Molecular signals of plasticity at the tetrapartite synapse. *Curr. Opin. Neurobiol.* 21, 353–359. doi: 10.1016/j.conb.2010.12.006

Dityatev, A., Schachner, M., and Sonderegger, P. (2010). The dual role of the extracellular matrix in synaptic plasticity and homeostasis. *Nat. Rev. Neurosci.* 11, 735–746. doi: 10.1038/nrn2898

Dodrill, C. B. (2002). Progressive cognitive decline in adolescents and adults with epilepsy. *Prog. Brain Res.* 135, 399–407. doi: 10.1016/s0079-6123(02)35037-4

Dziembowska, M., Milek, J., Janusz, A., Rejmak, E., Romanowska, E., Gorkiewicz, T., et al. (2012). Activity-dependent local translation of matrix metalloproteinase-9. *J. Neurosci.* 32, 14538–14547. doi: 10.1523/JNEUROSCI.6028-11.2012

Dziembowska, M., Pretto, D. I., Janusz, A., Kaczmarek, L., Leigh, M. J., Gabriel, N., et al. (2013). High MMP-9 activity levels in fragile X syndrome are lowered by minocycline. *Am. J. Med. Genet. A* 161A, 1897–1903. doi: 10.1002/ajmg.a.36023

Elger, C. E., Helmstaedter, C., and Kurthen, M. (2004). Chronic epilepsy and cognition. *Lancet Neurol.* 3, 663–672. doi: 10.1016/S1474-4422(04)00906-8

Ervasti, J. M., and Campbell, K. P. (1993). A role for the dystrophin-glycoprotein complex as a transmembrane linker between laminin and actin. *J. Cell Biol.* 122, 809–823. doi: 10.1083/jcb.122.4.809

Ethell, I. M., and Ethell, D. W. (2007). Matrix metalloproteinases in brain development and remodeling: synaptic functions and targets. *J. Neurosci. Res.* 85, 2813–2823. doi: 10.1002/jnr.21273

Faust, A., Waschkau, B., Waldeck, J., Höltke, C., Breyholz, H.-J., Wagner, S., et al. (2008). Synthesis and evaluation of a novel fluorescent photoprobe for imaging matrix metalloproteinases. *Bioconjug. Chem.* 19, 1001–1008. doi: 10.1021/bc700409j

Filippov, M. A., and Dityatev, A. (2012). Matrix metalloproteinase-9 and non-amyloidogenic pathway of amyloid precursor protein processing. *J. Neurochem.* 121, 181–183. doi: 10.1111/j.1471-4159.2011.07641.x

Fogel, A. I., Akins, M. R., Krupp, A. J., Stagi, M., Stein, V., and Biederer, T. (2007). SynCAMs organize synapses through heterophilic adhesion. *J. Neurosci.* 27, 12516–12530. doi: 10.1523/jneurosci.2739-07.2007

Foscarin, S., Ponchione, D., Pajaj, E., Leto, K., Gawlak, M., Wilczynski, G. M., et al. (2011). Experience-dependent plasticity and modulation of growth regulatory molecules at central synapses. *PLoS One* 6:e16666. doi: 10.1371/journal.pone.0016666

Freiman, T. M., Eismann-Schweimler, J., and Frotscher, M. (2011). Granule cell dispersion in temporal lobe epilepsy is associated with changes in dendritic orientation and spine distribution. *Exp. Neurol.* 229, 332–338. doi: 10.1016/j.expneurol.2011.02.017

Fudala, R., Ranjan, A. P., Mukerjee, A., Vishwanatha, J. K., Gryczynski, Z., Borejdo, J., et al. (2011). Fluorescence detection of MMP-9: I. MMP-9 selectively cleaves Lys-Gly-Pro-Arg-Ser-Leu-Ser-Gly-Lys peptide. *Curr. Pharm. Biotechnol.* 12, 834–838. doi: 10.2174/138920111795470967

Fukata, Y., Itoh, T. J., Kimura, T., Menager, C., Nishimura, T., Shiromizu, T., et al. (2002). CRMP-2 binds to tubulin heterodimers to promote microtubule assembly. *Nat. Cell Biol.* 4, 583–591. doi: 10.1038/ncb825

Gallyas, F., Kiglics, V., Baracskay, P., Juhasz, G., and Czurko, A. (2008). The mode of death of epilepsy-induced "dark" neurons is neither necrosis nor apoptosis: an electron-microscopic study. *Brain Res.* 1239, 207–215. doi: 10.1016/j.brainres.2008.08.069

Ganguly, K., Rejmak, E., Mikosz, M., Nikolaev, E., Knapska, E., and Kaczmarek, L. (2013). Matrix metalloproteinases (MMP) 9 transcription in mouse brain induced by fear learning. *J. Biol. Chem.* 288, 20978–20991. doi: 10.1074/jbc.m113.457903

Gawlak, M., Górkiewicz, T., Gorlewicz, A., Konopacki, F. A., Kaczmarek, L., and Wilczynski, G. M. (2009). High resolution in situ zymography reveals matrix metalloproteinase activity at glutamatergic synapses. *Neuroscience* 158, 167–176. doi: 10.1016/j.neuroscience.2008.05.045

Gee, S. H., Blacher, R. W., Douville, P. J., Provost, P. R., Yurchenco, P. D., and Carbonetto, S. (1993). Laminin-binding protein 120 from brain is closely related to the dystrophin-associated glycoprotein, dystroglycan and binds with high affinity to the major heparin binding domain of laminin. *J. Biol. Chem.* 268, 14972–14980.

Glausier, J. R., and Lewis, D. A. (2013). Dendritic spine pathology in schizophrenia. *Neuroscience* 251, 90–107. doi: 10.1016/j.neuroscience.2012.04.044

González-Burgos, I., López-Vázquez, M. A., and Beas-Zárate, C. (2004). Density, but not shape, of hippocampal dendritic spines varies after a seizure-inducing acute dose of monosodium glutamate in rats. *Neurosci. Lett.* 363, 22–24. doi: 10.1016/j.neulet.2004.03.035

Gorkiewicz, T., Szczuraszek, K., Wyrembek, P., Michaluk, P., Kaczmarek, L., and Mozrzymas, J. W. (2010). Matrix metalloproteinase-9 reversibly affects the time course of NMDA-induced currents in cultured rat hippocampal neurons. *Hippocampus* 20, 1105–1108. doi: 10.1002/hipo.20736

Grossetete, M., Phelps, J., Arko, L., Yonas, H., and Rosenberg, G. A. (2009). Elevation of matrix metalloproteinases 3 and 9 in cerebrospinal fluid and blood in patients with severe traumatic brain injury. *Neurosurgery* 65, 702–708. doi: 10.1227/01.neu.0000351768.11363.48

Gu, Y., and Ihara, Y. (2000). Evidence that collapsin response mediator protein-2 is involved in the dynamics of microtubules. *J. Biol. Chem.* 275, 17917–17920. doi: 10.1074/jbc.c000179200

Gustafson, J. A., Price, R. A., Frandsen, J., Henak, C. R., Cappello, J., and Ghandehari, H. (2013). Synthesis and characterization of a matrix-metalloproteinase responsive silk-elastinlike protein polymer. *Biomacromolecules* 14, 618–625. doi: 10.1021/bm3013692

Hadass, O., Tomlinson, B. N., Gooyit, M., Chen, S., Purdy, J. J., Walker, J. M., et al. (2013). Selective inhibition of matrix metalloproteinase-9 attenuates secondary damage resulting from severe traumatic brain injury. *PLoS One* 8:e76904. doi: 10.1371/journal.pone.0076904

Hagerman, R. J., Ono, M. Y., and Hagerman, P. J. (2005). Recent advances in fragile X: a model for autism and neurodegeneration. *Curr. Opin. Psychiatry* 18, 490–496. doi: 10.1097/01.yco.0000179485.39520.b0

Hahn-Dantona, E., Ruiz, J. F., Bornstein, P., and Strickland, D. K. (2001). The low density lipoprotein receptor-related protein modulates levels of matrix metalloproteinase 9 (MMP-9) by mediating its cellular catabolism. *J. Biol. Chem.* 276, 15498–15503. doi: 10.1074/jbc.m100121200

Hama, H., Kurokawa, H., Kawano, H., Ando, R., Shimogori, T., Noda, H., et al. (2011). Scale: a chemical approach for fluorescence imaging and reconstruction of transparent mouse brain. *Nat. Neurosci.* 14, 1481–1488. doi: 10.1038/nn.2928

Harris, K. M., and Stevens, J. K. (1989). Dendritic spines of CA1 pyramidal cells in the rat hippocampus: serial electron microscopy with reference to their biophysical characteristics. *J. Neurosci.* 9, 2982–2997.

Hasebe, Y., Egawa, K., Shibanuma, M., and Nose, K. (2007). Induction of matrix metalloproteinase gene expression in an endothelial cell line by direct interaction with malignant cells. *Cancer Sci.* 98, 58–67. doi: 10.1111/j.1349-7006.2006.00344.x

Helmstaedter, C. (2002). Effects of chronic epilepsy on declarative memory systems. *Prog. Brain Res.* 135, 439–453. doi: 10.1016/s0079-6123(02)35041-6

Henry, M. D., Satz, J. S., Brakebusch, C., Costell, M., Gustafsson, E., Fassler, R., et al. (2001). Distinct roles for dystroglycan, β1 integrin and perlecan in cell surface laminin organization. *J. Cell Sci.* 114, 1137–1144.

Hill, J. W., Poddar, R., Thompson, J. F., Rosenberg, G. A., and Yang, Y. (2012). Intranuclear matrix metalloproteinases promote DNA damage and apoptosis induced by oxygen-glucose deprivation in neurons. *Neuroscience* 220, 277–290. doi: 10.1016/j.neuroscience.2012.06.019

Hsieh, H. L., Chi, P. L., Lin, C. C., Yang, C. C., and Yang, C. M. (2014). Up-regulation of ROS-dependent matrix metalloproteinase-9 from high-glucose-challenged astrocytes contributes to the neuronal apoptosis. *Mol. Neurobiol.* in press. doi: 10.1007/s12035-013-8628-y. [Epub ahead of print].

Huntley, G. W. (2012). Synaptic circuit remodelling by matrix metalloproteinases in health and disease. *Nat. Rev. Neurosci.* 13, 743–757. doi: 10.1038/nrn3320

Hwang, J. J., Park, M. H., Choi, S. Y., and Koh, J. Y. (2005). Activation of the Trk signaling pathway by extracellular zinc: role of metalloproteinases. *J. Biol. Chem.* 280, 11995–12001. doi: 10.1074/jbc.m403172200

Inagaki, N., Chihara, K., Arimura, N., Menager, C., Kawano, Y., Matsuo, N., et al. (2001). CRMP-2 induces axons in cultured hippocampal neurons. *Nat. Neurosci.* 4, 781–782. doi: 10.1038/90476

Isokawa, M. (2000). Remodeling dendritic spines of dentate granule cells in temporal lobe epilepsy patients and the rat pilocarpine model. *Epilepsia* 41(Suppl. 6), S14–S17. doi: 10.1111/j.1528-1157.2000.tb01550.x

Jaworski, J., Biedermann, I. W., Lapinska, J., Szklarczyk, A., Figiel, I., Konopka, D., et al. (1999). Neuronal excitation-driven and AP-1-dependent activation of tissue inhibitor of metalloproteinases-1 gene expression in rodent hippocampus. *J. Biol. Chem.* 274, 28106–28112. doi: 10.1074/jbc.274.40.28106

Jiang, M., Lee, C. L., Smith, K. L., and Swann, J. W. (1998). Spine loss and other persistent alterations of hippocampal pyramidal cell dendrites in a model of early-onset epilepsy. *J. Neurosci.* 18, 8356–8368.

Jourquin, J., Tremblay, E., Decanis, N., Charton, G., Hanessian, S., Chollet, A. M., et al. (2003). Neuronal activity-dependent increase of net matrix metalloproteinase activity is associated with MMP-9 neurotoxicity after kainate. *Eur. J. Neurosci.* 18, 1507–1517. doi: 10.1046/j.1460-9568.2003.02876.x

Kaczmarek, L. (2013). MMP-9 inhibitors in the brain: can old bullets shoot new targets? *Curr. Pharm. Des.* 19, 1085–1089. doi: 10.2174/1381612811319060010

Kaczmarek, L., Lapinska-Dzwonek, J., and Szymczak, S. (2002). Matrix metalloproteinases in the adult brain physiology: a link between c-Fos, AP-1 and remodeling of neuronal connections? *EMBO J.* 21, 6643–6648. doi: 10.1093/emboj/cdf676

Kaijzel, E. L., Van Heijningen, P. M., Wielopolski, P. A., Vermeij, M., Koning, G. A., Van Cappellen, W. A., et al. (2010). Multimodality imaging reveals a gradual increase in matrix metalloproteinase activity at aneurysmal lesions in live fibulin-4 mice. *Circ. Cardiovasc. Imaging* 3, 567–577. doi: 10.1161/circimaging.109.933093

Kaliszewska, A., Bijata, M., Kaczmarek, L., and Kossut, M. (2012). Experience-dependent plasticity of the barrel cortex in mice observed with 2-DG brain mapping and c-Fos: effects of MMP-9 KO. *Cereb. Cortex* 22, 2160–2170. doi: 10.1093/cercor/bhr303

Kharazia, V. N., and Weinberg, R. J. (1999). Immunogold localization of AMPA and NMDA receptors in somatic sensory cortex of albino rat. *J. Comp. Neurol.* 412, 292–302. doi: 10.1002/(sici)1096-9861(19990920)412:2<292::aid-cne8>3.0.co;2-g

Kim, B. G., Dai, H. N., McAtee, M., Vicini, S., and Bregman, B. S. (2006). Remodeling of synaptic structure in the motor cortex following spinal cord injury. *Exp. Neurol.* 198, 401–415. doi: 10.1016/j.expneurol.2005.12.010

Kim, G. W., Kim, H. J., Cho, K. J., Kim, H. W., Cho, Y. J., and Lee, B. I. (2009). The role of MMP-9 in integrin-mediated hippocampal cell death after pilocarpine-induced status epilepticus. *Neurobiol. Dis.* 36, 169–180. doi: 10.1016/j.nbd.2009.07.008

Kim, Y. H., Kwon, H. J., and Kim, D. S. (2012). Matrix metalloproteinase 9 (MMP-9)-dependent processing of βig-h3 protein regulates cell migration, invasion and adhesion. *J. Biol. Chem.* 287, 38957–38969. doi: 10.1074/jbc.M112.357863

Kitaura, H., Hiraishi, T., Murakami, H., Masuda, H., Fukuda, M., Oishi, M., et al. (2011). Spatiotemporal dynamics of epileptiform propagations: imaging of human brain slices. *Neuroimage* 58, 50–59. doi: 10.1016/j.neuroimage.2011.05.046

Kjeldsen, L., Johnsen, A. H., Sengelov, H., and Borregaard, N. (1993). Isolation and primary structure of NGAL, a novel protein associated with human neutrophil gelatinase. *J. Biol. Chem.* 268, 10425–10432.

Klein, R. (2004). Eph/ephrin signaling in morphogenesis, neural development and plasticity. *Curr. Opin. Cell Biol.* 16, 580–589. doi: 10.1016/j.ceb.2004.07.002

Konopacki, F. A., Rylski, M., Wilczek, E., Amborska, R., Detka, D., Kaczmarek, L., et al. (2007). Synaptic localization of seizure-induced matrix metalloproteinase-9 mRNA. *Neuroscience* 150, 31–39. doi: 10.1016/j.neuroscience.2007.08.026

Konopka, A., Grajkowska, W., Ziemianska, K., Roszkowski, M., Daszkiewicz, P., Rysz, A., et al. (2013). Matrix metalloproteinase-9 (MMP-9) in human intractable epilepsy caused by focal cortical dysplasia. *Epilepsy Res.* 104, 45–58. doi: 10.1016/j.eplepsyres.2012.09.018

Kovács, Z., Kekesi, K. A., Baracskay, P., Juhasz, G., and Czurko, A. (2011). Doxycycline could aggravate the absence-like epileptic seizures of WAG/Rij rats via matrix metalloproteinase inhibition. *Neurochem. Int.* 59, 563–566. doi: 10.1016/j.neuint.2011.06.016

Kowluru, R. A., Mohammad, G., dos Santos, J. M., and Zhong, Q. (2011). Abrogation of MMP-9 gene protects against the development of retinopathy in diabetic mice by preventing mitochondrial damage. *Diabetes* 60, 3023–3033. doi: 10.2337/db11-0816

Kuzniewska, B., Rejmak, E., Malik, A. R., Jaworski, J., Kaczmarek, L., and Kalita, K. (2013). Brain-derived neurotrophic factor induces matrix metalloproteinases-9 expression in neurons via the the serum response factor/c-Fos pathway. *Mol. Cell. Biol.* 33, 2149–2162. doi: 10.1128/MCB.00008-13

Labrie, M., and St-Pierre, Y. (2013). Epigenetic regulation of *mmp-9* gene expression. *Cell. Mol. Life Sci.* 70, 3109–3124. doi: 10.5713/ajas.2012.12529

Larsen, P. H., Wells, J. E., Stallcup, W. B., Opdenakker, G., and Yong, V. W. (2003). Matrix metalloproteinase-9 facilitates remyelination in part by processing the inhibitory NG2 proteoglycan. *J. Neurosci.* 23, 11127–11135.

Lee, C. M., Jang, D., Cheong, S. J., Jeong, M. H., Kim, E. M., Kim, D. W., et al. (2012). Optical imaging of MMP expression and cancer progression in an inflammation-induced colon cancer model. *Int. J. Cancer* 131, 1846–1853. doi: 10.1002/ijc.27451

Leigh, M. J., Nguyen, D. V., Mu, Y., Winarni, T. I., Schneider, A., Chechi, T., et al. (2013). A randomized double-blind, placebo-controlled trial of minocycline in children and adolescents with fragile × syndrome. *J. Dev. Behav. Pediatr.* 34, 147–155. doi: 10.1097/DBP.0b013e318287cd17

Lin, K. T., Sloniowski, S., Ethell, D. W., and Ethell, I. M. (2008). Ephrin-B2-induced cleavage of EphB2 receptor is mediated by matrix metalloproteinases to trigger cell repulsion. *J. Biol. Chem.* 283, 28969–28979. doi: 10.1074/jbc.M804401200

Liu, Y., Brown, S., Shaikh, J., Fishback, J. A., and Matsumoto, R. R. (2008). Relationship between methamphetamine exposure and matrix metalloproteinase 9 expression. *Neuroreport* 19, 1407–1409. doi: 10.1097/WNR.0b013e32830dd606

Lonskaya, I., Partridge, J., Lalchandani, R. R., Chung, A., Lee, T., Vicini, S., et al. (2013). Soluble ICAM-5, a product of activity dependent proteolysis, increases mEPSC frequency and dendritic expression of GluA1. *PLoS One* 8:e69136. doi: 10.1371/journal.pone.0069136

Lukasiuk, K., Wilczynski, G. M., and Kaczmarek, L. (2011). Extracellular proteases in epilepsy. *Epilepsy Res.* 96, 191–206. doi: 10.1016/j.eplepsyres.2011.08.002

Meighan, S. E., Meighan, P. C., Choudhury, P., Davis, C. J., Olson, M. L., Zornes, P. A., et al. (2006). Effects of extracellular matrix-degrading proteases matrix metalloproteinases 3 and 9 on spatial learning and synaptic plasticity. *J. Neurochem.* 96, 1227–1241. doi: 10.1111/j.1471-4159.2005.03565.x

Meyer, D., Bonhoeffer, T., and Scheuss, V. (2014). Balance and stability of synaptic structures during synaptic plasticity. *Neuron* 82, 430–443. doi: 10.1016/j.neuron.2014.02.031

Michaluk, P., and Kaczmarek, L. (2007). Matrix metalloproteinase-9 in glutamate-dependent adult brain function and dysfunction. *Cell Death Differ.* 14, 1255–1258. doi: 10.1038/sj.cdd.4402141

Michaluk, P., Kolodziej, L., Mioduszewska, B., Wilczynski, G. M., Dzwonek, J., Jaworski, J., et al. (2007). β-dystroglycan as a target for MMP-9, in response to enhanced neuronal activity. *J. Biol. Chem.* 282, 16036–16041. doi: 10.1074/jbc.m700641200

Michaluk, P., Mikasova, L., Groc, L., Frischknecht, R., Choquet, D., and Kaczmarek, L. (2009). Matrix metalloproteinase-9 controls NMDA receptor surface diffusion through integrin beta1 signaling. *J. Neurosci.* 29, 6007–6012. doi: 10.1523/JNEUROSCI.5346-08.2009

Michaluk, P., Wawrzyniak, M., Alot, P., Szczot, M., Wyrembek, P., Mercik, K., et al. (2011). Influence of matrix metalloproteinase MMP-9 on dendritic spine morphology. *J. Cell Sci.* 124, 3369–3380. doi: 10.1242/jcs.090852

Mizoguchi, H., Nakade, J., Tachibana, M., Ibi, D., Someya, E., Koike, H., et al. (2011a). Matrix metalloproteinase-9 contributes to kindled seizure development in pentylenetetrazole-treated mice by converting pro-BDNF to mature BDNF in the hippocampus. *J. Neurosci.* 31, 12963–12971. doi: 10.1523/JNEUROSCI.3118-11.2011

Mizoguchi, H., Yamada, K., and Nabeshima, T. (2011b). Matrix metalloproteinases contribute to neuronal dysfunction in animal models of drug dependence, Alzheimer's disease and epilepsy. *Biochem. Res. Int.* 2011:681385. doi: 10.1155/2011/681385

Mollayeva, T., Colantonio, A., Mollayeva, S., and Shapiro, C. M. (2013). Screening for sleep dysfunction after traumatic brain injury. *Sleep Med.* 14, 1235–1246. doi: 10.1016/j.sleep.2013.07.009

Morrison, C. J., Butler, G. S., Rodriguez, D., and Overall, C. M. (2009). Matrix metalloproteinase proteomics: substrates, targets and therapy. *Curr. Opin. Cell Biol.* 21, 645–653. doi: 10.1016/j.ceb.2009.06.006

Multani, P., Myers, R. H., Blume, H. W., Schomer, D. L., and Sotrel, A. (1994). Neocortical dendritic pathology in human partial epilepsy: a quantitative Golgi study. *Epilepsia* 35, 728–736. doi: 10.1111/j.1528-1157.1994.tb02503.x

Murai, K. K., and Pasquale, E. B. (2004). Eph receptors, ephrins and synaptic function. *Neuroscientist* 10, 304–314. doi: 10.1177/1073858403262221

Nagase, H., and Woessner, J. F. Jr. (1999). Matrix metalloproteinases. *J. Biol. Chem.* 274, 21491–21494. doi: 10.1074/jbc.274.31.21491

Nagy, V., Bozdagi, O., Matynia, A., Balcerzyk, M., Okulski, P., Dzwonek, J., et al. (2006). Matrix metalloproteinase-9 is required for hippocampal late-phase long-term potentiation and memory. *J. Neurosci.* 26, 1923–1934. doi: 10.1523/jneurosci.4359-05.2006

Nakamura, H., Fujii, Y., Inoki, I., Sugimoto, K., Tanzawa, K., Matsuki, H., et al. (2000). Brevican is degraded by matrix metalloproteinases and aggrecanase-1 (ADAMTS4) at different sites. *J. Biol. Chem.* 275, 38885–38890. doi: 10.1074/jbc.m003875200

Nedivi, E., Hevroni, D., Naot, D., Israeli, D., and Citri, Y. (1993). Numerous candidate plasticity-related genes revealed by differential cDNA cloning. *Nature* 363, 718–722. doi: 10.1038/363718a0

Nusser, Z., Lujan, R., Laube, G., Roberts, J. D., Molnar, E., and Somogyi, P. (1998). Cell type and pathway dependence of synaptic AMPA receptor number and variability in the hippocampus. *Neuron* 21, 545–559. doi: 10.1016/s0896-6273(00)80565-6

Okulski, P., Jay, T. M., Jaworski, J., Duniec, K., Dzwonek, J., Konopacki, F. A., et al. (2007). TIMP-1 abolishes MMP-9-dependent long-lasting long-term potentiation in the prefrontal cortex. *Biol. Psychiatry* 62, 359–362. doi: 10.1016/j.biopsych.2006.09.012

Overall, C. M. (2002). Molecular determinants of metalloproteinase substrate specificity: matrix metalloproteinase substrate binding domains, modules and exosites. *Mol. Biotechnol.* 22, 51–86. doi: 10.1385/mb:22:1:051

Pal-Ghosh, S., Blanco, T., Tadvalkar, G., Pajoohesh-Ganji, A., Parthasarathy, A., Zieske, J. D., et al. (2011). MMP9 cleavage of the β4 integrin ectodomain leads to recurrent epithelial erosions in mice. *J. Cell Sci.* 124, 2666–2675. doi: 10.1242/jcs.085480

Paribello, C., Tao, L., Folino, A., Berry-Kravis, E., Tranfaglia, M., Ethell, I. M., et al. (2010). Open-label add-on treatment trial of minocycline in fragile × syndrome. *BMC Neurol.* 10:91. doi: 10.1186/1471-2377-10-91

Peixoto, R. T., Kunz, P. A., Kwon, H., Mabb, A. M., Sabatini, B. L., Philpot, B. D., et al. (2012). Transsynaptic signaling by activity-dependent cleavage of neuroligin-1. *Neuron* 76, 396–409. doi: 10.1016/j.neuron.2012.07.006

Peng, H. B., Ali, A. A., Daggett, D. F., Rauvala, H., Hassell, J. R., and Smalheiser, N. R. (1998). The relationship between perlecan and dystroglycan and its implication in the formation of the neuromuscular junction. *Cell Adhes. Commun.* 5, 475–489. doi: 10.3109/15419069809005605

Penzes, P., Cahill, M. E., Jones, K. A., VanLeeuwen, J.-E., and Woolfrey, K. M. (2011). Dendritic spine pathology in neuropsychiatric disorders. *Nat. Neurosci.* 14, 285–293. doi: 10.1038/nn.2741

Pirici, D., Pirici, I., Mogoanta, L., Margaritescu, O., Tudorica, V., Margaritescu, C., et al. (2012). Matrix metalloproteinase-9 expression in the nuclear compartment of neurons and glial cells in aging and stroke. *Neuropathology* 32, 492–504. doi: 10.1111/j.1440-1789.2011.01279.x

Ramón y Cajal, S. (1888). Estructura de los centros nerviosos de las aves. *Rev. Trim. Histol. Norm. Pat.* 1, 1–10.

Ramón y Cajal, S. (1891). Sur la structure de l'écorce cérébrale de quelques mamifères. *Cellule* 7, 124–176.

Ramón y Cajal, S. (1893). Neue darstellung vom histologischen bau des centralnervensystem. *Arch. Anat. Entwick. Anat. Abt. Suppl.* 1893, 319–428.

Ramón y Cajal, S. (1899). Estudios sobre la cortexa cerebral humana: corteza visual. *Rev. Trim. Microgr.* 4, 1–63.

Represa, A., Jorquera, I., Le Gal La Salle, G., and Ben-Ari, Y. (1993). Epilepsy induced collateral sprouting of hippocampal mossy fibers: does it induce the development of ectopic synapses with granule cell dendrites? *Hippocampus* 3, 257–268. doi: 10.1002/hipo.450030303

Rezaei, S., Asgari, K., Yousefzadeh, S., Moosavi, H. A., and Kazemnejad, E. (2012). Effects of neurosurgical treatment and severity of head injury on cognitive functioning, general health and incidence of mental disorders in patients with traumatic brain injury. *Arch. Trauma Res.* 1, 93–100. doi: 10.5812/atr.6546

Rivera, S., Khrestchatisky, M., Kaczmarek, L., Rosenberg, G. A., and Jaworski, D. M. (2010). Metzincin proteases and their inhibitors: foes or friends in nervous system physiology? *J. Neurosci.* 30, 15337–15357. doi: 10.1523/JNEUROSCI.3467-10.2010

Roghani, M., Becherer, J. D., Moss, M. L., Atherton, R. E., Erdjument-Bromage, H., Arribas, J., et al. (1999). Metalloprotease-disintegrin MDC9: intracellular maturation and catalytic activity. *J. Biol. Chem.* 274, 3531–3540. doi: 10.1074/jbc.274.6.3531

Rosenblum, G., Van Den Steen, P. E., Cohen, S. R., Grossmann, J. G., Frenkel, J., Sertchook, R., et al. (2007). Insights into the structure and domain flexibility of full-length pro-matrix metalloproteinase-9/gelatinase B. *Structure* 15, 1227–1236. doi: 10.1016/j.str.2007.07.019

Roy, R., Zurakowski, D., Pories, S., Moss, M. L., and Moses, M. A. (2011). Potential of fluorescent metalloproteinase substrates for cancer detection. *Clin. Biochem.* 44, 1434–1439. doi: 10.1016/j.clinbiochem.2011.09.016

Rudelli, R. D., Brown, W. T., Wisniewski, K., Jenkins, E. C., Laure-Kamionowska, M., Connell, F., et al. (1985). Adult fragile X syndrome: clinico-neuropathologic findings. *Acta Neuropathol.* 67, 289–295. doi: 10.1007/bf00687814

Rybakowski, J. K., Remlinger-Molenda, A., Czech-Kucharska, A., Wojcicka, M., Michalak, M., and Losy, J. (2013). Increased serum matrix metalloproteinase-9 (MMP-9) levels in young patients during bipolar depression. *J. Affect. Disord.* 146, 286–289. doi: 10.1016/j.jad.2012.07.019

Rylski, M., Amborska, R., Zybura, K., Michaluk, P., Bielinska, B., Konopacki, F. A., et al. (2009). JunB is a repressor of MMP-9 transcription in depolarized rat brain neurons. *Mol. Cell. Neurosci.* 40, 98–110. doi: 10.1016/j.mcn.2008.09.005

Rylski, M., Amborska, R., Zybura, K., Mioduszewska, B., Michaluk, P., Jaworski, J., et al. (2008). Yin Yang 1 is a critical repressor of matrix metalloproteinase-9 expression in brain neurons. *J. Biol. Chem.* 283, 35140–35153. doi: 10.1074/jbc.M804540200

Sala, C., and Segal, M. (2014). The locus of structural and functional plasticity. *Physiol. Rev.* 94, 141–188. doi: 10.1152/physrev.00012.2013

Samochowiec, A., Grzywacz, A., Kaczmarek, L., Bienkowski, P., Samochowiec, J., Mierzejewski, P., et al. (2010). Functional polymorphism of matrix metalloproteinase-9 (MMP-9) gene in alcohol dependence: family and case control study. *Brain Res.* 1327, 103–106. doi: 10.1016/j.brainres.2010.02.072

Sarkisova, K., and van Luijtelaar, G. (2011). The WAG/Rij strain: a genetic animal model of absence epilepsy with comorbidity of depression [corrected]. *Prog. Neuropsychopharmacol. Biol. Psychiatry* 35, 854–876. doi: 10.1016/j.pnpbp.2010.11.010

Sbai, O., Ferhat, L., Bernard, A., Gueye, Y., Ould-Yahoui, A., Thiolloy, S., et al. (2008). Vesicular trafficking and secretion of matrix metalloproteinases-2, -9 and tissue inhibitor of metalloproteinases-1 in neuronal cells. *Mol. Cell. Neurosci.* 39, 549–568. doi: 10.1016/j.mcn.2008.08.004

Sbai, O., Ould-Yahoui, A., Ferhat, L., Gueye, Y., Bernard, A., Charrat, E., et al. (2010). Differential vesicular distribution and trafficking of MMP-2, MMP-9 and their inhibitors in astrocytes. *Glia* 58, 344–366. doi: 10.1002/glia.20927

Scharfman, H. E. (2002). Epilepsy as an example of neural plasticity. *Neuroscientist* 8, 154–173. doi: 10.1177/107385840200800211

Scherer, R., Mcintyre, J. O., and Matrisian, L. (2008). Imaging matrix metalloproteinases in cancer. *Cancer Metastasis Rev.* 27, 679–690. doi: 10.1007/s10555-008-9152-9

Schonbeck, U., Mach, F., and Libby, P. (1998). Generation of biologically active IL-1β by matrix metalloproteinases: a novel caspase-1-independent pathway of IL-1β processing. *J. Immunol.* 161, 3340–3346.

Shen, H. W., Toda, S., Moussawi, K., Bouknight, A., Zahm, D. S., and Kalivas, P. W. (2009). Altered dendritic spine elasticity in cocaine-withdrawn rats. *J. Neurosci.* 29, 2876–2884. doi: 10.1523/JNEUROSCI.5638-08.2009

Sheu, B. C., Hsu, S. M., Ho, H. N., Lien, H. C., Huang, S. C., and Lin, R. H. (2001). A novel role of metalloproteinase in cancer-mediated immunosuppression. *Cancer Res.* 61, 237–242.

Spolidoro, M., Putignano, E., Munafo, C., Maffei, L., and Pizzorusso, T. (2012). Inhibition of matrix metalloproteinases prevents the potentiation of nondeprived-eye responses after monocular deprivation in juvenile rats. *Cereb. Cortex* 22, 725–734. doi: 10.1093/cercor/bhr158

Stawarski, M., Rutkowska-Wlodarczyk, I., Zeug, A., Bijata, M., Madej, H., Kaczmarek, L., et al. (2014). Genetically encoded FRET-based biosensor for imaging MMP-9 activity. *Biomaterials* 35, 1402–1410. doi: 10.1016/j.biomaterials.2013.11.033

Stute, J., Pourmotabbed, T., and Tschesche, H. (2003). Kinetic analysis of the binding of hemopexin-like domain of gelatinase B cloned and expressed in Pichia pastoris to tissue inhibitor of metalloproteinases-1. *J. Protein Chem.* 22, 509–514. doi: 10.1023/b:jopc.0000005499.51466.50

Suenaga, N., Ichiyama, T., Kubota, M., Isumi, H., Tohyama, J., and Furukawa, S. (2008). Roles of matrix metalloproteinase-9 and tissue inhibitors of metalloproteinases 1 in acute encephalopathy following prolonged febrile seizures. *J. Neurol. Sci.* 266, 126–130. doi: 10.1016/j.jns.2007.09.011

Sugita, S., Saito, F., Tang, J., Satz, J., Campbell, K., and Sudhof, T. C. (2001). A stoichiometric complex of neurexins and dystroglycan in brain. *J. Cell Biol.* 154, 435–445. doi: 10.1083/jcb.200105003

Susaki, E. A., Tainaka, K., Perrin, D., Kishino, F., Tawara, T., Watanabe, T. M., et al. (2014). Whole-brain imaging with single-cell resolution using chemical cocktails and computational analysis. *Cell* 157, 726–739. doi: 10.1016/j.cell.2014.03.042

Suzuki, F., Makiura, Y., Guilhem, D., Sorensen, J. C., and Onteniente, B. (1997). Correlated axonal sprouting and dendritic spine formation during kainate-induced neuronal morphogenesis in the dentate gyrus of adult mice. *Exp. Neurol.* 145, 203–213. doi: 10.1006/exnr.1997.6469

Swann, J. W., Al-Noori, S., Jiang, M., and Lee, C. L. (2000). Spine loss and other dendritic abnormalities in epilepsy. *Hippocampus* 10, 617–625. doi: 10.1002/1098-1063(2000)10:5<617::aid-hipo13>3.3.co;2-i

Szepesi, Z., Bijata, M., Ruszczycki, B., Kaczmarek, L., and Wlodarczyk, J. (2013). Matrix metalloproteinases regulate the formation of dendritic spine head protrusions during chemically induced long-term potentiation. *PLoS One* 8:e63314. doi: 10.1371/journal.pone.0063314

Szepesi, Z., Hosy, E., Ruszczycki, B., Bijata, M., Pyskaty, M., Bikbaev, A., et al. (2014). Synaptically released matrix metalloproteinases activity in control of structural plasticity and the cel surface distribution of GluA1-AMPA receptors. *PLoS One* 9:e98274. doi: 10.1371/journal.pone.0098274

Szklarczyk, A., Lapinska, J., Rylski, M., McKay, R. D., and Kaczmarek, L. (2002). Matrix metalloproteinase-9 undergoes expression and activation during dendritic remodeling in adult hippocampus. *J. Neurosci.* 22, 920–930.

Takacs, E., Nyilas, R., Szepesi, Z., Baracskay, P., Karlsen, B., Rosvold, T., et al. (2010). Matrix metalloproteinase-9 activity increased by two different types of epileptic seizures that do not induce neuronal death: a possible role in homeostatic synaptic plasticity. *Neurochem. Int.* 56, 799–809. doi: 10.1016/j.neuint.2010.03.003

Takumi, Y., Ramirez-Leon, V., Laake, P., Rinvik, E., and Ottersen, O. P. (1999). Different modes of expression of AMPA and NMDA receptors in hippocampal synapses. *Nat. Neurosci.* 2, 618–624. doi: 10.1038/10172

Tian, L., Stefanidakis, M., Ning, L., Van Lint, P., Nyman-Huttunen, H., Libert, C., et al. (2007). Activation of NMDA receptors promotes dendritic spine development through MMP-mediated ICAM-5 cleavage. *J. Cell Biol.* 178, 687–700. doi: 10.1083/jcb.200612097

Tønnesen, J., Katona, G., Rózsa, B., and Nägerl, U. V. (2014). Spine neck plasticity regulates compartmentalization of synapses. *Nat. Neurosci.* 17, 678–685. doi: 10.1038/nn.3682

Tsien, R. Y. (2013). Very long-term memories may be stored in the pattern of holes in the perineuronal net. *Proc. Natl. Acad. Sci. U S A* 110, 12456–12461. doi: 10.1073/pnas.1310158110

Uchida, Y., and Goshima, Y. (2005). [Molecular mechanism of axon guidance mediated by phosphorylation of CRMP2]. *Seikagaku* 77, 1424–1427.

Utari, A., Chonchaiya, W., Rivera, S. M., Schneider, A., Hagerman, R. J., Faradz, S. M., et al. (2010). Side effects of minocycline treatment in patients with fragile X syndrome and exploration of outcome measures. *Am. J. Intellect. Dev. Disabil.* 115, 433–443. doi: 10.1352/1944-7558-115.5.433

Vaisar, T., Kassim, S. Y., Gomez, I. G., Green, P. S., Hargarten, S., Gough, P. J., et al. (2009). MMP-9 sheds the β_2 integrin subunit (CD18) from macrophages. *Mol. Cell Proteomics* 8, 1044–1060. doi: 10.1074/mcp.m800449-mcp200

Van den Steen, P. E., Proost, P., Wuyts, A., Van Damme, J., and Opdenakker, G. (2000). Neutrophil gelatinase B potentiates interleukin-8 tenfold by aminoterminal processing, whereas it degrades CTAP-III, PF-4 and GRO-α and leaves RANTES and MCP-2 intact. *Blood* 96, 2673–2681.

Van den Steen, P. E., Van Aelst, I., Hvidberg, V., Piccard, H., Fiten, P., Jacobsen, C., et al. (2006). The hemopexin and O-glycosylated domains tune gelatinase B/MMP-9 bioavailability via inhibition and binding to cargo receptors. *J. Biol. Chem.* 281, 18626–18637. doi: 10.1074/jbc.m512308200

Van Wart, H. E., and Birkedal-Hansen, H. (1990). The cysteine switch: a principle of regulation of metalloproteinase activity with potential applicability to the entire matrix metalloproteinase gene family. *Proc. Natl. Acad. Sci. U S A* 87, 5578–5582. doi: 10.1073/pnas.87.14.5578

Vandooren, J., Van den Steen, P. E., and Opdenakker, G. (2013). Biochemistry and molecular biology of gelatinase B or matrix metalloproteinase-9 (MMP-9): the next decade. *Crit. Rev. Biochem. Mol. Biol.* 48, 222–272. doi: 10.3109/10409238.2013.770819

Verslegers, M., Lemmens, K., Van Hove, I., and Moons, L. (2013). Matrix metalloproteinase-2 and -9 as promising benefactors in development, plasticity and repair of the nervous system. *Prog. Neurobiol.* 105, 60–78. doi: 10.1016/j.pneurobio.2013.03.004

Wallis de Vries, B. M., Hillebrands, J. L., Van Dam, G. M., Tio, R. A., De Jong, J. S., Slart, R. H. J. A., et al. (2009). Multispectral near-infrared fluorescence molecular imaging of matrix metalloproteinases in a human carotid plaque using a matrix-degrading metalloproteinase-sensitive activatable fluorescent probe. *Circulation* 119, e534–e536. doi: 10.1161/circulationaha.108.821389

Wang, X., Jung, J., Asahi, M., Chwang, W., Russo, L., Moskowitz, M. A., et al. (2000). Effects of matrix metalloproteinase-9 gene knock-out on morphological and motor outcomes after traumatic brain injury. *J. Neurosci.* 20, 7037–7042.

Wang, X. B., Bozdagi, O., Nikitczuk, J. S., Zhai, Z. W., Zhou, Q., and Huntley, G. W. (2008). Extracellular proteolysis by matrix metalloproteinase-9 drives dendritic spine enlargement and long-term potentiation coordinately. *Proc. Natl. Acad. Sci. U S A* 105, 19520–19525. doi: 10.1073/pnas.0807248105

Wang, X. Q., Sun, P., and Paller, A. S. (2003). Ganglioside GM3 inhibits matrix metalloproteinase-9 activation and disrupts its association with integrin. *J. Biol. Chem.* 278, 25591–25599. doi: 10.1074/jbc.m302211200

Wiera, G., Wójtowicz, T., Lebida, K., Piotrowska, A., Drulis-Fajdasz, D., Gomułkiewicz, A., et al. (2012). Long term potentiation affects intracellular metalloproteinases activity in the mossy fiber-CA3 pathway. *Mol. Cell. Neurosci.* 50, 147–159. doi: 10.1016/j.mcn.2012.04.005

Wiera, G., Wozniak, G., Bajor, M., Kaczmarek, L., and Mozrzymas, J. W. (2013). Maintenance of long-term potentiation in hippocampal mossy fiber-CA3 pathway requires fine-tuned MMP-9 proteolytic activity. *Hippocampus* 23, 529–543. doi: 10.1002/hipo.22112

Wilczynski, G. M., Konopacki, F. A, Wilczek, E., Lasiecka, Z., Gorlewicz, A., Michaluk, P., et al. (2008). Important role of matrix metalloproteinase 9 in epileptogenesis. *J. Cell Biol.* 180, 1021–1035. doi: 10.1083/jcb.200708213

Williams, J. (2003). Learning and behavior in children with epilepsy. *Epilepsy Behav.* 4, 107–111. doi: 10.1016/s1525-5050(03)00024-6

Wlodarczyk, J., Mukhina, I., Kaczmarek, L., and Dityatev, A. (2011). Extracellular matrix molecules, their receptors and secreted proteases in synaptic plasticity. *Dev. Neurobiol.* 71, 1040–1053. doi: 10.1002/dneu.20958

Wong, M. (2005). Modulation of dendritic spines in epilepsy: cellular mechanisms and functional implications. *Epilepsy Behav.* 7, 569–577. doi: 10.1016/j.yebeh.2005.08.007

Wong, M., and Guo, D. (2013). Dendritic spine pathology in epilepsy: cause or consequence? *Neuroscience* 251, 141–150. doi: 10.1016/j.neuroscience.2012.03.048

Yan, P., Hu, X., Song, H., Yin, K., Bateman, R. J., Cirrito, J. R., et al. (2006). Matrix metalloproteinase-9 degrades amyloid-β fibrils *in vitro* and compact plaques *in situ*. *J. Biol. Chem.* 281, 24566–24574. doi: 10.1074/jbc.m602440200

Yang, Y., Candelario-Jalil, E., Thompson, J. F., Cuadrado, E., Estrada, E. Y., Rosell, A., et al. (2010). Increased intranuclear matrix metalloproteinase activity in neurons interferes with oxidative DNA repair in focal cerebral ischemia. *J. Neurochem.* 112, 134–149. doi: 10.1111/j.1471-4159.2009.06433.x

Ye, S. (2000). Polymorphism in matrix metalloproteinase gene promoters: implication in regulation of gene expression and susceptibility of various diseases. *Matrix Biol.* 19, 623–629. doi: 10.1016/s0945-053x(00)00102-5

Yeghiazaryan, M., Żybura-Broda, K., Cabaj, A., Włodarczyk, J., Sławinska, U., Rylski, M., et al. (2012). Fine-structural distribution of MMP-2 and MMP-9 activities in the rat skeletal muscle upon training: a study by high-resolution in situ zymography. *Histochem. Cell Biol.* 138, 75–87. doi: 10.1007/s00418-012-0940-5

Yoshimura, T., Kawano, Y., Arimura, N., Kawabata, S., Kikuchi, A., and Kaibuchi, K. (2005). GSK-3β regulates phosphorylation of CRMP-2 and neuronal polarity. *Cell* 120, 137–149. doi: 10.1016/j.cell.2004.11.012

Yu, Q., and Stamenkovic, I. (2000). Cell surface-localized matrix metalloproteinase-9 proteolytically activates TGF-β and promotes tumor invasion and angiogenesis. *Genes Dev.* 14, 163–176.

Yuan, M., Zhan, Q., Duan, X., Song, B., Zeng, S., Chen, X., et al. (2013). A functional polymorphism at miR-491–5p binding site in the 3'-UTR of MMP-9 gene confers increased risk for atherosclerotic cerebral infarction in a Chinese population. *Atherosclerosis* 226, 447–452. doi: 10.1016/j.atherosclerosis.2012.11.026

Zagulska-Szymczak, S., Filipkowski, R. K., and Kaczmarek, L. (2001). Kainate-induced genes in the hippocampus: lessons from expression patterns. *Neurochem. Int.* 38, 485–501. doi: 10.1016/s0197-0186(00)00101-7

Zhang, J. W., Deb, S., and Gottschall, P. E. (2000). Regional and age-related expression of gelatinases in the brains of young and old rats after treatment with kainic acid. *Neurosci. Lett.* 295, 9–12. doi: 10.1016/s0304-3940(00)01582-2

Zhou, F. C., Anthony, B., Dunn, K. W., Lindquist, W. B., Xu, Z. C., and Deng, P. (2007). Chronic alcohol drinking alters neuronal dendritic spines in the brain reward center nucleus accumbens. *Brain Res.* 1134, 148–161. doi: 10.1016/j.brainres.2006.11.046

Zhu, D., Larin, K. V., Luo, Q., and Tuchin, V. V. (2013). Recent progress in tissue optical clearing. *Laser Photon. Rev.* 7, 732–757. doi: 10.1002/lpor.201200056

Zimowska, M., Swierczynska, M., and Ciemerych, M. A. (2013). Nuclear MMP-9 role in the regulation of rat skeletal myoblasts proliferation. *Biol. Cell* 105, 334–344. doi: 10.1111/boc.201300020

3

Pyramidal cell development: postnatal spinogenesis, dendritic growth, axon growth and electrophysiology

Guy N. Elston[1]* and Ichiro Fujita[2]

[1] *Centre for Cognitive Neuroscience, Sunshine Coast, QLD, Australia*
[2] *Graduate School of Frontier Biosciences and Center for Information and Neural Networks, Osaka University and National Institute of Communication Technology, Suita, Japan*

Correspondence:
Guy N. Elston, Centre for Cognitive Neuroscience, 60 Duke Rd., Doonan, Sunshine Coast, QLD 4562, Australia
e-mail: guyelston@yahoo.com

Here we review recent findings related to postnatal spinogenesis, dendritic and axon growth, pruning and electrophysiology of neocortical pyramidal cells in the developing primate brain. Pyramidal cells in sensory, association and executive cortex grow dendrites, spines and axons at different rates, and vary in the degree of pruning. Of particular note is the fact that pyramidal cells in primary visual area (V1) prune more spines than they grow during postnatal development, whereas those in inferotemporal (TEO and TE) and granular prefrontal cortex (gPFC; Brodmann's area 12) grow more than they prune. Moreover, pyramidal cells in TEO, TE and the gPFC continue to grow larger dendritic territories from birth into adulthood, replete with spines, whereas those in V1 become smaller during this time. The developmental profile of intrinsic axons also varies between cortical areas: those in V1, for example, undergo an early proliferation followed by pruning and local consolidation into adulthood, whereas those in area TE tend to establish their territory and consolidate it into adulthood with little pruning. We correlate the anatomical findings with the electrophysiological properties of cells in the different cortical areas, including membrane time constant, depolarizing sag, duration of individual action potentials, and spike-frequency adaptation. All of the electrophysiological variables ramped up before 7 months of age in V1, but continued to ramp up over a protracted period of time in area TE. These data suggest that the anatomical and electrophysiological profiles of pyramidal cells vary among cortical areas at birth, and continue to diverge into adulthood. Moreover, the data reveal that the "use it or lose it" notion of synaptic reinforcement may speak to only part of the story, "use it but you still might lose it" may be just as prevalent in the cerebral cortex.

Keywords: synaptogenesis, axon, dendrite, spine, bouton, cortex, human, macaque

INTRODUCTION

Two opposing theories on postnatal synaptogenesis have dominated over the past two and a half decades. One theory posits that circuitry in all cortical areas matures concurrently (Rakic et al., 1986), whereas the other states that circuitry in different cortical areas mature at different rates (Huttenlocher and Dabholkar, 1997). Both theories have been derived from electronmicroscopic study of the cortical neuropil. In the former hypothesis, the maximum synaptic connectivity is achieved at approximately three and a half months of age, after which there is a net reduction in the number of synaptic connections in cortex (**Figure 1**). Data were sampled from visual (V1), somatosensory (SI), motor (M1) and prefrontal cortices. In the latter hypothesis, synaptic density in the neuropil may continue to increase over an extended period of time (**Figure 2**). Data were sampled from V1, auditory (A1) and granular prefrontal cortex (middle frontal gyrus). On the face of it, these hypotheses appear to be irreconcilable. However, these two theories were based on data obtained from different species, data leading to the former view were obtained from the macaque monkey whereas those supporting the later view were obtained from the human brain. Furthermore, these data were sampled from a select few cortical areas, and were not corrected for cell death, changes in myelination nor cortical growth (see Guillery, 2005 for a review). More recent studies, which accounted for changes in myelination and blood vessels, revealed laminar differences in the developmental profiles of synaptogenesis (Bourgeois et al., 1989; Huttenlocher, 1990; Zecevic and Rakic, 1991; Bourgeois and Rakic, 1993; Granger et al., 1995), but do not reconcile the different theories.

A number of other groups have investigated the issue by using a different approach—that of studying the growth of the dendritic trees of neurons. The results are less clear cut than the above interpretations, and vary with neuron type, cortical layer and cortical area. For example, Lund and colleagues, by studying thalamocortial recipient neurons in V1 of the macaque monkey, concluded that dendritic growth is not concurrent (temporally coincident) in different populations of cells, but, rather, there is a temporal disjoin between neurons in the magno- and

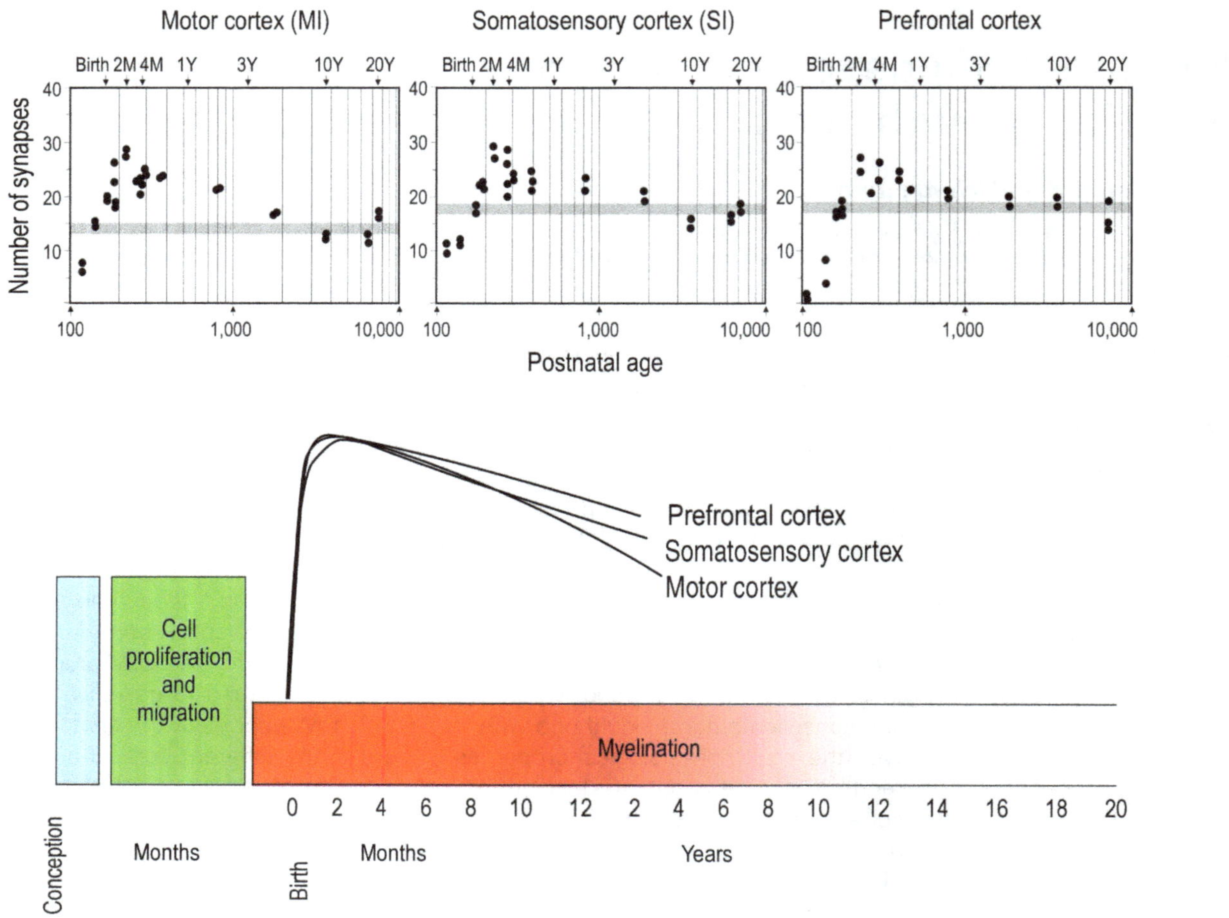

FIGURE 1 | Concurrent synaptogenesis. Plots illustrating the density of synapses per 100 μm of cortical neuropil in the primary motor (MI) and somatosensory (SI) areas and ventrolateral prefrontal cortex (Brodmann's area 12) of the macaque monkey. The average synaptic density observed in the adult in each cortical area is represented by gray stipple. Note that in all cortical areas the maximum synapse density is recorded at approximately 2 months of age. Modified from Rakic et al. (1986).

parvocellular pathways (Lund and Holbach, 1991). Moreover, the study revealed that the basal dendritic trees of pyramidal cells in V1 may continue to grow up to 9 months of age, despite a general trend for a decrease in the number of dendritic spines, the site of excitatory synaptic inputs, after 2 months of age (Boothe et al., 1979; Mates and Lund, 1983a,b). O'Kusky and Colonnier (1982) reported an increase in neuronal connectivity (as revealed by relative neuronal density, synaptic density and cortical thickness) from birth to 6 months of age in V1 of the macaque monkey, being most pronounced in supragranular layers. Becker et al. (1984) reported progressive dendritic growth and branching in the dendritic trees of supragranular pyramidal cells from conception until 2 years of age in human V1. Data reported at 2 years of age was greater than that reported in adults, but, it is difficult to determine at what age the dendritic trees stopped growing and began to retract to the size reported in the adult. Cupp and Uemura (1980) reported continued dendritic growth in pyramidal cells in the superior frontal gyrus of the macaque monkey up to 28 years of age. Koenderink et al. (1994) suggest continued growth of the dendritic trees of infragranular pyramidal cells up to at least 15 years of age in the human gPFC. Studies in the human and chimpanzee cortex reveal postnatal growth of the dendritic trees of pyramidal cells in the gPFC outstrip those in V1: in both species the dendritic trees of cells in the gPFC are small and sparsely branched at birth compared to those in V1, whereas in the adult they are markedly larger and more branched (Travis et al., 2005; Bianchi et al., 2012, 2013). Despite the variability in the results, the current view is that dendritic trees of some neurons may continue to grow well beyond the peak in synaptogenesis. The variability may reflect the different cortical areas, and species, that have been studied.

While the studies of dendritic growth provide significant insights into how the developmental profiles of neurons may vary among cortical areas, they are difficult to interpret because one must compare data sampled from one cortical area of a given species with another cortical area of a different species, or from one cortical layer with another. In addition, all of these studies

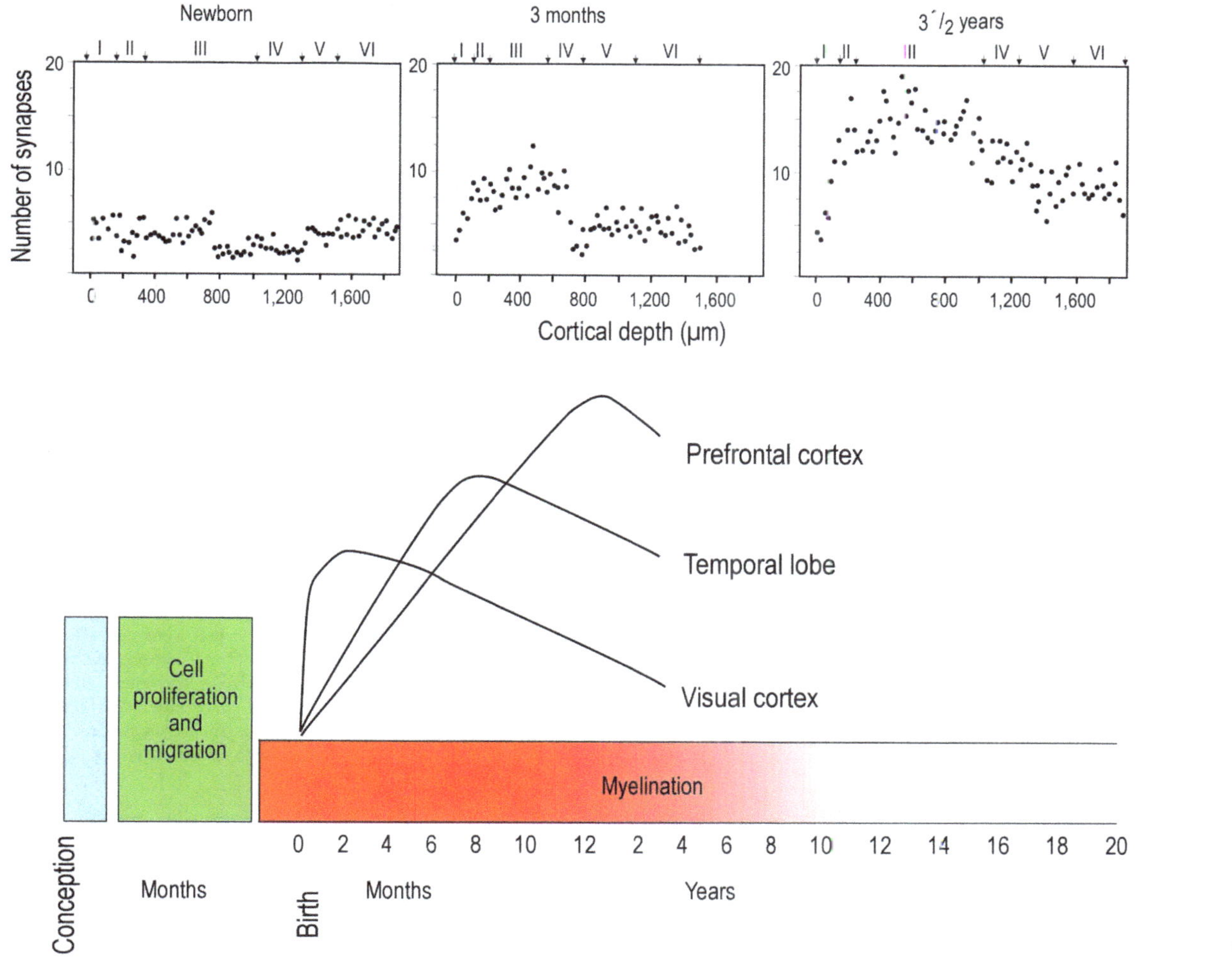

FIGURE 2 | Hierarchical synaptogenesis. Plots illustrating the density of synapses per 100 µm of cortical neuropil in human left middle frontal gyrus in the newborn, 3 month old and in the three and a half year old postnatal brain. Note that the maximum synapse density at three and a half years of age is greater than that at 3 months of age. Note also the relative differences in synapse densities in the different cortical layers at the different ages illustrated. Modified from Huttenlocher and Dabholkar (1997).

relied on the use of Golgi method. As discussed elsewhere (Elston et al., 2011b), this methodology only allows reconstruction of part of the dendritic tree (**Figure 3**). To visualize the entire basal dendritic tree of pyramidal cells in the human temporal lobe, for example, the sections would have to be at least 600 µm thick. Even then, only neurons with their cell body located some 300 µm into the section could be included for analyses otherwise some dendrites would be clipped (cf. Elston et al., 2001). Thus, while the Golgi method has been used to great effect for more than 100 years and it is fair to say that the field of neuroanatomy was built on this methodology (e.g., refer to the works of Santiago Ramon y Cajal, Karl Retzius, J LeRoy Conel, and Jennifer Lund to mention a few) and is still being used to great effect (e.g., Jacobs et al., 1997, 2001, 2014; Travis et al., 2005; Petanjek et al., 2008; Bianchi et al., 2012, 2013), a different approach was needed to test for area-specific differences in pyramidal cell structure.

A DIFFERENT WAY OF LOOKING AT IT

Intracellular injection of neurons in slices cut tangential to the cortical surface allows the visualization of the entire basal dendritic tree of large numbers of individual cells (>1000) in a single brain allowing an uninterrupted reconstruction of even the longest dendrites (**Figure 4**) that may project more than 300 µm from the cell body (e.g., Elston et al., 2001) yielding sufficient data to allow robust statistical comparisons. Neurons can be injected randomly, or specific populations of cells can be injected, such as corticocortical projecting or subcortical projecting cells (Vercelli and Innocenti, 1993; Matsubara et al., 1996; Elston and Rosa, 2006). In addition, all of the spines along a dendrite can be visualized with the aid of a high power objective and there is no need to attempt to correct for spines hidden by the Golgi precipitate (e.g., Feldman and Peters, 1979) as the DAB precipitate is less electron dense than the Golgi precipitate and the viewer is able to focus through the DAB precipitate under intense illumination

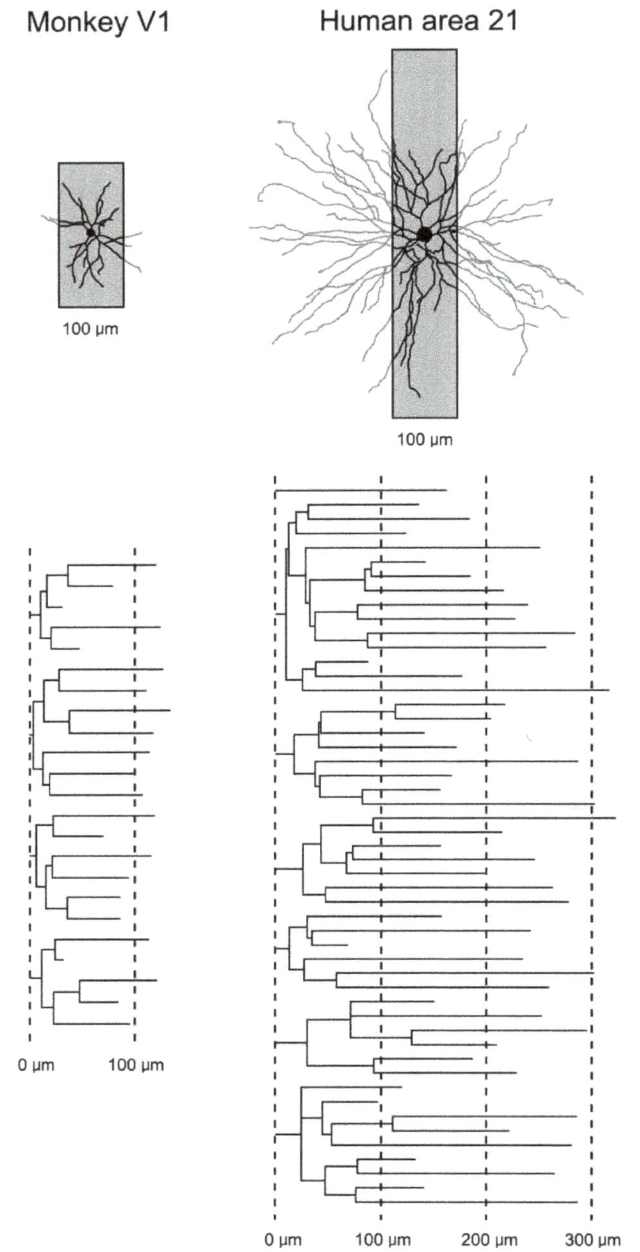

FIGURE 3 | Transverse vs. tangential plane. Schematic illustrating how the study of pyramidal cell morphology in the transverse plane may bias for uniformity in structure. Illustrated are two cells sampled from the primary visual area (V1) of the macaque monkey and Brodmann's area 21 of the temporal lobe of human (Brodmann, 1909). The basal dendritic trees of the two cells are shown in the tangential plane. Superimposed on each cell is a 100 µm gray box representing the thickness of section routinely used in Golgi studies. In black is the part of the dendritic tree that would be seen in a Golgi study. In gray is the part of the dendritic tree that would have been clipped off during sectioning and thus invisible to the observer. Below are illustrated the dendrograms of each of the two cells, which resulted from reconstruction of the complete basal dendritic tree as seen in the tangential plane. Based on our observations in the human temporal lobe (Elston et al., 2001), transverse sections used in Golgi studies would have to be > 600 µm thick, and the cell body located in the center of the section, to be able to visualize all dendrites.

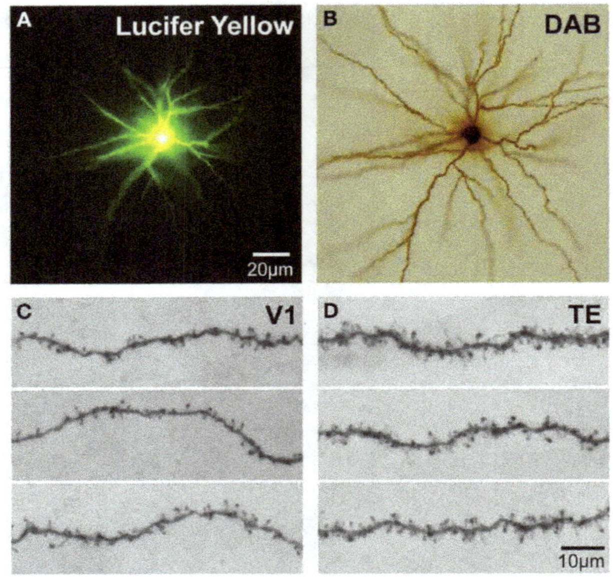

FIGURE 4 | Cell injection. (A) Low power photomicrographs of Lucifer Yellow-injected layer III pyramidal cells that were injected in tangential sections taken from the granular prefrontal cortex of the macaque monkey (area 12vl) and processed for a DAB reaction product. **(B) (C,D)** Higher power photos of primary visual (V1) and inferotemporal (TE) cortical cells as viewed through a ×100 oil-immersion Zeiss objective, revealing aspects of their fine structure including dendritic spines. Scale bar = 20 µm in **(A,B)** and 10 µm in **(C,D)**.

by standard light microscopy (see Elston and Rosa, 1997 for a discussion). Over the past 10 years we have applied this methodology to the study of pyramidal cell development in the cerebral cortex.

DENDRITIC GROWTH IN POSTNATAL DEVELOPMENT

The application of the cell injection method in flat-mount sections taken from the macaque monkey revealed systematic differences in the growth profiles of pyramidal cells among cortical areas (**Figure 5**). Notably, the basal dendritic trees of supragranular pyramidal cells continue to grow into adulthood in high level cortical areas such as visual association areas TEO, and TEpd whereas those in V1 attain their greatest postnatal size around birth (Boothe et al., 1979; Elston et al., 2010a). In granular prefrontal cortex (Brodmann's area 12), the basal dendritic trees of layer III pyramidal cells attain their largest size in adulthood (Elston et al., 2009; see also Cupp and Uemura, 1980; Anderson et al., 1995). The dendritic trees of pyramidal cells in V2 and V4 attain their greatest size at 3.5 months of age, and then decrease in size to their adult type (Elston et al., 2010a). A different profile again has been reported for cells in the primary auditory cortex (A1) in macaque, where cells grow larger dendritic trees from birth until at least 7 months of age, before decreasing in size to their adult form (Elston et al., 2010b).

Comparison of these data with previous Golgi data, and emerging cell injection data in other species, reveals potential species differences in the postnatal growth profiles of pyramidal cells in the cerebral cortex. The trend observed here in pyramidal cell growth in V1 of the macaque monkey is consistent with that

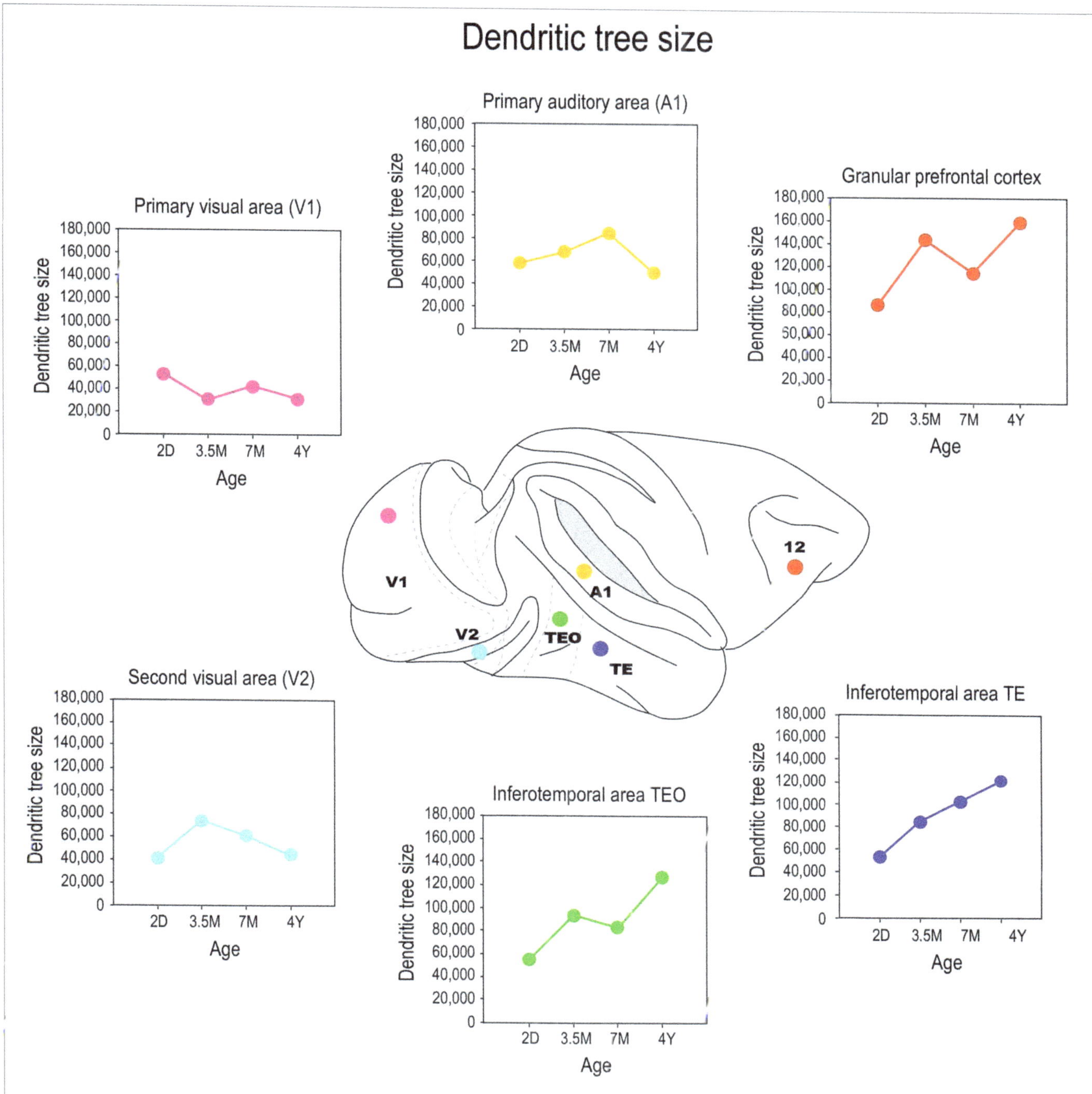

FIGURE 5 | Growth profiles. Plots of the size of the basal dendritic trees of layer III pyramidal neurons sampled from primary visual area (V1), the second visual area (V2), the primary auditory cortex (A1), the posterior and anterior portion of the inferotemporal cortex (TEO and TEpd, respectively) and prefrontal cortex (Brodmann's area 12) at postnatal day two (2D), three and a half months of age (3.5M), seven months of age (7M) and four and a half years (4Y) of age. Data taken from Elston et al. (2009, 2010a,b).

reported in human: cells become smaller after birth (Becker et al., 1984). The extended period of growth of the dendritic trees of cells in association areas of the temporal lobe and the granular prefrontal cortex in macaque is consistent with that reported in human (Conel, 1941, 1947, 1955, 1959, 1963, 1967; Elston et al., 2009, 2010a,b, 2011a). However studies in the New World marmoset monkey reveal that pyramidal cells in V1 are larger in the adult than in the newborn (Oga et al., 2013). Clearly, further comparative investigations are required.

BRANCHING

Differences were also observed in the branching profiles of the dendritic trees of pyramidal cells among cortical areas during postnatal development (**Figure 6**). Contrary to what might be

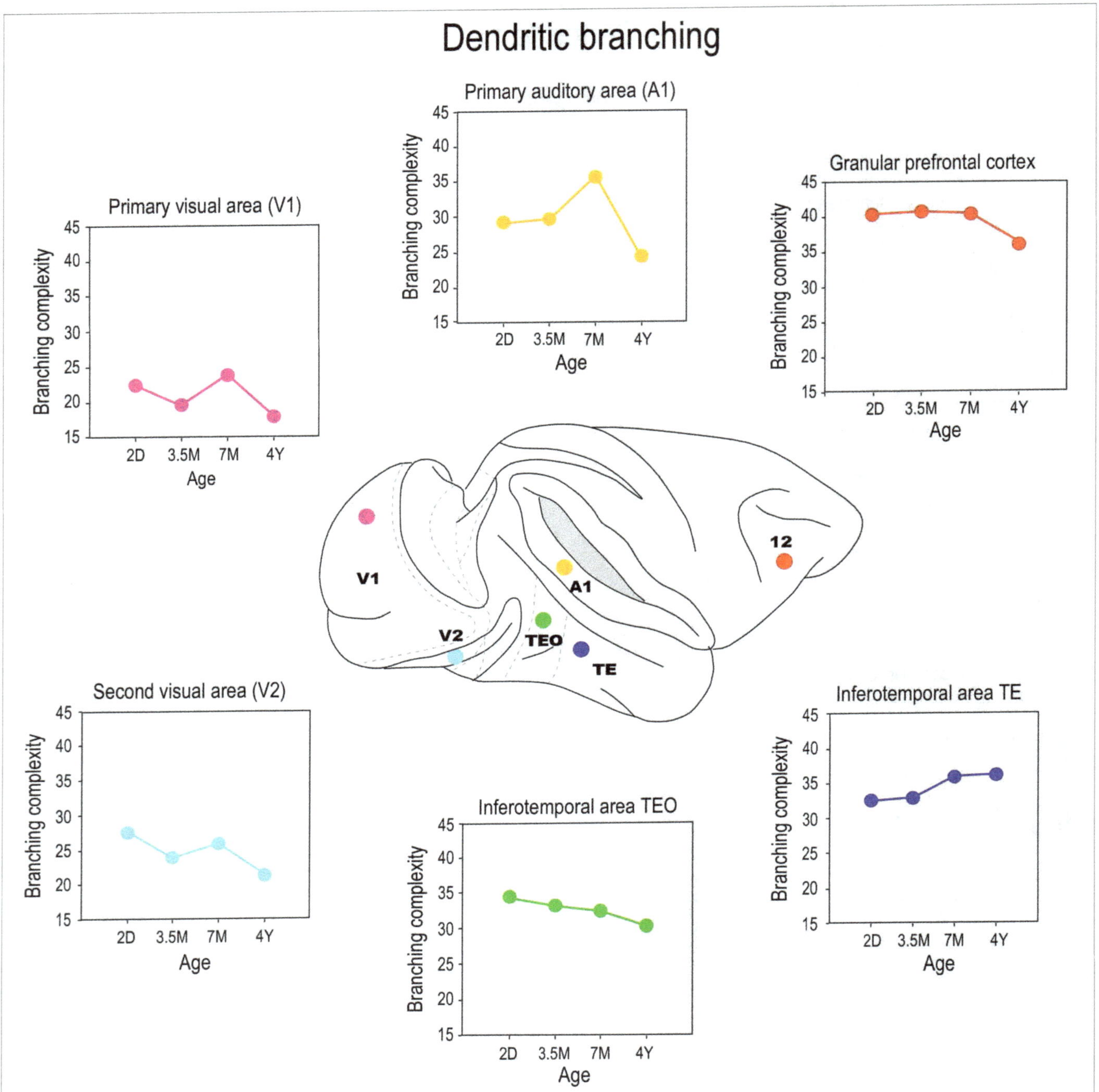

FIGURE 6 | Branching profiles. Plots of the branching structure of the basal dendritic trees of layer III pyramidal neurons sampled from primary visual area (V1), the second visual area (V2), the primary auditory cortex (A1), the posterior and anterior portion of the inferior temporal cortex (TEO and TEav, respectively) and prefrontal cortex (Brodmann's area 12) at postnatal day two (2D), three and a half months of age (3.5M), seven months of age (7M) and four and a half years (4Y) of age. Note that both the size and branching structure of the dendritic trees may share similar developmental profiles, or diverge independently (compare **Figure 5**). Data taken from Elston et al. (2009, 2010a,b, 2011a).

expected from the size, the dendritic trees of layer III pyramidal cells in area TEO of the macaque monkey were most branched at birth, and became less branched through juvenile and adolescent stages into adulthood (Elston et al., 2010a). In V1, V2, and V4, the most branched dendritic trees were observed at PND2 and the least branched dendritic trees were observed in the adult (Elston et al., 2010a). In A1, the dendritic trees of layer III pyramidal cells became increasingly more branched from PND2 to 3.5–7 months of age before declining to their adult values (Elston et al., 2010b). Cells in granular prefrontal area

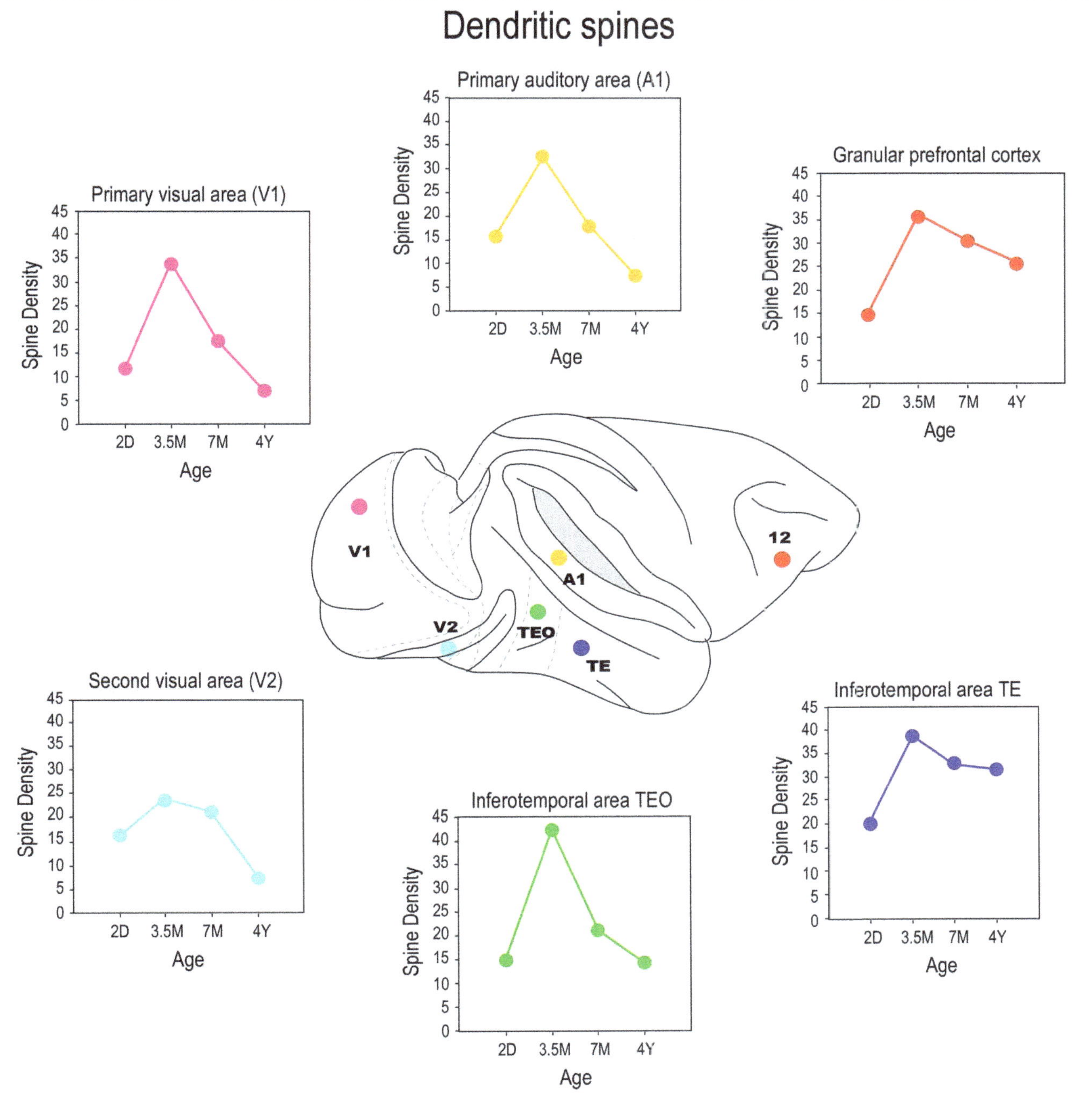

FIGURE 7 | Spinogenesis. Plots of the peak spine density (defined as the average of the maximum spine density observed in all 10 μm segments of dendrite from the soma to the distal tips of the dendrites of all cells quantified for any given age) of layer III pyramidal cells sampled in the primary visual area (V1), the second visual area (V2), the primary auditory area (A1), the posterior and anterior portion of the inferior temporal cortex (TEO and TE, respectively) and prefrontal cortex (Brodmann's area 12) at postnatal day two (2D), three and a half months of age (3.5M), seven months of age (7M) and adults (AD). Note that in V1, V2, and A1 there is a net reduction in the number of spines in the dendritic trees of pyramidal cells from birth to adulthood whereas in TEO, TE and area 12 there is a net increase in the number of spines over the same period. That is to say, the total number of spines grown in V1, V2, and A1 following the onset of sensory experience is, on balance, lost with increasing sensory experience, but is stabilized, to varying degrees, with increasing associative and executive function in TEpd, TEav and area 12. Data taken from Elston et al. (2009, 2010a,b, 2011a).

12, on the other hand, have relatively stable branching structure from birth to adolescence, then become less branched into adulthood, whereas those in area 46 become increasingly more branched from birth to >4.5 years of age (Anderson et al., 1995). While seemingly contradictory, pyramidal cells in different areas within the mature gPFC of the macaque differ in size, branching structure and spine densities (Elston et al., 2011a). In the marmoset monkey, pyramidal cells in V1, TE, and area 12 are more branched in the adult than in the newborn (Oga et al., 2013).

These data make it tolerably clear that mechanisms that modulate postnatal dendritic growth and dendritic branching are not inextricably coupled *in situ*. For example, although the dendritic trees of pyramidal cells in V1 of the macaque were at their largest at 2D, they were most branched at 3 weeks of age. Cells in TEO and posterior TEpd in the macaque attain their greatest branching complexity at 3 weeks and 7 months of age, respectively, yet these cells are characterized by continual dendritic growth from PND2 to adulthood (Elston et al., 2010a). Cells in TEav are most branched in the adult, but attain their greatest size at 7 months of age (Elston et al., 2011b). Moreover, the mechanisms modulating growth and branching may exert their influence for different periods of time in different cortical areas. For example, in V2 the greatest branching complexity was observed in the dendritic trees at 3 weeks of age, whereas in V4 the greatest branching complexity occurred at 3½ months of age (Elston et al., 2010a). In A1 the greatest branching complexity was observed at 7 months of age (Elston et al., 2010b). Growth of the dendritic tree and branching also show a degree of disjoin in the marmoset monkey: pyramidal cells in TE and area 12, in particular, are characterized by a marked increase in branching complexity from 2 months to 4.5 years of age while there is only a modest increase in the size of the trees during this same time (Oga et al., 2013). Recent detailed studies of pyramidal cell development in rodent somatosensory cortex also reveal different temporal profiles for growth, branching and spinogenesis (Romand et al., 2011). The authors found fast growth during the early postnatal period and the slow localized growth at latter ages, which they interpret as supporting functional compartmental development. Indeed, different compartments within the dendritic trees of pyramidal cells were shown to grow independently of each other (Romand et al., 2011).

SPINOGENESIS

By injecting cells in thick cortical slices, cut in the tangential plane, it is possible to reconstruct the entire basal dendritic trees of individual neurons. Thus, it is possible to draw and tally spines along the entire extent of dendrites, from the cell bodies to the distal tips, and determine the spine density as a function of distance from the soma (Eayrs and Goodhead, 1959; Valverde, 1967; Elston, 2001). Consistent with Pasco Rakic's findings for synapses (1986), we found that maximum peak spine density (defined as the average of the maximum spine density observed in all 10 µm segments of dendrite from the soma to the distal tips of the dendrites of all cells quantified for any given age) was greatest in all cortical areas at approximately 3.5 months (**Figure 7**). The maximum peak spine density among cells in the different cortical areas were remarkably similar at 3.5 months of age (approximately 30 spines per 10 micrometers). However, the rate of spine loss in the dendritic trees of pyramidal cells in the different cortical areas varies considerably such that those in V1, for example, prune to a maximum peak spine density of approximately 6 spines per 10 micrometers whereas those in the gPFC prune to a peak of approximately 25 spines per 10 micrometers. Likewise, the maximum peak spine density was observed at approximately 3.5 months of age in the marmoset

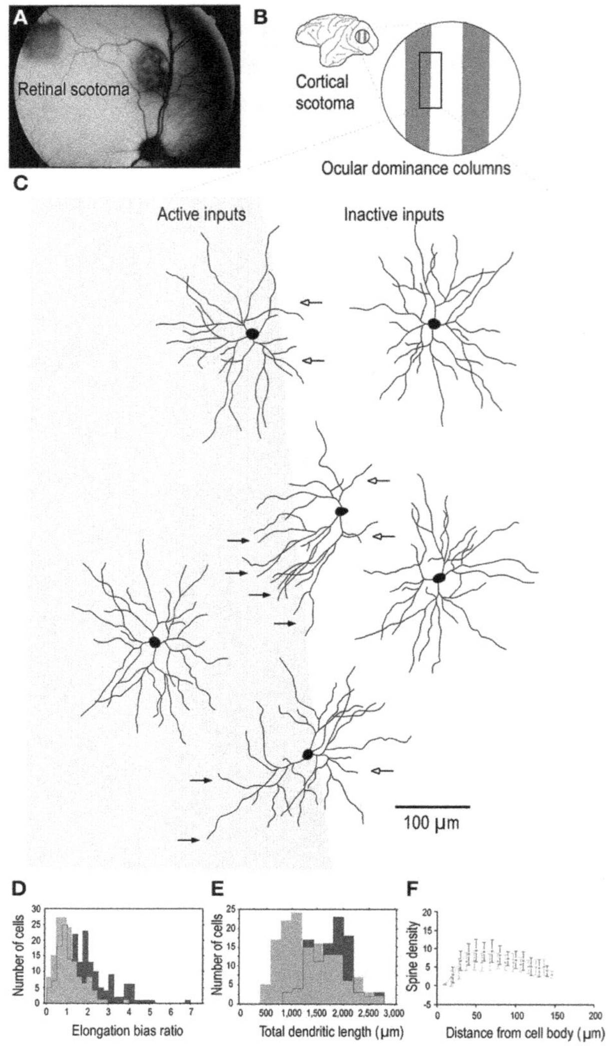

FIGURE 8 | Adult dendritic growth. Schematic illustrating placement of a retinal scotoma (laser lesion) **(A)** in the adult macaque monkey, and the corresponding region of the contralateral V1 **(B)**, in which individual neurons were injected across occular dominance columns **(C)**. Cells located near a border of an ocular dominance column appeared to show a regression of dendrites which projected toward the center of the CO-poor column (open arrows) and an elongation of dendrites toward the CO-rich column (closed arrows). Cells located in the centers of the OD columns appeared to be relatively symmetrical. Comparison of over 400 layer III pyramidal cells intracellularly injected in 3 adult monkeys in which we placed monocular retinal lesions, and 5 age/gender/ hemisphere/layer-matched controls, revealed that the basal dendritic trees of layer III pyramidal neurons within the portion of V1 corresponding to the retinal lesion (the lesion projection zone, LPZ) undergo dendritic growth **(D, E)** and spinogenesis **(F)**. Cells in the OD column corresponding to the non-lesioned eye within the LPZ have 65% more spines in their dendritic trees than those in the OD columns corresponding to the lesioned eye. The structural changes are not limited to cells within the LPZ in V1. Neurons in the region of cortex immediately surrounding the LPZ in V1 (the peri-LPZ) are considerably larger and more spinous than those within the LPZ. These cells have double the number of spines in their dendritic trees as compared with those in age/gender/hemisphere/layer-matched controls. Others have also reported perturbations in the peri-LPZ in V1, including marked changes

(Continued)

FIGURE 8 | Continued
in the expression of receptor subunits (Arckens et al., 2000) and expansion in receptive field sizes (Kaas et al., 1990; Chino et al., 1992; Schmid et al., 1996; Calford et al., 1999). In conjunction, these data suggest that anatomical and functional reorganization in the peri-LPZ differs in magnitude to that observed within the LPZ. Figure modified from Elston and DeFelipe (2002).

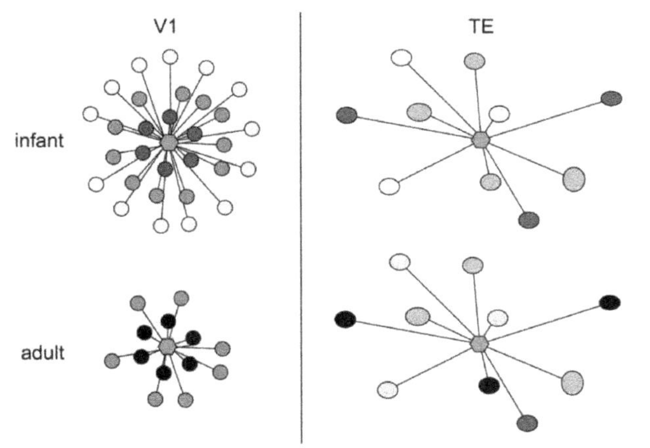

FIGURE 9 | Axon growth in development. Schematic illustration of the postnatal development of intrinsic axon patches in the primary visual area (V1) and visual association area TE in the macaque monkey. At center in each representation is a hexagon representing a single injection site. The shaded circles represent the intrinsic patches labeled by the single injection site. The intensity of labeling varied among patches, illustrated as varying shades of gray. Note that labeled patches were observed both in TE and V1 at 1 week of age (infant). Even at this age the size, interpatch distance and distribution pattern differ between the two cortical areas. The patterns of connectivity then diverge, resulting in qualitatively and quantitatively different patterns in the adult. In particular, the number and the maximal lateral extent of patches are reduced during postnatal development in V1, whereas in TE the number of patches remains constant and connectivity among these patches strengthens with aging. Based on data from Wang et al. (1998).

monkey: approximately 30–40 spines per 10 micrometers (Oga et al., 2013; Sasaki et al., 2014).

In previous studies an estimate of the number of synapses per neuron were made at different ages by dividing the density of synapses in the neuropil with the number of neurons (Huttenlocher, 1979, 1990). These calculations made no distinction between asymmetrical and symmetrical synapses, nor between the different neuronal types (pyramidal vs. spiny stellate), nor compartmentalization within the dendritic trees (e.g., apical vs. basal dendrites). By studying the morphology of individual neurons, it is possible to calculate an estimate of the total number of excitatory synapses to that cell by quantifying the number of dendritic spines [i.e., each dendritic spine receives at least one excitatory input (DeFelipe et al., 1988; Petralia et al., 1994a,b,c; Arellano et al., 2007)]. By multiplying the spine density at a given increment along the dendrites with the number of branches at the corresponding distance it is possible to obtain a better estimate of the total number of excitatory synapses received by individual identified neurons.

These calculations revealed that different numbers of spines were grown in the dendritic trees of cells among these cortical areas, and then subsequently pruned. There was a net decrease in the number of spines in the dendritic trees of cells in V1, V2, V4, and A1 from birth to adulthood, whereas there was a net increase in the number of spines in the dendritic trees of cells in TEO, TE and prefrontal cortex area 12 during this same period (Elston et al., 2009, 2010a,b). In other words, pruning exceeds spinogenesis in V1, V2, V4, and A1 (early and middle sensory areas), whereas spinogenesis exceeds pruning in TEO, TE and prefrontal cortex (higher visual cortex and multimodal association cortex), during the normal course of postnatal development. It is worth noting that, on average, layer III pyramidal cells in prefrontal cortex grew 4 times the number of spines in their basal dendritic trees as did those in V1 (15,900 and 3900, respectively). The number of spines then pruned from cells in gPFC into adulthood (7400) equates to >8 times the total number of spines observed in the dendritic trees of pyramidal cells in V1 of the adult (600–900) (Elston et al., 2009). In the marmoset monkey, spinogenesis greatly exceeded pruning in areas TE and gPFC whereas in V1 spinogenesis slightly outweighed pruning in V1 (Oga et al., 2013).

One interpretation of these findings may be that all synaptic connections to the dendritic trees of pyramidal cells are formed by 3.5 months of age, some of which are then pruned into adulthood. However, such an interpretation can't account for the presence of dendritic spines throughout the entire dendritic trees of cells that continue to grow in size beyond 3.5 months of age. Nor can it account for the fact that where cells continue to increase in branching complexity beyond the peak in spinogenesis, spines are found studded along all dendrites. A more parsimonious interpretation is that although there may be net reduction in spine density in the dendritic trees of cells from 3.5 months of age into adulthood, new spines are continually grown through this period. What is revealed then in our data is a snapshot of the absolute number of dendritic spines accounting for new spine growth and spine loss. While such spinogenesis, dendrite growth and axogenesis has been demonstrated in the adult cortex following injury (**Figure 8**; e.g., Jones and Schallert, 1992; Darian-Smith and Gilbert, 1994; Jones et al., 1996; Elston and DeFelipe, 2002; Trachtenberg et al., 2002; Matsuzaki et al., 2004; Knott et al., 2006; Keck et al., 2008; Knott and Holtmaat, 2008; Sala et al., 2008), our data suggest adult spinogenesis is a feature of the normal healthy growing brain, that a percentage of spines are continually turned over, the average number per neuron varying among cortical areas. That is to say, dendrites and spines of pyramidal cells continue to grow throughout the entire life cycle, including infancy, childhood, adolescence, adulthood and senescence, as a normal process without the necessity of occasioning a trigger such as injury to the peripheral or central nervous system. At times there will be a net increase in neurite (dendrite, axon, spine) growth, at times there will be a net reduction in neurite growth.

AXON PROJECTIONS

The above data give us some insights into postnatal changes in the postsyanpatic matrix (dendritic spines and dendrites) in cortical circuitry, what then of the development of the presynaptic matrix (axons and axon boutons)? While it has been well documented that presynaptic matrix is characterized by a patchwork or lattice-like structure in the adult cortex, and that the size and pattern of these patches vary among cortical areas (Rockland and Lund, 1982, 1983; Amir et al., 1993; Lund et al., 1993; Fujita and Fujita, 1996; Melchitzky et al., 1998, 2001; Tanigawa et al., 1998, 2005; González-Burgos et al., 2000), little is known of their development. Fujita and colleagues quantified the postnatal development of these axonal patches from birth to adulthood in areas V1 and TE of the macaque monkey (Wang et al., 1998). The axon patches are present at birth (PND7) and follow divergent maturation profiles with the onset of visual experience, with some shared characteristics. Of particular note was the decrease in the number of the patches is observed in V1 from PND7 to adulthood as compared with the trend in area TE where the number of patches remained consistent (**Figure 9**). There was also a decrease in the horizontal extent of the patches in V1 from PND7 to adulthood as compared with TE where the horizontal extent of axon patch labeling was maintained over the same period.

At the level of individual axons, in both V1 and TE axons within the patches were relatively straight at birth, and developed increasingly more varicosities with increasing postnatal age. In both TE and V1, the density of boutons along axons located within the patches increased with age, at least from infants. These data reveal that axonal branches and boutons within the patches in area TE continue to develop over many months, with connections being strengthened with aging. Previous studies revealed that the horizontal axons form this patchy pattern in V1 of the macaque monkey at least 3 weeks prior to birth (Coogan and Van Essen, 1996). Likewise, ipsilateral (Barone et al., 1996; Coogan and Van Essen, 1996) and callosal (Meissirel et al., 1991; Schwartz and Goldman-Rakic, 1991) corticocortical projections in macaque V1 are initially diffuse and then become patchy before birth. Although little is known of the patches in prenatal TE, and further studies are obviously needed, the maturity of horizontal axons at PND 7 (injection at PND 4) suggests that a patchy projection pattern is also established *in utero* in TE. Thus, patch formation does not likely require visual experience in either the striate cortex or extrastriate cortex, at least, in monkeys (see Schwartz and Goldman-Rakic, 1990, for a review).

NEURONAL PHYSIOLOGY: DEVELOPMENTAL CHANGES AND AREAL SPECIALIZATION

To test whether changes in the morphology of pyramidal cells during development outlined above influences cell physiology, Fujita and colleagues made intracellular whole-cell clamp recordings of pyramidal cells in V1 and TE from animals aged 10 days to 6 years of age (Maruyama et al., 2007). A number of physiological properties were quantified, including resting potential, firing threshold, membrane time constant, depolarizing sag, duration of individual action potentials, and spike-frequency adaptation. Most notably, membrane time constant, depolarizing sag, duration of individual action potentials, and spike-frequency adaptation ramped up until 7 months of age in cells in V1, but continued to ramp up over a protracted period of time in cells in TE. By contrast, the depolarizing sag increased through all ages in V1, but did not change until 1 year of age in TE. In addition to these changes in intrinsic membrane properties of individual neurons, synaptic transimission properites also change postnatally. For example, the excitatory postsynaptic currents recorded in layer III pyramidal cells at 15 months of age in the gPFC are considerably different to those recorded at 3 months of age (Gonzalez-Burgos et al., 2008) (**Figure 10**). These developmental differences in the electrophysiological signatures of pyramidal cells result in different, arguably specialized, functional signatures in the adult cortex. For example, Luebke and colleagues recently demonstrated in an elegant study that pyramidal cells in V1 have a significantly higher input resistance, depolarized resting membrane potential, higher action potential (AP) firing rates, lower spontaneous postsynaptic currents and faster kinetics

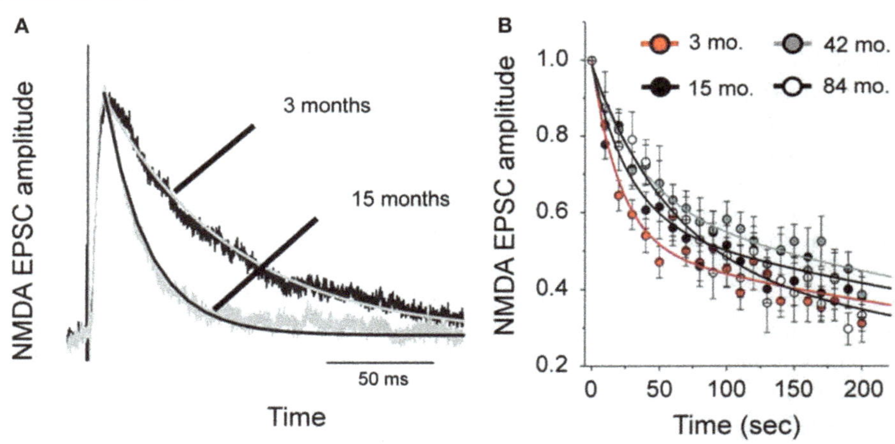

FIGURE 10 | Age differences in cell physiology. Plots of the difference in NMDA-mediated excitatory postsynaptic currents (NMDA-EPSCs) in pyramidal cells sampled from the prefrontal cortex of 3 and 15 month old macaque monkeys. **(A)** Examples of average NMDA-EPSCs scaled to the same peak amplitude illustrating the exponential functions fit to the traces. Note the differences in duration. **(B)** The amplitude of NMDA-EPSCs was normalized relative to that of the first response recorded after resuming stimulation in the presence of an NMDA antagonist, MK801. The lines represent double-exponential functions fit to the data from animals of different ages by non-linear regression. Modified from Gonzalez-Burgos et al. (2008).

than those in granular PFC (Amatrudo et al., 2012) (**Figure 11**). Moreover, pyramidal cells in V1 and TE of the mature brain show a diametrically opposed reaction to extrinsic tetanic stimulation: extracellular stimulation (20–40 pulses at 40–100 Hz, applied every 4 s for 3–5 min) of intrinsic horizontal connections of layers 2 and 3 results in long term depression (LTD) of extracellular potentials in V1 and long term potentiation (LTP) in TE (Murayama et al., 1997). Although Luebke and colleagues were unable to demonstrate such changes in the electrophysiological properties in V1 by *in vitro* recording (Luebke et al., 2013), on balance, we suggest the above data reveal that the anatomical and electrophysiological profiles of pyramidal cells vary among cortical areas at birth, and continue to diverge into adulthood.

Comparison of the results of studies in primates with those in rodents reveals some interesting differences in their electrophysiological properties with aging. For example, whereas resting potential of layer III pyramidal cells remained unchanged in V1 and TE of the macaque monkey, there is a significant change in these same cells in A1 of the mouse (Oswald and Reyes, 2008; Romand et al., 2011). Input resistance of layer III pyramidal cell differed between V1 and TE of the macaque monkey remained unchanged with age. In mouse A1, the input resistance of layer III pyramidal cells decreased with aging (Metherate and Aramakis, 1999; Oswald and Reyes, 2008). Neuronal discharge following an intracellularly applied electrical pulse increased with age in layer III pyramidal cells in mouse A1, as was the case in macaque V1, but decreased in macaque TE. Discharge with

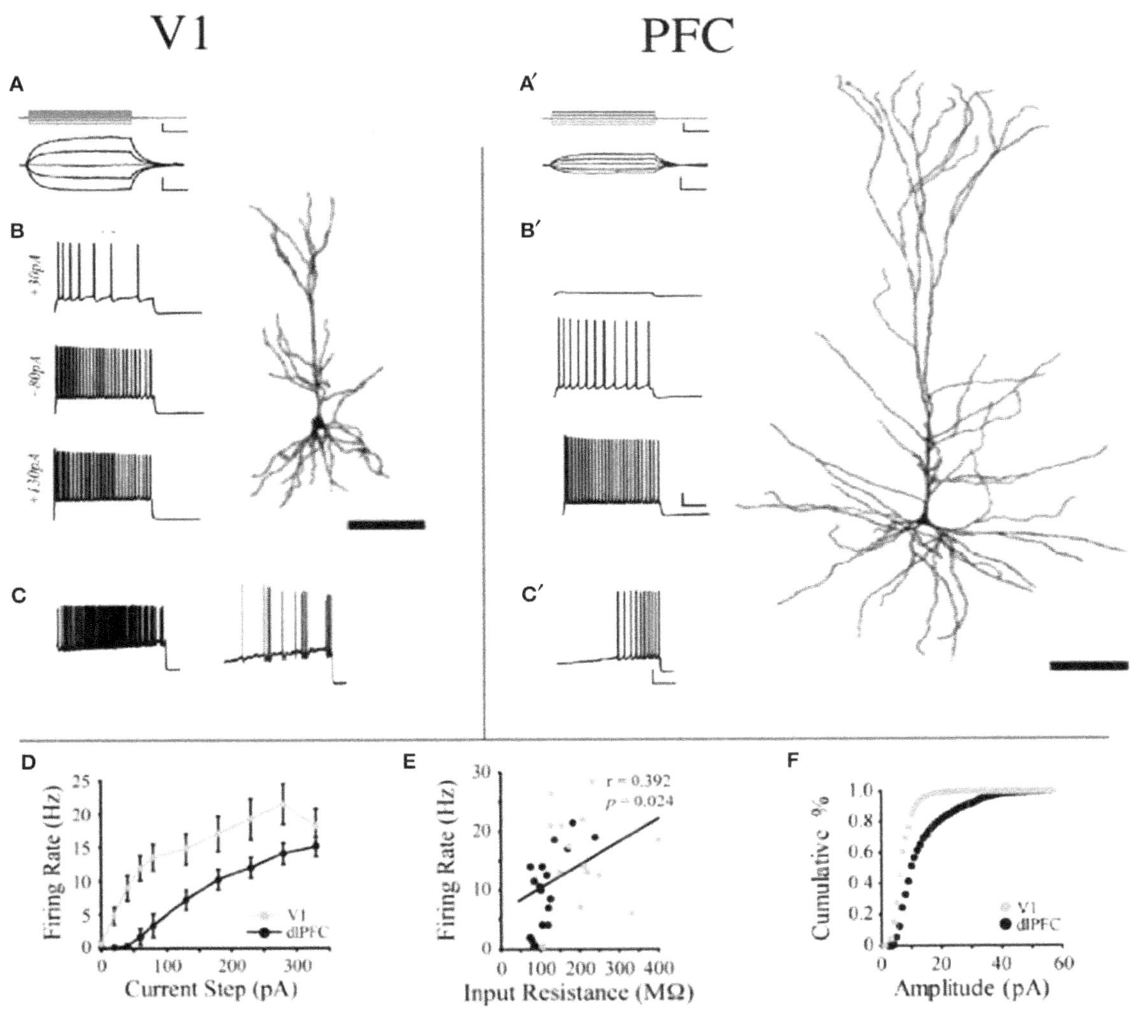

FIGURE 11 | Area differences in cell physiology. Reconstructions of layer III pyramidal cells sampled in the adult primary visual area (V1) and granular dorsolateral prefrontal cortex (PFC) and schematics illustrating their voltage responses to **(A,A¹)** 200-ms current pulses (−40 to +40 pA) and **(B,B¹)** 2-s current steps of +30, +80, and +130 pA and their firing patterns in response to a current ramp protocol resulting in phasic and tonic discharge **(C,C¹)**. **(D)** Mean firing rates of V1 vs. PFC neurons are illustrated in response to a series of depolarizing current steps. V1 was significantly different from PFC at steps +20 to +280 pA ($p < 0.05$) **(E)** Relationship between input resistance and firing rate is illustrated in response to a −130 pA current step for all V1 and dlPFC neurons. Linear regression (black line) demonstrates a significant positive correlation. **(F)** Cumulative frequency histograms of sEPSC amplitudes (1 pA bins) in V1 and PFC neurons. Modified from Amatrudo et al. (2012).

increasing age also increased in layer V pyramidal cells in rat prelimbic cortex (Zhang, 2004). Zhang (2004) also reported a decrease in input resistance, resting potential and time constant with aging, as also reported in layer V pyramidal cells in rat visual and somatosensory cortex (McCormick and Prince, 1987; Kasper et al., 1994). Clearly then, the electrophysiological properties of pyramidal cells may vary independently among different cortical layers, different cortical areas and different species.

It is worth remembering that while pyramidal cells vary in size and branching complexity among cortical areas in some rodents (Benavides-Piccione et al., 2002, 2006; Ballesteros-Yáñez et al., 2006; Elston et al., 2006b), the extent of this variation is but a small fraction of that reported in higher primates. For example, in the mouse there is a 2-fold difference in the number of dendritic spines in the basal dendritic trees of layer III pyramidal cells across the adult cortical mantle. In adult primates, there is a 23-fold difference in the number of dendritic spines in the basal dendritic trees of layer III pyramidal cells between V1 and the gPFC (see Elston, 2003a, for a review). Accordingly, differences in the postnatal developmental profiles of pyramidal cell electrophysiology reported in rodents may well to underscore that evident in primates.

NEURONAL RECEPTIVE FIELD PROPERTIES IN POSTNATAL DEVELOPMENT

Movshon et al. (1999, 2000) demonstrated that receptive field sizes of neurons located in the central 5 degrees of the visual representation in V1 decrease in size from early postnatal development to adulthood. In addition, they demonstrated that the spatial resolution of cells in V1 (the highest spatial frequency at which cells give a response of at least 10% of its maximum) increases from birth to adulthood. There is also a general trend for increasing surround suppression from birth to adulthood (Kiorpes and Movshon, 2003; Chino et al., 2004) and facilitation develops slowly over the first year after birth (Li et al., 2013). These changes in receptive field size, spatial acuity and surround suppression could plausibly be attributed to changes in the geometrical sampling of neurons as their dendritic trees change shape (Sholl, 1955; Ferster, 1998; Taylor et al., 2000; Taylor and Vaney, 2002). Specifically, as the dendritic trees of neurons decrease in size with maturation they may sample a progressively smaller portion of the visuotopically organized afferent projection and thus have progressively smaller receptive fields. The developmental time course of sensivity to global form and motion and visual texture modulation have been shown to be measured in years, rather than months (Kiorpes and Movshon, 2004; El-Shamayleh et al., 2010; Kiorpes et al., 2012). In conjunction these data suggested a protracted developmental profile for neurons in V1, both morphologically and functionally, that extends well beyond the peak synaptogeneses demonstrated relatively early in development (**Figure 12**).

Chino and colleagues (Zhang et al., 2008) reported that in V2, receptive fields of neurons mature later than those in V1 neurons, consistent with our finding that the dendritic trees of pyramidal cells in V2 continue to grow from 2D to 3½ months of age while those in V1 become smaller during this time. Although they report that by 4 weeks of age the spatial receptive field structure in V2 is as complex as in adults (Zhang et al., 2013), but their ability to discriminate fine disparity differences was significantly reduced compared with adults (Maruko et al., 2008). V2 neurons of 8-week-old monkeys had significantly lower optimal temporal frequencies and resolutions than those of adults (Zheng et al., 2007). Neurons in area TE do not develop their adult-like response properties until even later in development (Rodman et al., 1993), consistent with our findings of continued growth and branching from birth. Furthermore, anatomical connections of TE undergo a protracted period of refinement from birth to adulthood compared to other visual areas (Webster et al.,

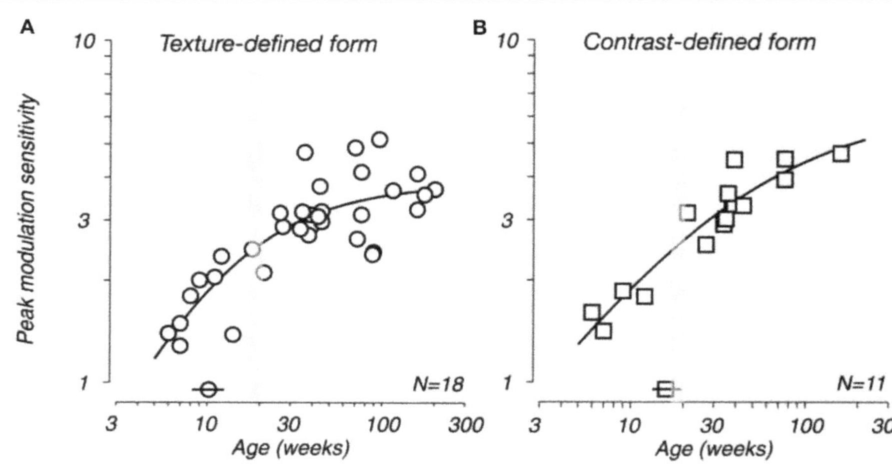

FIGURE 12 | Developing visual sensitivity. Plots illustrating the developmental time course of peak behavioral modulation sensitivity for **(A)** texture-defined and **(B)** contrast-defined form as a function of age. Isolated symbols intersected by horizontal bars (above the x-axis) indicate the age at which modulation sensitivity reached half of adult levels (10 and 17 weeks for **A,B**, respectively). *N* indicates the number of monkeys tested. Because many of these subjects were tested longitudinally, each plot contains more data points than the indicated population size. Note that the peak spine and synapse density occurs at approximately 3.5 months of age (gray shading). Modified from El-Shamayleh et al. (2010).

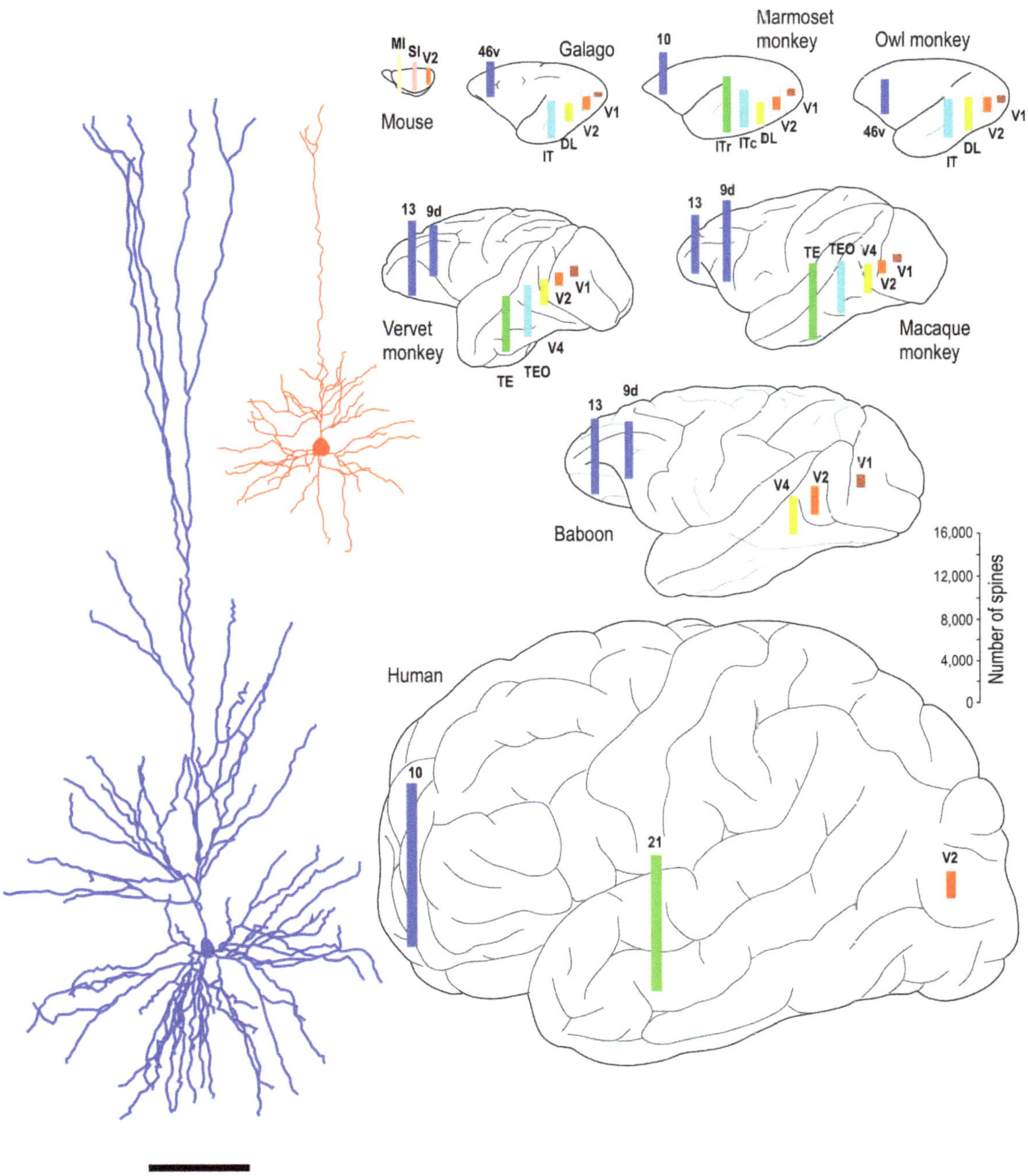

FIGURE 13 | Specialization in pyramidal cell structure in the adult brain. Schematic illustrating regional and species differences in pyramidal cell structure. At left are illustrated two individual layer III cells sampled from the primary visual area (V1) and the inferotemporal cortical area TEpd of the adult macaque monkey. Note the difference in thickness of layer III between the two cortical areas, the tangential extent of both the basal and apical dendritic trees. Illustrated at right are the estimates of the total number of spines in the basal dendritic trees of layer III pyramidal cells in visual areas V1, V2, V4 (DL), TEO (ITc), TE (ITr), and prefrontal cortex (areas 9d, 10, 13, and 46v of Preuss and Goldman-Rakic, 1991). Prefrontal cortex refers as originally defined by Brodmann (1913) as granular cortex anterior to the central sulcus (see Elston and Garey, 2004, for a translation). Bars are color coded for homology, that is, homologous/analagous cortical areas are illustrated by a single color. The bars representing the number of spines are not necessarily located in the exact position from which the cells were sampled, but have been positioned for aesthetic balance. Schematics of the different brains are not drawn to scale. Data taken from the mouse (Ballesteros-Yáñez et al., 2006), galago (Elston et al., 2005b,c), owl monkey (Elston, 2003b,c), marmoset monkey (Elston et al., 1999b, 2001), vervet monkey (Elston et al., 2005d, 2011b), macaque monkey (Elston and Rosa, 1997, 1998; Elston et al., 1999a, 2001, 2011b; Elston, 2000), baboon (Elston et al., 2005e, 2011b) and human (Elston et al., 2001). Systematic differences have also been demonstrated in the total number of spines in the basal dendritic trees of layer III pyramidal cells in sensorimotor and cingunalte cortex in all species studied to date, including the adult vervet monkey, macaque monkey and baboon (Elston and Rockland, 2002; Elston et al., 2005a,f,g,h,i) (not illustrated).

1991, 1994, 1995; Rodman and Consuelos, 1994; Barone et al., 1996; Coogan and Van Essen, 1996) and this region becomes myelinated much later in development than V1 (Rodman, 1994). The anatomical data in TEO and TE, which reveal progressively larger dendritic trees from birth to adulthood, parallel the physiological data for increasing receptive field size during postnatal maturation.

In addition to the size of the dendritic trees, their branching structure may influence aspects of cellular function. Considerable work has been done in the retina relating neuronal branching structure to functional qualities such as direction selectivity (see Vaney et al., 2012, for a review). Although less well studied, it has been proposed that dendrtic branching structure may be important in V1, for example, in determining orientation and direction selectivity (Pettigrew, 1974; Tieman and Hirsch, 1982; Elston and Rosa, 1997; Ferster, 1998; Livingstone, 1998). Moreover, the onset of form discrimination at 3 weeks of age (Zimmermann, 1961) occurs at the time when cells are most branched. Could the increase in the number of branches facilitate compartmentalization of processing within the dendritic tree (Poirazi and Mel, 2001; Chklovskii et al., 2004) and allow detection of inputs associated with asymmetric features throughout the dendritic tree?

SPECIALIZED PYRAMIDAL CELL GROWTH PROFILES RESULT IN SPECIALIZED CORTICAL CIRCUITS IN THE MATURE BRAIN

Whatever the explanation, the different developmental profiles result in marked differences in pyramidal cell structure among cortical areas in the mature brain (**Figure 13**). Cells become increasingly larger and more spinous with anterior progression through visual areas V1, V2, V4, TEO, and TE (Elston and Rosa, 1997, 1998; Elston et al., 1999b, 2005b,d,e; Elston, 2003b). Likewise, cells become increasingly larger and more spinous with progression through somatosensory areas 3b, 5, and 7 (Elston and Rockland, 2002; Elston et al., 2005h,i). Those in polysensory cortex, such as the superior temporal polysensory area (STP) are larger and more spinous than those in TE (Elston et al., 1999a). Those in cingulate cortex are larger and more spinous than those in sensory and sensory association cortex (Elston et al., 2005a,f,g), and those in prefrontal cortex are among the most spinous of all pyramidal cells in the cerebral cortex (Elston et al., 2001, 2011b; Jacobs et al., 2001; Bianchi et al., 2012). It has also been demonstrated that pyramidal cells are increasingly more complex in structure and more spinous in primate species with increasingly larger granular prefrontal cortex (Elston et al., 2005c, 2006a, 2011b). Pyramidal cells in the adult brain of rodents and primates appear also to be influenced by different developmental and phylogenetic controls (Elston and Manger, 2014). Pyramidal cells in V1 of adult rodents vary considerably among species, being larger, more branched and more spinous with increasing size of V1, whereas that in adult primate V1 is relatively constant, irrespective of the size of V1 (**Figure 14**).

These structural differences potentially influence the number of inputs received by pyramidal cells in any given cortical area, the manner in which these inputs are integrated within the dendritic trees, and the degree of interconnectivity between neurons

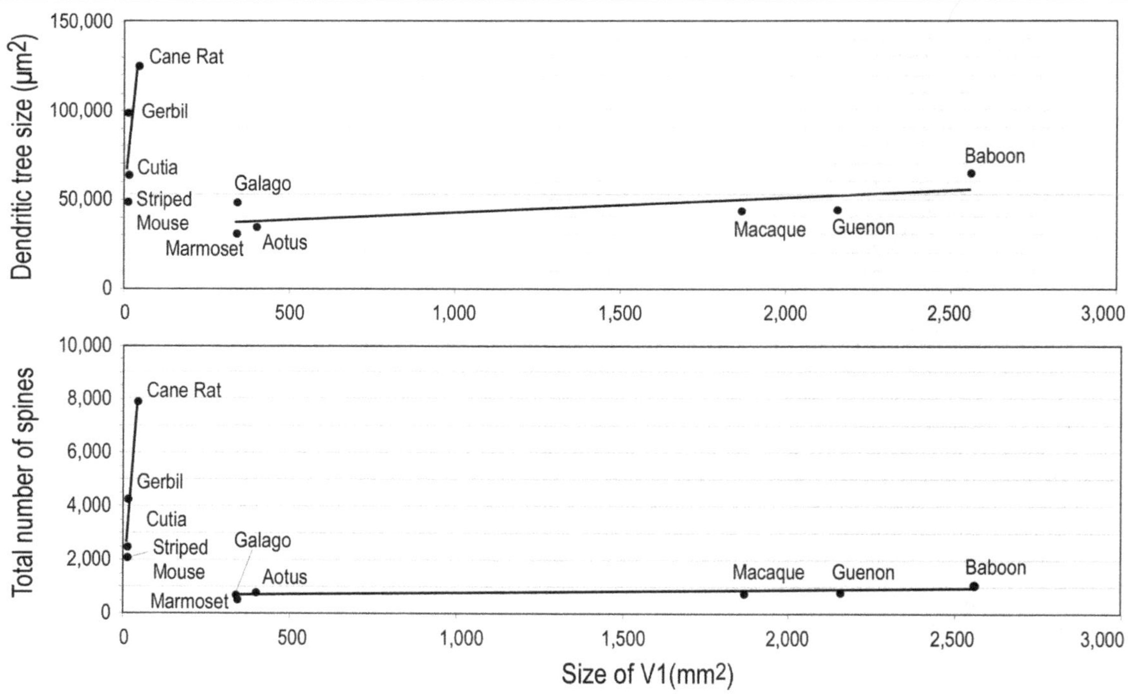

FIGURE 14 | Neuron growth and cortical size. Graphs illustrating phylogentic differences in the trends between pyramidal cell structure and size of the of the primary visual area (V1) in rodents and primates. Illustrated are the size of, and number of dendritic spines in, the "average" pyramidal cell vs. the size V1 in the cane rat, bushvelt gerbil, striped mouse, agouti (cutia), tree shrew, galago, marmoset monkey, owl monkey, guenon (vervet monkey), macaque monkey, and baboon. Separate trend lines (linear regressions) are illustrated for the rodent and primate data (reproduced from Elston and Manger, 2014).

within cortical circuits (Jacobs and Scheibel, 2002; Elston, 2003a, 2007; London and Häusser, 2005; Spruston, 2008). In V1, the differences in the size of the dendritic trees, in the tangential plane, influence the portion of the visutopic representation sampled by individual cells (**Figure 15**). Both the functional capacity of neurons and their potential for plastic change have been correlated with their morphological complexity (Poirazi and Mel, 2001; Chklovskii et al., 2004). Moreover, the different structural complexity of pyramidal cells in sensory, association and executive cortex may provide an anatomical platform for tonic vs. phasic sampling, believed to be important for memory (Miller and Cohen, 2001; Funahashi and Takeda, 2002; Elston, 2007).

In addition, differences have also been reported in inhibitory circuitry among cortical areas in the adult brain. Specifically, the density and connectivity of interneurons may differ among cortical areas (Hof and Nimchinsky, 1992; Kritzer et al., 1992; Kondo et al., 1994; Hof and Morrison, 1995; DeFelipe et al., 1999; Elston and González-Albo, 2003; Yáñez et al., 2005; Benavides-Piccione and DeFelipe, 2007; Freire et al., 2010, 2012). The different types of interneurons, such as Chandelier cells, Martinotti cells and basket cells, project to different compartments of pyramidal cells, including the soma, axon initial segment and dendrites (see DeFelipe, 1993; Somogyi et al., 1998; DeFelipe et al., 2002 for reviews). The differences in both the density and distribution of interneurons, and pyramidal cell structure, among cortical areas result in quantifiably different patterns of connectivity (DeFelipe et al., 1999; Elston et al., 1999d; Blazquez-Llorca et al., 2010; da Rocha et al., 2012). In future studies it will be of particular interest to determine the developmental profiles of inhibitory neurons (e.g., Anderson et al., 1995), especially in view of the different types of neuronal migration during development: radial and tangential (see Rakic, 1990; Nakajima, 2007; Jones, 2009; Chédotal, 2010; Govek et al., 2011 for reviews). It will also be of great importance to expand the scope of research to identify possible species differences in postnatal development of cortical circuitry, particularly in human prefrontal cortex which is disproportionately large compared with that in other primates (Brodmann, 1913) translated by Elston and Garey (2004), to better comprehend the development of the neural substrate for cognitive functions (see Fuster, 1997; Goldman-Rakic, 1999; Preuss, 2000; Elston, 2007; Rakic, 2009 for reviews).

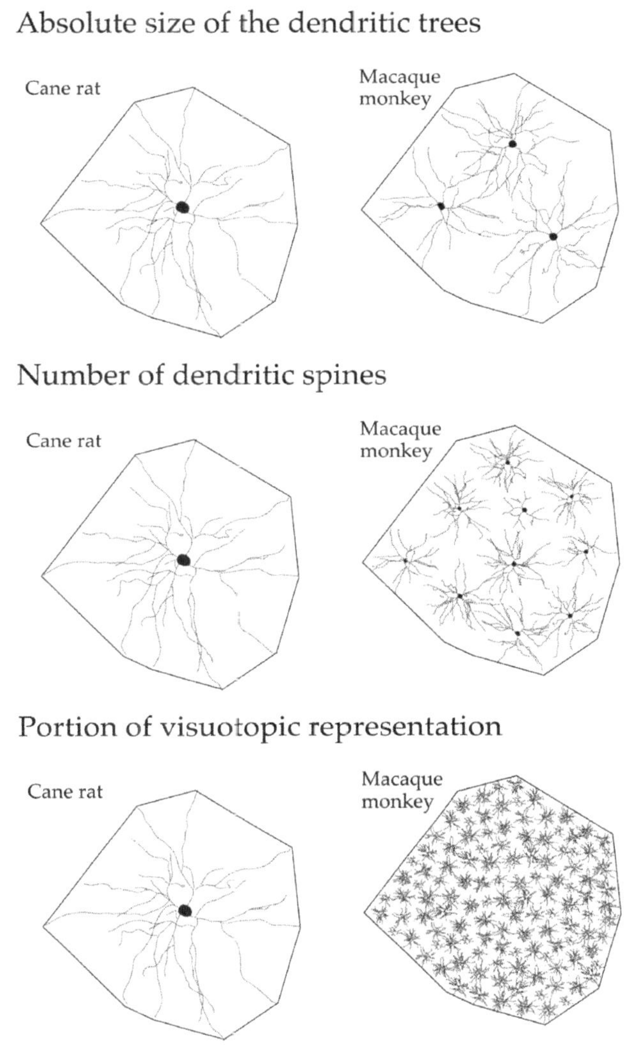

FIGURE 15 | Neuron structure and cortical connectivity. Schematic, not drawn to scale, illustrating the dendritic tree of the "average" layer III pyramidal cell in V1 of the adult cane rat and macaque monkey: that in the cane rat is, on average, three times the size of that in the macaque monkey. Differences in the size, branching structure and spine density result in a more than 10-fold difference in the estimate of the total number of spines, putative excitatory inputs, in the basal dendritic tree of the "average" layer III pyramidal cell between the two species. As V1 in the adult macaque is, on average, more than 40 times the size of V1 in the adult cane rat, the dendritic trees of cells in the adult cane rat sample a portion of the visuotopic field approximately 120 times larger than do those in the adult monkey. Thus, 120 cells are required in the macaque monkey V1 to achieve the spatial coverage of a single cell in the cane rat. One hundred and twenty cells in the adult macaque V1 have, on average, a sum total of more than 88,000 spines (120 × 743), being more than 110 times the number of spines in an individual cell in the adult cane rat. (reproduced from Elston and Manger, 2014).

CONCLUSIONS

Recent cell injection studies reveal variation in the developmental profiles of pyramidal cells among different cortical areas in the primate brain. The different growth profiles of pyramidal cells among cortical areas potentially influence the number of inputs received by neurons in any given cortical area, the manner in which these inputs are integrated within the dendritic trees, and the degree of connectivity between neurons. Together, these features may influence the physiological properties of the cells, and the circuitry they compose. Moreover, the data reveal that spine loss in the developing cortex does not result solely from the pruning of existing spines observed at the peak (approximately 3 months of age) but, rather, by the net reduction of existing and newly acquired spines (both those formed by 3 months of age and in the more mature cortex). Furthermore, the rate of spine loss in the dendritic trees of pyramidal cells varies among cortical areas in both absolute and relative terms. The "use it or lose it" principle may belie the diversity of mechanisms that drive synapse stabilization or elimination in the developing and mature cerebral cortex.

Use it but you may still lose it may prove to be just as, if not more, prevalent in the developing brain.

FUNDING

This work was supported by an RD Wright Fellowship from the National Health and Medical Research Council of Australia (210341: GNE) and grants from the Japan Science and Technology Agency (Core Research for Evolutional Science and Technology), the Ministry of Education, Science, Sports, and Culture (Japan; grant number 17022025), Osaka University, and the I Hear Innovation Foundation (Australia) and the Sunshine Coast Regional Council (Australia).

ACKNOWLEDGMENT

We thank Tomofumi Oga and Hirosato Aoi for assistance with preparing some of the figures.

REFERENCES

Amatrudo, J. M., Weaver, C. M., Crimins, J. L., Hof, P. R., Rosene, D. L., and Luebke, J. I. (2012). Influence of highly distinctive structural properties on the excitability of pyramidal neurons in monkey visual and prefrontal cortices. *J. Neurosci.* 32, 13644–13660. doi: 10.1523/JNEUROSCI.2581-12.2012

Amir, Y., Harel, M., and Malach, R. (1993). Cortical hierarchy reflected in the organization of intrinsic connections in macaque monkey visual cortex. *J. Comp. Neurol.* 334, 19–46. doi: 10.1002/cne.903340103

Anderson, S. A., Classey, J. D., Condé, F., Lund, J. S., and Lewis, D. A. (1995). Synchronous development of pyramidal neuron dendritic spines and parvalbumin immunoreactive chandelier neuron axon terminals in layer III of monkey prefrontal cortex. *Neuroscience* 67, 7–22. doi: 10.1016/0306-4522(95)00051-J

Arckens, L., van der Gucht, E., Eysel, T. H., Orban, G., and Vandesande, F. (2000). Investigation of cortical reorganization in area 17 and nine extrastriate visual areas through the detection of changes in immediate early gene expression as induced by retinal lesions. *J. Comp. Neurol.* 425, 531–544. doi: 10.1002/1096-9861(20001002)425:4%3C531::AID-CNE5%3E3.0.CO;2-J

Arellano, J. I., Espinosa, A., Fairén, A., Yuste, R., and DeFelipe, J. (2007). Non-synaptic dendritic spines in neocortex. *Neuroscience* 145, 464–469. doi: 10.1016/j.neuroscience.2006.12.015

Ballesteros-Yáñez, I., Benavides-Piccione, R., Elston, G. N., Yuste, R., and DeFelipe, J. (2006). Density and morphology of pyramidal cell dendritic spines in the mouse neocortex. *Neuroscience* 138, 403–409. doi: 10.1016/j.neuroscience.2005.11.038

Barone, P., Dehay, C., Berland, M., and Kennedy, H. (1996). Role of directed growth and target selection in the formation of cortical pathways: prenatal development of the projection of area V2 to V4 in the monkey. *J. Comp. Neurol.* 374, 1–20.

Becker, L. E., Armstrong, D. L., Chan, F., and Wood, M. M. (1984). Dendritic development in human occipital cortical networks. *Devel Brain Res.* 13, 117–124. doi: 10.1016/0165-3806(84)90083-X

Benavides-Piccione, R., Ballesteros-Yáñez, I., DeFelipe, J., and Yuste, R. (2002). Cortical area and species differences in dendritic spine morphology. *J. Neurocytol.* 31, 337–346. doi: 10.1023/A:1024134312173

Benavides-Piccione, R., and DeFelipe, J. (2007). Distribution of neurons expressing tyrosine hydroxylase in the human cerebral cortex. *J. Anat.* 211, 212–222. doi: 10.1111/j.1469-7580.2007.00760.x

Benavides-Piccione, R., Hamzei-Sichani, F., Ballesteros-Yáñez, I., DeFelipe DeFelipe, J., and Yuste, R. (2006). Dendritic size of pyramidal neurons differs among mouse cortical regions. *Cereb. Cortex* 16, 990–1001. doi: 10.1093/cercor/bhj041

Bianchi, S., Stimpson, C. D., Bauernfeind, A. L., Schapiro, S. J., Baze, W. B., McArthur, M. J., et al. (2012). Dendritic morphology of pyramidal neurons in the chimpanzee neocortex: regional specializations and comparison to humans. *Cereb. Cortex* 23: 2429–2436. doi: 10.1093/cercor/bhs239

Bianchi, S., Stimpson, C. D., Duka, T., Larsen, M. D., Janssen, W. G. M., Collins, Z., et al. (2013). Synaptogenesis and development of pyramidal neuron dendritic morphology in the chimpanzee neocortex resembles humans. *Proc. Natl. Acad. Sci. U.S.A.* 110(Suppl. 2), 10395–10401. doi: 10.1073/pnas.1301224110

Blazquez-Llorca, L., García-Marín, V., and DeFelipe, J. (2010). GABAergic complex basket formations in the human neocortex. *J. Comp. Neurol.* 518, 4917–4937. doi: 10.1002/cne.22496

Boothe, R. G., Greenough, W. T., Lund, J. S., and Wrege, K. (1979). A quantitative investigation of spine and dendrite development of neurons in visual cortex (area 17) of *Macaca nemistrina* monkeys. *J. Comp. Neurol.* 186, 473–490. doi: 10.1002/cne.901860310

Bourgeois, J.-P., Jastreboff, P. J., and Rakic, P. (1989). Synaptogenesis in visual cortex of normal and preterm monkeys: evidence for intrinsic regulation of synaptic overproduction. *Proc. Natl. Acad. Sci. U.S.A.* 86, 4297–4301. doi: 10.1073/pnas.86.11.4297

Bourgeois, J.-P., and Rakic, P. (1993). Changes of synaptic density in the primary visual cortex of the macaque monkey from fetal to adult stage. *J. Neurosci.* 13, 2801–2820.

Brodmann, K. (1909). *Vergleichende Lokalisationslehre der Großhirnrinde.* Leipzig: Johann Ambrosius Barth.

Brodmann, K. (1913). Neue Forschungsergebnisse der Grosshirnrindenanatomie mit besonderer Berücksichtigung anthropologischer Fragen. *Geselsch Deuts Naturf Artze* 85, 200–240.

Calford, M. B., Schmid, L. M., and Rosa, M. G. P. (1999). Monocular focal retinal lesions induce short-term topographic plasticity in adult cat visual cortex. *Proc. R. Soc. B Biol. Ser.* 266, 499–507.

Chédotal, A. (2010). Should I stay or should I go? Becoming a granule cell. *Trends Neurosci.* 33, 163–172. doi: 10.1016/j.tins.2010.01.004

Chino, Y. M., Bi, M., and Zhang, B. (2004). "Normal and abnormal development of the neuronal response properties in primate visual cortex," in *The Primate Visual System,* eds J. H. Kaas and C. Collins (Boca Raton, FL: CRC Press), 81–108.

Chino, Y. M., Kaas, J. H., Smith, E. L. III., Langston, A. L., and Cheng, H. (1992). Rapid reorganization of cortical maps in adult cats following restricted deafferentation in retina. *Vision Res.* 32, 789–796. doi: 10.1016/0042-6989(92)90021-A

Chklovskii, D. B., Mel, B. W., and Svoboda, K. (2004). Cortical rewiring and information storage. *Nature* 431, 782–788. doi: 10.1038/nature03012

Conel, J. L. (1941). "The cortex of a one month old infant," in *The Post Natal Development of the Human Cerebral Cortex* (Cambridge: Harvard University Press). doi: 10.4159/harvard.9780674187658

Conel, J. L. (1947). "The cortex of a three month old infant," in *The Post Natal Development of the Human Cerebral Cortex* (Cambridge: Harvard University Press). doi: 10.4159/harvard.9780674187672

Conel, J. L. (1955). "The cortex of a fifteen month old infant," in *The Post Natal Development of the Human Cerebral Cortex* (Cambridge: Harvard University Press). doi: 10.4159/harvard.9780674187696

Conel, J. L. (1959). "The cortex of a twenty-four month old infant," in *The Post Natal Development of the Human Cerebral Cortex* (Cambridge: Harvard University Press). doi: 10.4159/harvard.9780674187702

Conel, J. L. (1963). "The cortex of a four year old child," in *The Post Natal Development of the Human Cerebral Cortex* (Cambridge: Harvard University Press). doi: 10.4159/harvard.9780674187719

Conel, J. L. (1967). "The cortex of a six year old child," in *The Post Natal Development of the Human Cerebral Cortex* (Cambridge: Harvard University Press). doi: 10.4159/harvard.9780674187733

Coogan, T. A., and Van Essen, D. C. (1996). Development of connections within and between areas V1 and V2 of macaque monkeys. *J. Comp. Neurol.* 372, 327–342.

Cupp, C. J., and Uemura, E. (1980). Age-related changes in the prefrontal cortex of *Macaca mulatta*: quantitative analysis of dendritic branching patterns. *Exp. Neurol.* 69, 143–163. doi: 10.1016/0014-4886(80)90150-8

Darian-Smith, C., and Gilbert, C. D. (1994). Axonal sprouting accompanies functional reorganization in adult striate cortex. *Nature* 368, 737–740. doi: 10.1038/368737a0

da Rocha, E. G., Freire, M. A. M., Bahia, C. P., Pereira, A., Sosthenes, M. C. K., Silveira, L. C. L., et al. (2012). Dendritic structure varies as a function of eccentricity in V1: a quantitative study of NADPH diaphorase neurons in the diurnal South American rodent agouti, *Dasyprocta prymnolopha.* *Neuroscience* 216, 94–102. doi: 10.1016/j.neuroscience.2012.04.042

DeFelipe, J. (1993). Neocortical neuronal diversity: chemical heterogeneity revealed by colocalization studies of classic neurotransmitters, neuropeptides, calcium-binding proteins, and cell surface molecules. *Cereb. Cortex* 3, 273–289. doi: 10.1093/cercor/3.4.273

DeFelipe, J., Alonso-Nanclares, L., and Arellano, J. I. (2002). Microstructure of the neocortex: comparative aspects. *J. Neurocytol.* 31, 299–316. doi: 10.1023/A:1024130211265

DeFelipe, J., Conti, F., Van Eyck, S. L., and Manzoni, T. (1988). Demonstration of glutamate-positive axon terminals forming asymmetric synapses in cat neocortex. *Brain Res.* 455, 162–165. doi: 10.1016/0006-8993(88)90127-8

DeFelipe, J., del Río, M. R., González-Albo, M. C., and Elston, G. N. (1999). Distribution and patterns of connectivity of interneurons containing calbindin, calretinin and parvalbumin in visual areas of the occipital and temporal lobes of the macaque monkey. *J. Comp. Neurol.* 412, 515–526.

Eayrs, J. T., and Goodhead, B. (1959). Postnatal development of the cerebral cortex in the rat. *J. Anat.* 93, 385–402.

El-Shamayleh, Y., Movshon, J. A., and Kiorpes, L. (2010). Development of sensitivity to visual texture modulation in macaque monkeys. *J. Vis.* 10, 11. doi: 10.1167/10.11.11

Elston, G. N. (2000). Pyramidal cells of the frontal lobe: all the more spinous to think with. *J. Neurosci.* 20, RC95.

Elston, G. N. (2001). Interlaminar differences in the pyramidal cell phenotype in areas 7m and STP (the superior temporal polysensory area) of the macaque monkey. *Exp. Brain Res.* 138, 141–152. doi: 10.1007/s002210100705

Elston, G. N. (2003a). Cortex, cognition and the cell: new insights into the pyramidal neuron and prefrontal function. *Cereb. Cortex* 13, 1124–1138. doi: 10.1093/cercor/bhg093

Elston, G. N. (2003b). Pyramidal cell heterogeneity in the visual cortex of the nocturnal New World owl monkey (*Aotus trivirgatus*). *Neuroscience* 117, 213–219. doi: 10.1016/S0306-4522(02)00806-0

Elston, G. N. (2003c). The pyramidal neuron in occipital, temporal and prefrontal cortex of the owl monkey (*Aotus trivirgatus*): regional specialization in cell structure. *Eur. J. Neurosci.* 17, 1313–1318. doi: 10.1046/j.1460-9568.2003.02552.x

Elston, G. N. (2007). "Specializations in pyramidal cell structure during primate evolution," in *Evolution of Nervous Systems,* eds J. H. Kaas and T. M. Preuss (Oxford: Academic Press), 191–242.

Elston, G. N., Benavides-Piccione, R., and DeFelipe, J. (2001). The pyramidal cell in cognition: a comparative study in human and monkey. *J. Neurosci.* 21, RC163.

Elston, G. N., Benavides-Piccione, R., and DeFelipe, J. (2005a). A study of pyramidal cell structure in the cingulate cortex of the macaque monkey with comparative notes on inferotemporal and primary visual cortex. *Cereb. Cortex* 15, 64–73. doi: 10.1093/cercor/bhh109

Elston, G. N., Benavides-Piccione, R., Elston, A., DeFelipe, J., and Manger, P. (2005e). Pyramidal cell specialization in the occipitotemporal cortex of the Chacma baboon (*Papio ursinus*). *Exp. Brain Res.* 167, 496–503. doi: 10.1007/s00221-005-0057-3

Elston, G. N., Benavides-Piccione, R., Elston, A., DeFelipe, J., and Manger, P. (2005g). Specialization in pyramidal cell structure in the cingulate cortex of the Chacma baboon (*Papio ursinus*): an intracellular injection study of the posterior and anterior cingulate gyrus with comparative notes on macaque and vervet monkeys. *Neurosci. Lett.* 387, 130–135. doi: 10.1016/j.neulet.2005.06.010

Elston, G. N., Benavides-Piccione, R., Elston, A., DeFelipe, J., and Manger, P. (2005h). Specialization in pyramidal cell structure in the sensory-motor cortex of the vervet monkey (*Cercopithecus pygerythrus*). *Neuroscience* 134, 1057–1068. doi: 10.1016/j.neuroscience.2005.04.054

Elston, G. N., Benavides-Piccione, R., Elston, A., Manger, P., and DeFelipe, J. (2005d). Pyramidal cell specialization in the occipitotemporal cortex of the vervet monkey (*Cercopithecus pygerythrus*). *Neuroreport* 16, 967–970. doi: 10.1097/00001756-200506210-00017

Elston, G. N., Benavides-Piccione, R., Elston, A., Manger, P., and DeFelipe, J. (2005f). Regional specialization in pyramidal cell structure in the limbic cortex of the vervet monkey (*Cercopithecus pygerythrus*): an intracellular injection study of the anterior and posterior cingulate gyrus. *Exp. Brain Res.* 167, 315–323. doi: 10.1007/s00221-005-0043-9

Elston, G. N., Benavides-Piccione, R., Elston, A., Manger, P., and DeFelipe, J. (2005i). Specialization in pyramidal cell structure in the sensory-motor cortex of the Chacma baboon (*Papio ursinus*) with comparative notes on the macaque monkey. *Anat. Rec.* 286, 854–865. doi: 10.1002/ar.a.20217

Elston, G. N., Benavides-Piccione, R., Elston, A., Manger, P., and DeFelipe, J. (2011b). Pyramidal cells in prefrontal cortex: comparative observations reveal unparalleled specializations in neuronal structure among primate species. *Front. Neuroanat.* 5:2. doi: 10.3389/fnana.2011.00002

Elston, G. N., Benavides-Piccione, R., Elston, A., Zietsch, B., DeFelipe, J., Manger, P., et al. (2006a). Specializations of the granular prefrontal cortex of primates: implications for cognitive processing. *Anat. Rec.* 288A, 26–35. doi: 10.1002/ar.a.20278

Elston, G. N., and DeFelipe, J. (2002). "Spine distribution in neocortical pyramidal cells: a common organizational principle across species," in *Progress in Brain Research,* eds E. C. Azmitia, J. DeFelipe, E G. Jones, P. Rakic, and C. E. Ribak (Amsterdam: Elsevier), 109–133.

Elston, G. N., DeFelipe, J., Arellano, J. I., González-Albo, M. C., and Rosa, M. G. P. (1999d). Variation in the spatial relationship between parvalbumin immunoreactive interneurones and pyramidal neurones in rat somatosensory cortex. *Neuroreport* 10, 2975–2979. doi: 10.1097/00001756-199909290-00019

Elston, G. N., Elston, A., Aurelio-Freire, M., Gomes Leal, W., Amaral Dias, I., Pereira, A. Jr., et al. (2006b). Specialization of pyramidal cell structure in the visual areas V1, V2 and V3 of the South American rodent, *Dasyprocta primnolopha. Brain Res.* 1106, 99–110. doi: 10.1016/j.brainres.2006.05.100

Elston, G. N., Elston, A., Casagrande, V. A., and Kaas, J. H. (2005c). Pyramidal neurons of granular prefrontal cortex the galago: complexity in the evolution of the psychic cell. *Anat. Rec.* 285, 610–618. doi: 10.1002/ar.a.20198

Elston, G. N., Elston, A., Kaas, J., and Casagrande, V. A. (2005b). Regional specialization in pyramidal cell structure in the visual cortex of the galago. an intracellular injection study with comparative notes on New World and Old World monkeys. *Brain Behav. Evol.* 66, 10–21. doi: 10.1159/000085044

Elston, G. N., and Garey, L. J. (2004). *New Research Findings on the Anatomy of the Cerebral Cortex of Special Relevance to Anthropological Questions.* Brisbane, QLD: University of Queensland Printery.

Elston, G. N., and González-Albo, M. C. (2003). Parvalbumin-, calbindin- and calretinin- immunoreactive neurons in the prefrontal cortex of the owl monkey (*Aotus trivirgatus*): a standardized quantitative comparison with sensory and motor cortex. *Brain Behav. Evol.* 62: 19–30. doi: 10.1159/000071957

Elston, G. N., and Manger, P. R. (2014). Pyramidal cells in V1 of African rodents are bigger more branched and more spiny than those in primates. *Front. Neuroanat.* 8:4. doi: 10.3389/fnana.2014.00004

Elston, G. N., Oga, T., and Fujita, I. (2009). Spinogenesis and pruning scales across functional hierarchies. *J. Neurosci.* 29, 3271–3275. doi: 10.1523/JNEUROSCI.5216-08.2009

Elston, G. N., Oga, T., Okamoto, T., and Fujita, I. (2010a). Spinogenesis and pruning from early visual onset to adulthood: an intracellular injection study of layer III pyramidal cells in the ventral visual cortical pathway of the macaque monkey. *Cereb. Cortex* 20, 1398–1408. doi: 10.1093/cercor/bhp203

Elston, G. N., Oga, T., Okamoto, T., and Fujita, I. (2011a). Spinogenesis and pruning in the anterior ventral inferotemporal cortex of the macaque monkey: an intracellular injection study of layer III pyramidal cells. *Front. Neuroanat.* 5:42. doi: 10.3389/fnana.2011.00042

Elston, G. N., Okamoto, T., Oga, T., Dornan, D., and Fujita, I. (2010b). Spinogenesis and pruning in the primary auditory cortex of the macaque monkey (*Macaca fascicularis*): An intracellular injection study of layer III pyramidal cells. *Brain Res.* 1316, 35–42. doi: 10.1016/j.brainres.2009.12.056

Elston, G. N., and Rockland, K. (2002). The pyramidal cell of the sensorimotor cortex of the macaque monkey: phenotypic variation. *Cereb. Cortex* 12, 1071–1078. doi: 10.1093/cercor/12.10.1071

Elston, G. N., and Rosa, M. G. P. (1997). The occipitoparietal pathway of the macaque monkey: comparison of pyramidal cell morphology in layer III of functionally related cortical visual areas. *Cereb. Cortex* 7, 432–452. doi: 10.1093/cercor/7.5.432

Elston, G. N., and Rosa, M. G. P. (1998). Morphological variation of layer III pyramidal neurones in the occipitotemporal pathway of the macaque monkey visual cortex. *Cereb. Cortex* 8, 278–294. doi: 10.1093/cercor/8.3.278

Elston, G. N., and Rosa, M. G. P. (2006). Ipsilateral corticocortical projections to the primary and middle temporal visual areas of the primate cerebral cortex: area-specific variations in the morphology of connectionally identified pyramidal cells. *Eur. J. Neurosci.* 23, 3337–3345. doi: 10.1111/j.1460-9568.2006.04847.x

Elston, G. N., Tweedale, R., and Rosa, M. G. P. (1999a). Cortical integration in the visual system of the macaque monkey: large scale morphological differences of pyramidal neurones in the occipital, parietal and temporal lobes. *Proc. R. Soc. Lond. Ser. B* 266, 1367–1374. doi: 10.1098/rspb.1999.0789

Elston, G. N., Tweedale, R., and Rosa, M. G. P. (1999b). Cellular heterogeneity in cerebral cortex. A study of the morphology of pyramidal neurones in visual areas of the marmoset monkey. *J. Comp. Neurol.* 415, 33–51.

Feldman, M. L., and Peters, A. (1979). A technique for estimating total spine numbers on Golgi-impregnated dendrites. *J. Comp. Neurol.* 188, 527–542. doi: 10.1002/cne.901880403

Ferster, D. (1998). A sense of direction. *Nature* 392, 433–434. doi: 10.1038/33005

Freire, M. A. M., Faber, J., Picanço-Diniz, C. W., Franca, J. G., and Pereira, A. (2012). Morphometric variability of nicotinamide adenine dinucleotide phosphate diaphorase neurons in the primary sensory areas of the rat. *Neuroscience* 205, 140–153. doi: 10.1016/j.neuroscience.2011.12.029

Freire, M. A. M., Rocha, E. G., Oliveira, J. L. F., Guimarães, J. S., Silveira, L. C. L., Elston, G. N., et al. (2010). Morphological variability of NADPH diaphorase neurons across areas V1, V2, and V3 of the common agouti. *Brain Res.* 1318, 52–63. doi: 10.1016/j.brainres.2009.12.045

Fujita, I., and Fujita, T. (1996). Intrinsic connections in the macaque inferior temporal cortex. *J. Comp. Neurol.* 368, 467–486.

Funahashi, S., and Takeda, K. (2002). Information processes in the primate prefrontal cortex in relation to working memory processes. *Rev. Neurosci.* 13, 313–345. doi: 10.1515/REVNEURO.2002.13.4.313

Fuster, J. M. (1997). *The Prefrontal Cortex: Anatomy, Physiology, and Neuropsychology of the Frontal Lobe.* Philadelphia, PA: Lippincott-Raven.

Goldman-Rakic, P. S. (1999). The "psychic" neuron of the cerebral cortex. *Ann. N.Y. Acad. Sci.* 868, 13–26. doi: 10.1111/j.1749-6632.1999.tb11270.x

González-Burgos, G., Barrionuevo, G., and Lewis, D. A. (2000). Horizontal synaptic connections in monkey prefrontal cortex: an *in vitro* electrophysiological study. *Cereb. Cortex* 10, 82–92. doi: 10.1093/cercor/10.1.82

Gonzalez-Burgos, G., Kroener, S., Zaitsev, A. V., Povysheva, N. V., Krimer, L. S., Barrionuevo, G., et al. (2008). Functional maturation of excitatory synapses in layer 3 pyramidal neurons during postnatal development of the primate prefrontal cortex. *Cereb. Cortex* 18, 626–637. doi: 10.1093/cercor/bhm095

Govek, E. E., Hatten, M. E., and Van Aelst, L. (2011). The role of Rho GTPase proteins in CNS neuronal migration. *Dev. Neurobiol.* 71, 528–553. doi: 10.1002/dneu.20850

Granger, B., Tekaia, F., Le Sourd, A. M., Rakic, P., and Bourgeois, J. P. (1995). Tempo of neurogenesis and synaptogenesis in the primate cingulate mesocortex: comparison with the neocortex. *J. Comp. Neurol.* 360, 363–376. doi: 10.1002/cne.903600212

Guillery, R. W. (2005). Is postnatal neocortical maturation hierarchical? *Trends Neurosci.* 28, 512–517. doi: 10.1016/j.tins.2005.08.006

Hof, P. R., and Morrison, J. H. (1995). Neurofilament protein defines regional patterns of cortical organization in the macaque monkey visual system: a quantitative immunohistochemical analysis. *J. Comp. Neurol.* 352, 161–186. doi: 10.1002/cne.903520202

Hof, P. R., and Nimchinsky, E. A. (1992). Regional distribution of neurofilament and calcium-binding proteins in the cingulate cortex of the macaque monkey. *Cereb. Cortex* 2, 456–467. doi: 10.1093/cercor/2.6.456

Huttenlocher, P. R. (1979). Synaptic density in human frontal cortex- developmental changes and effects of aging. *Brain Res.* 163, 195–205. doi: 10.1016/0006-8993(79)90349-4

Huttenlocher, P. R. (1990). Morphometric study of human cerebral cortex development. *Neuropsychologia* 28, 517–527. doi: 10.1016/0028-3932(90)90031-I

Huttenlocher, P. R., and Dabholkar, A. S. (1997). Regional differences in synaptogenesis in human cerebral cortex. *J. Comp. Neurol.* 387, 167–178.

Jacobs, B., Driscoll, L., and Schall, M. (1997). Life-span dendritic and spine changes in areas 10 and 18 of human cortex: a quantitative Golgi study. *J. Comp. Neurol.* 386, 661–680.

Jacobs, B., Johnson, N. L., Wahl, D., Schall, M., Maseko, B. C., Lewandowski, A., et al. (2014). Comparative neuronal morphology of the cerebellar cortex in afrotherians, carnivores, cetartiodactyls, and primates. *Front. Neuroanat.* 8:24. doi: 10.3389/fnana.2014.00024

Jacobs, B., Schall, M., Prather, M., Kapler, E., Driscoll, L., Baca, S., et al. (2001). Regional dendritic and spine variation in human cerebral cortex: a quantitative study. *Cereb. Cortex* 11, 558–571. doi: 10.1093/cercor/11.6.558

Jacobs, B., and Scheibel, A. B. (2002). "Regional dendritic variation in primate cortical pyramidal cells," in *Cortical Areas: Unity And Diversity,* eds A. Schüz and R. Miller (London: Taylor and Francis), 111–131. doi: 10.1201/9780203299296.pt2

Jones, E. G. (2009). The origins of cortical interneurons: mouse versus monkey and human. *Cereb. Cortex* 19, 1953–1956. doi: 10.1093/cercor/bhp088

Jones, T. A., Kleim, J. A., and Greenough, W. T. (1996). Synaptogenesis and dendritic growth in cortex opposite unilateral sensorimotor cortex damage in adult rats: a quantitative electron microscopic examination. *Brain Res.* 733, 142–148. doi: 10.1016/0006-8993(96)00792-5

Jones, T. A., and Schallert, T. (1992). Overgrowth and pruning of dendrites in adult rats recovering from neocortical damage. *Brain Res.* 581, 156–160. doi: 10.1016/0006-8993(92)90356-E

Kaas, J. H., Krubitzer, L. A., Chino, Y. M., Langston, A. L., Polley, E. H., and Blair, N. (1990). Reorganization of retinotopic cortical maps in adult mammals after lesions of the retina. *Science* 248, 229–231. doi: 10.1126/science.2326637

Kasper, E. M., Larkman, A. U., Lübke, J., and Blakemore, C. (1994). Pyramidal neurons in layer 5 of the rat visual cortex. II. Development of electrophysiological properties. *J. Comp. Neurol.* 339, 475–494. doi: 10.1002/cne.903390403

Keck, T., Mrsic-Flogel, T. D., Vaz Afonso, M., Eysel, U. T., Bonhoeffer, T., and Hübener, M. (2008). Massive restructuring of neuronal circuits during functional reorganization of adult visual cortex. *Nat. Neurosci.* 11, 1162–1167. doi: 10.1038/nn.2181

Kiorpes, L., and Movshon, J. A. (2003). "Neural limitations on visual development in primates," in *The Visual Neurosciences,* eds L. M. Chalupa and J. S.Werner (New York, NY: The MIT Press), 159–173.

Kiorpes, L., and Movshon, J. A. (2004). Development of sensitivity to visual motion in macaque monkeys. *Vis. Neurosci.* 21, 851–859. doi: 10.1017/S0952523804216054

Kiorpes, L., Price, T., Hall-Haro, C., and Movshon, J. A. (2012). Development of sensitivity to global form and motion in macaque monkeys (*Macaca nemestrina*). *Vision Res.* 63, 34–42. doi: 10.1016/j.visres.2012.04.018

Knott, G., and Holtmaat, A. (2008). Dendritic spine plasticity–current understanding from *in vivo* studies. *Brain Res. Rev.* 58, 282–289. doi: 10.1016/j.brainresrev.2008.01.002

Knott, G. W., Holtmaat, A., Wilbrecht, L., Welker, E., and Svoboda, K. (2006). Spine growth precedes synapse formation in the adult neocortex *in vivo*. *Nat. Neurosci.* 9, 1117–1124. doi: 10.1038/nn1747

Koenderink, M. J., Uylings, H. B., and Mrzljak, L. (1994). Postnatal maturation of the layer III pyramidal neurons in the human prefrontal cortex: a quantitative Golgi analysis. *Brain Res.* 653, 173–182. doi: 10.1016/0006-8993(94)90387-5

Kondo, H. T., Hashikawa, T., Tanaka, K., and Jones, E. G. (1994). Neurochemical gradient along the monkey occipito-temporal cortical pathway. *Neuroreport* 5, 613–616. doi: 10.1097/00001756-199401000-00020

Kritzer, M. F., Cowey, A., and Somogyi, P. (1992). Patterns of inter- and intralaminar GABAergic connections distinguish striate (V1) and extrastriate (V2, V4) visual cortices and their functionally specialized subdivisions in the rhesus monkeys. *J. Neurosci.* 12, 4545–4564.

Li, D.-P., Hagan, M. A., and Kiorpes, L. (2013). Linking structure and function: development of lateral spatial interactions in macaque monkeys. *Vis. Neurosci.* 30, 263–270. doi: 10.1017/S0952523813000394

Livingstone, M. S. (1998). Mechanisms of direction selectivity in macaque V1. *Neuron* 20, 509–526. doi: 10.1016/S0896-6273(00)80991-5

London, M., and Häusser, M. (2005). Dendritic computation. *Annu. Rev. Neurosci.* 28, 503–532. doi: 10.1146/annurev.neuro.28.061604.135703

Luebke, J. I., Medalla, M., Amatrudo, J. M., Weaver, C. M., Crimins, J. L., Hunt, B., et al. (2013). Age-related changes to layer 3 pyramidal cells in the rhesus monkey visual cortex. *Cereb. Cortex.* doi: 10.1093/cercor/bht336. [Epub ahead of print].

Lund, J. S., and Holbach, S. M. (1991). Postnatal development of thalamic recipient neurons in the striate cortex: I. comparison of spine acquisition and dendrite growth of layer 4C alpha and beta spiny stellate neurons. *J. Comp. Neurol.* 309, 115–128. doi: 10.1002/cne.903090108

Lund, J. S., Yoshioka, T., and Levitt, J. B. (1993). Comparison of intrinsic connectivity in different areas of macaque monkey cerebral cortex. *Cereb. Cortex* 3, 148–162. doi: 10.1093/cercor/3.2.148

Maruko, I., Zhang, B., Tao, X., Tong, J., Smith, E. L., and Chino, Y. M. (2008). Postnatal development of disparity sensitivity in visual area 2 (V2) of macaque monkeys. *J. Neurophysiol.* 100, 2486–2495. doi: 10.1152/jn.90397.2008

Maruyama, A., Ishikawa, A., Hosoyama, D., Yoshimura, Y., Tamura, H., Sato, H., et al. (2007). Development of membrane properties of layer III pyramidal neurons in macaque visual cortical areas V1 and TE. *Soc. Neurosci. Abstr.* 279, 10.

Mates, S. L., and Lund, J. S. (1983a). Neuronal composition and development in lamina 4C of monkey striate cortex. *J. Comp. Neurol.* 221, 60–90. doi: 10.1002/cne.902210106

Mates, S. L., and Lund, J. S. (1983b). Spine formation and maturation of type 1 synapses on spiny stellate neurons in primate visual cortex. *J. Comp. Neurol.* 221, 91–97. doi: 10.1002/cne.902210107

Matsubara, J. A., Chase, R., and Thejomayen, M. (1996). Comparative morphology of three types of projection-identified pyramidal neurons in the superficial layers of cat visual cortex. *J. Comp. Neurol.* 366, 93–108.

Matsuzaki, M., Honkura, N., Ellis-Davis, G. C., and Kasai, H. (2004). Structural basis of long-term potentiation in single dendritic spines. *Nature* 429, 761–766. doi: 10.1038/nature02617

McCormick, D. A., and Prince, D. A. (1987). Post-natal development of electrophysiological properties of rat cerebral cortical pyramidal neurones. *J. Physiol. (Lond.)* 393, 743–762.

Meissirel, C., Dehay, C., Berland, M., and Kennedy, H. (1991). Segregation of callosal and association pathways during development in the visual cortex of the primate. *J. Neurosci.* 11, 3297–3316.

Melchitzky, D. S., González-Burgos, G., Barrionuevo, G., and Lewis, D. A. (2001). Synaptic targets of the intrinsic axon collaterals of supragranular pyramidal neurons in monkey prefrontal cortex. *J. Comp. Neurol.* 430, 209–221. doi: 10.1002/1096-9861(20010205)430:2%3C209::AID-CNE1026%3E3.0.CO;2-%23

Melchitzky, D. S., Sesack, S. R., Pucak, M. L., and Lewis, D. A. (1998). Synaptic targets of pyramidal neurons providing intrinsic horizontal connections in monkey prefrontal cortex. *J. Comp. Neurol.* 390, 211–224.

Metherate, R., and Aramakis, V. B. (1999). Intrinsic electrophysiology of neurons in thalamorecipient layers of developing rat auditory cortex. *Brain Res. Dev. Brain Res.* 115, 131–144. doi: 10.1016/S0165-3806(99)00058-9

Miller, E. K., and Cohen, J. D. (2001). An integrative theory of prefrontal cortex. *Annu. Rev. Neurosci.* 24, 167–202. doi: 10.1146/annurev.neuro.24.1.167

Movshon, J. A., Kiorpes, L., Cavanaugh, J. R., and Hawken, M. J. (1999). Receptive field properties and surround interactions in V1 neurons in infant macaque monkeys. *Soc. Neurosci. Abstr.* 25, 1048.

Movshon, J. A., Kiorpes, L., Cavanaugh, J. R., and Hawken, M. J. (2000). Developmental reorganization of receptive field surrounds in V1 neurons in infant macaque monkeys. *Invest. Ophthalmol. Vis. Sci.* 41, 333.

Murayama, Y., Fujita, I., and Kato, M. (1997). Contrasting forms of synaptic plasticity in monkey inferotemporal and primary visual cortices. *Neuroreport* 8, 1503–1508. doi: 10.1097/00001756-199704140-00036

Nakajima, K. (2007). Control of tangential/non-radial migration of neurons in the developing cerebral cortex. *Neurochem. Int.* 51, 121–131. doi: 10.1016/j.neuint.2007.05.006

Oga, T., Aoi, H., Sasaki, T., Fujita, I., and Ichinohe, N. (2013). Postnatal development of layer III pyramidal cells in the primary visual, inferior temporal, and prefrontal cortices of the marmoset. *Front. Neural Circuits* 7:31. doi: 10.3389/fncir.2013.00031

O'Kusky, J., and Colonnier, M. (1982). Postnatal changes in the number of neurons and synapses in the visual cortex (area 17) of the macaque monkey: a stereological analysis in normal and monocularly deprived animals. *J. Comp. Neurol.* 210, 291–306. doi: 10.1002/cne.902100308

Oswald, A.-M., and Reyes, A. D. (2008). Maturation of intrinsic and synaptic properties of layer 2/3 pyramidal neurons in mouse auditory cortex. *J. Neurophysiol.* 99, 2998–3008. doi: 10.1152/jn.01160.2007

Petanjek, Z., Judas, M., Kostovic, I., and Uylings, H. B. M. (2008). Lifespan alterations of basal dendritic trees of pyramidal neurons in the human prefrontal cortex: a layer-specific pattern. *Cereb. Cortex* 18, 915–929. doi: 10.1093/cercor/bhm124

Petralia, R. S., Wang, Y. X., and Wenthold, R. J. (1994b). The NMDA receptor subunits NR2A and NR2B show histological and ultrastructural localization patterns similar to those of NR1. *J. Neurosci.* 14, 6102–6120.

Petralia, R. S., Wang, Y.-X., and Wenthold, R. J. (1994c). Histological and ultrastructural localization of kainate receptor subunits, KA2 and GluR6/7, in the rat nervous system using selective antipeptide antibodies. *J. Comp. Neurol.* 349, 85–110. doi: 10.1002/cne.903490107

Petralia, R. S., Yokotani, N., and Wenthold, R. J. (1994a). Light and electron microscope distribution of the NMDA receptor subunit NMDAR1 in the rat nervous system using a selective antipeptide antibody. *J. Neurosci.* 14, 667–696.

Pettigrew, J. D. (1974). The effect of visual experience on the development of stimulus specificity by kitten cortical neurones. *J. Physiol. (Lond.)* 237, 49–74.

Poirazi, P., and Mel, B. W. (2001). Impact of active dendrites and structural plasticity on the memory capacity of neural tissue. *Neuron* 29, 779–796. doi: 10.1016/S0896-6273(01)00252-5

Preuss, T. M. (2000). "What's human about the human brain?," in *The New Cognitive Neurosciences,* ed M. S. Gazzaniga (Cambridge, MA: MIT Press), 1219–1234.

Preuss, T. M., and Goldman-Rakic, P. S. (1991). Architectonics of the parietal and temporal association cortex in the strepsirhine primate *Galago* compared to the anthropoid *Macaca*. *J. Comp. Neurol.* 310, 475–506. doi: 10.1002/cne.903100403

Rakic, P. (1990). Principles of neuronal cell migration. *Experientia* 46, 882–891. doi: 10.1007/BF01939380

Rakic, P. (2009). Evolution of the neocortex: a perspective from developmental biology. *Nat. Rev. Neurosci.* 10, 724–735. doi: 10.1038/nrn2719

Rakic, P., Bourgeois, J.-P., Eckenhoff, M. F., Zecevic, N., and Goldman-Rakic, P. S. (1986). Concurrent overproduction of synapses in diverse regions of the primate cerebral cortex. *Science* 232, 232–235. doi: 10.1126/science.3952506

Rockland, K. S., and Lund, J. S. (1982). Widespread periodic intrinsic connections in the tree shrew visual cortex. *Science* 215, 1532–1534. doi: 10.1126/science.7063863

Rockland, K. S., and Lund, J. S. (1983). Intrinsic laminar lattice connections in primate visual cortex. *J. Comp. Neurol.* 216, 303–318. doi: 10.1002/cne.902160307

Rodman, H. R. (1994). Development of inferior temporal cortex in monkey. *Cereb. Cortex* 5, 484–498. doi: 10.1093/cercor/4.5.484

Rodman, H. R., and Consuelos, M. J. (1994). Cortical projections to anterior inferior temporal cortex in infant macaque monkeys. *Vis. Neurosci.* 11, 119–133. doi: 10.1017/S0952523800011160

Rodman, H. R., Scalaidhe, S. P., and Gross, G. C. (1993). Response properties of neurons in temporal cortical visual areas of infant monkeys. *J. Neurophysiol.* 70, 1115–1136.

Romand, S., Wang, Y., Toledo-Rodriguez, M., and Markram, H. (2011). Morphological development of thick-tufted layer V pyramidal cells in the rat smoatosensory cortex. *Front. Neuroanat.* 5:5. doi: 10.3389/fnana.2011.00005

Sala, C., Cambianica, I., and Rossi, F. (2008). Molecular mechanisms of dendritic spine development and maintenance. *Acta Neurobiol. Exp. (Wars)* 68, 289–304.

Sasaki, T., Aoi, H., Oga, T., Fujita, I., and Ichinohe, N. (2014). Postnatal development of dendritic structure of layer III pyramidal neurons in the medial prefrontal cortices of the marmoset. *Brain. Struct. Funct.* [Epub ahead of print].

Schmid, L. M., Rosa, M. G. P., Calford, M. B., and Ambler, J. S. (1996). Visuotopic reorganisation in the primary visual cortex of adult cats following monocular and binocular retinal lesions. *Cereb. Cortex* 6, 388–405. doi: 10.1093/cercor/6.3.388

Schwartz, M. L., and Goldman-Rakic, P. (1990). Development and plasticity of the primate cerebral cortex. *Clin. Perinatol.* 17, 83–102.

Schwartz, M. L., and Goldman-Rakic, P. S. (1991). Prenatal specification of callosal connections in rhesus monkey. *J. Comp. Neurol.* 307, 142–162. doi: 10.1002/cne.903070113

Sholl, D. A. (1955). The surface area of cortical neurons. *J. Anat.* 89, 571–572.

Somogyi, P., Tamas, G., Lujan, R., and Buhl, E. H. (1998). Salient features of synaptic organisation in the cerebral cortex. *Brain Res. Brain Res. Rev.* 26, 113–135. doi: 10.1016/S0165-0173(97)00061-1

Spruston, N. (2008). Pyramidal neurons: dendritic structure and synaptic integration. *Nat. Rev. Neurosci.* 9, 206–221. doi: 10.1038/nrn2286

Tanigawa, H., Fujita, I., Kato, M., and Ojima, H. (1998). Distribution, morphology, and γ-aminobutyric acid immunoreactivity of horizontally projecting neurons in the inferior temporal cortex. *J. Comp. Neurol.* 401, 129–143.

Tanigawa, H., Wang, Q.-X., and Fujita, I. (2005). Organization of horizontal axons in the inferior temporal cortex and primary visual cortex of the macaque monkey. *Cereb. Cortex* 15, 1887–1899. doi: 10.1093/cercor/bhi067

Taylor, W. R., He, S., Levick, W R., and Vaney, D. I. (2000). Dendritic computation of direction selectivity by retinal ganglion cells. *Science* 289, 2347–2350. doi: 10.1126/science.289.5488.2347

Taylor, W. R., and Vaney, D. I. (2002). Diverse synaptic mechanisms generate direction selectivity in the rabbit retina. *J. Neurosci.* 22, 7712–7720.

Tieman, S. B., and Hirsch, H. V. B. (1982). Exposure to lines of only one orientation modifies dendritic morphology of cells in visual cortex of the cat. *J. Comp. Neurol.* 211, 353–362. doi: 10.1002/cne.902110403

Trachtenberg, J. T., Chen, B. E., Knott, G. W., Feng, G. P., Sanes, J. R., Welker, E., et al. (2002). Long-term *in vivo* imaging of experience-dependent synaptic plasticity in adult cortex. *Nature* 420, 788–794. doi: 10.1038/nature01273

Travis, K., Ford, K., and Jacobs, B. (2005). Regional dendritic variation in neonatal human cortex: a quantitative Golgi study. *Dev. Neurosci.* 27, 277–287. doi: 10.1159/000086707

Valverde, F. (1967). Apical dendritic spines of the visual cortex and light deprivation in the mouse. *Exp. Brain Res.* 3, 337–352. doi: 10.1007/BF00237559

Vaney, D. I., Sivyer, B., and Taylor, W. R. (2012). Direction selectivity in the retina: symmetry and asymmetry in structure and function. *Nat. Rev. Neurosci.* 13, 194–208. doi: 10.1038/nrn3165

Vercelli, A., and Innocenti, G. M. (1993). Morphology of visual callosal neurons with different locations, contralateral targets or patterns of development. *Exp. Brain Res.* 94, 393–404. doi: 10.1007/BF00230198

Wang, Q. W., Tanigawa, H., and Fujita, I. (1998). Postnatal development of horizontal axons in the inferior temporal and primary visual cortices in the monkey. *Soc. Neurosci. Abstr.* 24, 900.

Webster, M. J., Bachevalier, J., and Ungerleider, L. G. (1994). Connections of inferior temporal areas TEO and TE with parietal and frontal cortex in macaque monkeys. *Cereb. Cortex* 4, 470–483. doi: 10.1093/cercor/4.5.470

Webster, M. J., Bachevalier, J., and Ungerleider, L. G. (1995). Transient subcortical connections of inferior temporal areas TEO and TE in infant macaque monkeys. *J. Comp. Neurol.* 352, 213–226. doi: 10.1002/cne.903520205

Webster, M. J., Ungerleider, L. G., and Bachevalier, J. (1991). Connections of inferior temporal areas TE and TEO with medial temporal-lobe structures in infant and adult monkeys. *J. Neurosci.* 11, 1095–1116.

Yáñez, I. B., Muñoz, A., Contreras, J., Gonzalez, J., Rodriguez-Veiga, E., and DeFelipe, J. (2005). Double bouquet cell in the human cerebral cortex and a comparison with other mammals. *J. Comp. Neurol.* 486, 344–360. doi: 10.1002/cne.20533

Zecevic, N., and Rakic, P. (1991). Synaptogenesis in monkey somatosensory cortex. *Cereb. Cortex* 1, 510–523. doi: 10.1093/cercor/1.6.510

Zhang, B., Smith, E. L. R., and Chino, Y. M. (2008). Postnatal development of onset transient responses in macaque V1 and V2 neurons. *J. Neurophysiol.* 100, 1476–1487. doi: 10.1152/jn.90446.2008

Zhang, B., Tao, X., Shen, G., Smith, E. R., Ohzawa, I., and Chino, Y. M. (2013). Receptive-field subfields of V2 neurons in macaque monkeys are adult-like near birth. *J. Neurosci.* 33, 2639–2649. doi: 10.1523/JNEUROSCI.4377-12.2013

Zhang, Z. W. (2004). Maturation of layer V pyramidal neurons in the rat prefrontal cortex: intrinsic properties and synaptic function. *J. Neurophysiol.* 91, 1171–1182. doi: 10.1152/jn.00855.2003

Zheng, J., Zhang, B., Bi, H., Maruko, I., Watanabe, I., Nakatsuka, C., et al. (2007). Development of temporal response properties and contrast sensitivity of V1 and V2 neurons in macaque monkeys. *J. Neurophysiol.* 97, 3905–3916. doi: 10.1152/jn.01320.2006

Zimmermann, R. R. (1961). Analysis of discrimination learning capacities in the infant Rhesus monkey. *J. Comp. Physiol. Psychol.* 54, 1–10. doi: 10.1037/h0042320

4

The "addicted" spine

Saturnino Spiga[1], Giovanna Mulas[1,2], Francesca Piras[1,3] and Marco Diana[2]*

[1] Department of Animal Biology and Ecology, University of Cagliari, Cagliari, Italy
[2] "G.Minardi" Laboratory of Cognitive Neuroscience, Department of Chemistry and Pharmacy, University of Sassari, Sassari, Italy
[3] Department of Natural Science and the Territory, University of Sassari, Sassari, Italy

***Correspondence:**
Marco Diana, "G.Minardi" Laboratory of Cognitive Neuroscience, Department of Chemistry and Pharmacy, University of Sassari, Via Muroni 23, 07100, Sassari, Italy
e-mail: dsfdiana@uniss.it

Units of dendritic branches called dendritic spines represent more than simply decorative appendages of the neuron and actively participate in integrative functions of "spinous" nerve cells thereby contributing to the general phenomenon of synaptic plasticity. In animal models of drug addiction, spines are profoundly affected by treatments with drugs of abuse and represent important sub cellular markers which interfere deeply into the physiology of the neuron thereby providing an example of the burgeoning and rapidly increasing interest in "structural plasticity". Medium Spiny Neurons (MSNs) of the Nucleus Accumbens (Nacc) show a reduced number of dendritic spines and a decrease in TH-positive terminals upon withdrawal from opiates, cannabinoids and alcohol. The reduction is localized "strictly" to second order dendritic branches where dopamine (DA)-containing terminals, impinging upon spines, make synaptic contacts. In addition, long-thin spines seems preferentially affected raising the possibility that cellular learning of these neurons may be selectively hampered. These findings suggest that dendritic spines are affected by drugs widely abused by humans and provide yet another example of drug-induced aberrant neural plasticity with marked reflections on the physiology of synapses, system structural organization, and neuronal circuitry remodeling.

Keywords: spines, long thin, learning, dopamine, nucleus accumbens

INTRODUCTION

Dendritic spines have been recognized, described and named, for the first time by Ramón y Cajal on the surface of Purkinje cells using the Golgi staining method (Cajal, 1888, 1891). While other investigators and even Golgi himself, disregarded spines as artifacts, Gray (1959) unambiguously showed that spines were sites of synaptic contact. It is now clear that dendritic spines are the main postsynaptic compartments of excitatory synapses in the brain with peculiar and distinctive morphological features.

Dendritic spines are heterogeneous in size and shape but, mostly mature ones, consist of a bulbous head and a thinner neck that connects the spine to the dendritic shaft (Wilson et al., 1983; Svoboda et al., 1996). This morphological configuration is particularly important for synaptic efficacy. In particular, dimensions of the spine head (Kirov and Harris, 1999; Holtmaat and Svoboda, 2009), rather than the neck, realistically reflect the observed differences in synaptic strength (Harris and Stevens, 1988). The neck constriction might serve to isolate metabolic events in the vicinity of activated synapses without significantly influencing the transfer of synaptic charge to the parent dendrite (Harris and Stevens, 1988) and thus favoring "local" changes in the number and shape of spines during synaptic plasticity (Engert and Bonhoeffer, 1999). Indeed, individual spines may represent partially autonomous compartments with a cytoskeleton composed mostly of F-actin, and may hold numerous specialized organelle such as the smooth endoplasmic reticulum, which in the largest spines forms the "spine apparatus" (Gray, 1959) with polyribosomes, near the base of the spine (Steward and Levy, 1982) offering the possibility of local protein synthesis.

At the ultrastructural level, the spine head is characterized by an electron-dense matrix of receptors and supporting proteins collectively known as the postsynaptic density (PSD; Yamauchi, 2002). This complex assembly, made of hundreds of distinct proteins (Moon et al., 1994), dynamically changes its structure and composition during development and in response to synaptic activity. The PSD contains signaling molecules including the subunits of the *N*-methyl-D-aspartate (NMDA) glutamate receptors, the a-amino-3-hydroxy-5-methyl-4-isoxazolepropionic-acid (AMPA), the subunits of Ca21/calmodulin-dependent protein kinase II (CaMKII; Kennedy et al., 1983) and synGAP, a ras GTPase-activating protein phosphorylated by CaMKII and dopamine (DA) receptors (Zhang et al., 2007). Other prominent PSD proteins are scaffold molecules, including the PSD-95 family (Cho et al., 1992), that link receptors to signaling proteins or to the cytoskeleton, thus helping organize the structure of PSDs (Kornau et al., 1995).

CLASSIFICATION

Spine development is a dynamic process which includes transition from small dendritic formations to large spines and vice versa, through a series of sophisticated structural refinements (Calabrese et al., 2006). The continuous and rapid change in shape of dendritic spines is essential for short and long term plasticity (Kasai et al., 2003, 2010) and different shapes may reflect dynamically different functions (Hering and Sheng, 2001).

A pioneering classification was proposed by Peters and Kaiserman-Abramof (1970), where they distinguished three categories: stubby, thin, and mushroom spines. However, it was necessary to introduce the dendritic filopodia in this classification. In some cases, following establishment of contact with an afferent fiber, these transient structures can become a spine (Ziv and Smith, 1996; Fiala et al., 1998; Sorra and Harris, 2000). On the other hand, some author prefers to distinguish mature spines into two broad categories: large and small considering the head size (Kasai et al., 2003, 2010) emphasizing spine function.

The confocal microscope is able to detect sufficient details of the Golgi-Cox-stained neurons. In this case is possible to extract numerical information from 3D recontruction and to establish an unambiguous criterion of classification (**Figure 1**) which was recently introduced (Spiga et al., 2014).

THE SPINE OF THE NUCLEUS ACCUMBENS

The Medium Spiny Neuron (MSN) of the Nucleus Accumbens (Nacc) plays a central role in the integration of cortical, thalamic and mesencephalic afferents and MSNs (accounting for 90–95% of the total striatal complex) are involved in various behavioral sequelae including movement control (Björklund and Dunnett, 2007; Pissadaki and Bolam, 2013), motivation (Ostlund et al., 2014) and addiction (Diana, 2011). Terminals of DA containing neurons from the ventral tegmentum (VTA) are jumbled in a dense network of connections in many forebrain regions. Although the number of these neurons is relatively small, the projections from individual neurons are very extensive having a total axonal length (including collaterals) of roughly 74 cm with 500,000 terminals (Björklund and Dunnett, 2007; Pissadaki and Bolam, 2013) forming, in the striatum, approximately 20% of all synapses (Zhou et al., 2002, 2003). Basically, in this area every MSN is innervated by a conspicuous number of DAergic axons (Yao et al., 2008). MSNs also receive glutamate inputs from the PFC, thalamus, hippocampus (Harris and Stevens, 1989), and amygdala (Bredt and Nicoll, 2003). Accordingly, the Nacc plays a central role in the integration of cortical and mesencephalic afferent systems. Cell body and different portions of dendrites of MSNs, are targeted by various inputs. Mainly the soma and most proximal dendrites receive recurrent collaterals from other MSN (Groves, 1983), while cortical and DAergic afferents synapse onto spines located more distally on the dendrite. On distal dendrites a significant subpopulation of spines shows a particular synaptic architecture, called "striatal microcircuit" or "synaptic triad" (Freund et al., 1984), that involves both DAergic and glutamatergic axons (**Figure 2**). Similar innervation architecture is also observed in pyramidal neurons in the cortex (Sesack and Pickel, 1992), hippocampus (Totterdell and Smith, 1989) and magnocellualar neurons of basolateral amygdala (Johnson et al., 1994). In this configuration, DAergic terminals make a symmetric synapse with the neck whereas cortical terminals form an asymmetric contact in the spine head (Bouyer et al., 1984; Freund et al., 1984; Smith et al., 1994). In other words, DArgic and prefrontal cortical terminals in the MSNs dually synapse on a common dendritic spine (Sesack and Pickel, 1992; Moss and Bolam, 2008). The significance of this heterosynaptic formation is not very clear but it seems to suggest that DA (Pascoli et al., 2011) is able to modulate the influence of cortical glutamatergic

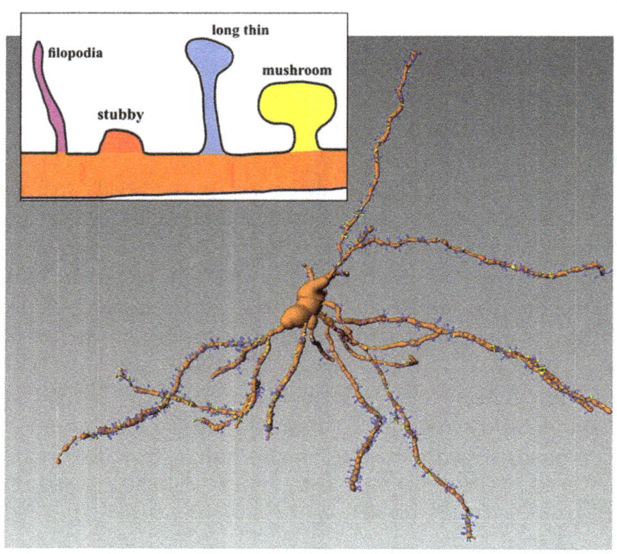

FIGURE 1 | Representative Golgi-Cox stained MSN with various spines types. Inset shows details of different morphologies. Image is color-coded. Reconstructed with filament tracer algorithm (Imaris 7.4). Note relative abundance of blu (long thin) spines which amount for 52% of all spines (see Spiga et al., 2014 for further details).

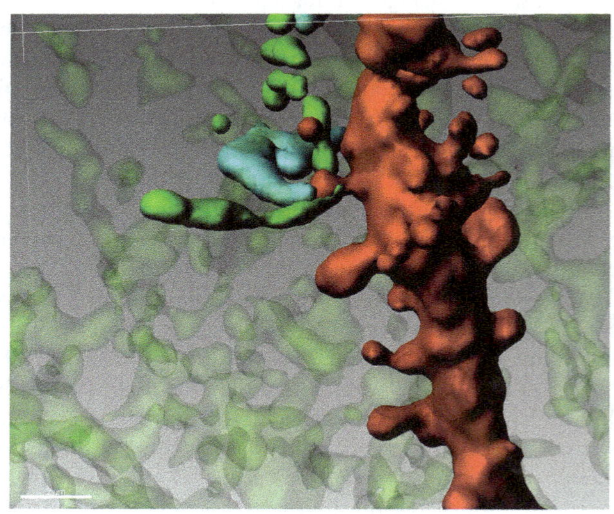

FIGURE 2 | Synaptic triad in the Nucleus Accumbens. Tyrosine Hydroxylase-positive terminals (green) are forming a putative contact with the neck of a spine on a second order dendritic trunk (red), while the head of the same spine is reached by a Golgi-Cox impregnated fiber (blue) from an adjacent neuron.

axons (see Spiga et al., 2014 for discussion on this point). This aspect is particularly important because, despite their distinct targets, all addictive drugs commonly abused by humans evoke variations on DA concentrations within the Nacc (Di Chiara and Imperato, 1988) and it may have a role in spine density, morphology and synaptic strength. Because of this particular synaptic configuration, even modest changes in the number of dendritic spines, can have major effects on the entire neuronal pathway. Accordingly, conditions of lowered DA tone such as morphine withdrawal has been associated with spine loss (Spiga et al., 2005). Similarly, cannabis-dependent subjects undergo spine pruning in the shell of the Nacc (Spiga et al., 2010) with a reduced MSN intrinsic excitability (Spiga et al., 2010) and alcohol-dependent rats show a DA-dependent selective loss of long thin spines associated with a lack of long term depression (Spiga et al., 2014).

ABNORMAL SPINE PLASTICITY AND ADDICTION

The number and shape of dendritic spines, during pathological events, are extremely variable. A broad variety of psychiatric diseases and neurological disorders are accompanied by patterns of spine disruption (Huttenlocher, 1970; Fiala et al., 2002) and changes in morphology (Irwin et al., 2000; Kaufmann and Moser, 2000). Schizophrenia, for example, is commonly associated with fewer spines and synapses in many brain areas and neuronal types (Garey et al., 1998; Glantz and Lewis, 2000; Lewis and Levitt, 2002). Further, neurodegenerative disorders such as Parkinson's disease are characterized by a loss of dendritic spines in striatal neurons (Villalba et al., 2009). Likewise, neural events related to chronic drug intake are linked to long-lasting drug-induced whole cell plasticity (Miller et al., 2012; Diana, 2013) and abnormal spine structure and density in critical brain areas (Robinson and Kolb, 2004; Russo et al., 2010). Four functionally connected structures of the brain: medial PFC, Nacc, lateral hypothalamus and the mesencephalic VTA, represent the neuroanatomical substrate of the so-called reward pathway (Koob, 1992; Melis et al., 2005). This fundamental system of regulation of complex behavior, influences rudimentary functions like food intake (Wise, 2006), sexual behavior (Robbins and Everitt, 1996), sensory perception (Berridge and Robinson, 1998), emotions (LeDoux, 2000), intellectual evaluations and processes of memory and learning (Robbins and Everitt, 2002; Hyman et al., 2006). Drugs of abuse "illegally" occupy this circuit over-stimulating the reward mechanism, causing cumulative impacts on neurotransmission. Addictive drugs, for example, can release 2–10 times the amount of DA (Di Chiara and Imperato, 1988) that natural rewards do and they do it more quickly and more reliably. Accordingly, addiction can be considered an example of experience-dependent plasticity (Robinson and Kolb, 2004).

Drug-induced structural plasticity of dendritic spines was first described by Kunz et al. (1976) and by Riley and Halkar (1978) in hippocampal pyramidal neurons following long-term alcohol consumption and is now an emerging field of investigation (Chen et al., 2010). While chronic administration of ethanol (Zhou et al., 2007) and morphine is accompanied by a decrease in the density of dendritic spines and dendritic branching of NAcc MSNs and mPFC pyramidal neurons (Robinson and Kolb, 1999b; Robinson et al., 2002), administration (or self administration) of amphetamine (Robinson and Kolb, 1997, 1999a; Heijtz et al., 2003; Kolb et al., 2003; Li et al., 2003; Crombag et al., 2005), cocaine (Robinson and Kolb, 1999a; Robinson et al., 2001; Li et al., 2003; Norrholm et al., 2003) and nicotine (Brown and Kolb, 2001; Gonzalez et al., 2005) increases spine density and dendritic branching on NAcc MSNs and pyramidal cells in the mPFC (Kolb et al., 2003). Indeed, a direct comparison among different substances is not easy because researchers use a wide variety of doses and ways of drug administration, producing, very often, divergent results on neuron morphology, during different phases of treatment with the same substance. In particular, the withdrawal syndrome after chronic drug administration seems to be a crucial point of the addictive process that is manifested by the induction of rapid changes in dendritic spine density and morphology and is thus experimentally appealing to gain insights when the drug is not on-board, to avoid possible confounds. Accordingly, we observed radical changes on spine density in accumbal MSNs during the early phases of abstinence of various drugs of abuse (Spiga et al., 2005, 2010). In fact, spontaneous and naloxone-induced morphine withdrawal, after 14 days of escalating chronic morphine administration, selectively alters spine density in the MSN second order dendrites of the NAcc shell (Spiga et al., 2005; Diana et al., 2006). Similar results we found when rats were subjected to a chronic treatment with two different cannabinoid agonists (Delta(9)-tetrahydrocannabinol and CP 55 940) and withdrawn spontaneously and pharmacologically with the CB1 antagonist SR141716A. Confocal analysis of Golgi-Cox-stained MSNs of the NAcc revealed a decrease in spine density in the shell, but not in the core only during withdrawal (both spontaneous and pharmacologically-precipitated) (Spiga et al., 2010). In contrast, no changes in the number of spines were observed during chronic morphine, cannabis and ethanol treatment, thereby suggesting that as long as the drug is "on-board" it supports spine persistence and function, whereas abrupt withdrawal discloses spine pruning and synaptic dysfunction. Interestingly, 3 weeks of daily cocaine administration did not seem to alter spine density in the core subregion of the Nacc (Shen et al., 2009) whereas other studies showed an increased spine density in the shell (Ren et al., 2010) 1–2 days after interruption of consecutive cocaine injections in mice. Further, increases were seen in the whole Nacc (Lee et al., 2006) and the core (Kim et al., 2009). However, there are no clear indications how and whether (and if) these additional spines participate in the network activity (but see Heck et al., 2014). These experiments cast doubt and urge caution on the notion that chronic cocaine or morphine treatments are unequivocally accompanied by an increase or a decrease of dendritic spines density in the NAcc, but suggest that the withdrawal itself might be the time-window in which to observe unequivocally the reported functional and morphological changes. Indeed, chronic treatment (*per se*) without exact dosing, regimen, degree of tolerance etc., cannot offer clear-cut results. On the other hand, it should be considered that withdrawal, after (not during) chronic drug intake, is one of the most powerful factor (negative reinforcement) driving dependence (Koob and Volkow, 2010). Accordingly, it is during this phase, to expect major changes at the neural level which in turn, will elicit behavioral changes and is considered the "driving force" in the transition from chronic drug intake to "addiction" (George et al., 2014). On the contrary, repeated exposure of drugs of abuse (drug on-board) likely alters the brain, but adaptive mechanisms intervened over the course of treatment may hide objective observations, potentially misleading judgement and spoiling conclusions (Kosten and George, 2002) because, mainly due to the wide variety of drugs, diverse treatment regimens, ample dosing, different pharmacokinetic properties, and various degrees of adaptive mechanisms such as tolerance, sensitization and others.

One possible explanation for these conflicting results, is provided by the particular nature of dendritic spines, relationships with afferents and their dynamic nature in changing size, shape and function (Kasai et al., 2010). For example, in the striatum the loss of DA terminals, in animal models of Parkinson disease (Schintu et al., 2009) and/or aging (Darbin, 2012), on the spine neck removes a modulatory influence that determines if cortically derived signals invade the dendritic shaft (Garcia et al., 2010). Conversely, a decrease in activity results in elongation of spines and a collapse of their heads (Segal, 2010) or a loss altogether (Nägerl et al., 2004). Remodeling in size and morphology of dendritic spines seems to be important at least as much as their changes in density on behavioral plasticity (Grutzendler et al., 2002; Trachtenberg et al., 2002). In drug addiction (Dumitriu et al., 2012) and schizophrenia (Faludi and Mirnics, 2011), in some brain areas, spines are approximately 30% smaller than controls (Roberts et al., 1996). Two spine types seem to be particularly involved in excitatory synaptic activity: long thin and mushroom. Mushroom are large and more stable spines that can persist for months (Bourne and Harris, 2007), whereas long thin seem to be "designed" for rapid responses to changes imposed by salient stimuli (Matsuzaki et al., 2004). Although long thin spines can change their volume even independently from synaptic activity, reflecting a native instability of these structures (Yasumatsu et al., 2008), the stimulation of a single spine cause a nearly immediate expansion of the spine head volume by 3–4-fold (Matsuzaki et al., 2004). During the course of cocaine treatment, spines shift from small to large (Shen et al., 2009) as a consequence of changes in synaptic strength (Bourne and Harris, 2007). On the contrary, thin spines shift toward smaller size in response to cocaine withdrawal with the addition of new thin spines (Dumitriu et al., 2012), perhaps immature, and silent synapses (Huang et al., 2009), that contain NMDA but few or no AMPA receptors (Russo et al., 2010). These newly formed spines appear to be highly "plastic", being able to retract or consolidate into larger spines (Shen et al., 2009). Therefore, the stabilization of heads enlargement of potentiated spines is associated with recruitment of additional AMPA-type glutamate receptors (Nusser et al., 1998; Kharazia and Weinberg, 1999) and an increase of protein synthesis as well as actin remodeling (Matsuzaki et al., 2004; Okamoto et al., 2004; Bramham, 2008; Honkura et al., 2008). In line with an active remodeling theory, by the introduction of a new staining method combining Golgi-Cox impregnation with immunofluorescence (Spiga et al., 2011), we recently found that the reduction in spine density in ethanol abstinent rats could be attributed almost entirely to long thin spines (while "mushroom" remains relatively unaffected) (Spiga et al., 2014). At the same time, PSD-95 and tyrosine hydroxilase (but not DA transporters) immunoreactivity were similarly reduced in association with ethanol withdrawal. These results show a close relationship between morphology and function of spines and reiterate on the trophic role of DA on spines in addictive states (Melis et al., 2005; Diana, 2011) and further support the "hypodopaminergic state" as a key element in animal models of addiction. On the other hand, long thin spines, in MSNs, could be strategically used as elements highly modifiable to support important modulatory roles in synaptic transmission (Jones, 2011).

It seems clear that even a single neuron respond differently as a result of exposure to different drugs and different modality of intake of the same drug in a sort of learned addictive behavior or "memory of addiction" (Mello, 1972; Kalant, 1973; Boening, 2001; Nestler, 2013; Dong and Nestler, 2014). This kind of "memory" may be similar to the long-term learning model supported by excitatory synapses located on dendritic spines (Kasai et al., 2010) of neurons in the dopaminoceptive areas such as PFC and hippocampus. This raises the possibility that long lasting changes in synapse formation and synaptic organization induced by drugs of abuse, may interact and hinder those produced by experience in the reward pathway. These drug-paired memories and the drug withdrawal-associated aversive feeling have been suggested to contribute to the high rate of relapse among addicts (Nestler, 2001; Hyman et al., 2006; Robbins et al., 2008). This wrong (aberrant) learning mechanism should be strongly related to synapse formation, changes in efficacy of synaptic transmission and morphology, modulated by DA tone in different cell types and brain regions. The resulting changes in neuronal connectivity are likely to contribute to hamper cognitive functions such as decision making and emotional rigidity typical of addicts.

ACKNOWLEDGMENTS

This work was supported, in part, by funds from Regione Autonoma della Sardegna (RAS), Progetti di ricerca di base—Bando 2008, to Marco Diana.

REFERENCES

Berridge, K. C., and Robinson, T. E. (1998). What is the role of dopamine in reward: hedonic impact, reward learning, or incentive salience? *Brain Res. Brain Res. Rev.* 28, 309–369. doi: 10.1016/s0165-0173(98)00019-8

Björklund, A., and Dunnett, S. B. (2007). Dopamine neuron systems in the brain: an update. *Trends Neurosci.* 5, 194–202. doi: 10.1016/j.tins.2007.03.006

Boening, J. A. (2001). Neurobiology of an addiction memory. *J. Neural Transm.* 108, 755–765. doi: 10.1007/s007020170050

Bourne, J., and Harris, K. M. (2007). Do thin spines learn to be mushroom spines that remember? *Curr. Opin. Neurobiol.* 17, 381–386. doi: 10.1016/j.conb.2007.04.009

Bouyer, J. J., Park, D. H., Joh, T. H., and Pickel, V. M. (1984). Chemical and structural analysis of the relation between cortical inputs and tyrosine hydroxylase-containing terminals in rat neostriatum. *Brain Res.* 302, 267–275. doi: 10.1016/0006-8993(84)90239-7

Bramham, C. R. (2008). Local protein synthesis, actin dynamics and LTP consolidation. *Curr. Opin. Neurobiol.* 18, 524–531. doi: 10.1016/j.conb.2008.09.013

Bredt, D. S., and Nicoll, R. A. (2003). AMPA receptor trafficking at excitatory synapses. *Neuron* 40, 361–379. doi: 10.1016/s0896-6273(03)00640-8

Brown, R. W., and Kolb, B. (2001). Nicotine sensitization increases dendritic length and spine density in the nucleus accumbens and cingulate cortex. *Brain Res.* 899, 94–100. doi: 10.1016/s0006-8993(01)02201-6

Cajal, S. (1888). Estructura de los centros nerviosos de las aves. *Rev. Trim. Histol. Norm. Patol.* 1, 1–10.

Cajal, S. (1891). Significación fisiológica de las expansiones protoplásmicas y nerviosas de las células de la sustancia gris. *Rev. Cienc. Méd. Barc.* 22, 23–37.

Calabrese, B., Wilson, M. S., and Halpain, S. (2006). Development and regulation of dendritic spine synapses. *Physiology (Bethesda)* 21, 38–47. doi: 10.1152/physiol.00042.2005

Chen, B. T., Hopf, F. W., and Bonci, A. (2010). Synaptic plasticity in the mesolimbic system: therapeutic implications for substance abuse. *Ann. N Y Acad. Sci.* 1187, 129–139. doi: 10.1111/j.1749-6632.2009.05154.x

Cho, K.-O., Hunt, C. A., and Kennedy, M. B. (1992). The rat brain postsynaptic density fraction contains a homolog of the Drosophila discs-large tumor suppressor protein. *Neuron* 9, 929–942. doi: 10.1016/0896-6273(92)90245-9

Crombag, H. S., Gorny, G., Li, Y., Kolb, B., and Robinson, T. E. (2005). Opposite effects of amphetamine self-administration experience on dendritic spines in the medial and orbital prefrontal cortex. *Cereb. Cortex* 3, 341–348. doi: 10.1093/cercor/bhh136

Darbin, O. (2012). The aging striatal dopamine function. *Parkinsonism Relat. Disord.* 18, 426–432. doi: 10.1016/j.parkreldis.2011.11.025

Diana, M. (2011). The dopamine hypothesis of drug addiction and its potential therapeutic value. *Front. Psychiatry* 2:64. doi: 10.3389/fpsyt.2011.00064

Diana, M. (2013). The addicted brain. *Front. Psychiatry* 4:40. doi: 10.3389/fpsyt.2013.00040

Diana, M., Spiga, S., and Acquas, E. (2006). Persistent and reversible morphine withdrawal-induced morphological changes in the nucleus accumbens. *Ann. N Y Acad. Sci.* 1074, 446–457. doi: 10.1196/annals.1369.045

Di Chiara, G., and Imperato, A. (1988). Drugs abused by humans preferentially increase synaptic dopamine concentrations in the mesolimbic system of freely moving rats. *Proc. Natl. Acad. Sci. U S A* 85, 5274–5278. doi: 10.1073/pnas.85.14.5274

Dong, Y., and Nestler, E. J. (2014). The neural rejuvenation hypothesis of cocaine addiction. *Trends Pharmacol. Sci.* 35, 374–383. doi: 10.1016/j.tips.2014.05.005

Dumitriu, D., LaPlant, Q., Grossman, Y. S., Dias, C., Janssen, W. G., Russo, S. J., et al. (2012). Subregional, dendritic compartment and spine subtype specificity in cocaine-regulation of dendritic spines in the nucleus accumbens. *J. Neurosci.* 20, 6957–6966. doi: 10.1523/JNEUROSCI.5718-11.2012

Engert, F., and Bonhoeffer, T. (1999). Dendritic spine changes associated with hippocampal long-term synaptic plasticity. *Nature* 399, 66–70. doi: 10.1038/19978

Faludi, G., and Mirnics, K. (2011). Synaptic changes in the brain of subjects with schizophrenia. *Int. J. Dev. Neurosci.* 29, 305–309. doi: 10.1016/j.ijdevneu.2011.02.013

Fiala, J. C., Feinberg, M., Popov, V., and Harris, K. M. (1998). Synaptogenesis via dendritic filopodia in developing hippocampal area CA1. *J. Neurosci.* 18, 8900–8911.

Fiala, J. C., Spacek, J., and Harris, K. M. (2002). Dendritic spine pathology: cause or consequence of neurological disorders? *Brain Res. Brain Res. Rev.* 39, 29–54. doi: 10.1016/s0165-0173(02)00158-3

Freund, T. F., Powell, J. F., and Smith, A. D. (1984). Tyrosine hydroxylase-immunoreactive boutons in synaptic contact with identified striatonigral neurons, with particular reference to dendritic spines. *Neuroscience* 13, 1189–1215. doi: 10.1016/0306-4522(84)90294-x

Garcia, B. G., Neely, M. D., and Deutch, A. Y. (2010). Cortical regulation of striatal medium spiny neuron dendritic remodeling in parkinsonism: modulation of glutamate release reverses dopamine depletion-induced dendritic spine loss. *Cereb. Cortex* 20, 2423–2432. doi: 10.1093/cercor/bhp317

Garey, L. J., Ong, W. Y., Patel, T. S., Kanani, M., Davis, A., Mortimer, A. M., et al. (1998). Reduced dendritic spine density on cerebral cortical pyramidal neurons in schizophrenia. *J. Neurol. Neurosurg. Psychiatry* 65, 446–453. doi: 10.1136/jnnp.65.4.446

George, O., Koob, G. F., and Vendruscolo, L. F. (2014). Negative reinforcement via motivational withdrawal is the driving force behind the transition to addiction. *Psychopharmacology (Berl)* 231, 3911–3917. doi: 10.1007/s00213-014-3623-1

Glantz, L. A., and Lewis, D. A. (2000). Decreased dendritic spine density on prefrontal cortical pyramidal neurons in schizophrenia. *Arch. Gen. Psychiatry* 57, 65–73. doi: 10.1001/archpsyc.57.1.65

Gonzalez, C. L. R., Gharbawie, O. A., Whishaw, I. Q., and Kolb, B. (2005). Nicotine stimulates dendritic arborization in motor cortex and improves concurrent motor skill but impairs subsequent motor learning. *Synapse* 55, 183–191. doi: 10.1002/syn.20106

Gray, E. G. (1959). Electron microscopy of synaptic contacts on dendritic spines of the cerebral cortex. *Nature* 183, 1592–1593. doi: 10.1038/1831592a0

Groves, P. M. (1983). A theory of the functional organization of the neostriatum and the neostriatal control of voluntary movement. *Brain Res.* 286, 109–132. doi: 10.1016/0165-0173(83)90011-5

Grutzendler, J., Kasthuri, N., and Gan, W. B. (2002). Long-term dendritic spine stability in the adult cortex. *Nature* 420, 812–816. doi: 10.1038/nature01276

Harris, K. M., and Stevens, J. K. (1988). Dendritic spines of rat cerebellar Purkinje cells: serial electron microscopy with reference to their biophysical characteristics. *J. Neurosci.* 8, 4455–4469.

Harris, K. M., and Stevens, J. K. (1989). Dendritic spines of CA 1 pyramidal cells in the rat hippocampus: serial electron microscopy with reference to their biophysical characteristics. *J. Neurosci.* 9, 2982–2997.

Heck, N., Dos Santos, M., Amairi, B., Salery, M., Besnard, A., Herzog, E., et al. (2014). A new automated 3D detection of synaptic contacts reveals the formation of cortico-striatal synapses upon cocaine treatment in vivo. *Brain Struct. Funct.* doi: 10.1007/s00429-014-0837-2. [Epub ahead of print].

Heijtz, R. D., Kolb, B., and Forssberg, H. (2003). Can a therapeutic dose of amphetamine during pre-adolescence modify the pattern of synaptic organization in the brain? *Eur. J. Neurosci.* 18, 3394–3399. doi: 10.1046/j.0953-816x.2003.03067.x

Hering, H., and Sheng, M. (2001). Dendritic spines: structure, dynamics and regulation. *Nat. Rev. Neurosci.* 2, 880–888. doi: 10.1038/35104061

Holtmaat, A., and Svoboda, K. (2009). Experience-dependent structural synaptic plasticity in the mammalian brain. *Nat. Rev. Neurosci.* 10, 64–758. doi: 10.1038/nrn2699

Honkura, N., Matsuzaki, M., Noguchi, J., Ellis-Davies, G. C., and Kasai, H. (2008). The subspine organization of actin fibers regulates the structure and plasticity of dendritic spines *Neuron* 57, 719–729. doi: 10.1016/j.neuron.2008.01.013

Huang, Y. H., Lin, Y., Mu, P., Lee, B. R., Brown, T. E., Wayman, G., et al. (2009). In vivo cocaine experience generates silent synapses. *Neuron* 1, 40–47. doi: 10.1016/j.neuron.2009.06.007

Huttenlocher, P. R. (1970). Dendritic development and mental defect. *Neurology* 20:381.

Hyman, S. E., Malenka, R. C., and Nestler, E. J. (2006). Neural mechanisms of addiction: the role of reward-related learning and memory. *Annu. Rev. Neurosci.* 29, 565–598. doi: 10.1146/annurev.neuro.29.051605.113009

Irwin, S. A., Galvez, R., and Greenough, W. T. (2000). Dendritic spine structural anomalies in fragile-X mental retardation syndrome. *Cereb. Cortex* 10, 1038–1044. doi: 10.1093/cercor/10.10.1038

Johnson, L. R., Aylward, R. L. M., Hussain, Z., and Totterdell, S. (1994). Input from the amygdala to the rat nucleus accumbens: its relationship with tyrosine hydroxylase immunoreactivity and identified neurons. *Neuroscience* 61, 851–865. doi: 10.1016/0306-4522(94)90408-1

Jones, S. (2011). "Dopamine—glutamate interactions in the basal ganglia," in *Frontiers in Neuroscience Series*, ed S. Jones (Switzerland: Taylor & Francis/CRC Press), 71–105.

Kalant, H. (1973). Relationship between psychological and physiological dependence and drug addiction. *Vie Med. Can. Fr.* 2, 766–774.

Kasai, H., Fukuda, M., Watanabe, S., Hayashi-Takagi, A., and Noguchi, J. (2010). Structural dynamics of dendritic spines in memory and cognition. *Trends Neurosci.* 33, 121–129. doi: 10.1016/j.tins.2010.01.001

Kasai, H., Matsuzaki, M., Noguchi, J., Yasumatsu, N., and Nakahara, H. (2003). Structure-stability-function relationships of dendritic spines. *Trends Neurosci.* 26, 360–368. doi: 10.1016/s0166-2236(03)00162-0

Kaufmann, W. E., and Moser, H. W. (2000). Dendritic anomalies in disorders associated with mental retardation. *Cereb. Cortex* 10, 981–991. doi: 10.1093/cercor/10.10.981

Kennedy, M. B., McGuinness, T., and Greengard, P. (1983). A calcium/calmodulin-dependent protein kinase from mammalian brain that phosphorylates synapsin I: partial purification and characterization. *J. Neurosci.* 3, 818–831.

Kharazia, V. N., and Weinberg, R. J. (1999). Immunogold localization of AMPA and NMDA receptors in somatic sensory cortex of albino rat. *J. Comp. Neurol.* 412, 292–302. doi: 10.1002/(sici)1096-9861(19990920)412:2<292::aid-cne8>3.0.co;2-g

Kim, Y., Teylan, M. A., Baron, M., Sands, A., Nairn, A. C., and Greengard, P. (2009). Methylphenidate-induced dendritic spine formation and DeltaFosB expression in nucleus accumbens. *Proc. Natl. Acad. Sci. U S A* 106, 2915–2920. doi: 10.1073/pnas.0813179106

Kirov, S. A., and Harris, K. M. (1999). Dendrites are more spiny on mature hippocampal neurons when synapses are inactivated. *Nat. Neurosci.* 2, 878–883. doi: 10.1038/13178

Kolb, B., Gorny, G., Li, Y., Samaha, A. N., and Robinson, T. E. (2003). Amphetamine or cocaine limits the ability of later experience to promote structural plasticity in the neocortex and nucleus accumbens. *Proc. Natl. Acad. Sci. U S A* 100, 10523–10528. doi: 10.1073/pnas.1834271100

Koob, G. F. (1992). Drugs of abuse: anatomy, pharmacology and function of reward pathways. *Trends Pharmacol. Sci.* 13, 177–184. doi: 10.1016/0165-6147(92)90060-j

Koob, G. F., and Volkow, N. D. (2010). Neurocircuitry of addiction. *Neuropsychopharmacology* 35, 217–238. doi: 10.1038/npp.2009.110

Kornau, H.-C., Schenker, L. T., Kennedy, M. B., and Seeburg, P. H. (1995). Domain interaction between NMDA receptor subunits and the postsynaptic density protein PSD-95. *Science* 269, 1737–1740. doi: 10.1126/science.7569905

Kosten, T. R., and George, T. P. (2002). The neurobiology of opioid dependence: implications for treatment. *Sci. Pract. Perspect.* 1, 13–20. doi: 10.1151/spp021113

Kunz, G., Englisch, H. J., and Wenzel, J. (1976). Spine-distribution of pyramidal neurons of the CAl-region of the rat hippocampus following long-term oral alcohol administration. *J. Hirnforsch.* 17, 351–363.

LeDoux, J. E. (2000). Emotion circuits in the brain. *Annu. Rev. Neurosci.* 23, 155–184. doi: 10.1146/annurev.neuro.23.1.155

Lee, K. W., Kim, Y., Kim, A. M., Helmin, K., Nairn, A. C., and Greengard, P. (2006). Cocaine-induced dendritic spine formation in D1 and D2 dopamine receptor-containing medium spiny neurons in nucleus accumbens. *Proc. Natl. Acad. Sci. U S A* 103, 3399–3404. doi: 10.1073/pnas.0511244103

Lewis, D. A., and Levitt, P. (2002). Schizophrenia as a disorder of neurodevelopment. *Annu. Rev. Neurosci.* 25, 409–432. doi: 10.1146/annurev.neuro.25.112701.142754

Li, Y., Kolb, B., and Robinson, T. E. (2003). The location of persistent amphetamine-induced changes in the density of dendritic spines on medium spiny neurons in the nucleus accumbens and caudate putamen. *Neuropsychopharmacology* 238, 1082–1085. doi: 10.1038/sj.npp.1300115

Matsuzaki, M., Honkura, N., Ellis-Davies, G. C., and Kasai, H. (2004). Structural basis of long-term potentiationin single dendritic spines. *Nature* 429, 761–766. doi: 10.1038/nature02617

Melis, M., Spiga, S., and Diana, M. (2005). The dopamine hypothesis of drug addiction: hypodopaminergic state. *Int. Rev. Neurobiol.* 63, 101–154. doi: 10.1016/s0074-7742(05)63005-x

Mello, N. K. (1972). "Behavioral studies of alcoholism," in *Biology of Alcoholism*, eds B. Kissin and H. Begleiter (New York: Plenum Press), 210–219.

Miller, E. C., Zhang, L., Dummer, B. W., Cariveau, D. R., Loh, H., Law, P. Y., et al. (2012). Differential modulation of drug-induced structural and functional plasticity of dendritic spines. *Mol. Pharmacol.* 82, 333–343. doi: 10.1124/mol.112.078162

Moon, I. S., Apperson, M. L., and Kennedy, M. B. (1994). The major tyrosine-phosphorylated protein in the postsynaptic density fraction is N-methyl-D-aspartate receptor subunit 2B. *Proc. Natl. Acad. Sci. U S A* 91, 3954–3958. doi: 10.1073/pnas.91.9.3954

Moss, J., and Bolam, J. P. (2008). A dopaminergic axon lattice in the striatum and its relationship with cortical and thalamic terminals. *J. Neurosci.* 28, 11221–11230. doi: 10.1523/JNEUROSCI.2780-08.2008

Nägerl, U. V., Eberhorn, N., Cambridge, S. B., and Bonhoeffer, T. (2004). Bidirectional activity-dependent morphological plasticity in hippocampal neurons. *Neuron* 44, 759–767. doi: 10.1016/j.neuron.2004.11.016

Nestler, E. J. (2001). Neurobiology. Total recall-the memory of addiction. *Science* 292, 2266–2267. doi: 10.1126/science.1063024

Nestler, E. J. (2013). Cellular basis of memory for addiction. *Dialogues Clin. Neurosci.* 4, 431–443.

Norrholm, S. D., Bibb, J. A., Nestler, E. J., Ouimet, C. C., Taylor, J. R., and Greengard, P. (2003). Cocaine-induced proliferation of dendritic spines in nucleus accumbens is dependent on the activity of cyclin-dependent kinase-5. *Neuroscience* 116, 19–22. doi: 10.1016/s0306-4522(02)00560-2

Nusser, Z., Lujan, R., Laube, G., Roberts, J. D., Molnar, E., and Somogyi, P. (1998). Cell type and pathway dependence of synaptic AMPA receptor number and variability in the hippocampus. *Neuron* 1, 545–559. doi: 10.1016/s0896-6273(00)80565-6

Okamoto, K., Nagai, T., Miyawaki, A., and Hayashi, Y. (2004). Rapid and persistent modulation of actin dynamics regulates postsynaptic reorganization underlying bidirectional plasticity. *Nat. Neurosci.* 7, 1104–1112. doi: 10.1038/nn1311

Ostlund, S. B., LeBlanc, K. H., Kosheleff, A. R., Wassum, K. M., and Maidment, N. T. (2014). Phasic mesolimbic dopamine signaling encodes the facilitation of incentive motivation produced by repeated cocaine exposure. *Neuropsychopharmacology* 39, 2441–2449. doi: 10.1038/npp.2014.96

Pascoli, V., Turiault, M., and Lüscher, C. (2011). Reversal of cocaine-evoked synaptic potentiation resets drug-induced adaptive behaviour. *Nature* 481, 71–75. doi: 10.1038/nature10709

Peters, A., and Kaiserman-Abramof, I. R. (1970). The small pyramidal neuron of the rat cerebral cortex. The perikaryon, dendrites and spines. *Am. J. Anat.* 127, 321–355. doi: 10.1002/aja.1001270402

Pissadaki, E. K., and Bolam, J. P. (2013). The energy cost of action potential propagation in dopamine neurons: clues to susceptibility in Parkinson's disease. *Front. Comput. Neurosci.* 7:13. doi: 10.3389/fncom.2013.00013

Ren, Z., Sun, W. L., Jiao, H., Zhang, D., Kong, H., Wang, X., et al. (2010). Dopamine D1 and N-methyl-d-aspartate receptors and extracellular signal-regulated kinase mediate neuronal morphological changes induced by repeated cocaine administration. *Neuroscience* 168, 48–60. doi: 10.1016/j.neuroscience.2010.03.034

Riley, J. N., and Halkar, D.-W. (1978). Morphological alterations in hippocampus after long-term alcohol consumption in mice. *Science* 210, 646–648. doi: 10.1126/science.566953

Robbins, T. W., Ersche, K. D., and Everitt, B. J. (2008). Drug addiction and the memory systems of the brain. *Ann. N Y Acad. Sci.* 1141, 1–21. doi: 10.1196/annals.1441.020

Robbins, T. W., and Everitt, B. J. (1996). Neurobehavioural mechanisms of reward and motivation. *Curr. Opin. Neurobiol.* 6, 228–236. doi: 10.1016/s0959-4388(96)80077-8

Robbins, T. W., and Everitt, B. J. (2002). Limbic-striatal memory systems and drug addiction. *Neurobiol. Learn. Mem.* 78, 625–636. doi: 10.1006/nlme.2002.4103

Roberts, R. C., Conley, R., Kung, L., Peretti, F. J., and Chute, D. J. (1996). Reduced striatal spine size in schizophrenia: a postmortem ultrastructural study. *Neuroreport* 7, 1214–1218. doi: 10.1097/00001756-199604260-00024

Robinson, T. E., Gorny, G., Mitton, E., and Kolb, B. (2001). Cocaine self-administration alters the morphology of dendrites and dendritic spines in the nucleus accumbens and neocortex. *Synapse* 39, 257–266. doi: 10.1002/1098-2396(20010301)39:3<257::aid-syn1007>3.3.co;2-t

Robinson, T. E., Gorny, G., Savage, V. R., and Kolb, B. (2002). Widespread but regionally specific effects of experimenter- versus self-administered morphine on dendritic spines in the nucleus accumbens, hippocampus and neocortex of adult rats. *Synapse* 46, 271–279. doi: 10.1002/syn.10146

Robinson, T. E., and Kolb, B. (1997). Persistent structural modifications in nucleus accumbens and prefrontal cortex neurons produced by previous experience with amphetamine. *J. Neurosci.* 17, 8491–8497.

Robinson, T. E., and Kolb, B. (1999a). Alterations in the morphology of dendrites and dendritic spines in the nucleus accumbens and prefrontal cortex following repeated treatment with amphetamine or cocaine. *Eur. J. Neurosci.* 11, 1598–1604. doi: 10.1046/j.1460-9568.1999.00576.x

Robinson, T. E., and Kolb, B. (1999b). Morphine alters the structure of neurons in the nucleus accumbens and neocortex of rats. *Synapse* 33, 160–162. doi: 10.1002/(sici)1098-2396(199908)33:2<160::aid-syn6>3.3.co;2-j

Robinson, T. E., and Kolb, B. (2004). Structural plasticity associated with exposure to drugs of abuse. *Neuropharmacology* 47, 33–46. doi: 10.1016/j.neuropharm.2004.06.025

Russo, S. J., Dietz, D. M., Dumitriu, D., Morrison, J. H., Malenka, R. C., and Nestler, E. J. (2010). The addicted synapse: mechanisms of synaptic and structural plasticity in nucleus accumbens. *Trends Neurosci.* 33, 267–276. doi: 10.1016/j.tins.2010.02.002

Schintu, N., Frau, L., Ibba, M., Garau, A., Carboni, E., and Carta, A. R. (2009). Progressive dopaminergic degeneration in the chronic MPTPp mouse model of Parkinson's disease. *Neurotox. Res.* 16, 127–139. doi: 10.1007/s12640-009-9061-x

Segal, M. (2010). Dendritic spines, synaptic plasticity and neuronal survival: activity shapes dendritic spines toenhance neuronal viability. *Eur. J. Neurosci.* 31, 2178–2184. doi: 10.1111/j.1460-9568.2010.07270.x

Sesack, S. R., and Pickel, V. M. (1992). Prefrontal cortical efferents in the rat synapse on unlabeled neuronal targets of catecholamine terminals in the nucleus accumbens septi and on dopamine neurons in the ventral tegmental area. *J. Comp. Neurol.* 320, 145–160. doi: 10.1002/cne.903200202

Shen, H. W., Toda, S., Moussawi, K., Bouknight, A., Zahm, D. S., and Kalivas, P. W. (2009). Altered dendritic spine plasticity in cocaine-withdrawn rats. *J. Neurosci.* 29, 2876–2884. doi: 10.1523/JNEUROSCI.5638-08.2009

Smith, Y., Bennett, B. D., Bolam, J. P., Parent, A., and Sadikot, A. F. (1994). Synaptic relationships between dopaminergic afferents and cortical or thalamic input in the sensorimotor territory of the striatum in monkey. *J. Comp. Neurol.* 344, 1–19. doi: 10.1002/cne.903440102

Sorra, K. E., and Harris, K. M. (2000). Overview on the structure, composition, function, development and plasticity of hippocampal dendritic spines. *Hippocampus* 10, 501–511. doi: 10.1002/1098-1063(2000)10:5<501::aid-hipo1>3.3.co;2-k

Spiga, S., Acquas, E., Puddu, M. C., Mulas, G., Lintas, A., Diana, M., et al. (2011). Simultaneous Golgi-Cox and immunofluorescence using confocal microscopy. *Brain Struct. Funct.* 216, 171–182. doi: 10.1007/s00429-011-0312-2

Spiga, S., Lintas, A., Migliore, M., and Diana, M. (2010). Altered architecture and functional consequences of the mesolimbic dopamine system in cannabis dependence. *Addict. Biol.* 15, 266–276. doi: 10.1111/j.1369-1600.2010.00218.x

Spiga, S., Puddu, M. C., Pisano, M., and Diana, M. (2005). Morphine withdrawal-induced morphological changes in the nucleus accumbens. *Eur. J. Neurosci.* 22, 2332–2340. doi: 10.1111/j.1460-9568.2005.04416.x

Spiga, S., Talani, G., Mulas, G., Licheri, V., Fois, G. R., Muggironi, G., et al. (2014). Hampered LTD formation and thin spine loss in the nucleus accumbens of ethanol dependent rats. *Proc. Natl. Acad. Sci. U S A* 111, E3745–E3754. doi: 10.1073/pnas.1406768111

Steward, O., and Levy, W. B. (1982). Preferential localization of polyribosomes under the base of dendritic spines in granule cells of the dentate gyrus. *J. Neurosci.* 2, 284–291.

Svoboda, K., Tank, D. W., and Denk, W. (1996). Direct measurement of coupling between dendritic spines and shafts. *Science* 272, 716–719. doi: 10.1126/science.272.5262.716

Totterdell, S., and Smith, A. S. (1989). Convergence of hippocampal and DA-ergic input onto identified neurons in the nucleus accumbens of the rat. *J. Chem. Neuroanat.* 2, 285–298.

Trachtenberg, J. T., Chen, B. E., Knott, G. W., Feng, G., Sanes, J. R., Welker, E., et al. (2002). Long-term in vivo imaging of experience-dependent synaptic plasticity in adult cortex. *Nature* 420, 788–794. doi: 10.1038/nature01273

Villalba, R. M., Lee, H., and Smith, Y. (2009). Dopaminergic denervation and spine loss in the striatum of MPTP-treated monkeys. *Exp. Neurol.* 215, 220–227. doi: 10.1016/j.expneurol.2008.09.025

Wilson, C. J., Groves, P. M., Kitai, S. T., and Linder, J. C. (1983). Three-dimensional structure of dendritic spines in the rat neostriatum. *J. Neurosci.* 3, 383–398.

Wise, R. (2006). Role of brain dopamine in food reward and reinforcement. *Philos. Trans. R. Soc. Lond. B Biol. Sci.* 361, 1149–1158. doi: 10.1098/rstb.2006.1854

Yamauchi, T. (2002). Molecular constituents and phosphorylation dependent regulation of the post-synaptic density. *Mass Spectrom. Rev.* 21, 266–286. doi: 10.1002/mas.10033

Yao, W. D., Spealman, R. D., and Zhang, J. (2008). Dopaminergic signaling in dendritic spines. *Biochem. Pharmacol.* 75, 2055–2069. doi: 10.1016/j.bcp.2008.01.018

Yasumatsu, N., Matsuzaki, M., Miyazaki, T., Noguchi, J., and Kasai, H. (2008). Principles of long-term dynamics of dendritic spines. *J. Neurosci.* 28, 13592–13608. doi: 10.1523/JNEUROSCI.0603-08.2008

Zhang, J., Vinuela, A., Neely, M. H., Hallett, P. J., Grant, S. G., Miller, G. M., et al. (2007). Inhibition of the dopamine D1 receptor signaling by PSD-95. *J. Biol. Chem.* 282, 15778–15789. doi: 10.1074/jbc.m611485200

Zhou, F. C., Anthony, B., Dunn, K. W., Lindquist, W. B., Xu, Z. C., and Deng, P. (2007). Chronic alcohol drinking alters neuronal dendritic spines in the brain reward center nucleus accumbens. *Brain Res.* 1134, 148–161. doi: 10.1016/j.brainres.2006.11.046

Zhou, F. M., Wilson, C. J., and Dani, J. A. (2002). Cholinergic interneuron characteristics and nicotinic properties in the striatum. *J. Neurobiol.* 53, 590–605. doi: 10.1002/neu.10150

Zhou, F. M., Wilson, C. J., and Dani, J. A. (2003). Muscarinic and nicotinic cholinergic mechanisms in the mesostriatal dopamine systems. *Neuroscientist* 9, 23–36. doi: 10.1177/1073858402239588

Ziv, N. E., and Smith, S. J. (1996). Evidence for a role of dendritic filopodia in synaptogenesis and spine formation. *Neuron* 17, 91–102. doi: 10.1016/s0896-6273(00)80283-4

5

Lipid dynamics at dendritic spines

Carlos Gerardo Dotti *, Jose Antonio Esteban and María Dolores Ledesma *

Centro Biología Molecular Severo Ochoa, CSIC-UAM, Madrid, Spain

Correspondence:
Carlos Gerardo Dotti and María Dolores Ledesma, Centro Biología Molecular Severo Ochoa, CSIC-UAM, Nicolás Cabrera 1, Madrid 28049, Spain
e-mail: cdotti@cbm.csic.es; dledesma@cbm.csic.es

Dynamic changes in the structure and composition of the membrane protrusions forming dendritic spines underlie memory and learning processes. In recent years a great effort has been made to characterize in detail the protein machinery that controls spine plasticity. However, we know much less about the involvement of lipids, despite being major membrane components and structure determinants. Moreover, protein complexes that regulate spine plasticity depend on specific interactions with membrane lipids for proper function and accurate intracellular signaling. In this review we gather information available on the lipid composition at dendritic spine membranes and on its dynamics. We pay particular attention to the influence that spine lipid dynamism has on glutamate receptors, which are key regulators of synaptic plasticity.

Keywords: dendritic spines, cholesterol, sphingolipids, phosphoinositides, glutamate receptors, synaptic plasticity

INTRODUCTION

At most excitatory synapses in the Central Nervous System, presynaptic boutons synapse onto small membrane protrusions that emerge from the dendritic shaft: the dendritic spines. Changes in dendritic spine number, size and shape contribute to determine the strength of excitatory synaptic transmission (Yuste and Bonhoeffer, 2001; Carlisle and Kennedy, 2005). The remodeling of these membrane protrusions in response to stimuli depends on lipids, which are major components of the membrane with the ability to shape it and modify protein activities within. However, only recently the contribution of spine lipids has attracted similar attention to that of spine proteins. Pioneer work showing the requirement of glial cholesterol for synapse formation (Mauch et al., 2001) and the elimination of spines upon reduction of cholesterol or sphingolipids (Hering et al., 2003) triggered research in this field. Technical progress facilitates today the not so long ago impossible analysis of the subtle changes in lipid composition and of the topographical distribution of individual lipid species in cellular compartments. Probes have been developed to label lipid molecules such as new generation fluorescent tags (Eggeling et al., 2009) or modified toxins with specific lipid binding abilities such as the theta-toxin or lysenin, which bind cholesterol or sphingomyelin, respectively (Abe et al., 2012). These probes together with advanced microscopy techniques that achieve sub-diffraction optical resolution (i.e., near-field scanning optical microscopy (NSOM), photoactivated localization microscopy (PALM) stochastic optical reconstruction microscopy (STORM) or stimulated depletion (STED) fluorescent microscopy) allow the direct observation of the nanoscale dynamics of membrane lipids in a living cell (Eggeling et al., 2009; van Zanten et al., 2010; Castro et al., 2013). As we gain insight on how lipids and their metabolic enzymes regulate dendritic spine shape and protein function their importance is confirmed and strengthened. We aim here to review this knowledge focusing the attention on the dynamic lipidomics of dendritic spines. We will also discuss about how this influences synaptic plasticity through the modulation of glutamate receptors of the AMPA and NMDA-type (AMPARc and NMDARc). These receptors are instrumental to elicit Long Term Potentiation (LTP) and Long Term Depression (LTD), which are considered the molecular mechanisms underlying learning and memory (Neves et al., 2008; Collingridge et al., 2010).

LIPID COMPOSITION AT DENDRITIC SPINES

A relevant question about spine physiology is whether spine membrane lipid composition and organization is different to that of the dendritic shaft membranes from which these protrusions emerge. A systematic analysis of spine lipid composition is lacking due to technical limitations. However, accumulating evidence indicates it differs from that of the shaft. This raises questions such as why this specificity is necessary and how it is achieved, maintained or modulated upon stimuli. Until now, most of the information on synaptic lipid composition comes from the biochemical analysis of synaptosomal preparations. Functional studies have also highlighted the relevant contribution of certain lipids to spine physiology. From these two types of approaches we now know that cholesterol and sphingolipids are enriched in spines. Because of their chemical affinity these lipids form highly dynamic and heterogeneous membrane nanodomains, the so called rafts, which can be stabilized to form larger platforms by protein-protein or protein-lipid interactions (Pike, 2006). Rafts compartmentalize cellular processes contributing to the accurate spatial and temporal organization of molecules required at dendritic spines (Allen et al., 2007).

Neurotrophin and neurotransmitter receptors (NTRcs) are recruited from extrasynaptic to synaptic sites through association to lipid rafts, which reduce receptor lateral mobility at the synaptic space (Nagappan and Lu, 2005; Fernandes et al., 2010). In fact, the post synapse has been proposed as a lipid raft-enriched territory and certain key structural proteins such as the postsynaptic density protein 95 (PSD95) as well as AMPARc dynamically associate to these domains (Perez and Bredt, 1998; Suzuki, 2002; Hering et al., 2003; Suzuki et al., 2011). The tight control of the turnover of phosphoinositides and their derivatives plays also a central role in spine plasticity. We next describe data available on the presence of the aforementioned lipids in spines and on their contribution to spine physiology. Hopefully, the already mentioned imaging techniques based on advanced lipid probes and super-resolution microscopy together with most sensitive quantitative measurements (i.e., liquid chromatography coupled with tandem mass spectrometry) would contribute to more precisely define the lipid composition of spines and its changes in real time in living cells.

CHOLESTEROL

Pharmacological extraction of cholesterol or inhibition of its synthesis led to the disappearance of dendritic spines in cultured hippocampal neurons, probably mediated by disruption of the actin cytoskeleton (Hering et al., 2003). This finding defined cholesterol as a core component of spines. A series of functional reports have demonstrated the relevance of this lipid for synaptic plasticity. Pioneer work showed that acute cyclodextrin-mediated removal of membrane cholesterol blocks LTP in the hippocampus (Koudinov and Koudinova, 2001; Frank et al., 2008). On the other hand, excitatory neurotransmission, chronic and acute, induces cholesterol loss from synapses, which is recovered after stimuli (Sodero et al., 2011, 2012). In the aging brain, lifelong lasting synaptic activity and concomitant metabolic stress contributes to a moderate but irreversible loss of membrane cholesterol (Sodero et al., 2011), which is thought to underlie cognitive deficits present at this stage of life (Martin et al., 2014). In agreement, cholesterol replenishment restores LTD in hippocampal slices from aged mice and improves their learning and memory abilities (Martin et al., 2014). The molecular mechanisms by which cholesterol influences postsynaptic plasticity are just beginning to be understood. Thus, impaired LTD in the old produced as consequence of lower membrane cholesterol can be explained, to a certain extent, by sustained activity of the PI3K/Akt pathway, in turn leading to inactivation of GSK3β and reduced AMPAR internalization (Martin et al., 2014). The broad effect of cholesterol on the biophysical properties of the membrane bilayer (i.e., viscosity, Renner et al., 2009) may affect the molecular flow in and out of synapses and therefore the mobility and interactions of NTRc (Fantini and Barrantes, 2009). Changes in the amount of cholesterol at spines might also exert functional effects through cholesterol metabolites. Thus, the most abundant in the brain, 24(S)-hydroxycholesterol, is a potent and selective positive modulator of NMDARc and enhances LTP (Paul et al., 2013).

SPHINGOLIPIDS

Long term stability and dynamic changes in dendritic spines are intimately linked to the actin cytoskeleton, which is particularly enriched in these structures (Hotulainen and Hoogenraad, 2010; Koleske, 2013). Changes in the amount of filamentous actin (F-actin) mediate long-lasting alterations in spine size and synaptic efficacy. The repetitive firing of synapses that occurs during high-frequency stimulation to induce LTP, promotes actin polymerization and spine enlargement (Matsuzaki et al., 2004; Okamoto et al., 2004). Conversely, treatment that weakens synaptic efficacy, such as low-frequency stimulation that results in LTD, causes F-actin loss and dendritic spine shrinkage (Okamoto et al., 2004; Zhou et al., 2004). Enlargement and shrinkage of the spine requires the coordination of the actin cytoskeleton with the membrane. Recent work shows that the most abundant sphingolipid in neuronal membranes, sphingomyelin (SM), plays a relevant role in the spine membrane-cytoskeleton crosstalk by modulating membrane binding and activity of main regulators of the actin cytoskeleton at synapses: the Rho GTPases. Hence, high SM levels lower the amount of type I metabotropic glutamate receptors (mGluRs) at the cell surface impairing membrane attachment, and therefore activity, of the small GTPase RhoA concomitantly with the inhibition of its effectors ROCK and Profilin IIa. This seems to be the mechanism leading to reduced F-actin content and smaller size of spines in mice lacking the acid sphingomyelinase (ASM) gene (Arroyo et al., 2014). Conversely, low SM levels in postsynaptic membranes are responsible for the enhanced activity of the RhoA-ROCK-Profilin I pathway resulting in increased actin polymerization and dendritic spine size in mice lacking the actin related protein WIP (Franco-Villanueva et al., 2014). Moreover, the dynamic partitioning of RhoA into raft membrane domains, which is enhanced upon stimuli, is dependent on the maintenance of appropriate SM levels at the synaptic membrane (Franco-Villanueva et al., 2014).

Ceramide is another major sphingolipid contributing to spine plasticity by virtue of its capacity to favor membrane fusogenicity promoting receptor clustering (Krönke, 1999). The rapid generation of ceramide modulates excitatory postsynaptic currents by controlling the insertion and clustering of NMDARc (Wheeler et al., 2009). In agreement, direct additions of synthetic cell-permeable ceramide analogs increase excitatory postsynaptic currents without affecting presynaptic plasticity (Coogan et al., 1999; Fasano et al., 2003). The ceramide-associated enhancement of excitatory currents is often transient and is followed by sustained depression of excitatory postsynaptic currents (Coogan et al., 1999; Yang, 2000; Davis et al., 2006). These findings support complex roles for the spatial and temporal production of ceramide in regulating neuronal excitability. In addition, ceramide contributes to spine maturation by promoting the transformation of dendritic fillopodia into mature spines (Carrasco et al., 2012).

PHOSPHOINOSITIDES AND DERIVATIVES

Despite phosphoinositides (PIPs) are minor components of synaptic membranes, their exceptional high rate of metabolic turnover and their compartmentalization make them key players in postsynaptic excitability (Hammond and Schiavo, 2007). The presence at dendritic spines of the enzymes that interconvert different PIPs supports a relevant role for these lipids in the dynamics of these structures.

Continuous synthesis and availability of phosphatidylinositol(3,4,5) triphosphate (PIP3) at the postsynaptic terminal is necessary for sustaining synaptic function in rat hippocampal neurons (Arendt et al., 2010). PIP3 shows greater accumulation in spines than in dendritic shafts under basal conditions. Interestingly, glutamate stimulation promotes spine enlargement and the appearance of filopodia-like protrusions (spinules) projecting from spines (Richards et al., 2005) to which PIP3 redistributes (Ueda and Hayashi, 2013). Consistent with a key role for PIP3 in spinule formation, blockage or inhibition of this lipid prevent their appearance (Ueda and Hayashi, 2013). The biological significance of spinules is not yet established. However, trans-endocytosis of these protrusions by presynaptic buttons may aid postsynaptic membrane remodeling by removing the excess membrane at postsynaptic sites (Spacek and Harris, 2004). It was also proposed that PIP3 signaling at spinules enables new synapses to form with functional presynaptic boutons contributing to the change in synaptic connectivity. PIP3 could also mediate membrane-cytoskeleton crosstalk at spines by virtue of its capacity to regulate the activity of multiple Rho GTPase effectors (Yin and Janmey, 2003). Additionally, PIP3 is the upstream regulator of the Akt-mTOR pathway, which signals activity-dependent regulation of protein synthesis (Kelleher et al., 2004) and participates in dendritic and spine morphogenesis (Kumar et al., 2005).

Appropriate levels and clustering of phosphatidylinositol(4,5) diphosphate (PIP2) at the postsynaptic membrane, which are modulated by the activities of Phospholipase γ (PLCγ) and PIP5K, are important for synaptic plasticity, both LTP (Trovò et al., 2013) and LTD (Unoki et al., 2012). The PIP2-clustering molecule myristoylated alanine-rich C kinase substrate (MARCKS) critically contributes to this requirement. The effector domain of MARCKS reversibly sequesters PIP2 on the plasma membrane, which can be released in response to local increases in intracellular calcium (McLaughlin and Murray, 2005). Low levels of this protein, leading to PIP2 paucity at the membrane, promote the age-related impairment of synaptic plasticity (**Figure 1**). Hence, its overexpression in the hippocampus of old mice or intraventricular perfusion of MARCKS peptide result in enhanced LTP and improved memory (Trovò et al., 2013). On the other hand, MARCKs appears to be a key molecule in spine morphogenesis promoting the transition from thin immature dendritic spines to larger, more stable mushroom by controlling actin cytoskeleton (Calabrese and Halpain, 2005). In agreement, MARCKs deficient mice show impaired LTP and spatial cognition (McNamara et al., 1998; Hussain et al., 2006). Association of MARCKS to the membrane is necessary for its ability to crosslink F-actin (Calabrese and Halpain, 2005). Membrane levels of cholesterol, to which MARCKs can bind, would mediate this association. Evidence suggests that indeed defective MARCKs-induced PIP2 clustering in old synaptic membranes responds to the reduction of cholesterol levels during aging (Trovò et al., 2013; Martin et al., 2014; **Figure 1**).

Besides PIPs themselves, PIP derived second messengers such as Diacylglycerol (DAG) and 1,4,5-triphosphate (IP3) generated by the hydrolysis of PIP2 by PLC, are also important in dendritic spine organization and function. Unlike IP3, which is released into the spine cytoplasm, DAG is embedded in the membrane and recruits and activates DAG effectors (among them PKC), which have been involved in spine maintenance (Brose et al., 2004). DAG molecules are produced in dendritic spines through activation of postsynaptic receptors, including those of the NMDA type. It has been proposed that the rapid and focal generation of DAG, together with ceramide, triggers the fusion of vesicles and insertion of NMDARc subunits into lipid rafts. Based on the biophysical properties of DAG, it is likely that the generation of this lipid serves to destabilize the membranes to create fusion points at the postsynapse (Wheeler et al., 2009). In turn, phosphatidic acid (PA) that is generated by DAG phosphorylation, also regulates spines together with its effectors. Among them, the alpha-p-21-activated kinase PAK1 promotes spine formation by stabilizing actin filaments through myosin phosphorylation (Zhang et al., 2005).

DYNAMISM OF THE LIPID COMPOSITION AT DENDRITIC SPINES: THE ROLE OF LIPID METABOLIC ENZYMES

The aforementioned evidences highlight not only the wealth and specificity of the lipid composition at spines but also its dynamism and panoply of biological roles. The question remains on how this lipid composition is achieved and maintained, or changed, in different physiological situations. While still being an open question, local recruitment and removal of the different metabolic enzymes is a reasonable possibility. In fact, a number of these enzymes have been localized in dendritic spines, change their activity upon synaptic stimuli and/or have the ability to modulate NTRc trafficking and function. While the recruitment of certain enzymes occurs in response to stimuli others are constitutively present at postsynapses. In the following section we describe examples of the contribution of lipid metabolic enzymes to spine physiology.

CHOLESTEROL 24-HYDROXYLASE

The cytochrome P450 enzyme, cholesterol 24-hydroxylase (Cyp46A1) is selectively expressed in the brain, where it is responsible for cholesterol oxidation and eventual excretion to the general circulation (Lund et al., 1999). Pyramidal neurons of the hippocampus and cortex, Purkinje cells of the cerebellum, and hippocampal and cerebellar interneurons show particularly high levels of this enzyme, which is preferentially localized in the endoplasmic reticulum (ER) of dendrites and cell bodies (Ramirez et al., 2008). Cyp46A1 contribution to synaptic plasticity is supported by the observations that mice lacking this enzyme present impaired learning and hippocampal LTP (Kotti et al., 2006) while mice overexpressing human Cyp46A1 present improved spatial memory (Maioli et al., 2013). Increased levels of Cyp46A1 parallel the mild but significant cholesterol reduction in membranes of the hippocampus of old rodents and of hippocampal neurons aged in culture (Martin et al., 2008; Sodero et al., 2011). In turn, knockdown of the enzyme prevents glutamate-mediated cholesterol loss (Sodero et al., 2012), supporting a cause-effect relationship between cholesterol reduction in the aged and Cyp46A1 increased activity. Biotinylation, electron microscopy and TIRF analysis indicated that Cyp46A1 is present in spines of hippocampal neurons and that, upon stimulation, a close approximation occurs between the site of residence of

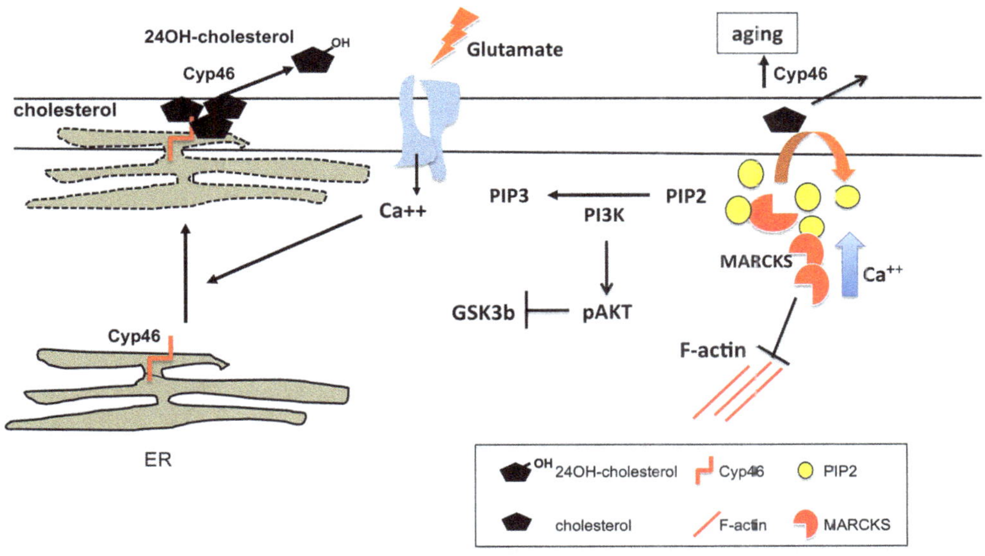

FIGURE 1 | Cholesterol regulation at spines upon glutamate stimulation. Acute glutamate stimulatory conditions lead to loss of membrane cholesterol. The mechanism proposed involves glutamate induced rise in intracellular Ca++ leading to the approximation/apposition of ER membranes to the synaptic plasma membrane. This allows Cyp46A1, whose active site is in the lumenal side of the ER, to oxidize cholesterol present in the exoplasmic leaflet that is released as hydroxycholesterol. In the aging context, constitutive high intracellular calcium and irreversible cholesterol loss due to lifelong lasting synaptic activity leads to reduced membrane-associated MARCKS, which affects synaptic plasticity by several mechanisms: (1) impaired MARCKS-mediated actin dynamics; (2) reduced membrane clustering of PIP2; and (3) high PI3K activity resulting in reduced glutamate-mediated Akt dephosphorylation and GSK3β activation. The later contributes to the impaired AMPARc internalization and LTD in aged neurons.

the enzyme (the ER) and the plasma membrane, suggesting that this could be the mechanism by which cholesterol is removed from the plasma membrane (Sodero et al., 2012). The increase in surface Cyp46A1 after stimulation supports this notion, and the higher production of its metabolite 24S-hydroxycholesterol in stimulated neurons indicates that the pool of the enzyme that increase at the plasma membrane is active. Not surprisingly for an ER-resident protein, the process of Cyp46A1 mediated cholesterol loss requires high levels of intracellular Ca^{2+} and a functional ER-plasma membrane communication via the stromal interaction molecule 2 (STIM2; Sodero et al., 2012). It has been proposed that high levels of Ca^{2+} elicit such communication bypassing the Golgi apparatus. This process would be consistent with the observation that the distance between the ER and the plasma membrane can be as small as 10 nm (Pichler et al., 2001; Lebiedzinska et al., 2009) and that NMDARc stimulation produces a transient and reversible fission of ER tubules (Kucharz et al., 2009). This mechanism provides an efficient, temporally and spatially controlled, mean to change postsynaptic membrane lipid composition (**Figure 1**). Whether lipid metabolic enzymes other than Cyp46A1 follow the same mechanism is unknown.

NEUTRAL SPHINGOMYELINASE-2

Among the sphingolipid metabolic enzymes the Neutral sphingomeylinase-2 (NSM) has been directly related to spine size and to postsynaptic function. NSM is the main responsible of SM degradation and conversion to ceramide at the plasma membrane (Stoffel, 1999). Its rapid kinetics and location enriched in hippocampus made it a likely candidate to modulate plasticity (Hofmann et al., 2000). In support, abundant NSM has been found in synaptic membranes (Arroyo et al., 2014). The rapid generation of ceramide by NSM modulates excitatory postsynaptic currents by controlling the insertion and clustering of NMDARc (Wheeler et al., 2009). In addition recent work shows the ability of this enzyme to modulate spine actin cytoskeleton. Hence, activation of NSM corrects the abnormally low size and F-actin content of dendritic spines in mice lacking the acid sphingomyelinase, which present high SM synaptic levels, by enhancing the RhoA pathway (Arroyo et al., 2014). Conversely, NSM inhibition restores normal RhoA activity and diminishes the abnormally increased size and F-actin levels of spines in neurons of mice lacking WIP (Franco-Villanueva et al., 2014; **Figure 2**). This actin-related protein has the ability to sense the levels of F-actin to which it can bind. It has been proposed that WIP modulates SM amount at the spine membrane by RhoA mediated transcriptional control of the NSM, thus controlling the spine response to actin polymerization stimuli (Franco-Villanueva et al., 2014). This places NSM at a key position to mediate membrane-cytoskeleton crosstalk at spines. It remains to be determined whether the enzyme levels and activity could be modulated at synapses by a local transcriptional control mechanism. The observation that activation of NSM with dexamethasone corrects actin related anomalies in isolated synaptosomes argues in favor of this possibility (Arroyo et al., 2014). If true, the question arises on whether, similar to those of many actin related proteins, mRNAs of lipid metabolic enzymes are present at synapses to facilitate the immediate spine

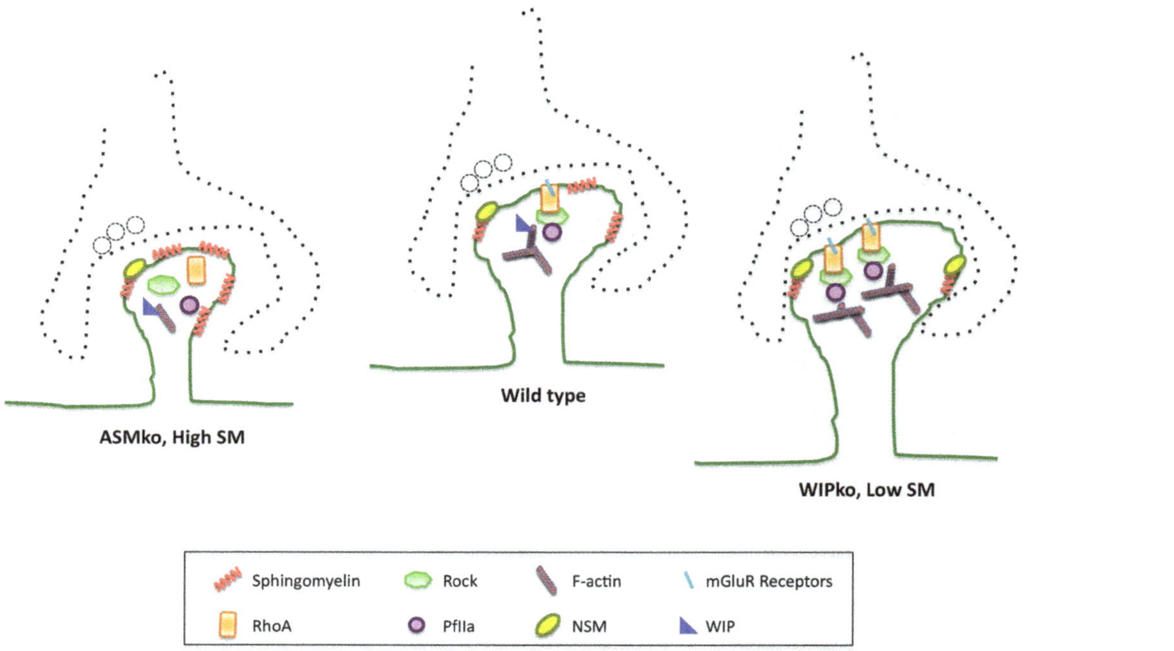

FIGURE 2 | SM and its catabolic enzymes in dendritic spine physiology and pathology. SM levels at the postsynaptic membrane modulate membrane binding and activation of the small GTPase RhoA, which in turn modulates F-actin content through its effectors ROCK and profillin 2A. This molecular mechanism controls dendritic spine size. The SM catabolic enzymes ASM and NSM are involved in this process. Hence, mice lacking ASM show abnormally high SM levels in their postsynaptic membranes that lower the amount of cell surface mGluRs. This impairs RhoA membrane binding and pathway activation, which diminish spine F-actin content and size. These anomalies can be corrected by NSM activation. Conversely, mice lacking the actin related protein WIP show constitutively active NSM leading to reduced SM levels, which enhance RhoA membrane binding and pathway activation resulting in bigger dendritic spines with higher F-actin content. Spine anomalies could explain the cognitive deficits observed in ASMko mice, which are a model for Niemann Pick disease type A, and those of individuals carrying mutations in the region encoding for WIP.

remodeling in response to stimuli. Alternatively, NSM would translocate to the synaptic plasma membrane upon stimulation. This is supported by evidences in non-neuronal cells showing that a stress-mediated PKC mechanism induces the appearance of the enzyme at the plasma membrane (Clarke et al., 2008). The possibility that not only NSM but also its analog enzyme, ASM, regulates SM levels at the postsynaptic membrane is not yet clarified. The presence of ASM in spines has not been reported. However, the observations that lack of this enzyme leads to reduced spine size and F-actin content (Arroyo et al., 2014) and that it can function at neutral pH (Schissel et al., 1998) or in acidified microenvironments that may exist at the cell surface (Bourguignon et al., 2004), support the regulated action of the two sphingomyelinases to control spine SM levels and actin cytoskeleton (**Figure 2**).

CARNITINE PALMITOYLTRANSFERASE 1C (CPT1C)

The brain specific isoform of Carnitine Palmitoyltransferase 1 (CPT1C), modulates ceramide levels in hippocampal neurons where it is especially enriched (Carrasco et al., 2012). CPT1C is located in the ER and has been recently found inside dendritic spines. The mechanism by which this enzyme, which facilitates fatty acid transport across intracellular membranes (Wolfgang et al., 2006), modulates ceramide levels is still unknown. Activation of *de novo* synthesis of the lipid has been discarded. Instead, CPT1C may influence the generation of ceramide from the sphingosine pool through the salvage pathway and/or on its degradation. CPT1C deficiency increases immature filopodia and reduces mature mushroom and stubby spines, while not affecting total spine number or spine head area. These effects on spine maturation can be restored by ceramide addition (Carrasco et al., 2012). Consistent with the role of CPT1C on the transformation of dendritic filopodia into mature spines, mice lacking this enzyme show defects in hippocampus dependent learning abilities (Carrasco et al., 2012).

PHOSPHOINOSITIDE METABOLIC ENZYMES

Several enzymes tightly control PIP turnover at dendritic spines (**Figure 3**). Biochemical and imaging experiments demonstrated that the phosphatase and tensin homolog deleted on chromosome ten (PTEN), which converts PIP3 into PIP2 (Maehama and Dixon, 1999), is recruited to dendritic spines upon NMDARc but not AMPARc activation (Jurado et al., 2010). NMDARc activation triggers a biphasic regulation of PTEN mobility in dendritic spines. First, there is a rapid and transient increase in mobility independent from PTEN interactions through its PDZ motif. A longer-lasting and PDZ-dependent anchoring of PTEN to the postsynaptic density follows this phase. This regulated mechanism of recruitment of PTEN may provide means to achieve synapse-specific modulation of PIP3 signaling during

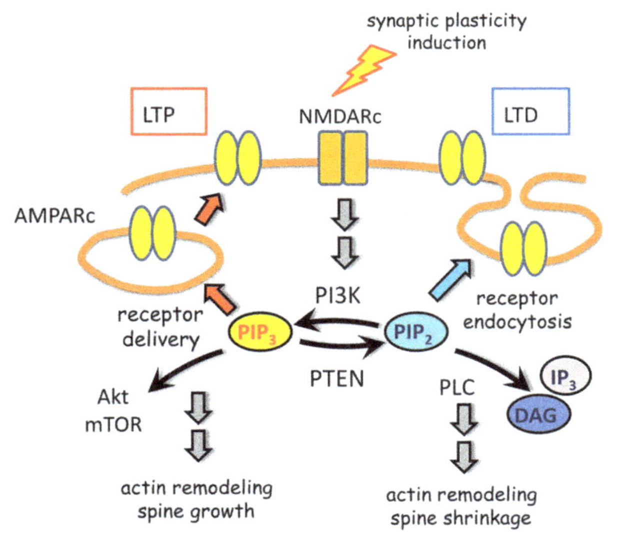

FIGURE 3 | PIP metabolism in spine plasticity. Activation of NMDARc modulate AMPARc trafficking through spatially and timely controlled activity of PIPs and their metabolic enzymes. On one hand, PI3K association with AMPARc is required for receptor cell surface delivery during LTP. On the other hand, PTEN activity leading to PIP3 downregulation promotes migration of AMPARc from the postsynaptic density to the perisynaptic membrane. This depresses AMPARc synaptic responses by promoting receptor endocytosis during LTD. Moreover, signaling pathways initiated by PIP3 or PIP2, in which Akt/mTOR, DAG and IP3 are involved, contribute to actin remodeling and spine changes in size.

plasticity. The enhancement of PTEN lipid phosphatase activity is able to drive depression of AMPARc-mediated synaptic responses (Jurado et al., 2010). Consistently, mice with altered PTEN expression show multiple impairments in synaptic function including LTP and LTD (Wang et al., 2006; Fraser et al., 2008).

The class I phosphatydilinsositol-3-kinase (PI3K) constitutively localizes at synapses by means of a direct interaction between its p85 subunit and the AMPARc (Man et al., 2003). By converting PIP2 into PIP3 this kinase ensures the delivery of new AMPARc into spines in response to NMDARc activation (Man et al., 2003) and the maintenance of AMPARc clustering at the postsynaptic membrane (Arendt et al., 2010; **Figure 3**).

The major PIP2 producing enzyme in the brain, the phosphatidylinositol-4-phosphate 5-kinaseγ661 (PIP5Kγ661), becomes dephosphorylated and associates with the clathrin adaptor protein complex AP-2 at postsynapses upon NMDA receptor activation (Unoki et al., 2012). This event is necessary to elicit AMPARc endocytosis and LTD. PLC, which catalyzes hydrolysis of PIP2, is enriched in spine heads and primarily localized in a thin border around the postsynaptic density (Yoshida et al., 2006). PLC activity is enhanced by NMDARc stimulation and its blockage impairs LTD (Reyes-Harde and Stanton, 1998). This activity is required for changes in postsynaptic structure by depolymerizing spine actin and decreasing PSD95 levels. This in turn promotes AMPARc internalization during LTD (Horne and Dell'Acqua, 2007). PLC has been also related to the termination of synaptic stimuli. It has been proposed that lipid signals (i.e., 2-arachidonoylglycerol) generated at dendritic spines by PLC activity, upon activation of type I metabotropic glutamate receptors (mGluRs), diffuse across the synaptic cleft and activate cannabinoid receptors, reducing presynaptic Ca^{2+} channel activity and inhibiting further glutamate release (Chevaleyre et al., 2006).

DAG KINASES

Evidence accumulates in support of the notion that DAG-metabolizing enzymes DAG kinases (DGK), which are coupled to synaptic scaffolding proteins, tightly control synaptic DAG concentrations (Kim et al., 2010). Activation of NTRc, including mGluR and NMDARc, induce the production of DAG and its phosphorylation by DGKs, converting DAG into PA. The DGKζ isoform has been critically involved in spine maintenance. DGKζ is targeted to excitatory synapses through its direct interaction with the postsynaptic scaffold protein PSD-95. Overexpression of DGKζ in cultured neurons increases the number of dendritic spines in a manner requiring its catalytic activity and PSD-95 binding. Conversely, DGKζ knockdown reduces spine density (Kim et al., 2009). In agreement, mice deficient in DGKζ expression show reduced spine density and excitatory synaptic transmission. Time-lapse imaging indicates that DGKζ is required for spine maintenance but not formation (Kim et al., 2009). It has been proposed that DAG and PA signaling pathways are integrated within synaptic multi-protein complexes that intersect with small GTPases controlling actin cytoskeleton (Tada and Sheng, 2006; Kim et al., 2010).

INFLUENCE OF MEMBRANE LIPIDS ON GLUTAMATE RECEPTOR FUNCTION AT DENDRITIC SPINES

Modifications in the number and complement of glutamate-sensing receptors in the postsynaptic membrane are key mechanisms to adjust strength in excitatory synapses. AMPA and NMDA-type glutamate receptors are ligand-gated ion channels critical for synaptic plasticity (Barria and Malinow, 2002; Malinow and Malenka, 2002; Washbourne et al., 2004). Although the identification and characterization of proteins involved in the regulation of these receptors has been a productive area of research, there has been less progress in understanding how changes in membrane lipids affect their function. Lipids could modulate glutamate receptor affinity or capacity to bind their ligands by influencing receptor conformation, orientation, subunit composition or oligomerization. Lipids could as well alter the properties of the channels themselves. Lateral movement and endo-exocytic trafficking of NTRcs are essential for glutamate signaling. Lipids are also good candidates to regulate these membrane dependent events. Although we still lack accurate information about the differences in lipid composition between synaptic and extrasynaptic sites, specific lipid changes (i.e., cholesterol or PIP3 loss) affect the synaptic but not the extrasynaptic pool of AMPARc (Arendt et al., 2010; Martin et al., 2014). Hence, lipids could contribute to the balance between synaptic and extrasynaptic glutamate receptor activity, which is key for synaptic plasticity. Accumulating evidence supports the view that lipid rafts provide both a spatial and a temporal meeting point for receptors and proteins involved in a common pathway facilitating their intracellular signaling (Allen et al., 2007). Supporting the relevance of rafts for glutamate receptor function, different subunits of NMDARc (GluN1A, GluN2A, GluN2B) and AMPARc (GluA1, 2/3 and 4) have been localized to these membrane domains (Hering et al., 2003; Allen et al., 2007). Because of their localization in spines and importance for postsynaptic excitatory transmission we will next comment examples of particular lipids influencing AMPARc and NMDARc function.

LIPID INFLUENCE ON AMPARc

AMPARc mediate most excitatory transmission in the brain, and their regulated addition and removal from the postsynaptic membrane leads to long lasting forms of synaptic plasticity such as LTP and LTD (Malinow and Malenka, 2002). In addition, AMPARc continuously cycle in and out the synaptic membrane independently of synaptic activity. This constitutive trafficking involves both exocytic delivery from intracellular compartments (Gerges et al., 2006), fast exchange with surface extra-synaptic receptors via lateral diffusion (Tardin et al., 2003) and internalization of the displaced receptors by endocytosis, which is essential to sustain LTD (Carroll et al., 1999; Beattie et al., 2000). Although for most of these effects the specific molecular mechanism has not yet been elucidated, experimental modulation of lipids in brain slices or cultured neurons lead to changes in AMPARc localization and electrophysiological behavior. As we next describe, some of these effects received *in vivo* confirmation in mouse models with genetically or experimentally altered lipid content.

Cholesterol depletion reduces early-AMPA-mediated calcium influx (Frank et al., 2008). It was proposed that this effect was not due to a direct influence on the AMPARc channel kinetics but to altered surface expression of at least a subpopulation of AMPARc. Indeed, cholesterol levels have been shown to modulate AMPARc surface mobility (Renner et al., 2009) as well as endosomal dynamics (Hering et al., 2003; Hou et al., 2008). The loss of cholesterol in synaptic membranes of aged neurons impairs AMPARc internalization due to PI3K/Akt activation, which precludes Akt dephosphorylation required for GSK3β activation-mediated glutamate receptor endocytosis (Martin et al., 2014). Quantum-dot-based single molecule tracking analysis showed that reduction of cholesterol also affects GluR2-AMPARc lateral diffusion. These alterations lead to the impaired LTD typical of old neurons. Consistently, increasing cholesterol levels *in vitro* or *in vivo* by chronic infusion of the lipid restores LTD and cognitive deficits in the old mice (Martin et al., 2014).

Little is known about the influence of membrane shingolipids in AMPARc function. A positive role for the signaling sphingolipid Sphingosine-1-phosphate (S1P) in AMPARc-mediated miniature excitatory postsynaptic currents has been reported in hippocampal slices. Inhibition of sphingosine kinase (SphK) impaired LTP that was fully restored by S1P addition. Consistently, mice lacking SphK show poor memory performance (Kanno et al., 2010). However, it has been proposed that these effects do not take place in spines but correlate with the S1P-induced translocation of S1P receptors to presynaptic terminals thereby facilitating S1P receptor-mediated signals towards glutamate release.

Different studies indicate that AMPARc trafficking depends on PIP metabolism (**Figure 3**). Direct association of AMPARc with PI3K is required for receptor cell surface insertion and expression during LTP (Man et al., 2003). It has been proposed that the mobility of synaptic but not extra-synaptic AMPA receptors during LTD requires PIP3 depletion (Arendt et al., 2010). Hence, down-regulation of PIP3, either by overexpression of its pleckstrin homology (PH) domain or by inhibiting PI3K, impairs PSD-95 accumulation in spines and promotes AMPARc mobility leading to their migration from the postsynaptic density, where excitatory transmission occurs, towards the perisynaptic membrane within the spine, enabling synaptic depression (Arendt et al., 2010). PIP3 effects are specific for synaptic AMPARc, since it does not affect NMDARc nor extrasynaptic AMPARc. Given PIP3 contribution to the accumulation of PSD95 at spines, it has been proposed that the lipid favors AMPARc retention via modulation of the PSD95 synaptic scaffold. Complementary, enhancement of PTEN lipid phosphatase activity, which turns PIP3 into PIP2, is able to drive depression of AMPA receptor-mediated synaptic responses. This activity is specifically required for NMDARc-dependent LTD but not for LTP or mGluR-dependent LTD (Jurado et al., 2010). Further turnover of PIP2 by PLC favors synaptic actin depolymerization and PSD95 degradation, also contributing to the reduction of surface AMPARc expression and spine remodeling (Horne and Dell'Acqua, 2007).

LIPID INFLUENCE ON NMDARc

NMDARc are heterotetrameric ion channels directly implicated in LTP and LTD being the predominant molecular device for controlling synaptic plasticity and memory function (Bashir et al., 1991; Cui et al., 2004; Li and Tsien, 2009). Studies performed with purified NMDARc reconstituted in liposomes showed that membrane stretch reduce Mg^{2+} blockade of NMDA channel enhancing ion currents (Kloda et al., 2007). As these results were obtained in a minimal system that lacks cellular proteins, they unambiguously demonstrate that mechanical deformation of the lipid bilayer is sufficient to modulate the gating properties of NMDA channels (Piomelli et al., 2007). Experimental evidence suggests that as much as 60% of NMDARc are located in lipid rafts (Besshoh et al., 2005), which by virtue of their particular physical properties might dynamically regulate NMDARc subunit composition and trafficking. In support of this possibility, changes in cholesterol content inhibit NMDA-stimulated influx of calcium in hippocampal cells in culture (Frank et al., 2004). Cholesterol reduction redistributes the NMDARc GluN2B subunit, from rafts to non-raft membrane fractions (Abulrob et al., 2005). On the other hand, the cholesterol metabolite 24(S)-hydroxycholesterol has been recently identified as a potent and highly selective positive modulator of NMDARc. This hydroxysterol enhances NMDARc currents and LTP and restores behavioral and cognitive deficits in rodents treated with NMDARc channel blockers (Paul et al., 2013). It appears that the mechanism underlying these effects does not involve receptor insertion or transcription but direct binding of the lipid to a modulatory site in the receptor.

Dysregulation of brain sphingolipid balance following inhibition of NSM alters the subunit composition of NMDARc that might account for memory impairment following long-term inhibition of NSM (Tabatadze et al., 2010). NSM activity modulates the phosphorylation of the NMDARc subunit GluN1 on serine 896 promoting the clustering of these modified subunits into lipid rafts. It has been proposed that the rapid and focal generation of ceramide upon NSM activation shifts the composition of membrane lipids to bring into close proximity GluN1 and its kinases PKC and PKA (Wheeler et al., 2009). However, it is not clear if these events are the result of lateral diffusion of the kinases and membrane docked receptors or a translocation to the plasma membrane.

More work is needed to determine the influence of PIPs in NMDARc. The already mentioned observation that activation of these receptors recruits the PIP3 degrading enzyme, PTEN, to dendritic spines mediating NMDA dependent but not mGluR dependent LTD (Jurado et al., 2010), indicates a close relationship between PIP dynamics and NMDARc function. Moreover, blockade of the PIP3 synthesizing enzyme PI3K impairs forms of memory formation and LTP in the hippocampus (Chen et al., 2005). Whether and how this affects NMDARc is not known.

CONCLUDING REMARKS

We are still far from having a detailed picture of how lipids participate in dendritic spine physiology. However, research in recent years has started to unveil that they are not simple structural bystanders but play relevant roles in neurotransmission, through the control of spine architecture and by modulating neurotransmitter receptor function. As key components of postsynaptic membranes, lipids affect synaptic plasticity by shaping the membrane and modulating the levels, compartmentalization, interactions, trafficking and signaling properties of many proteins that are essential for synaptic function. By these means lipids regulate glutamate receptor function and actin cytoskeleton dynamics, which are instrumental features for postsynaptic plasticity. The application to the study of synapses of new generation fluorescent probes to label lipids, modified toxins that specifically identify them, different kinds of super-resolution microscopy and more sensitive quantitative methodologies will allow us to further dissect how spine lipids precisely function. As we know more on spine lipids the traditional view of the static role for these molecules fades away and is replaced by that of a remarkable dynamism. The activity of lipid metabolic enzymes at dendritic spines guarantees this dynamism. Some of these enzymes are constitutive components of these structures that change activity or get closer to their substrates upon stimulation. Others find different ways to reach the spine membrane when required. Deep insight on the role of lipids in dendritic spines and on how lipid pathways are topologically and temporally regulated will help to understand how we learn and keep our memories. Moreover, this will unveil the reasons behind the cognitive impairment occurring during aging and in diseases like many genetic lipidosis and neurodegenerative disorders where brain lipid imbalances have been reported. These investigations could yield novel therapeutics relying on lipid based drugs that readily cross the blood-brain barrier.

ACKNOWLEDGMENTS

The authors thank the support of the Ministerio Español de Ciencia e Innovacion (SAF2011-24550 to María Dolores Ledesma, SAF2013-45392-R to Carlos Gerardo Dotti, SAF2011-24730 to Jose Antonio Esteban, and Consolider Grant CSD2010-00045 to Carlos Gerardo Dotti, María Dolores Ledesma and Jose Antonio Esteban).

REFERENCES

Abe, M., Makino, A., Hullin-Matsuda, F., Kamijo, K., Ohno-Iwashita, Y., Hanada, K., et al. (2012). A role for sphingomyelin-rich lipid domains in the accumulation of phosphatidylinositol-4,5-bisphosphate to the cleavage furrow during cytokinesis. *Mol. Cell. Biol.* 32, 1396–1407. doi: 10.1128/MCB.06113-11

Abulrob, A., Tauskela, J. S., Mealing, G., Brunette, E., Faid, K., and Stanimirovic, D. (2005). Protection by cholesterol-extracting cyclodextrins: a role for N-methyl-D-aspartate receptor redistribution. *J. Neurochem.* 92, 1477–1486. doi: 10.1111/j.1471-4159.2005.03001.x

Allen, J. A., Halverson-Tamboli, R. A., and Rasenick, M. M. (2007). Lipid raft microdomains and neurotransmitter signalling. *Nat. Rev. Neurosci.* 8, 128–140. doi: 10.1038/nrn2059

Arendt, K. L., Royo, M., Fernández-Monreal, M., Knafo, S., Petrok, C. N., Martens, J. R., et al. (2010). PIP3 controls synaptic function by maintaining AMPA receptor clustering at the postsynaptic membrane. *Nat. Neurosci.* 13, 36–44. doi: 10.1038/nn.2462

Arroyo, A. I., Camoletto, P. G., Morando, L., Sassoe-Pognetto, M., Giustetto, M., Van Veldhoven, P. P., et al. (2014). Pharmacological reversion of sphingomyelin-induced dendritic spine anomalies in a Niemann pick disease type a mouse model. *EMBO Mol. Med.* 6, 398–413. doi: 10.1002/emmm.201302649

Barria, A., and Malinow, R. (2002). Subunit-specific NMDA receptor trafficking to synapses. *Neuron* 35, 345–353. doi: 10.1016/s0896-6273(02)00776-6

Bashir, Z. I., Alford, S., Davies, S. N., Randall, A. D., and Collingridge, G. L. (1991). Long-term potentiation of NMDA receptor-mediated synaptic transmission in the hippocampus. *Nature* 349, 156–158. doi: 10.1038/349156a0

Beattie, E. C., Carroll, R. C., Yu, X., Morishita, W., Yasuda, H., von Zastrow, M., et al. (2000). Regulation of AMPA receptor endocytosis by a signaling mechanism shared with LTD. *Nat Neurosci.* 3, 1291–1300. doi: 10.1038/81823

Besshoh, S., Bawa, D., Teves, L., Wallace, M. C., and Gurd, J. W. (2005). Increased phosphorylation and redistribution of NMDA receptors between synaptic lipid rafts and post-synaptic densities following transient global ischemia in the rat brain. *J. Neurochem.* 93, 186–194. doi: 10.1111/j.1471-4159.2004.03009.x

Bourguignon, L. Y., Singleton, P. A., Diedrich, F., Stern, R., and Gilad, E. (2004). CD44 interaction with Na+-H+ exchanger (NHE1) creates acidic microenvironments leading to hyaluronidase-2 and cathepsin B activation and breast tumor cell invasion. *J. Biol. Chem.* 279, 26991–27007. doi: 10.1074/jbc.m311838200

Brose, N., Betz, A., and Wegmeyer, H. (2004). Divergent and convergent signaling by the diacylglycerol second messenger pathway in mammals. *Curr. Opin. Neurobiol.* 14, 328–340. doi: 10.1016/s0959-4388(04)00073-x

Calabrese, B., and Halpain, S. (2005). Essential role for the PKC target MARCKS in maintaining dendritic spine morphology. *Neuron* 48, 77–90. doi: 10.1016/j.neuron.2005.08.027

Carlisle, H. J., and Kennedy, M. B. (2005). Spine architecture and synaptic plasticity. *Trends Neurosci.* 28, 182–187. doi: 10.1016/j.tins.2005.01.008

Carrasco, P., Sahún, I., McDonald, J., Ramírez, S., Jacas, J., Gratacós, E., et al. (2012). Ceramide levels regulated by carnitine palmitoyltransferase 1C control dendritic spine maturation and cognition. *J. Biol. Chem.* 287, 21224–21232. doi: 10.1074/jbc.M111.337493

Carroll, R. C., Lissin, D. V, von Zastrow, M., Nicoll, R. A., and Malenka, R. C. (1999). Rapid redistribution of glutamate receptors contributes to long-term depression in hippocampal cultures. *Nat. Neurosci.* 2, 454–460. doi: 10.1038/8123

Castro, B. M., Torreno-Piña, J. A., van Zanten, T. S., and Gracia-Parajo, M. F. (2013). Biochemical and imaging methods to study receptor membrane organization and association with lipid rafts. *Methods Cell Biol.* 117, 105–122. doi: 10.1016/b978-0-12-408143-7.00006-2

Chen, X., Garelick, M. G., Wang, H., Lil, V., Athos, J., and Storm, D. R. (2005). PI3 kinase signaling is required for retrieval and extinction of contextual memory. *Nat. Neurosci.* 8, 925–931. doi: 10.1038/nn1482

Chevaleyre, V., Takahashi, K. A., and Castillo, P. E. (2006). Endocannabinoid-mediated synaptic plasticity in the CNS. *Annu. Rev. Neurosci.* 29, 37–76. doi: 10.1146/annurev.neuro.29.051605.112834

Clarke, C. J., Guthrie, J. M., and Hannun, Y. A. (2008). Regulation of neutral sphingomyelinase-2 (nSMase2) by tumor necrosis factor-alpha involves protein kinase C-delta in lung epithelial cells. *Mol. Pharmacol.* 74, 1022–1032. doi: 10.1124/mol.108.046250

Collingridge, G. L., Peineau, S., Howland, J. G., and Wang, Y. T. (2010). Long-term depression in the CNS. *Nat. Rev. Neurosci.* 11, 459–473. doi: 10.1038/nrn2867

Coogan, A. N., O'Neill, L. A., and O'Connor, J. J. (1999). The P38 mitogen-activated protein kinase inhibitor SB203580 antagonizes the inhibitory effects of interleukin-1beta on long-term potentiation in the rat dentate gyrus in vitro. *Neuroscience* 93, 57–69. doi: 10.1016/s0306-4522(99)00100-1

Cui, Z., Wang, H., Tan, Y., Zaia, K. A., Zhang, S., and Tsien, J. Z. (2004). Inducible and reversible NR1 knockout reveals crucial role of the NMDA receptor in preserving remote memories in the brain. *Neuron* 41, 781–793. doi: 10.1016/s0896-6273(04)00072-8

Davis, C. N., Tabarean, I., Gaidarova, S., Behrens, M. M., and Bartfai, T. (2006). IL-1beta induces a MyD88-dependent and ceramide-mediated activation of Src in anterior hypothalamic neurons. *J. Neurochem.* 98, 1379–1389. doi: 10.1111/j.1471-4159.2006.03951.x

Eggeling, C., Ringemann, C., Medda, R., Schwarzmann, G., Sandhoff, K., Polyakova, S., et al. (2009). Direct observation of the nanoscale dynamics of membrane lipids in a living cell. *Nature* 457, 1159–1162. doi: 10.1038/nature07596

Fantini, J., and Barrantes, F. J. (2009). Sphingolipid/cholesterol regulation of neurotransmitter receptor conformation and function. *Biochim. Biophys. Acta* 1788, 2345–2361. doi: 10.1016/j.bbamem.2009.08.016

Fasano, C., Miolan, J. P., and Niel, J. P. (2003). Modulation by C2 ceramide of the nicotinic transmission within the coeliac ganglion in the rabbit. *Neuroscience* 116, 753–759. doi: 10.1016/s0306-4522(02)00760-1

Fernandes, C. C., Berg, D. K., and Gómez-Varela, D. (2010). Lateral mobility of nicotinic acetylcholine receptors on neurons is determined by receptor composition, local domain and cell type. *J. Neurosci.* 30, 8841–8851. doi: 10.1523/JNEUROSCI.6236-09.2010

Franco-Villanueva, A., Fernández-López, E., Gabandé-Rodríguez, E., Bañón-Rodríguez, I., Esteban, J. A., Antón, I. M., et al. (2014). WIP modulates dendritic spine actin cytoskeleton by transcriptional control of lipid metabolic enzymes. *Hum. Mol. Genet.* 16, 4383–4395. doi: 10.1093/hmg/ddu155

Frank, C., Giammarioli, A. M., Pepponi, R., Fiorentini, C., and Rufini, S. (2004). Cholesterol perturbing agents inhibit NMDA-dependent calcium influx in rat hippocampal primary culture. *FEBS Lett.* 566, 25–29. doi: 10.1016/j.febslet.2004.03.113

Frank, C., Rufini, S., Tancredi, V., Forcina, R., Grossi, D., and D'Arcangelo, G. (2008). Cholesterol depletion inhibits synaptic transmission and synaptic plasticity in rat hippocampus. *Exp. Neurol.* 212, 407–414. doi: 10.1016/j.expneurol.2008.04.019

Fraser, M. M., Bayazitov, I. T., Zakharenko, S. S., and Baker, S. J. (2008). Phosphatase and tensin homolog, deleted on chromosome 10 deficiency in brain causes defects in synaptic structure, transmission and plasticity and myelination abnormalities. *Neuroscience* 151, 476–488. doi: 10.1016/j.neuroscience.2007.10.048

Gerges, N. Z., Backos, D. S., Rupasinghe, C. N., Spaller, M. R., and Esteban, J. A. (2006). Dual role of the exocyst in AMPA receptor targeting and insertion into the postsynaptic membrane. *EMBO J.* 25, 1623–1634. doi: 10.1038/sj.emboj.7601065

Hammond, G. R., and Schiavo, G. (2007). Polyphosphoinositol lipids: under-PPInning synaptic function in health and disease. *Dev. Neurobiol.* 67, 1232–1247. doi: 10.1002/dneu.20509

Hering, H., Lin, C. C., and Sheng, M. (2003). Lipid rafts in the maintenance of synapses, dendritic spines and surface AMPA receptor stability. *J. Neurosci.* 23, 3262–3271.

Hofmann, K., Tomiuk, S., Wolff, G., and Stoffel, W. (2000). Cloning and characterization of the mammalian brain-specific, Mg2+-dependent neutral sphingomyelinase. *Proc. Natl. Acad. Sci. U S A* 97, 5895–5900. doi: 10.1073/pnas.97.11.5895

Horne, E. A., and Dell'Acqua, M. L. (2007). Phospholipase C is required for changes in postsynaptic structure and function associated with NMDA receptor-dependent long-term depression. *J. Neurosci.* 27, 3523–3534. doi: 10.1523/jneurosci.4340-06.2007

Hotulainen, P., and Hoogenraad, C. C. (2010). Actin in dendritic spines: connecting dynamics to function. *J. Cell Biol.* 189, 619–629. doi: 10.1083/jcb.201003008

Hou, Q., Huang, Y., Amato, S., Snyder, S. H., Huganir, R. L., and Man, H. Y. (2008). Regulation of AMPA receptor localization in lipid rafts. *Mol. Cell. Neurosci.* 38, 213–223. doi: 10.1016/j.mcn.2008.02.010

Hussain, R. J., Stumpo, D. J., Blackshear, P. J., Lenox, R. H., Abel, T., and McNamara, R. K. (2006). Myristoylated alanine rich C kinase substrate (MARCKS) heterozygous mutant mice exhibit deficits in hippocampal mossy fiber-CA3 long-term potentiation. *Hippocampus* 16, 495–503. doi: 10.1002/hipo.20177

Jurado, S., Benoist, M., Lario, A., Knafo, S., Petrok, C. N., and Esteban, J. A. (2010). PTEN is recruited to the postsynaptic terminal for NMDA receptor-dependent long-term depression. *EMBO J.* 29, 2827–2840. doi: 10.1038/emboj.2010.160

Kanno, T., Nishizaki, T., Proia, R. L., Kajimoto, T., Jahangeer, S., Okada, T., et al. (2010). Regulation of synaptic strength by sphingosine 1-phosphate in the hippocampus. *Neuroscience* 171, 973–980. doi: 10.1016/j.neuroscience.2010.10.021

Kelleher, R. J. 3rd, Govindarajan, A., and Tonegawa, S. (2004). Translational regulatory mechanisms in persistent forms of synaptic plasticity. *Neuron* 44, 59–73. doi: 10.1016/j.neuron.2004.09.013

Kim, K., Yang, J., and Kim, E. (2010). Diacylglycerol kinases in the regulation of dendritic spines. *J. Neurochem.* 112, 577–587. doi: 10.1111/j.1471-4159.2009.06499.x

Kim, K., Yang, J., Zhong, X. P., Kim, M. H., Kim, Y. S., Lee, H. W., et al. (2009). Synaptic removal of diacylglycerol by DGKzeta and PSD-95 regulates dendritic spine maintenance. *EMBO J.* 28, 1170–1179. doi: 10.1038/emboj.2009.44

Kloda, A., Lua, L., Hall, R., Adams, D. J., and Martinac, B. (2007). Liposome reconstitution and modulation of recombinant N-methyl-D-aspartate receptor channels by membrane stretch. *Proc. Natl. Acad. Sci. U S A* 104, 1540–1545. doi: 10.1073/pnas.0609649104

Koleske, A. J. (2013). Molecular mechanisms of dendrite stability. *Nat. Rev. Neurosci.* 14, 536–550. doi: 10.1038/nrn3486

Kotti, T. J., Ramirez, D. M., Pfeiffer, B. E., Huber, K. M., and Russell, D. W. (2006). Brain cholesterol turnover required for geranylgeraniol production and learning in mice. *Proc. Natl. Acad. Sci. U S A* 103, 3869–3874. doi: 10.1073/pnas.0600316103

Koudinov, A. R., and Koudinova, N. V. (2001). Essential role for cholesterol in synaptic plasticity and neuronal degeneration. *FASEB J.* 15, 1858–1860. doi: 10.1096/fj.00-0815fje

Krönke, M. (1999). Biophysics of ceramide signaling: interaction with proteins and phase transition of membranes. *Chem. Phys. Lipids.* 101, 109–121. doi: 10.1016/s0009-3084(99)00059-6

Kucharz, K., Krogh, M., Ng, A. N., and Toresson, H. (2009). NMDA receptor stimulation induces reversible fission of the neuronal endoplasmic reticulum. *PLoS One* 4:e5250. doi: 10.1371/journal.pone.0005250

Kumar, V., Zhang, M. X., Swank, M. W., Kunz, J., and Wu, G. Y. (2005). Regulation of dendritic morphogenesis by Ras-PI3K-Akt-mTOR and Ras-MAPK signaling pathways. *J. Neurosci.* 25, 11288–11299. doi: 10.1523/jneurosci.2284-05.2005

Lebiedzinska, M., Szabadkai, G., Jones, A. W., Duszynski, J., and Wieckowski, M. R. (2009). Interactions between the endoplasmic reticulum, mitochondria, plasma membrane and other subcellular organelles. *Int. J. Biochem. Cell Biol.* 41, 1805–1816. doi: 10.1016/j.biocel.2009.02.017

Li, F., and Tsien, J. Z. (2009). Memory and the NMDA receptors. *N. Engl. J. Med.* 361, 302–303. doi: 10.1056/NEJMcibr0902052

Lund, E. G., Guileyardo, J. M., and Russell, D. W. (1999). cDNA cloning of cholesterol 24-hydroxylase, a mediator of cholesterol homeostasis in the brain. *Proc. Natl. Acad. Sci. U S A* 96, 7238–7243. doi: 10.1073/pnas.96.13.7238

Maehama, T., and Dixon, J. E. (1999). PTEN: a tumour suppressor that functions as a phospholipid phosphatase. *Trends Cell Biol.* 9, 125–128. doi: 10.1016/s0962-8924(99)01519-6

Maioli, S., Båvner, A., Ali, Z., Heverin, M., Ismail, M. A., Puerta, E., et al. (2013). Is it possible to improve memory function by upregulation of the cholesterol 24S-hydroxylase (CYP46A1) in the brain? *PLoS One* 8:e68534. doi: 10.1371/journal.pone.0068534

Malinow, R., and Malenka, R. C. (2002). AMPA receptor trafficking and synaptic plasticity. *Annu. Rev. Neurosci.* 25, 103–126. doi: 10.1146/annurev.neuro.25.112701.142758

Man, H. Y., Wang, Q., Lu, W. Y., Ju, W., Ahmadian, G., Liu, L., et al. (2003). Activation of PI3-kinase is required for AMPA receptor insertion during LTP of mEPSCs in cultured hippocampal neurons. *Neuron* 38, 611–624. doi: 10.1016/s0896-6273(03)00228-9

Martin, M. G., Ahmed, T., Korovaichuk, A., Venero, C., Menchón, S. A., Salas, I., et al. (2014). Constitutive hippocampal cholesterol loss underlies poor cognition in old rodents. *EMBO Mol. Med.* 30, 902–917. doi: 10.15252/emmm.201303711

Martin, M. G., Perga, S., Trovò, L., Rasola, A., Holm, P., Rantamäki, T., et al. (2008). Cholesterol loss enhances TrkB signaling in hippocampal neurons aging in vitro. *Mol. Biol. Cell* 19, 2101–2112. doi: 10.1091/mbc.E07-09-0897

Matsuzaki, M., Honkura, N., Ellis-Davies, G. C., and Kasai, H. (2004). Structural basis of long-term potentiation in single dendritic spines. *Nature* 429, 761–766. doi: 10.1038/nature02617

Mauch, D. H., Nägler, K., Schumacher, S., Göritz, C., Müller, E. C., Otto, A., et al. (2001). CNS synaptogenesis promoted by glia-derived cholesterol. *Science* 294, 1354–1357. doi: 10.1126/science.294.5545.1354

McLaughlin, S., and Murray, D. (2005). Plasma membrane phosphoinositide organization by protein electrostatics. *Nature* 438, 605–611. doi: 10.1038/nature04398

McNamara, R. K., Stumpo, D. J., Morel, L. M., Lewis, M. H., Wakeland, E. K., Blackshear, P. J., et al. (1998). Effect of reduced myristoylated alanine-rich C kinase substrate expression on hippocampal mossy fiber development and spatial learning in mutant mice: transgenic rescue and interactions with gene background. *Proc. Natl. Acad. Sci. U S A* 95, 14517–14522. doi: 10.1073/pnas.95.24.14517

Nagappan, G., and Lu, B. (2005). Activity-dependent modulation of the BDNF receptor TrkB: mechanisms and implications. *Trends Neurosci.* 28, 464–471. doi: 10.1016/j.tins.2005.07.003

Neves, G., Cooke, S. F., and Bliss, T. V. (2008). Synaptic plasticity, memory and the hippocampus: a neural network approach to causality. *Nat. Rev. Neurosci.* 9, 65–75. doi: 10.1038/nrn2303

Okamoto, K., Nagai, T., Miyawaki, A., and Hayashi, Y. (2004). Rapid and persistent modulation of actin dynamics regulates postsynaptic reorganization underlying bidirectional plasticity. *Nat. Neurosci.* 7, 1104–1112. doi: 10.1038/nn1311

Paul, S. M., Doherty, J. J., Robichaud, A. J., Belfort, G. M., Chow, B. Y., Hammond, R. S., et al. (2013). The major brain cholesterol metabolite 24(S)-hydroxycholesterol is a potent allosteric modulator of N-methyl-D-aspartate receptors. *J. Neurosci.* 33, 17290–17300. doi: 10.1523/JNEUROSCI.2619-13.2013

Perez, A. S., and Bredt, D. S. (1998). The N-terminal PDZ-containing region of postsynaptic density-95 mediates association with caveolar-like lipid domains. *Neurosci. Lett.* 258, 121–123. doi: 10.1016/s0304-3940(98)00846-5

Pichler, H., Gaigg, B., Hrastnik, C., Achleitner, G., Kohlwein, S. D., Zellnig, G., et al. (2001). A subfraction of the yeast endoplasmic reticulum associates with the plasma membrane and has a high capacity to synthesize lipids. *Eur. J. Biochem.* 268, 2351–2361. doi: 10.1046/j.1432-1327.2001.02116.x

Pike, L. J. (2006). Rafts defined: a report on the keystone symposium on lipid rafts and cell function. *J. Lipid Res.* 47, 1597–1598. doi: 10.1194/jlr.e600002-jlr200

Piomelli, D., Astarita, G., and Rapaka, R. (2007). A neuroscientist's guide to lipidomics. *Nat. Rev. Neurosci.* 8, 743–754. doi: 10.1038/nrn2233

Ramirez, D. M., Andersson, S., and Russell, D. W. (2008). Neuronal expression and subcellular localization of cholesterol 24-hydroxylase in the mouse brain. *J. Comp. Neurol.* 507, 1676–1693. doi: 10.1002/cne.21605

Renner, M., Choquet, D., and Triller, A. (2009). Control of the postsynaptic membrane viscosity. *J. Neurosci.* 29, 2926–2937. doi: 10.1523/JNEUROSCI.4445-08.2009

Reyes-Harde, M., and Stanton, P. K. (1998). Postsynaptic phospholipase C activity is required for the induction of homosynaptic long-term depression in rat hippocampus. *Neurosci. Lett.* 252, 155–158. doi: 10.1016/s0304-3940(98)00496-0

Richards, D. A., Mateos, J. M., Hugel, S., de Paola, V., Caroni, P., Gähwiler, B. H., et al. (2005). Glutamate induces the rapid formation of spine head protrusions in hippocampal slice cultures. *Proc. Natl. Acad. Sci. U S A* 102, 6166–6171. doi: 10.1073/pnas.0501881102

Schissel, S. L., Jiang, X., Tweedie-Hardman, J., Jeong, T., Camejo, E. H., Najib, J., et al. (1998). Secretory sphingomyelinase, a product of the acid sphingomyelinase gene, can hydrolyze atherogenic lipoproteins at neutral pH. Implications for atherosclerotic lesion development. *J. Biol. Chem.* 273, 2738–2746. doi: 10.1074/jbc.273.5.2738

Sodero, A. O., Vriens, J., Ghosh, D., Stegner, D., Brachet, A., Pallotto, M., et al. (2012). Cholesterol loss during glutamate-mediated excitotoxicity. *EMBO J.* 31, 1764–1773. doi: 10.1038/emboj.2012.31

Sodero, A. O., Weissmann, C., Ledesma, M. D., and Dotti, C. G. (2011). Cellular stress from excitatory neurotransmission contributes to cholesterol loss in hippocampal neurons aging in vitro. *Neurobiol. Aging* 32, 1043–1053. doi: 10.1016/j.neurobiolaging.2010.06.001

Spacek, J., and Harris, K. M. (2004). Trans-endocytosis via spinules in adult rat hippocampus. *J. Neurosci.* 24, 4233–4241. doi: 10.1523/jneurosci.0287-04.2004

Stoffel, W. (1999). Functional analysis of acid and neutral sphingomyelinases in vitro and in vivo. *Chem Phys. Lipids.* 102, 107–121. doi: 10.1016/s0009-3084(99)00079-1

Suzuki, T. (2002). Lipid rafts at postsynaptic sites: distribution, function and linkage to postsynaptic density. *Neurosci. Res.* 44, 1–9. doi: 10.1016/S0168-0102(02)00080-9

Suzuki, T., Zhang, J., Miyazawa, S., Liu, Q., Farzan, M. R., and Yao, W. D. (2011). Association of membrane rafts and postsynaptic density: proteomics, biochemical and ultrastructural analyses. *J. Neurochem.* 119, 64–77. doi: 10.1111/j.1471-4159.2011.07404.x

Tabatadze, N., Savonenko, A., Song, H., Bandaru, V. V., Chu, M., and Haughey, N. J. (2010). Inhibition of neutral sphingomyelinase-2 perturbs brain sphingolipid balance and spatial memory in mice. *J. Neurosci. Res.* 88, 2940–2951. doi: 10.1002/jnr.22438

Tada, T., and Sheng, M. (2006). Molecular mechanisms of dendritic spine morphogenesis. *Curr. Opin. Neurobiol.* 16, 95–101. doi: 10.1016/j.conb.2005.12.001

Tardin, C., Cognet, L., Bats, C., Lounis, B., and Choquet, D. (2003). Direct imaging of lateral movements of AMPA receptors inside synapses. *EMBO J.* 22, 4656–4665. doi: 10.1093/emboj/cdg463

Trovò, L., Ahmed, T., Callaerts-Vegh, Z., Buzzi, A., Bagni, C., Chuah, M., et al. (2013). Low hippocampal PI(4,5)P_2 contributes to reduced cognition in old mice as a result of loss of MARCKS. *Nat. Neurosci.* 16, 449–455. doi: 10.1038/nn.3342

Ueda, Y., and Hayashi, Y. (2013). PIP_3 regulates spinule formation in dendritic spines during structural long-term potentiation. *J. Neurosci.* 33, 11040–11047. doi: 10.1523/JNEUROSCI.3122-12.2013

Unoki, T., Matsuda, S., Kakegawa, W., Van, N. T., Kohda, K., Suzuki, A., et al. (2012). NMDA receptor-mediated PIP5K activation to produce PI(4,5)P_2 is essential for AMPA receptor endocytosis during LTD. *Neuron* 73, 135–148. doi: 10.1016/j.neuron.2011.09.034

van Zanten, T. S., Gómez, J., Manzo, C., Cambi, A., Buceta, J., Reigada, R., et al. (2010). Direct mapping of nanoscale compositional connectivity on intact cell membranes. *Proc. Natl. Acad. Sci. U S A* 107, 15437–15442. doi: 10.1073/pnas.1003876107

Wang, Y., Cheng, A., and Mattson, M. P. (2006). The PTEN phosphatase is essential for long-term depression of hippocampal synapses. *Neuromolecular Med.* 8, 329–336. doi: 10.1385/nmm:8:3:329

Washbourne, P., Liu, X. B., Jones, E. G., and McAllister, A. K. (2004). Cycling of NMDA receptors during trafficking in neurons before synapse formation. *J. Neurosci.* 24, 8253–8264. doi: 10.1523/jneurosci.2555-04.2004

Wheeler, D., Knapp, E., Bandaru, V. V., Wang, Y., Knorr, D., Poirier, C., et al. (2009). Tumor necrosis factor-alpha-induced neutral sphingomyelinase-2 modulates synaptic plasticity by controlling the membrane insertion of NMDA receptors. *J. Neurochem.* 109, 1237–1249. doi: 10.1111/j.1471-4159.2009.06038.x

Wolfgang, M. J., Kurama, T., Dai, Y., Suwa, A., Asaumi, M., Matsumoto, S., et al. (2006). The brain-specific carnitine palmitoyltransferase-1c regulates energy homeostasis. *Proc. Natl. Acad. Sci. U S A* 103, 7282–7287. doi: 10.1073/pnas.0602205103

Yang, S. N. (2000). Ceramide-induced sustained depression of synaptic currents mediated by ionotropic glutamate receptors in the hippocampus: an essential role of postsynaptic protein phosphatases. *Neuroscience* 96, 253–258. doi: 10.1016/s0306-4522(99)00582-5

Yin, H. L., and Janmey, P. A. (2003). Phosphoinositide regulation of the actin cytoskeleton. *Annu. Rev. Physiol.* 65, 761–789. doi: 10.1146/annurev.physiol.65.092101.142517

Yoshida, T., Fukaya, M., Uchigashima, M., Miura, E., Kamiya, H., Kano, M., et al. (2006). Localization of diacylglycerol lipase-alpha around postsynaptic spine suggests close proximity between production site of an endocannabinoid, 2-arachidonoyl-glycerol and presynaptic cannabinoid CB1 receptor. *J. Neurosci.* 26, 4740–4751. doi: 10.1523/jneurosci.0054-06.2006

Yuste, R., and Bonhoeffer, T. (2001). Morphological changes in dendritic spines associated with long-term synaptic plasticity. *Annu. Rev. Neurosci.* 24, 1071–1089. doi: 10.1146/annurev.neuro.24.1.1071

Zhang, H., Webb, D. J., Asmussen, H., Niu, S., and Horwitz, A. F. (2005). A GIT1/PIX/Rac/PAK signaling module regulates spine morphogenesis and synapse formation through MLC. *J. Neurosci.* 25, 3379–3388. doi: 10.1523/jneurosci.3553-04.2005

Zhou, Q., Homma, K. J., and Poo, M. M. (2004). Shrinkage of dendritic spines associated with long-term depression of hippocampal synapses. *Neuron* 44, 749–757. doi: 10.1016/j.neuron.2004.11.011

6

Dendritic spine dysgenesis in Rett syndrome

Xin Xu, Eric C. Miller and Lucas Pozzo-Miller*

Department of Neurobiology, Civitan International Research Center, The University of Alabama at Birmingham, Birmingham, AL, USA

Correspondence:
Lucas Pozzo-Miller, Department of Neurobiology, Civitan International Research Center, The University of Alabama at Birmingham, SHEL-1002, 1825 University Boulevard, Birmingham, AL, 35294-2182, USA
e-mail: lucaspm@uab.edu

Spines are small cytoplasmic extensions of dendrites that form the postsynaptic compartment of the majority of excitatory synapses in the mammalian brain. Alterations in the numerical density, size, and shape of dendritic spines have been correlated with neuronal dysfunction in several neurological and neurodevelopmental disorders associated with intellectual disability, including Rett syndrome (RTT). RTT is a progressive neurodevelopmental disorder associated with intellectual disability that is caused by loss of function mutations in the transcriptional regulator methyl CpG-binding protein 2 (*MECP2*). Here, we review the evidence demonstrating that principal neurons in RTT individuals and *Mecp2*-based experimental models exhibit alterations in the number and morphology of dendritic spines. We also discuss the exciting possibility that signaling pathways downstream of brain-derived neurotrophic factor (BDNF), which is transcriptionally regulated by MeCP2, offer promising therapeutic options for modulating dendritic spine development and plasticity in RTT and other *MECP2*-associated neurodevelopmental disorders.

Keywords: MeCP2, BDNF, excitatory synapse, spine density, hippocampus, organotypic slice cultures, TrkB, autism spectrum disorder

INTRODUCTION

Espinas dendríticas are small cytoplasmic extensions emerging from the dendrites of neurons that were first described in the cerebellum and cerebrum of birds and mammals by Santiago Ramón y Cajal at the end of the 19th century (Ramón y Cajal, 1888, 1891b, 1896; as cited in Yuste, 2010). Cajal had already envisioned that dendritic spines are contacted by axons at synapses (Ramón y Cajal, 1891a, 1894), and used this arrangement as the main example in support of his *Neuronal Doctrine* (Ramón y Cajal, 1933). With the aid of electron microscopy and confocal fluorescence microscopy, it is now well established that spines are the postsynaptic sites of most excitatory synapses in the brain, receiving inputs from glutamatergic axons (Bhatt et al., 2009; Yuste, 2010; Shirao and Gonzalez-Billault, 2013). Despite their small size ($\sim$1 μm in diameter), proper dendritic spine formation is critical for brain function. Numerous proteins, including neurotransmitter and neuropeptide receptors, signaling kinases, and phosphatases, as well as ion channels are expressed in dendritic spines, where they participate in excitatory synaptic transmission and activity-dependent synaptic plasticity, and ultimately in learning and memory (Sala and Segal, 2014). During development and throughout adulthood, the numerical density and morphology of individual spines are critical for the fine-tuning of neuronal and synaptic excitability, allowing the initial establishment and activity-dependent remodeling of connectivity of neuronal circuits (Luebke et al., 2010).

The morphology of dendritic spines is highly variable, and by defining the biochemical and electrical properties of the postsynaptic compartment, it contributes to the strength and plasticity of excitatory synapses (Luebke et al., 2010). Spines have been broadly classified into three morphological types: stubby, mushroom and thin (Peters and Kaiserman-Abramof, 1969). Mushroom spines have a large head that is connected to the parent dendrite through a narrow neck. Stubby spines do not have a noticeable neck and are most common during postnatal development (Chapleau et al., 2009b; Rochefort and Konnerth, 2012). These two types of large spines are referred to as "memory spines," because they are stable, persist for longer periods of time, and are the postsynaptic side of strong excitatory synapses (Trachtenberg et al., 2002; Kasai et al., 2003). Conversely, thin spines have a thin, long neck, and a small bulbous head, are highly motile, unstable, and often short-lived, usually representing weak or silent synapses (Rochefort and Konnerth, 2012). Because thin spines are more plastic than large spines and have the potential to become stable spines, they have been dubbed "learning spines" (Grutzendler et al., 2002; Trachtenberg et al., 2002; Kasai et al., 2003; Holtmaat et al., 2005). It should be noted that thin protrusions longer than thin spines and without a noticeable head are called dendritic filopodia, and are more numerous than spines in developing neurons. Dendritic filopodia are transient and highly motile protrusions that can receive synaptic input and develop into mature spines, thus initiating synaptogenesis (Fiala et al., 1998; Luebke et al., 2010).

Following the well-known relationship between form and function in biological systems, recent *in vitro* and *in vivo* studies have demonstrated that the morphology of spines relates closely to the function and plasticity of the synapses they belong to (Yuste et al., 2000; Trachtenberg et al., 2002; Mizrahi et al., 2004; Segal, 2005; Kasai et al., 2010). For example, the volume of the spine head is directly proportional to the area of the postsynaptic density and the number of synaptic vesicles docked at the presynaptic active zone (Harris and Stevens, 1989; Schikorski and Stevens, 1999), the number of postsynaptic receptors (Nusser et al., 1998), and hence to the size of synaptic currents and synaptic strength (Yuste and Bonhoeffer, 2001; Luebke et al., 2010). Two-photon uncaging of glutamate on large spines evoked larger postsynaptic currents mediated by AMPA receptors than uncaging on small spines (Matsuzaki et al., 2001; Kasai et al., 2010). Such a structure-function relationship is also evident in the intracellular Ca^{2+} signals within spines triggered by afferent synaptic activity (Yuste et al., 2000; Nimchinsky et al., 2002; Bloodgood and Sabatini, 2007). Together with structural changes in response to afferent synaptic stimulation (Murphy and Segal, 1996; Srivastava and Penzes, 2011), all these findings support the long held view that dendritic spines are the morphological substrate of neuronal plasticity and learning and memory (Sala and Segal, 2014). In support of this notion, induction of long-term potentiation (LTP) leads to spine enlargement (Matsuzaki et al., 2004; Park et al., 2006), whereas long-term depression (LTD) causes spine shrinkage (Nagerl et al., 2004; Zhou et al., 2004; Hoogenraad and Akhmanova, 2010; Penzes et al., 2011b).

The relationship between dendritic spines and cognitive abilities was noted in early studies, when the term "spine dysgenesis" was coined by Dominick Purpura (Huttenlocher, 1970; Marin-Padilla, 1972; Purpura, 1974). Such anomalies in the morphology – and likely function – of dendritic spines have been described in several neurological disorders associated with cognitive decline, including typical aging, Alzheimer's and Huntington diseases, schizophrenia, neurodevelopmental intellectual disabilities, and autism spectrum disorders (Fiala et al., 2002; Fukuda et al., 2005; Zhao et al., 2007; Bourgeron, 2009; Chapleau et al., 2009b; Garey, 2010; Penzes et al., 2011a; Levenga and Willemsen, 2012).

DENDRITIC SPINE DYSGENESIS IN RETT SYNDROME

Rett syndrome (RTT) is an X-linked progressive autism spectrum disorder associated with intellectual disability that affects girls during early childhood (~1:15,000 birth worldwide; Neul and Zoghbi, 2004; Chapleau et al., 2009b). The disorder is characterized by a seemingly typical development for 6 to 18 months followed by regression and onset of a variety of neurological features, including motor impairments, loss of acquired language, intellectual disability, seizures, and anxiety (Chahrour and Zoghbi, 2007). The majority of RTT individuals carry loss-of-function mutations in *MECP2*, the gene encoding methyl CpG-binding protein 2 (MeCP2), a global transcriptional regulator that binds to methylated CpG sites in promoter regions of DNA (Amir et al., 1999; Chahrour et al., 2008). Emerging evidence indicates that RTT results from a deficit in synaptic maturation in the brain, and that MeCP2 plays a critical role in neuronal and synaptic maturation and pruning during development (Cohen et al., 2003; Calfa et al., 2011b), as well as in the function of established neuronal networks in adulthood (McGraw et al., 2011).

Pyramidal neurons in the cortex and hippocampus of RTT individuals have dendrites with atypical morphology (Belichenko et al., 1994; Armstrong et al., 1995; Chapleau et al., 2009a; **Figure 1A**). Two different mouse models lacking *Mecp2* (Chen et al., 2001; Guy et al., 2001) have reduced dendritic complexity (Fukuda et al., 2005; Nguyen et al., 2012; Stuss et al., 2012), and decreased dendritic spine density and motility in cortical and hippocampal neurons (Belichenko et al., 2009; Tropea et al., 2009; Landi et al., 2011; Chapleau et al., 2012; Castro et al., 2014). On the other hand, *Mecp2*^{308} mice expressing truncated MeCP2 (Shahbazian et al., 2002), which have impaired synaptic plasticity and hippocampal-dependent learning and memory and other RTT-related neurological deficits, do not show any dendritic or synaptic anomalies neither in cortical nor hippocampal neurons (Moretti et al., 2006). The reduced dendritic spine density, along with a decrease in the proportion of mushroom spines, is also present in primary hippocampal neurons (Chao et al., 2007; Baj et al., 2014) and hippocampal slice cultures (**Figure 1B**) prepared from newborn *Mecp2* knockout (KO) pups, as well as in neurons derived from induced pluripotent stem cells obtained from RTT individuals (Marchetto et al., 2010).

The spine dysgenesis phenotype in pyramidal neurons of the hippocampus in *Mecp2* KO mice has revealed unexpected complexities. CA1 and CA3 pyramidal neurons have lower spine density only in neonatal (postnatal day-7) *Mecp2* KOs, well before excitatory synapse expansion. Spine density reaches wildtype (WT) levels a week later (postnatal day-15), and is maintained at WT levels throughout the symptomatic stage (postnatal day-40 to 60). Quantitative electron microscopy confirmed that the density of asymmetric spine synapses in CA1 *stratum radiatum* of *Mecp2* KOs is comparable to that of WT mice (Calfa et al., 2011a; Chapleau et al., 2012). This developmental progression of the spine density phenotype is also reflected in the density of excitatory synapses imaged as VGLUT1-PSD95 immunofluorescent puncta, which is lower in area CA1 of 2 week-old *Mecp2* null mice, but comparable to WT levels at 5 weeks of age (Chao et al., 2007). Altogether, these data demonstrate that proper MeCP2 functioning is required for dendritic spine formation during early postnatal development, and that a secondary compensatory mechanism seems to take place during atypical development in *Mecp2* KOs. A couple of possibilities exist as to the extent of the compensatory mechanisms necessary to bring spine density to WT levels in hippocampal neurons. One possibility is that enhanced hippocampal network activity in *Mecp2* KOs promotes dendritic spine formation (Calfa et al., 2011a). A second possibility is that deranged homeostatic plasticity promotes spinogenesis, while still affecting pyramidal neuron function (Blackman et al., 2012; Qiu et al., 2012).

Consistent with a model that tightly regulated MeCP2 levels are necessary during brain development and adulthood, overexpression of *Mecp2 in vitro* or in the *MECP2* duplication mouse model (*Mecp2*^{Tg1}) either increased (Jugloff et al., 2005; Chao et al., 2007; Jiang et al., 2013) or decreased (Zhou et al., 2006; Chapleau et al., 2009a; Cheng et al., 2014) dendritic complexity, spine density, and the density of excitatory synapses. **Table 1** sumarizes all the published work on dendritic spines in RTT and experimenal models based on MeCP2 loss-of-function.

ROLE OF BDNF IN DENDRITIC SPINE FORMATION AND PLASTICITY: A POTENTIAL THERAPY FOR RTT

MeCP2 regulates the expression of thousands of genes, including brain-derived neurotrophic factor (*Bdnf*; Chen et al., 2003; Martinowich et al., 2003; Zhou et al., 2006). BDNF is well known to promote neuronal and synaptic maturation (Carvalho et al., 2008), increase dendritic spine density, and enhance synaptic plasticity and learning and memory (Figurov et al., 1996; Luine and

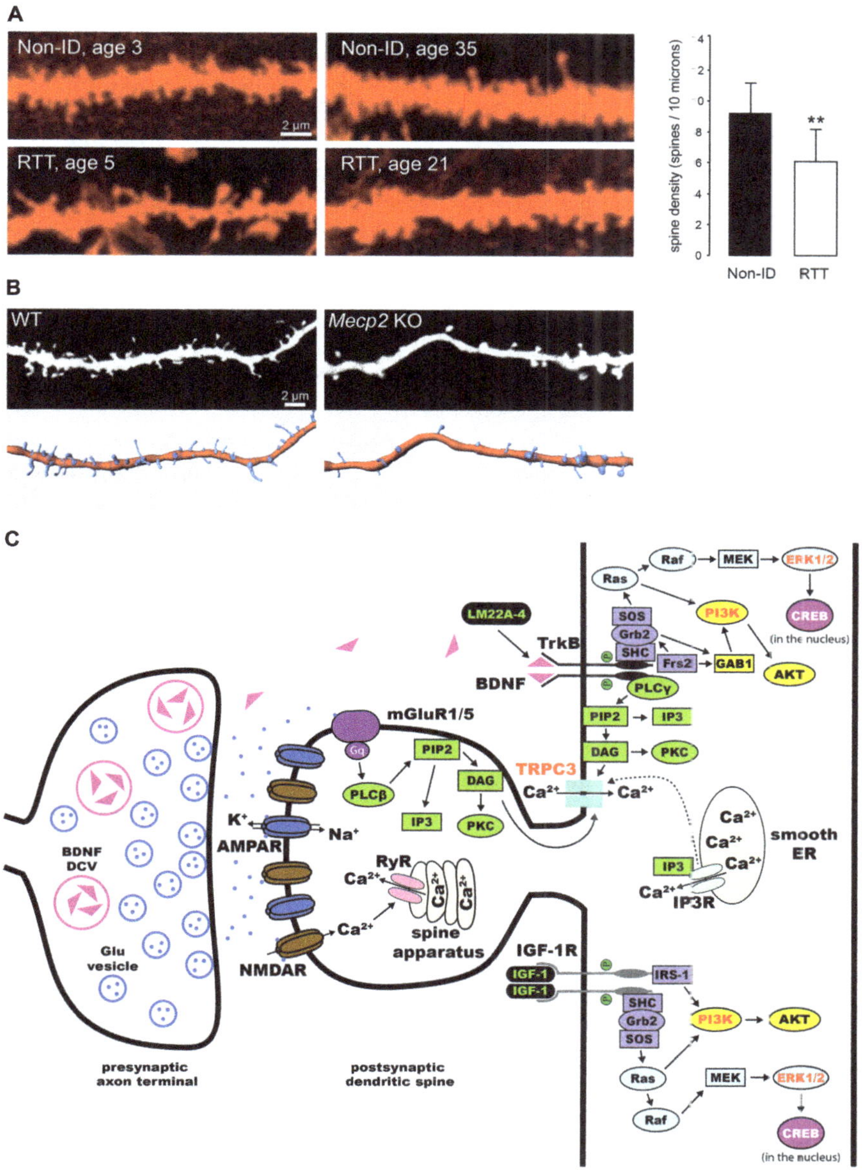

FIGURE 1 | Dendritic spine dysgenesis in Rett syndrome, and intracellular signaling cascades involved in spine plasticity mediated by BDNF and IGF-1. (A) Confocal images of human CA1 pyramidal neurons in hippocampal sections from autopsy material labeled with DiI. Neurons from RTT individuals have lower dendritic spine density than those from typically developing individuals (Non-ID, non-intellectually disabled). $^{**}P < 0.01$ (adapted from Chapleau et al., 2009a). **(B)** Confocal images of apical dendritic segments (top) of eYFP-expressing CA1 pyramidal neurons in 11 days *in vitro* hippocampal slice cultures prepared from postnatal day-5 wildtype (WT) and *Mecp2* knockout (KO) mice, and their corresponding surface-rendered reconstructions (bottom). **(C)** Schematic diagram of an exemplary excitatory synapse on a dendritic spine of a pyramidal neuron in the hippocampus. We highlight the intracellular signaling cascades that mediate the effects of BDNF and IGF-1 on structural plasticity of spines. TrkB receptors are activated upon binding of BDNF, leading to dimerization and auto-phosphorylation. This process allows for the binding of adaptor proteins to their intracellular domain, and the subsequent activation of Ras/ERK, PI3K, and PLCγ (reviewed by Huang and Reichardt, 2003). All these pathways have been implicated in the effects of BDNF on dendritic spines (highlighted in red, see text for references). Potential therapies for the treatment of RTT act on these pathways (highlighted in green, see text for details and references): LM22A-4 binds and activates TrkB receptors directly (Massa et al., 2010); activation of IGF-1 receptors triggers the PI3K and Ras/ERK signaling pathways (Zheng and Quirion, 2004). DCV, dense core vesicle; Glu, glutamate; AMPAR, α-amino-3-hydroxy-5-methyl-4-isoxazolepropionic acid receptor; NMDAR, *N*-methyl-D-aspartate receptor; mGluR, metabotropic glutamate receptor; ER, endoplasmic reticulum; RyR, ryanodine receptor; PIP2, phosphatidylinositol 4,5 bisphosphate; DAG, diacylglycerol; IP3, inositol triphosphate; IP3R, IP3 receptor; PKC, protein kinase C; SH-2, src homology domain 2; SHC, SH-2-containing protein; Grb2, growth factor receptor-binding protein 2; GAB1, Grb2-associated-binding protein 1; SOS, nucleotide exchange factor *son-of-sevenless*; Frs2, fibroblast growth factor receptor substrate 2; AKT, protein kinase B; Ras, rat sarcoma proto-oncogenic G-protein; Raf, proto-oncogenic serine/threonine protein kinase; MAPK, mitogen-activated protein kinase; MEK, MAPK kinase; cAMP, cyclic adenosine monophosphate; CREB, cAMP response element-binding protein; IGF-1R, IGF-1 receptor; IRS-1, insulin receptor substrate 1.

Table 1 | Dendritic spine dysgenesis in RTT individuals and MeCP2-deficient cells and mice.

Source	Brain region	Preparation	Alterations in dendrites and dendritic spines	Reference
RTT individuals	Cerebral cortex	Fixed postmortem brain (layer II and III at 2.9–35 years old)	↓Dendritic complexity ↓Dendritic spine density	Belichenko et al. (1994), Armstrong et al. (1995)
	Hippocampus	Fixed postmortem brain (CA1 region at 1–42 years old)	↓Dendritic spine density	Chapleau et al. (2009a)
	Induced pluripotent stem cells	Fibroblasts from patients' dermal biopsies (DIV56)	↓Excitatory synapse number ↓Dendritic spine density	Marchetto et al. (2010)
Mecp2$^{tm.1.1Bird}$	Cortex	Fixed brain (layer II/III motor cortex at P21)	↓Dendritic spine density	Belichenko et al. (2009)
		Fixed brain (layer II/III somatosensory cortex at P42)	↓Dendritic complexity ↓Dendritic spine density	Fukuda et al. (2005)
	Hippocampus	Autaptic culture (DIV7–9)	↓Excitatory synapse number	Chao et al. (2007)
		Primary culture (DIV9–15)	↓Excitatory synapse number ↓Dendritic complexity ↓Dendritic spine density ↓Mushroom spines ↑Stubby spines	Baj et al. (2014)
		Fixed brain (CA1 region at P21)	↓Dendritic spine density	Belichenko et al. (2009)
		Fixed brain (CA1 region at P42)	↓Dendritic complexity ↓Dendritic spine density	Nguyen et al. (2012)
	Fascia dentata	Fixed brain (P21)	↓Dendritic spine density	Belichenko et al. (2009)
Mecp2$^{tm.1.1Jae}$	Cortex	*In vivo* and fixed brain (layer V somatosensory cortex at P25, P40)	↓Dendritic spine density altered spine dynamics	Landi et al. (2011)
		Fixed brain (layer V motor cortex at P40)	↓Dendritic complexity ↓Dendritic spine density	Stuss et al. (2012)
		Fixed brain (layer II/III visual cortex at P42)	↓Dendritic spine density	Castro et al. (2014)
		Fixed brain (layer V motor cortex at P60)	↓Dendritic spine density	Tropea et al. (2009)
	Hippocampus	Fixed brain (CA1 region at P7)	↓Dendritic spine density	Chapleau et al. (2012)
		Fixed brain (CA1 region at P21)	↓Dendritic spine density	Belichenko et al. (2009)
		Fixed brain (newly matured DG neurons at P56)	↓Dendritic spine density	Smrt et al. (2007)
Mecp2 knockdown	Cortex	Primary culture (layer II/III visual cortex at DIV7-9)	↓Excitatory synapse number	Blackman et al. (2012)
	Hippocampus	Slice culture (CA1 region at DIV11)	↓Dendritic spine density ↓Mature spines	Chapleau et al. (2009a)
Mecp2^{Tg1}	Cortex	*In vivo* (layer V somatosensory cortex at P56)	↑Dendritic spine density	Jiang et al. (2013)
	Hippocampus	Autaptic culture (DIV7–9)	↑Excitatory synapse number	Chao et al. (2007)
Overexpression of *MECP2*	Cortex	Primary culture (DIV6)	↑Dendritic complexity	Jugloff et al. (2005)
		Primary culture (DIV6)	↓Dendritic complexity	Cheng et al. (2014)
	Hippocampus	Slice culture (pyramidal neurons at DIV7)	↓Dendritic complexity ↑Thin spines	Zhou et al. (2006)
		Slice culture (pyramidal neurons at DIV9)	↓Dendritic complexity ↓Dendritic spine density	Cheng et al. (2014)
		Slice culture (CA1 region at DIV9)	↓Dendritic spine density ↓Mature spines	Chapleau et al. (2009a)
Overexpression of *MECP2* mutations (R106W and T158M)	Hippocampus	Slice culture (CA1 region at DIV9–11)	↓Dendritic spine density ↓Mature spines	Chapleau et al. (2009a)

Frankfurt, 2013). MeCP2 binds to the *Bdnf* promoter and modulates *Bdnf* expression in an activity-dependent manner (Chen et al., 2003; Martinowich et al., 2003; Zhou et al., 2006; Chahrour and Zoghbi, 2007). Lower *Bdnf* mRNA and BDNF protein levels, as well as impaired BDNF trafficking and activity-dependent release, have been highlighted as pathophysiological mechanisms of RTT disease progression (Chang et al., 2006; Wang et al., 2006; Ogier et al., 2007; Li et al., 2012; Xu et al., 2014). Indeed, overexpression of BDNF rescues several cellular and behavioral deficits in *Mecp2* KO mice (Chang et al., 2006; Chahrour and Zoghbi, 2007). These studies indicate that BDNF plays a critical role in neurological impairments in MeCP2-deficient mice.

Several studies have demonstrated that BDNF participates in synaptic plasticity, and is critical for dendritic spine formation and maturation during development (Poo, 2001; Tyler et al., 2002a; Tanaka et al., 2008; Cohen-Cory et al., 2010; Vigers et al., 2012). For example, exogenously applied BDNF increases spine density in cultured hippocampal neurons and CA1 pyramidal neurons in slice cultures (Tyler and Pozzo-Miller, 2001; Ji et al., 2005). In addition, BDNF shifts the proportions of morphological types of spines in hippocampal slice cultures (Tyler and Pozzo-Miller, 2003; Chapleau et al., 2008). Moreover, overexpression of the *Bdnf* gene in cultured hippocampal neurons rescued the dendritic atrophy caused by shRNA-mediated *Mecp2* knockdown (Larimore et al., 2009). These effects of BDNF on dendritic spines are mediated by the tropomyosin related kinase B (TrkB) receptor (Tyler and Pozzo-Miller, 2001), and subsequent activation of extracellular signal-regulated kinase (ERK; Alonso et al., 2004), phosphatidylinositol 3-kinase (PI3K; Kumar et al., 2005), and phospholipase C-γ (PLC-γ), which leads to the opening of canonical transient receptor potential (TRPC) channels containing the TRPC3 subunit (Amaral and Pozzo-Miller, 2007; Chapleau et al., 2009b; Li et al., 2012; Luine and Frankfurt, 2013; **Figure 1C**).

Activity-dependent release of endogenously expressed (native) BDNF also modulates spine morphology in conjunction with spontaneous neurotransmitter release (Tyler et al., 2002b; Tyler and Pozzo-Miller, 2003; Tanaka et al., 2008). In addition, proper secretory trafficking of BDNF is essential for its actions on dendritic spine development and plasticity. The human *BDNF* gene has a single nucleotide polymorphism – a methionine (met) substitution for valine (val) at codon 66 – that impairs BDNF trafficking and its activity-dependent release, resulting in cognitive dysfunction in the general population (Egan et al., 2003; Chen et al., 2004), as well as more severe neurological symptoms in RTT individuals (Zeev et al., 2009). Consistently, dendritic complexity is reduced in dentate granule cells of Val66Met knock-in mice (Chen et al., 2006). Therefore, expression of this *BDNF* polymorphism might lead to deleterious effects on dendritic spine density and morphology.

The main limitation of BDNF-based therapies for neurological disorders, including RTT, is its poor blood-brain barrier permeability. Synthetic BDNF-loop mimetics with selective TrkB agonist activity are exciting alternatives (Massa et al., 2010; Kajiya et al., 2014). Indeed, systemic treatment with LM22A-4 rescues respiratory deficits in female *Mecp2* heterozygous mice (Schmid et al., 2012), and prevents spine loss in striatal medium-spiny neurons in a mouse model of Huntington's, rescuing their motor deficits (Simmons et al., 2013).

Other intriguing substitutes for BDNF are insulin-like growth factor-1 (IGF-1) and its active tripeptide ([1–3]IGF-1, also known as glypromate, GPE), a hormone widely expressed in the CNS during brain development that promotes neuronal survival as well as synaptic maturation (D'Ercole, 1996; O'Kusky et al., 2000; Tropea et al., 2009). Indeed, systemic treatment of male *Mecp2* KO mice with [1–3]IGF-1 significantly increased activity of signaling pathways downstream of TrkB and improved several RTT-like symptoms and increased dendritic spine density in cortical neurons (Tropea et al., 2009), effects that are all recapitulated by full-length IGF-1 (Castro et al., 2014). These effects are due to the activation of IGF-1 receptors directly by IGF-1, and indirectly by [1–3]IGF-1, which does not bind to the IGF-1 receptor but rather increases the expression of IGF-1 (Carlsson-Skwirut et al., 1989; Corvin et al., 2012). It should be noted that full-length IGF-1 worsened a metabolic syndrome in *Mecp2* KO mice, and did not affect dendritic spine density in hippocampal neurons (Pitcher et al., 2013). The safety and efficacy of recombinant human full-length IGF-1 (mecasermin) in a Phase-1 clinical trial in RTT individuals have been recently reported (Khwaja et al., 2014). The [1–3]IGF-1 analog glycyl-L-methylprolyl-L-glutamic acid (NNZ-2566; Neuren Pharmaceuticals) is in a Phase-2 clinical trial in RTT individuals.

CONCLUSION

Activity-dependent plasticity of dendritic spines includes both the formation of new spines and their maturation from thin, filipodia-like protrusions to "memory spines" that accompany excitatory synapse formation during brain development, as well as the structural remodeling of already existing spines. Alterations in neuronal circuitry are due to, or at least reflected by, deficits in dendritic spine structure and function. Dendritic spine anomalies have been identified in multiple brain regions in RTT and *Mecp2*-based mouse models. Since BDNF promotes the formation, maintenance, and activity-dependent sculpting of dendritic spines, and plays a critical role in neurological dysfunction in RTT, it emerges as one of the most exciting therapeutic agents for RTT. Thus, treatments that target the BDNF receptor TrkB and/or its downstream signaling pathways stand out as strong candidates to improve not only the spine dysgenesis phenotype, but also other synaptic plasticity deficits in RTT and other neurodevelopmental disorders caused by impaired BDNF availability.

ACKNOWLEDGMENTS

This work was supported by NIH grants NS-065027 and HD-074418 (to Lucas Pozzo-Miller). We are indebted to Chris Chapleau, Wei Li, and Mary Phillips for thoughtful discussions.

REFERENCES

Alonso, M., Medina, J. H., and Pozzo-Miller, L. (2004). ERK1/2 activation is necessary for BDNF to increase dendritic spine density in hippocampal CA1 pyramidal neurons. *Learn. Mem.* 11, 172–178. doi: 10.1101/lm.67804

Amaral, M. D., and Pozzo-Miller, L. (2007). TRPC3 channels are necessary for brain-derived neurotrophic factor to activate a nonselective cationic current and to induce dendritic spine formation. *J. Neurosci.* 27, 5179–5189. doi: 10.1523/JNEUROSCI.5499-06.2007

Amir, R. E., Van Den Veyver, I. B., Wan, M., Tran, C. Q., Francke, U., and Zoghbi, H. Y. (1999). Rett syndrome is caused by mutations in X-linked MECP2, encoding methyl-CpG-binding protein 2. *Nat. Genet.* 23, 185–188. doi: 10.1038/13810

Armstrong, D., Dunn, J. K., Antalffy, B., and Trivedi, R. (1995). Selective dendritic alterations in the cortex of Rett syndrome. *J. Neuropathol. Exp. Neurol.* 54, 195–201. doi: 10.1097/00005072-199503000-00006

Baj, G., Patrizio, A., Montalbano, A., Sciancalepore, M., and Tongiorgi, E. (2014). Developmental and maintenance defects in Rett syndrome neurons identified by a new mouse staging system in vitro. *Front. Cell. Neurosci.* 8:18. doi: 10.3389/fncel.2014.00018

Belichenko, P. V., Oldfors, A., Hagberg, B., and Dahlstrom, A. (1994). Rett syndrome: 3-D confocal microscopy of cortical pyramidal dendrites and afferents. *Neuroreport* 5, 1509–1513. doi: 10.1097/00001756-199407000-00025

Belichenko, P. V., Wright, E. E., Belichenko, N. P., Masliah, E., Li, H. H., Mobley, W. C., et al. (2009). Widespread changes in dendritic and axonal morphology in Mecp2-mutant mouse models of Rett syndrome: evidence for disruption of neuronal networks. *J. Comp. Neurol.* 514, 240–258. doi: 10.1002/cne.22009

Bhatt, D. H., Zhang, S., and Gan, W. B. (2009). Dendritic spine dynamics. *Annu. Rev. Physiol.* 71, 261–282. doi: 10.1146/annurev.physiol.010908.163140

Blackman, M. P., Djukic, B., Nelson, S. B., and Turrigiano, G. G. (2012). A critical and cell-autonomous role for MeCP2 in synaptic scaling up. *J. Neurosci.* 32, 13529–13536. doi: 10.1523/JNEUROSCI.3077-12.2012

Bloodgood, B. L., and Sabatini, B. L. (2007). Ca^{2+} signaling in dendritic spines. *Curr. Opin. Neurobiol.* 17, 345–351. doi: 10.1016/j.conb.2007.04.003

Bourgeron, T. (2009). A synaptic trek to autism. *Curr. Opin. Neurobiol.* 19, 231–234. doi: 10.1016/j.conb.2009.06.003

Calfa, G., Hablitz, J. J., and Pozzo-Miller, L. (2011a). Network hyperexcitability in hippocampal slices from Mecp2 mutant mice revealed by voltage-sensitive dye imaging. *J. Neurophysiol.* 105, 1768–1784. doi: 10.1152/jn.00800.2010

Calfa, G., Percy, A. K., and Pozzo-Miller, L. (2011b). Experimental models of Rett syndrome based on Mecp2 dysfunction. *Exp. Biol. Med. (Maywood)* 236, 3–19. doi: 10.1258/ebm.2010.010261

Carlsson-Skwirut, C., Lake, M., Hartmanis, M., Hall, K., and Sara, V. R. (1989). A comparison of the biological activity of the recombinant intact and truncated insulin-like growth factor 1 (IGF-1). *Biochim. Biophys. Acta* 1011, 192–197. doi: 10.1016/0167-4889(89)90209-7

Carvalho, A. L., Caldeira, M. V., Santos, S. D., and Duarte, C. B. (2008). Role of the brain-derived neurotrophic factor at glutamatergic synapses. *Br. J. Pharmacol.* 153(Suppl. 1), S310–S324. doi: 10.1038/sj.bjp.0707509

Castro, J., Garcia, R. I., Kwok, S., Banerjee, A., Petravicz, J., Woodson, J., et al. (2014). Functional recovery with recombinant human IGF1 treatment in a mouse model of Rett Syndrome. *Proc. Natl. Acad. Sci. U.S.A.* 111, 9941–9946. doi: 10.1073/pnas.1311685111

Chahrour, M., Jung, S. Y., Shaw, C., Zhou, X., Wong, S. T., Qin, J., et al. (2008). MeCP2, a key contributor to neurological disease, activates and represses transcription. *Science* 320, 1224–1229. doi: 10.1126/science.1153252

Chahrour, M., and Zoghbi, H. Y. (2007). The story of Rett syndrome: from clinic to neurobiology. *Neuron* 56, 422–437. doi: 10.1016/j.neuron.2007.10.001

Chang, Q., Khare, G., Dani, V., Nelson, S., and Jaenisch, R. (2006). The disease progression of Mecp2 mutant mice is affected by the level of BDNF expression. *Neuron* 49, 341–348. doi: 10.1016/j.neuron.2005.12.027

Chao, H. T., Zoghbi, H. Y., and Rosenmund, C. (2007). MeCP2 controls excitatory synaptic strength by regulating glutamatergic synapse number. *Neuron* 56, 58–65. doi: 10.1016/j.neuron.2007.08.018

Chapleau, C. A., Boggio, E. M., Calfa, G., Percy, A. K., Giustetto, M., and Pozzo-Miller, L. (2012). Hippocampal CA1 pyramidal neurons of Mecp2 mutant mice show a dendritic spine phenotype only in the presymptomatic stage. *Neural Plast.* 2012, 976164. doi: 10.1155/2012/976164

Chapleau, C. A., Calfa, G. D., Lane, M. C., Albertson, A. J., Larimore, J. L., Kudo, S., et al. (2009a). Dendritic spine pathologies in hippocampal pyramidal neurons from Rett syndrome brain and after expression of Rett-associated MECP2 mutations. *Neurobiol. Dis.* 35, 219–233. doi: 10.1016/j.nbd.2009.05.001

Chapleau, C. A., Larimore, J. L., Theibert, A., and Pozzo-Miller, L. (2009b). Modulation of dendritic spine development and plasticity by BDNF and vesicular trafficking: fundamental roles in neurodevelopmental disorders associated with mental retardation and autism. *J. Neurodev. Disord* 1, 185–196. doi: 10.1007/s11689-009-9027-6

Chapleau, C. A., Carlo, M. E., Larimore, J. L., and Pozzo-Miller, L. (2008). The actions of BDNF on dendritic spine density and morphology in organotypic slice cultures depend on the presence of serum in culture media. *J. Neurosci. Methods* 169, 182–190. doi: 10.1016/j.jneumeth.2007.12.006

Chen, R. Z., Akbarian, S., Tudor, M., and Jaenisch, R. (2001). Deficiency of methyl-CpG binding protein-2 in CNS neurons results in a Rett-like phenotype in mice. *Nat. Genet.* 27, 327–331. doi: 10.1038/85906

Chen, W. G., Chang, Q., Lin, Y., Meissner, A., West, A. E., Griffith, E. C., et al. (2003). Derepression of BDNF transcription involves calcium-dependent phosphorylation of MeCP2. *Science* 302, 885–889. doi: 10.1126/science.1086446

Chen, Z. Y., Jing, D., Bath, K. G., Ieraci, A., Khan, T., Siao, C. J., et al. (2006). Genetic variant BDNF (Val66Met) polymorphism alters anxiety-related behavior. *Science* 314, 140–143. doi: 10.1126/science.1129663

Chen, Z. Y., Patel, P. D., Sant, G., Meng, C. X., Teng, K. K., Hempstead, B. L., et al. (2004). Variant brain-derived neurotrophic factor (BDNF) (Met66) alters the intracellular trafficking and activity-dependent secretion of wild-type BDNF in neurosecretory cells and cortical neurons. *J. Neurosci.* 24, 4401–4411. doi: 10.1523/JNEUROSCI.0348-04.2004

Cheng, T. L., Wang, Z., Liao, Q., Zhu, Y., Zhou, W. H., Xu, W., et al. (2014). MeCP2 suppresses nuclear microRNA processing and dendritic growth by regulating the DGCR8/Drosha complex. *Dev. Cell* 28, 547–560. doi: 10.1016/j.devcel.2014.01.032

Cohen, D. R., Matarazzo, V., Palmer, A. M., Tu, Y., Jeon, O. H., Pevsner, J., et al. (2003). Expression of MeCP2 in olfactory receptor neurons is developmentally regulated and occurs before synaptogenesis. *Mol. Cell. Neurosci.* 22, 417–429. doi: 10.1016/S1044-7431(03)00026-5

Cohen-Cory, S., Kidane, A. H., Shirkey, N. J., and Marshak, S. (2010). Brain-derived neurotrophic factor and the development of structural neuronal connectivity. *Dev. Neurobiol.* 70, 271–288. doi: 10.1002/dneu.20774

Corvin, A. P., Molinos, I., Little, G., Donohoe, G., Gill, M., Morris, D. W., et al. (2012). Insulin-like growth factor 1 (IGF1) and its active peptide (1-3)IGF1 enhance the expression of synaptic markers in neuronal circuits through different cellular mechanisms. *Neurosci. Lett.* 520, 51–56. doi: 10.1016/j.neulet.2012.05.029

D'Ercole, A. J. (1996). Insulin-like growth factors and their receptors in growth. *Endocrinol. Metab. Clin. North. Am.* 25, 573–590. doi: 10.1016/S0889-8529(05)70341-8

Egan, M. F., Kojima, M., Callicott, J. H., Goldberg, T. E., Kolachana, B. S., Bertolino, A., et al. (2003). The BDNF val66met polymorphism affects activity-dependent secretion of BDNF and human memory and hippocampal function. *Cell* 112, 257–269. doi: 10.1016/S0092-8674(03)00035-7

Fiala, J. C., Feinberg, M., Popov, V., and Harris, K. M. (1998). Synaptogenesis via dendritic filopodia in developing hippocampal area CA1. *J. Neurosci.* 18, 8900–8911.

Fiala, J. C., Spacek, J., and Harris, K. M. (2002). Dendritic spine pathology: cause or consequence of neurological disorders? *Brain Res. Brain Res. Rev.* 39, 29–54. doi: 10.1016/S0165-0173(02)00158-3

Figurov, A., Pozzo-Miller, L. D., Olafsson, P., Wang, T., and Lu, B. (1996). Regulation of synaptic responses to high-frequency stimulation and LTP by neurotrophins in the hippocampus. *Nature* 381, 706–709. doi: 10.1038/381706a0

Fukuda, T., Itoh, M., Ichikawa, T., Washiyama, K., and Goto, Y. (2005). Delayed maturation of neuronal architecture and synaptogenesis in cerebral cortex of Mecp2-deficient mice. *J. Neuropathol. Exp. Neurol.* 64, 537–544.

Garey, L. (2010). When cortical development goes wrong: schizophrenia as a neurodevelopmental disease of microcircuits. *J. Anat.* 217, 324–333. doi: 10.1111/j.1469-7580.2010.01231.x

Grutzendler, J., Kasthuri, N., and Gan, W. B. (2002). Long-term dendritic spine stability in the adult cortex. *Nature* 420, 812–816. doi: 10.1038/nature01276

Guy, J., Hendrich, B., Holmes, M., Martin, J. E., and Bird, A. (2001). A mouse Mecp2-null mutation causes neurological symptoms that mimic Rett syndrome. *Nat. Genet.* 27, 322–326. doi: 10.1038/85899

Harris, K. M., and Stevens, J. K. (1989). Dendritic spines of CA 1 pyramidal cells in the rat hippocampus: serial electron microscopy with reference to their biophysical characteristics. *J. Neurosci.* 9, 2982–2997.

Holtmaat, A. J., Trachtenberg, J. T., Wilbrecht, L., Shepherd, G. M., Zhang, X., Knott, G. W., et al. (2005). Transient and persistent dendritic spines in the neocortex in vivo. *Neuron* 45, 279–291. doi: 10.1016/j.neuron.2005.01.003

Hoogenraad, C. C., and Akhmanova, A. (2010). Dendritic spine plasticity: new regulatory roles of dynamic microtubules. *Neuroscientist* 16, 650–661. doi: 10.1177/1073858410386357

Huang, E. J., and Reichardt, L. F. (2003). Trk receptors: roles in neuronal signal transduction. *Annu. Rev. Biochem.* 72, 609–642. doi: 10.1146/annurev.biochem.72.121801.161629

Huttenlocher, P. R. (1970). Dendritic development and mental defect. *Neurology* 20, 381.

Ji, Y., Pang, P. T., Feng, L., and Lu, B. (2005). Cyclic AMP controls BDNF-induced TrkB phosphorylation and dendritic spine formation in mature hippocampal neurons. *Nat. Neurosci.* 8, 164–172. doi: 10.1038/nn1381

Jiang, M., Ash, R. T., Baker, S. A., Suter, B., Ferguson, A., Park, J., et al. (2013). Dendritic arborization and spine dynamics are abnormal in the mouse model of MECP2 duplication syndrome. *J. Neurosci.* 33, 19518–19533. doi: 10.1523/JNEUROSCI.1745-13.2013

Jugloff, D. G., Jung, B. P., Purushotham, D., Logan, R., and Eubanks, J. H. (2005). Increased dendritic complexity and axonal length in cultured mouse cortical neurons overexpressing methyl-CpG-binding protein MeCP2. *Neurobiol. Dis.* 19, 18–27. doi: 10.1016/j.nbd.2004.11.002

Kajiya, M., Takeshita, K., Kittaka, M., Matsuda, S., Ouhara, K., Takeda, K., et al. (2014). BDNF mimetic compound LM22A-4 regulates cementoblast differentiation via the TrkB-ERK/Akt signaling cascade. *Int. Immunopharmacol.* 19, 245–252. doi: 10.1016/j.intimp.2014.01.028

Kasai, H., Fukuda, M., Watanabe, S., Hayashi-Takagi, A., and Noguchi, J. (2010). Structural dynamics of dendritic spines in memory and cognition. *Trends Neurosci.* 33, 121–129. doi: 10.1016/j.tins.2010.01.001

Kasai, H., Matsuzaki, M., Noguchi, J., Yasumatsu, N., and Nakahara, H. (2003). Structure-stability-function relationships of dendritic spines. *Trends Neurosci.* 26, 360–368. doi: 10.1016/S0166-2236(03)00162-0

Khwaja, O. S., Ho, E., Barnes, K. V., O'Leary, H. M., Pereira, L. M., Finkelstein, Y., et al. (2014). Safety, pharmacokinetics, and preliminary assessment of efficacy of mecasermin (recombinant human IGF-1) for the treatment of Rett syndrome. *Proc. Natl. Acad. Sci. U.S.A.* 111, 4596–4601. doi: 10.1073/pnas.1311141111

Kumar, V., Zhang, M. X., Swank, M. W., Kunz, J., and Wu, G. Y. (2005). Regulation of dendritic morphogenesis by Ras-PI3K-Akt-mTOR and Ras-MAPK signaling pathways. *J. Neurosci.* 25, 11288–11299. doi: 10.1523/JNEUROSCI.2284-05.2005

Landi, S., Putignano, E., Boggio, E. M., Giustetto, M., Pizzorusso, T., and Ratto, G. M. (2011). The short-time structural plasticity of dendritic spines is altered in a model of Rett syndrome. *Sci. Rep.* 1, 45. doi: 10.1038/srep00045

Larimore, J. L., Chapleau, C. A., Kudo, S., Theibert, A., Percy, A. K., and Pozzo-Miller, L. (2009). Bdnf overexpression in hippocampal neurons prevents dendritic atrophy caused by Rett-associated MECP2 mutations. *Neurobiol. Dis.* 34, 199–211. doi: 10.1016/J.Nbd.2008.12.011

Levenga, J., and Willemsen, R. (2012). Perturbation of dendritic protrusions in intellectual disability. *Prog. Brain Res.* 197, 153–168. doi: 10.1016/B978-0-444-54299-1.00008-X

Li, W., Calfa, G., Larimore, J., and Pozzo-Miller, L. (2012). Activity-dependent BDNF release and TRPC signaling is impaired in hippocampal neurons of Mecp2 mutant mice. *Proc. Natl. Acad. Sci. U.S.A.* 109, 17087–17092. doi: 10.1073/pnas.1205271109

Luebke, J. I., Weaver, C. M., Rocher, A. B., Rodriguez, A., Crimins, J. L., Dickstein, D. L., et al. (2010). Dendritic vulnerability in neurodegenerative disease: insights from analyses of cortical pyramidal neurons in transgenic mouse models. *Brain Struct. Funct.* 214, 181–199. doi: 10.1007/s00429-010-0244-242

Luine, V., and Frankfurt, M. (2013). Interactions between estradiol, BDNF and dendritic spines in promoting memory. *Neuroscience* 239, 34–45. doi: 10.1016/j.neuroscience.2012.10.019

Marchetto, M. C., Carromeu, C., Acab, A., Yu, D., Yeo, G. W., Mu, Y., et al. (2010). A model for neural development and treatment of Rett syndrome using human induced pluripotent stem cells. *Cell* 143, 527–539. doi: 10.1016/j.cell.2010.10.016

Marin-Padilla, M. (1972). Structural abnormalities of the cerebral cortex in human chromosomal aberrations: a Golgi study. *Brain Res.* 44, 625–629. doi: 10.1016/0006-8993(72)90324-1

Martinowich, K., Hattori, D., Wu, H., Fouse, S., He, F., Hu, Y., et al. (2003). DNA methylation-related chromatin remodeling in activity-dependent BDNF gene regulation. *Science* 302, 890–893. doi: 10.1126/science.1090842

Massa, S. M., Yang, T., Xie, Y., Shi, J., Bilgen, M., Joyce, J. N., et al. (2010). Small molecule BDNF mimetics activate TrkB signaling and prevent neuronal degeneration in rodents. *J. Clin. Invest.* 120, 1774–1785. doi: 10.1172/JCI41356

Matsuzaki, M., Ellis-Davies, G. C., Nemoto, T., Miyashita, Y., Iino, M., and Kasai, H. (2001). Dendritic spine geometry is critical for AMPA receptor expression in hippocampal CA1 pyramidal neurons. *Nat. Neurosci.* 4, 1086–1092. doi: 10.1038/nn736

Matsuzaki, M., Honkura, N., Ellis-Davies, G. C., and Kasai, H. (2004). Structural basis of long-term potentiation in single dendritic spines. *Nature* 429, 761–766. doi: 10.1038/nature02617

McGraw, C. M., Samaco, R. C., and Zoghbi, H. Y. (2011). Adult neural function requires MeCP2. *Science* 333, 186. doi: 10.1126/science.1206593

Mizrahi, A., Crowley, J. C., Shtoyerman, E., and Katz, L. C. (2004). High-resolution in vivo imaging of hippocampal dendrites and spines. *J. Neurosci.* 24, 3147–3151. doi: 10.1523/JNEUROSCI.5218-03.2004

Moretti, P., Levenson, J. M., Battaglia, F., Atkinson, R., Teague, R., Antalffy, B., et al. (2006). Learning and memory and synaptic plasticity are impaired in a mouse model of Rett syndrome. *J. Neurosci.* 26, 319–327. doi: 10.1523/JNEUROSCI.2623-05.2006

Murphy, D. D., and Segal, M. (1996). Regulation of dendritic spine density in cultured rat hippocampal neurons by steroid hormones. *J. Neurosci.* 16, 4059–4068.

Nagerl, U. V., Eberhorn, N., Cambridge, S. B., and Bonhoeffer, T. (2004). Bidirectional activity-dependent morphological plasticity in hippocampal neurons. *Neuron* 44, 759–767. doi: 10.1016/j.neuron.2004.11.016

Neul, J. L., and Zoghbi, H. Y. (2004). Rett syndrome: a prototypical neurodevelopmental disorder. *Neuroscientist* 10, 118–128. doi: 10.1177/1073858403260995

Nguyen, M. V., Du, F., Felice, C. A., Shan, X., Nigam, A., Mandel, G., et al. (2012). MeCP2 is critical for maintaining mature neuronal networks and global brain anatomy during late stages of postnatal brain development and in the mature adult brain. *J. Neurosci.* 32, 10021–10034. doi: 10.1523/JNEUROSCI.1316-12.2012

Nimchinsky, E. A., Sabatini, B. L., and Svoboda, K. (2002). Structure and function of dendritic spines. *Annu. Rev. Physiol.* 64, 313–353. doi: 10.1146/annurev.physiol.64.081501.
160008

Nusser, Z., Lujan, R., Laube, G., Roberts, J. D., Molnar, E., and Somogyi, P. (1998). Cell type and pathway dependence of synaptic AMPA receptor number and variability in the hippocampus. *Neuron* 21, 545–559. doi: 10.1016/S0896-6273(00)80565-6

Ogier, M., Wang, H., Hong, E., Wang, Q., Greenberg, M. E., and Katz, D. M. (2007). Brain-derived neurotrophic factor expression and respiratory function improve after ampakine treatment in a mouse model of Rett syndrome. *J. Neurosci.* 27, 10912–10917. doi: 10.1523/JNEUROSCI.1869-07.2007

O'Kusky, J. R., Ye, P., and D'Ercole, A. J. (2000). Insulin-like growth factor-I promotes neurogenesis and synaptogenesis in the hippocampal dentate gyrus during postnatal development. *J. Neurosci.* 20, 8435–8442.

Park, M., Salgado, J. M., Ostroff, L., Helton, T. D., Robinson, C. G., Harris, K. M., et al. (2006). Plasticity-induced growth of dendritic spines by exocytic trafficking from recycling endosomes. *Neuron* 52, 817–830. doi: 10.1016/j.neuron.2006.09.040

Penzes, P., Cahill, M. E., Jones, K. A., Vanleeuwen, J. E., and Woolfrey, K. M. (2011a). Dendritic spine pathology in neuropsychiatric disorders. *Nat. Neurosci.* 14, 285–293. doi: 10.1038/nn.2741

Penzes, P., Woolfrey, K. M., and Srivastava, D. P. (2011b). Epac2-mediated dendritic spine remodeling: implications for disease. *Mol. Cell. Neurosci.* 46, 368–380. doi: 10.1016/j.mcn.2010.11.008

Peters, A., and Kaiserman-Abramof, I. R. (1969). The small pyramidal neuron of the rat cerebral cortex. The synapses upon dendritic spines. *Z. Zellforsch. Mikrosk. Anat.* 100, 487–506. doi: 10.1007/BF00344370

Pitcher, M. R., Ward, C. S., Arvide, E. M., Chapleau, C. A., Pozzo-Miller, L., Hoeflich, A., et al. (2013). Insulinotropic treatments exacerbate metabolic syndrome in mice lacking MeCP2 function. *Hum. Mol. Genet.* 22, 2626–2633. doi: 10.1093/hmg/ddt111

Poo, M. M. (2001). Neurotrophins as synaptic modulators. *Nat. Rev. Neurosci.* 2, 24–32. doi: 10.1038/35049004

Purpura, D. P. (1974). Dendritic spine "dysgenesis" and mental retardation. *Science* 186, 1126–1128. doi: 10.1126/science.186.4169.1126

Qiu, Z., Sylwestrak, E. L., Lieberman, D. N., Zhang, Y., Liu, X. Y., and Ghosh, A. (2012). The Rett syndrome protein MeCP2 regulates synaptic scaling. *J. Neurosci.* 32, 989–994. doi: 10.1523/JNEUROSCI.0175-11.2012

Ramón y Cajal, S. (1888). Estructura de los centros nerviosos de las aves. *Rev. Trim. Histol. Norm. Pat.* 1, 1–10.

Ramón y Cajal, S. (1891a). Significación fisiológica de las expansiones protoplásmicas y nerviosas de la sustancia gris. *Rev. De Cienc. Med. De Barc.* 22, 23.

Ramón y Cajal, S. (1891b). Sur la structure de l'ecorce cerebrale de quelques mamiferes. *La Cellule* 7, 124–176.

Ramón y Cajal, S. (1894). La fine structure des centres nerveaux. the Croonian Lecture. *Proc. R. Soc. Lond.* 55, 443–468. doi: 10.1098/rspl.1894.0063

Ramón y Cajal, S. (1896). Les espines collaterales des cellules du cerveau colorees au bleu de methylene. *Rev. Trim. Microgr.* 1, 5–19.

Ramón y Cajal, S. (1933). *Neuronismo o Reticularismo? Las Pruebas Objetivas De La Unidad Anatómica De Las Celulas Nerviosas.* Madrid: Instituto Cajal.

Rochefort, N. L., and Konnerth, A. (2012). Dendritic spines: from structure to in vivo function. *EMBO Rep.* 13, 699–708. doi: 10.1038/embor.2012.102

Sala, C., and Segal, M. (2014). Dendritic spines: the locus of structural and functional plasticity. *Physiol. Rev.* 94, 141–188. doi: 10.1152/physrev.00012.2013

Schikorski, T., and Stevens, C. F. (1999). Quantitative fine-structural analysis of olfactory cortical synapses. *Proc. Natl. Acad. Sci. U.S.A.* 96, 4107–4112. doi: 10.1073/pnas.96.7.4107

Schmid, D. A., Yang, T., Ogier, M., Adams, I., Mirakhur, Y., Wang, Q., et al. (2012). A TrkB small molecule partial agonist rescues TrkB phosphorylation deficits and improves respiratory function in a mouse model of Rett syndrome. *J. Neurosci.* 32, 1803–1810. doi: 10.1523/JNEUROSCI.0865-11.2012

Segal, M. (2005). Dendritic spines and long-term plasticity. *Nat. Rev. Neurosci.* 6, 277–284. doi: 10.1038/nrn1649

Shahbazian, M., Young, J., Yuva-Paylor, L., Spencer, C., Antalffy, B., Noebels, J., et al. (2002). Mice with truncated MeCP2 recapitulate many Rett syndrome features and display hyperacetylation of histone H3. *Neuron* 35, 243–254. doi: 10.1016/S0896-6273(02)00768-7

Shirao, T., and Gonzalez-Billault, C. (2013). Actin filaments and microtubules in dendritic spines. *J. Neurochem.* 126, 155–164. doi: 10.1111/jnc.12313

Simmons, D. A., Belichenko, N. P., Yang, T., Condon, C., Monbureau, M., Shamloo, M., et al. (2013). A small molecule TrkB ligand reduces motor impairment and neuropathology in R6/2 and BACHD mouse models of Huntington's disease. *J. Neurosci.* 33, 18712–18727. doi: 10.1523/JNEUROSCI.1310-13.2013

Smrt, R. D., Eaves-Egenes, J., Barkho, B. Z., Santistevan, N. J., Zhao, C., Aimone, J. B., et al. (2007). Mecp2 deficiency leads to delayed maturation and altered gene expression in hippocampal neurons. *Neurobiol. Dis.* 27, 77–89. doi: 10.1016/j.nbd.2007.04.005

Srivastava, D. P., and Penzes, P. (2011). Rapid estradiol modulation of neuronal connectivity and its implications for disease. *Front. Endocrinol. (Lausanne)* 2:77. doi: 10.3389/fendo.2011.00077

Stuss, D. P., Boyd, J. D., Levin, D. B., and Delaney, K. R. (2012). MeCP2 mutation results in compartment-specific reductions in dendritic branching and spine density in layer 5 motor cortical neurons of YFP-H mice. *PLoS ONE* 7:e31896. doi: 10.1371/journal.pone.0031896

Tanaka, J., Horiike, Y., Matsuzaki, M., Miyazaki, T., Ellis-Davies, G. C., and Kasai, H. (2008). Protein synthesis and neurotrophin-dependent structural plasticity of single dendritic spines. *Science* 319, 1683–1687. doi: 10.1126/science.1152864

Trachtenberg, J. T., Chen, B. E., Knott, G. W., Feng, G., Sanes, J. R., Welker, E., et al. (2002). Long-term in vivo imaging of experience-dependent synaptic plasticity in adult cortex. *Nature* 420, 788–794. doi: 10.1038/nature01273

Tropea, D., Giacometti, E., Wilson, N. R., Beard, C., Mccurry, C., Fu, D. D., et al. (2009). Partial reversal of Rett Syndrome-like symptoms in MeCP2 mutant mice. *Proc. Natl. Acad. Sci. U.S.A.* 106, 2029–2034. doi: 10.1073/pnas.0812394106

Tyler, W. J., Alonso, M., Bramham, C. R., and Pozzo-Miller, L. D. (2002a). From acquisition to consolidation: on the role of brain-derived neurotrophic factor signalining in hippocampal-dependent learning. *Learn. Mem.* 9, 224–237. doi: 10.1101/lm.51202

Tyler, W. J., Perrett, S. P., and Pozzo-Miller, L. D. (2002b). The role of neurotrophins in neurotransmitter release. *Neuroscientist* 8, 524–531. doi: 10.1177/1073858402238511

Tyler, W. J., and Pozzo-Miller, L. D. (2001). BDNF enhances quantal neurotransmitter release and increases the number of docked vesicles at the active zones of hippocampal excitatory synapses. *J. Neurosci.* 21, 4249–4258.

Tyler, W. J., and Pozzo-Miller, L. (2003). Miniature synaptic transmission and BDNF modulate dendritic spine growth and form in rat CA1 neurones. *J. Physiol.* 553, 497–509. doi: 10.1113/jphysiol.2003.052639

Vigers, A. J., Amin, D. S., Talley-Farnham, T., Gorski, J. A., Xu, B., and Jones, K. R. (2012). Sustained expression of brain-derived neurotrophic factor is required for maintenance of dendritic spines and normal behavior. *Neuroscience* 212, 1–18. doi: 10.1016/j.neuroscience.2012.03.031

Wang, H., Chan, S. A., Ogier, M., Hellard, D., Wang, Q., Smith, C., et al. (2006). Dysregulation of brain-derived neurotrophic factor expression and neurosecretory function in Mecp2 null mice. *J. Neurosci.* 26, 10911–10915. doi: 10.1523/JNEUROSCI.1810-06.2006

Xu, X., Kozikowski, A. P., and Pozzo-Miller, L. (2014). A selective histone deacetylase-6 inhibitor improves BDNF trafficking in hippocampal neurons from Mecp2 knockout mice: implications for Rett syndrome. *Front. Cell. Neurosci.* 8:68. doi: 10.3389/fncel.2014.00068

Yuste, R. (2010). *Dendritic Spines.* Cambridge, MA: The MIT Press. doi: 10.7551/mitpress/9780262013505.001.0001

Yuste, R., and Bonhoeffer, T. (2001). Morphological changes in dendritic spines associated with long-term synaptic plasticity. *Annu. Rev. Neurosci.* 24, 1071–1089. doi: 10.1146/annurev.neuro.24.1.1071

Yuste, R., Majewska, A., and Holthoff, K. (2000). From form to function: calcium compartmentalization in dendritic spines. *Nat. Neurosci.* 3, 653–659. doi: 10.1038/76609

Zeev, B. B., Bebbington, A., Ho, G., Leonard, H., De Klerk, N., Gak, E., et al. (2009). The common BDNF polymorphism may be a modifier of disease severity in Rett syndrome. *Neurology* 72, 1242–1247. doi: 10.1212/01.wnl.0000345664.72220.6a

Zhao, X., Pak, C., Smrt, R. D., and Jin, P. (2007). Epigenetics and Neural developmental disorders: Washington DC, September 18 and 19, 2006. *Epigenetics* 2, 126–134. doi: 10.4161/epi.2.2.4236

Zheng, W. H., and Quirion, R. (2004). Comparative signaling pathways of insulin-like growth factor-1 and brain-derived neurotrophic factor in hippocampal neurons and the role of the PI3 kinase pathway in cell survival. *J. Neurochem.* 89, 844–852. doi: 10.1111/j.1471-4159.2004.02350.x

Zhou, Q., Homma, K. J., and Poo, M. M. (2004). Shrinkage of dendritic spines associated with long-term depression of hippocampal synapses. *Neuron* 44, 749–757. doi: 10.1016/j.neuron.2004.11.011

Zhou, Z., Hong, E. J., Cohen, S., Zhao, W. N., Ho, H. Y., Schmidt, L., et al. (2006). Brain-specific phosphorylation of MeCP2 regulates activity-dependent Bdnf transcription, dendritic growth, and spine maturation. *Neuron* 52, 255–269. doi: 10.1016/j.neuron.2006.09.037

7

The effects of postnatal exposure to low-dose bisphenol-A on activity-dependent plasticity in the mouse sensory cortex

Emily A. Kelly[1]*, Lisa A. Opanashuk[2] and Ania K. Majewska[1]*

[1] Department of Neurobiology and Anatomy, Center for Visual Science, School of Medicine and Dentistry, University of Rochester, Rochester, NY, USA
[2] Department of Environmental Medicine, University of Rochester, Rochester, NY, USA

Correspondence:
Ania K. Majewska and Emily A. Kelly, Department of Neurobiology and Anatomy, Center for Visual Science, School of Medicine and Dentistry, University of Rochester, 601 Elmwood Avenue, P.O. Box 603, Rochester, NY 14642, USA
e-mail: ania_majewska@urmc.rochester.edu; emily_kelly@urmc.rochester.edu

Bisphenol-A (BPA) is a monomer used in the production of polycarbonate plastics, epoxies and resins and is present in many common household objects ranging from water bottles, can linings, baby bottles, and dental resins. BPA exposure has been linked to numerous negative health effects throughout the body, although the mechanisms of BPA action on the developing brain are still poorly understood. In this study, we sought to investigate whether low dose BPA exposure during a developmental phase when brain connectivity is being organized can cause long-term deleterious effects on brain function and plasticity that outlast the BPA exposure. Lactating dams were orally exposed to 25 μg/kg/day of BPA (one half the U.S. Environmental Protection Agency's 50 μg/kg/day rodent dose reference) or vehicle alone from postnatal day (P)5 to P21. Pups exposed to BPA in their mother's milk exhibited deficits in activity-dependent plasticity in the visual cortex during the visual critical period (P28). To determine the possible mechanisms underlying BPA action, we used immunohistochemistry to examine histological markers known to impact cortical maturity and developmental plasticity and quantified cortical dendritic spine density, morphology, and dynamics. While we saw no changes in parvalbumin neuron density, myelin basic protein expression or microglial density in BPA-exposed animals, we observed increases in spine density on apical dendrites in cortical layer five neurons but no significant alterations in other morphological parameters. Taken together our results suggest that exposure to very low levels of BPA during a critical period of brain development can have profound consequences for the normal wiring of sensory circuits and their plasticity later in life.

Keywords: bisphenol-A, dendrite, spine, plasticity, ocular dominance, S1, V1

INTRODUCTION

There is growing public awareness of the possible health impact of exposure to environmental toxicants. One of the most ubiquitous of these is bisphenol-A (BPA), a monomer used in the production of consumer materials such as water and baby bottles (Brede et al., 2003), can linings (Kang et al., 2003), and dental sealants (Suzuki et al., 2000; Joskow et al., 2006). Processes such as heat and pH level shifts are sufficient to trigger BPA migration out of everyday household items and into the surrounding environment (Kang et al., 2003). Emerging evidence indicates that BPA exposure is detrimental to human health; nevertheless, governing bodies continue to debate the interpretation of scientific results. The U.S. Environmental Protection Agency (EPA) has calculated an acceptable daily exposure level that "is likely to be without an appreciable risk of deleterious effects during a lifetime" (U.S. Food and Drug Administration, 2010). However, numerous studies on BPA exposure have described adverse outcomes with much lower doses than the EPA standard (Itoh et al., 2012; Rochester, 2013; Szychowski and Wojtowicz, 2013).

Research on the risks of BPA has focused on the effects of prenatal exposure on the development of the reproductive system; but studies examining brain structure and function suggest widespread negative consequences. Interestingly, BPA exposure during perinatal, postnatal and even during adult periods results in adverse effects on brain processes (Richter et al., 2007) at BPA levels below the current accepted daily exposure level (Hajszan and Leranth, 2010), targeting such mechanisms as synaptogenesis, memory consolidation, and dendritic development. Indeed, BPA has been shown to influence synaptic plasticity in the hippocampus and prefrontal cortex (MacLusky et al., 2005; Eilam-Stock et al., 2012) where the synaptic interface (including the synaptic cleft and presynaptic active zone) have been affected (Xu et al., 2013b). However, our understanding of *how* BPA affects brain development and subsequent function is still in its infancy.

Here, we examine the long lasting effects of low dose BPA exposure during brain development on subsequent activity-dependent remodeling of neural circuits. We used intrinsic signal optical imaging to assess changes in ocular dominance plasticity (ODP) in mice exposed to low-dose BPA during an intense period of synaptogenesis (P5–P21). Our findings show that early BPA exposure results in an attenuation of ODP following 4-day monocular deprivation (4d MD). Our results suggest that even very low dose exposure to BPA during a period of intense synaptogenesis can alter normal development and lead to long lasting changes in the brain.

MATERIALS AND METHODS

ANIMALS

Animals were treated in strict accordance with the University of Rochester Committee on Animal Resources and the 2011 NIH Guide for the care and use of laboratory animals. Mice were group housed with food and water available *ad libitum* and were housed under a fixed 12-h light/dark cycle. To prevent any endogenous exposure to BPA, animals were housed in BPA free conditions (Howdeshell et al., 2003). C57BL6 mice (Charles River Laboratories, Wilmington, MA, USA) and mice expressing green fluorescent protein (GFP-M; Feng et al., 2000) were housed in polysulfone cages on alpha-dri paper bedding and fed a phytoestrogen-free diet (2020X; Harlan Laboratories Inc.; USA) and reverse osmosis filtered water. Only glass containers were used for sample preparation and all cages and containers were washed in fresh non-recirculated water. For brain harvesting, mice were anesthetized with sodium pentobarbital (150 mg/kg; i.p.) at P32 and perfused through the aortic arch with ice-cold phosphate-buffered saline [0.1 M PBS, 0.9% NaCl in 50 mM phosphate buffer (pH 7.4)] followed by 4% paraformaldehyde (PFA; in 0.1 M PBS, pH 7.4). Brains were post-fixed in 4% PFA for 2 h and transferred to an increasing gradient of sucrose (10, 20, 30% in ultra-pure water) at 4°C. Brains were sectioned coronally at a 50 μm thickness on a freezing, sliding microtome. Both female and male mice were included in the study. No significant differences were observed between sexes in any of the analyses and data from both sexes were pooled. See **Table 1** for all animal numbers.

BPA EXPOSURE

Animals were exposed to BPA at two different time points; during an early period of cortical development [*early exposure*; postnatal day (P)5–P21; No MD BPA-early, 4d MD BPA-early, No MD Oil-early, and 4d MD Oil-early; **Figure 1C**] and a later period of cortical development (*late exposure;* P24–P32; critical period for rodent visual cortical plasticity; 4d MD BPA-late; **Figure 1C**). For the *early exposure* paradigm, lactating mouse dams were fed a 0.1 *g* portion of a vanilla wafer cookie (Back to Nature Foods Company; Madison, WI, USA) containing either BPA (25 μg/kg body weight/day; Sigma Aldrich CAT# 239658) dissolved in tocopherol-stripped corn oil (Sigma Aldrich CAT# C8267) or corn oil alone and pipetted onto the cookie at approximately the same time each day. For the *late exposure* paradigm, cookies containing BPA or oil were fed directly to weaned mice. Thus both the ingested dose and the route of BPA delivery differed across the *early* vs. *late* exposure groups (mothers milk vs. direct consumption).

INTRINSIC SIGNAL OPTICAL IMAGING

To examine the extent of ODP after BPA exposure, mice were monocularly deprived for 4 days at the height of the critical

Table 1 | Animal and tissue used.

Experiment	Treatment	*n*	Sections/animal	Spines	Figure
Optical imaging	NoMD oil	4			1
	4dMD oil	6			1
	NoMD BPA	6			1
	4dMD BPA early	6			1
	4dMD BPA late	5			1
Parvalbumin	Oil	5	4		2
	BPA	11	4		2
Cortical thickness	Oil	5	4		2
	BPA	9	4		2
Myelin basic protein	Oil	5	6		3
	BPA	5	6		3
Dendritic spine density	Oil	6	3	230	4
	BPA	6	3	375	4
Dendritic spine morphology	Oil	6	3	230	5
	BPA	6	3	375	5
Dendritic spine dynamics	Oil	3		365	6
	BPA	3		331	6
Microglial density analysis	Oil	4	3		7
	BPA	5	3		7
Microglial markers	Oil	3	4		8
	BPA	3	4		8

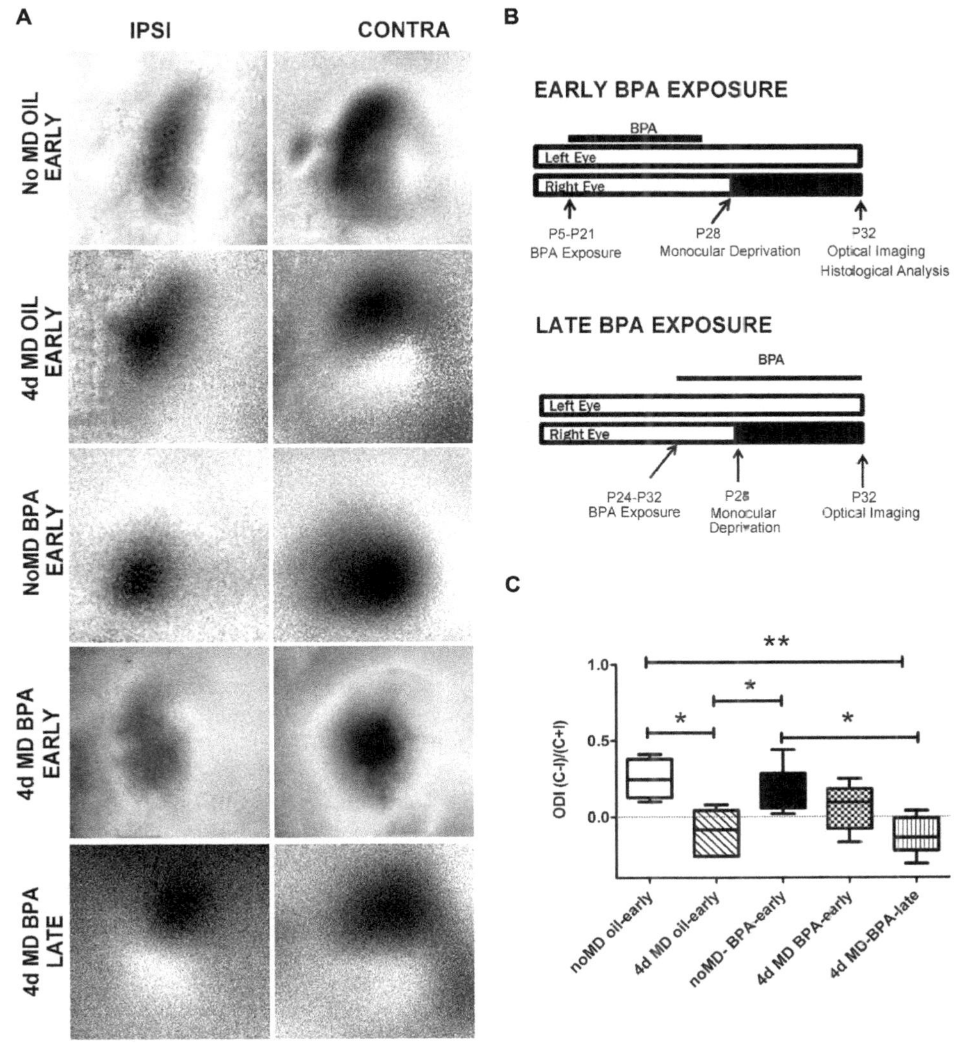

FIGURE 1 | Ocular dominance plasticity is attenuated in BPA-exposed mice. (A) Representative images of amplitude maps generated following intrinsic signal optical imaging (iOS). Non-deprived mice (No MD-early) showed an expected contralateral bias (strong contralateral amplitude when compared to ipsilateral amplitude; top panel). Following 4-days of monocular deprivation (4d MD-early), there was a shift in responsiveness toward the ipsilateral eye. NoMD BPA-early treated mice showed similar amplitude maps as NoMD Oil-early mice. Following 4d MD in early exposure BPA mice (4d MD BPA-early), maps retain a contralateral bias. A normal OD shift was observed after 4d MD in late exposure mice (4d MD BPA-late). **(B)** Treatment paradigms for *early exposure* (top schematic) and *late-exposure* BPA mice. **(C)** Ocular dominance index (ODI) results for BPA and Oil treated conditions. Values above 0 represent a contralateral ocular dominance bias (expected result in normal seeing mice). Values below 0 suggest an ipsilateral bias (expected result following monocular deprivation during the critical period). $*p < 0.05$; $**p < 0.01$.

period for cortical plasticity. Intrinsic signal optical imaging was performed using a DALSA 2M30 CCD camera (Kalatsky and Stryker, 2003). On P28 ± 2, lid margins were resected and lids sutured under isoflurane anesthesia (2–3%). After 4 days of MD, animals were anesthetized with isoflurane (2–3%) along with chlorprothixene (2 mg/kg) and the sutures removed for imaging. The skull over visual cortex was cleared, covered with agarose (1%) and a coverslip and illuminated with 700 nm light. Anesthetic level was maintained with isoflurane (0.75%) during imaging. An image of the vascular pattern was obtained through the skull by illumination with a green filter (550 nm). Intrinsic signal images were then captured using a red filter (700 nm). Visual stimuli consisting of white horizontal square-wave bars on a neutral background moving downward (270°) and upward (90°) for 6 min per run, were presented to each eye separately. The amplitude of the fast fourier transform component in the binocular visual cortex was analyzed offline using Matlab to determine ocular dominance (OD; Kalatsky and Stryker, 2003; Tropea et al., 2010). OD was compared between BPA exposed animals and oil exposed controls. An ocular dominance index (ODI) was calculated as (contralateral − ipsilateral)/(contralateral + ipsilateral) based on the average pixel intensities of the images obtained during visual stimulation of each eye. Positive ODI values indicate a contralateral bias; negative values indicate an ipsilateral bias.

IMMUNOHISTOCHEMISTRY

Fixed brain sections containing visual cortex were immersed in 0.1% sodium borohydride (in 0.1 M PBS) for 30 min at room temperature (RT), washed in 0.1 M PBS, and processed freely floating. Sections were blocked in a solution containing 0.5% bovine serum albuminin (BSA), 5% normal serum and 0.3% Triton-x for 2-h. Sections were then incubated for 24–48 h in either rabbit anti- Iba-1 [ionized calcium binding adaptor molecule-1; microglia- marker; 1:1000; Wako; (Imai et al., 1996)], or mouse anti-MBP [myelin basic protein (MBP); 1:1,000; Covance SMI-94]. Next, sections were incubated for 2-h in a solution containing either biotinylated goat anti-rabbit IgG or biotinylated goat anti-mouse IgG, respectively. Specific activity was detected using an ABC reagent (1:100; Vector Laboratories Inc, Burlington CA) and visualized with 3,3-diaminobenzidine (0.5 mg/ml) and hydrogen peroxide (0.03%) in buffer solution (DAB peroxidase kit; Vector Laboratories). Sections processed for fluorescent immunoreactivity were first preincubated in a blocking solution (as detailed above) and then incubated for 48-h in rabbit anti-parvalbumin [parvalbumin (PV);1:10,000; PA1-933; Affinity Bio Reagents], rat anti-MHC II (I-A/I-E; 1:5,000; Cat# 556999; BD Pharmingen), rabbit anti-Iba-1, or mouse anti-CD68 (ED-1; 1:800, ab31630; Abcam). Sections were washed in 0.1 M PBS and incubated for 2-h in a solution containing anti-rabbit Alexa 594 or 647 or anti-mouse Alexa 488 or anti-rat Alexa 488 (Invitrogen). Sections for light microscopy were mounted onto a microscope slide from a 1% gelatin solution (in 99% ethanol), dehydrated in ascending concentrations of ethanol, cleared in xylene and coverslipped with DPX mounting media (Electron Microscopy Sciences). Sections treated with immunofluorescence were coverslipped with Prolong Gold (Invitrogen) antifade media.

Epifluorescence microscopy images were taken on a BX51 Olympus scope at X 10 magnification (UPlanFL N; X 10/0.30; Olympus, Tokyo, Japan) and X 20 magnification (UPlanFL N; X 20/0.50; Olympus) mounted with a Spot Pursuit RT color digital camera (Diagnostic Instruments, Sterling Heights, MI, USA). Following image acquisition, images were analyzed using Image J software (freeware: http://rsb.info.nih.gov/ij/). For cell density analysis, all immunoreactive cell bodies were counted by hand, the cortical area was measured and densities were imported into Prism (Graphpad Software, Inc; La Jolla, CA, USA) for statistical analysis. For staining intensity analysis, the image was thresholded to encompass all immunoreactive regions. The intensity of pixels within the thresholded area was measured. To determine the laminar specific changes in MBP immunoreactivity, images were imported into Image J. Background intensity values were obtained from unstained portions of layer 1 within each image and subtracted from density averages obtained for each layer. Laminar densities were measured using the profile function of Image J as detailed by (McGee et al., 2005). Cortical thickness was assayed in sections from comparable rostro-caudal locations using the line tool in Image J.

DENDRITIC SPINE ANALYSIS

Green fluorescent protein-M mice were subject to *early exposure* of BPA or Oil as described above. Animals were perfused between P32 and P35. Brains were sectioned on a freezing sliding microtome to a 50 μm thickness. Sections were mounted out of a 0.1 M PBS solution and coverslipped with Prolong Gold (Invitrogen) antifade media. Confocal microscopy image acquisition and spine analysis was performed per (Bogart et al., 2011). Briefly, layers 2/3 within the primary somatosensory cortex (S1) were identified for imaging on a Zeiss LSM 510 confocal microscope (Care Zeiss, Thornwood, NY, USA). The distributions of imaged areas within S1 were similar between experimental conditions. GFP- labeled brain sections were excited at 488 nm and imaged through an HFT 514/633 dichroic and 530–600 nm band pass filter. Excitation power and settings for pinhole and detector gain were optimized to minimize photobleaching and utilize the full dynamic range of fluorophore emission intensity. High resolution (512 × 512 pixels) confocal image stacks of layer 5 apical dendritic branches located in layer 2/3 were collected using a 100x oil-immersion lens (NA 1.46), at a digital zoom factor 2 (pixel size 0.082 μm), and a z-step of 0.5 μm. Additional z-stacks were collected using lower power objectives to document the position of acquired images within the dendritic arbor stacks. Dendritic segments of the primary apical dendrite in layer 2/3 were located between 70 and 150 μm from the pial surface and were selected based on the quality of GFP expression and resulting signal-to-noise ratio, so that spines could be identified and measured as accurately as possible. Dendritic diameters were not statistically significantly different between groups (OIL: 1.65 ± 0.13 μm; BPA: 1.68 ± 0.13 μm; Student *t*-test; $p > 0.05$).

Following image acquisition, z-stacks were exported to TIF format using Zeiss's Axiovision software (release 4.6). Image analysis was then done using Image J. To quantify spine density, spines were identified by manually stepping through the z-stack, and definite spines were marked on the projected image. Specifically, only spines located in plane with their parent dendrite branch were marked and counted. Spines falling out of plane and those projecting from the parent dendritic branch in solely the z-dimension were systematically excluded from our counts even if they were visually identifiable as spines. Please note that for the purposes of this study we define spines as all visible dendritic protrusions and filopodia are included in the analysis. After all spines on a segment were marked, segment length was measured using the segmented line tool. 3D segment length was accounted for by measuring the absolute difference in depth between the two ends of the segment and using Pythagoras' theorem. Spine density was then computed as the number of spines per micron of dendrite. We also analyzed the dimensions of dendritic spines. Spine length was measured on maximum intensity projections using a segmented line tool to draw a line from the most distal point of the spine head to the base of the spine neck where it connects to the parent dendritic branch. Measurements of spine head and neck width were made based on fluorescence measurements. The fluorescence profile of a line placed along the center of the head and neck was determined and fit to Gaussian using custom-written algorithms in MATLAB (The MathWorks, Inc., Natick, MA, USA). The full-width half-max was taken as a measure of spine head width. This method may overestimate the size of small spines that fall under the limit of the resolution of our confocal microscope. The amplitude of the Gaussian fit to the spine neck fluorescence profile was normalized to the amplitude of the fit to the spine head profile as a relative measure of spine neck width. Background fluorescence was subtracted before fitting on a dendrite-by-dendrite basis. Great care was taken to avoid saturation in images, and saturated points were removed from the fluorescence profiles. Spines with more than two saturation points were removed from the analysis as it was determined that accurate fits were obtained if fewer than three points were omitted. This affected <2% of the population of spines.

TWO-PHOTON IMAGING AND DENDRITIC SPINE TURNOVER ANALYSIS

For two-photon imaging, mice were anesthetized with a fentanyl cocktail (fentanyl; 0.05 mg/kg of body weight; midazolam; 5 mg/kg; metatomadin; 0.5 mg/kg; i.p.); the skull was exposed, cleaned and glued to a thin metal plate. Primary somatosensory cortex (S1) was identified according to stereological coordinates. The skull above the imaged area was thinned with a dental drill. During surgery and imaging, the animal's temperature was kept constant with a heating pad and anesthesia was maintained with periodic administration of fentanyl. Imaging and data analysis were carried out as previously described (Majewska et al., 2006). A custom-made two-photon scanning microscope (Majewska et al., 2000) was employed, using a wavelength of 920 nm and a 20x 0.95 NA objective lens (Olympus, Melville, NY, USA) at 8.5x digital zoom. A map of the blood vessels was taken as a reference point. After image acquisition the animal's scalp was sutured and the animal was allowed to recover before being placed back in its home cage. Four days later, the animal was re-anesthetized and the skull re-exposed. The blood vessels map and dendritic architecture were used to identify the same imaging regions. Dendritic protrusions were identified as persistent if they were located within 0.5 μm laterally on the subsequent imaging session. Elimination and formation rates refer to the numbers of new spines and lost spines, respectively, observed on the second imaging time point divided by the total number of spines present in the first imaging session.

LIPOPOLYSACCHARIDE (LPS) CRANIAL INJECTIONS

As a positive control for microglial activations, we performed intracranial lipopolysaccharide (LPS) injections (Chugh et al., 2013) to induce focal inflammation in the brain ($n = 3$, C57B/6 mice, P32). Mice were anesthetized with a fentanyl cocktail (fentanyl; 0.05 mg/kg of body weight; midazolam; 5 mg/kg; metatomadin; 0.5 mg/kg; i.p.) and placed in a stereotaxic frame. The top of the head was swabbed with 70% ethanol and betadine before the skull was exposed. The surface of the skull was cleared and the injection coordinates (A/P −1.58, D/L +2.5) were calculated from bregma using The Mouse Brain atlas (Franklin and Paxinos, Third Edition). 2.5 mg/ml LPS (in saline, 1 ul total volume) was injected over 5 min in the left hemisphere. Following injections, the scalp was sutured and the animal was allowed to recover before being placed back in its home cage. Animals were sacrificed 24-h later (as described above) and the brains were harvested and sectioned for histological staining.

STATISTICAL ANALYSIS

Statistical analysis was performed using Prism (Graphpad Software, Inc; La Jolla, CA, USA). Significance was determined using two-tailed Mann Whitney test for comparison between two groups. For multi-group comparison, one-way ANOVA and Bonferroni *post hoc* test (for those data where the *p*-value of the ANOVA was <0.05) were performed to determine significance level. All data are reported as mean ± SEM.

RESULTS

OCULAR DOMINANCE PLASTICITY IS ATTENUATED IN MICE EXPOSED TO BPA EARLY IN DEVELOPMENT

While several studies have linked BPA exposure with changes in brain development and function, there is still a lack of understanding of how BPA exposure affects plastic processes that drive the remodeling of neural networks throughout life. We therefore set out to examine whether early life low-dose exposure to BPA would disrupt cortical synaptic plasticity. We chose to focus on a well described form of activity-dependent plasticity which is robustly elicited in the rodent binocular visual cortex following 4d MD during the visual critical period (Hubel and Wiesel, 1970). Under normal conditions (in the absence of visual manipulation; No MD Oil-early), the cortical response to visual stimulation of the contralateral eye is inherently higher than that of the ipsilateral eye resulting in a binocular response that is contralaterally biased (**Figure 1A**, No MD Oil-early). 4d MD during the visual critical period (~P28) results in a reduction of the response to visual stimulation of the now deprived contralateral eye and a subsequent increase in the response in the non-deprived ipsilateral eye (**Figure 1A**, 4d MD Oil-early). The resulting experience-dependent shift in responsiveness away from the contralateral eye is called ODP.

To determine how BPA exposure affects cortical synaptic plasticity, lactating dams were fed a vanilla cookie impregnated with either 25 μg/kg/day BPA or oil daily during the period that their pups were postnatal day 5 (P5) to P21. Animals had their contralateral eye monocular deprived on P28 and were assayed for ODP using intrinsic signal imaging on P32 (**Figure 1A**; No MD BPA-early, 4d MD BPA-early; **Figure 1B**, top panel). Notice that in this *early exposure paradigm*, the animals experience BPA during a developmental window which encompasses a period of rapid synaptogenesis and circuitry development, but that exposure ends a week before plasticity is induced.

To compare the difference in deprived and non-deprived eye responses across animals, an ODI was generated based on the response magnitudes obtained for each eye within the binocular visual cortex (**Figure 1C**; see methods). An ODI of −1 indicates that the animal's binocular zone responds only to stimulation of the ipsilateral eye, an ODI of +1 indicates responses to only the contralateral eye. An ODI of 0 would mean that the binocular zone responds equally to stimulation of the ipsilateral or contralateral eye. In normal development, MD elicits a shift from positive (contralaterally biased) toward negative ODI values indicative of ODP. Non-MD animals (no MD-oil early) imaged at P32 demonstrated a typical contralateral bias (**Figure 1C**, open bar). Consistent with previous findings, 4d MD resulted in a shift in OD toward the ipsilateral non-deprived eye in MD-oil control mice (**Figure 1C**, 4d MD Oil-early, diagonal filled bar). Results from animals treated with an early low-dose of BPA but not deprived were similar to control mice (**Figure 1C**, No MD BPA-early, solid bar). However, animals treated with BPA early during development (P5–P21), showed a reduced shift toward the ipsilateral eye following 4d MD which was not statistically significantly different from the ODI of non-MD animals (**Figure 1C**, 4d MD-BPA early checkerbox-filled bar), suggesting that ODP was impaired.

We therefore wondered if BPA could also affect plasticity acutely or whether its effects were limited to a specific developmental period. Therefore, we repeated the experiment in the *late exposure* group, where we sought to determine if exposing animals to BPA only during the critical period of visual cortical plasticity and development would have similar effects. Animals were fed vanilla cookies containing BPA or oil from P24-P32 and were assayed on P32 (**Figure 1B**, lower panel). In contrast to early exposure animals (4d MD-BPA-early), animals exposed to low-dose BPA during the critical period MD (4d MD-BPA-late), showed a significant shift in ODI indicative of normal ODP (**Figure 1C**, 4d MD-BPA-late, vertical line-filled bar). It is important to note however, that the doses were not the same for the early and late group due to the delivery route (lactation vs. direct ingestion, respectively). While this result may suggest that low dose exposure to BPA can affect the long term plasticity of the brain, but that its effects are limited to critical periods of brain development, more work is needed to fully understand how the dose and timing of BPA exposure affect plasticity.

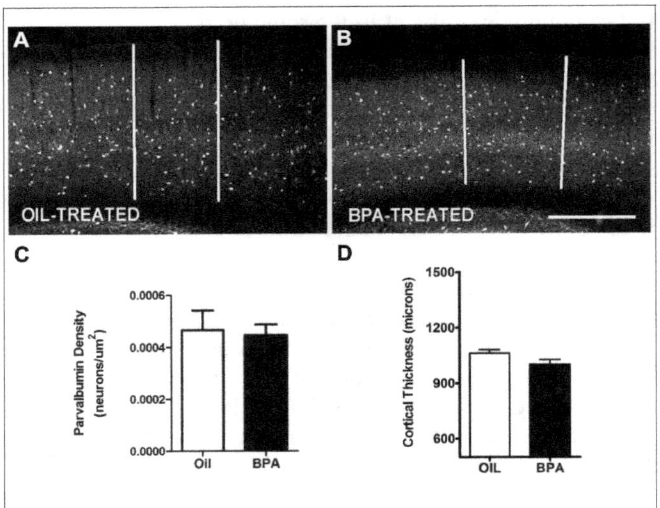

FIGURE 2 | Parvalbumin expression is unchanged in BPA exposed mice. Representative examples of anti-parvalbumin immunoreactivity in mice treated with oil **(A)** or low-dose BPA **(B)**. Notice that PV cells are distributed throughout the cortical layers. White vertical bars demarcate the binocular visual cortex, in the coronal plane, where measurements were taken. **(C)** Quantitative analysis of parvalbumin immuno-labeled cell density in the binocular visual cortex. **(D)** Cortical thickness measurement in oil-treated and BPA-treated mice. Scale bar = 200 μm.

PARVALBUMIN NEURON DENSITY AND MYELIN BASIC PROTEIN EXPRESSION ARE NOT AFFECTED BY BPA EXPOSURE

Ocular dominance plasticity requires the initial maturation of cortical circuitry and the regulated expression of specific cellular and network properties (Hensch, 2005). Both inhibitory neuron maturation and myelination play a considerable role in cortical development and are critical regulators of ODP. We sought to determine if low-dose BPA exposure during early development affects the maturation of cortical inhibitory networks and myelination which could in turn dampen plasticity during the visual critical period.

Parvalbumin is a calcium binding protein that co-localizes with GABAergic interneurons (Celio, 1986) and has previously been shown to be regulated during periods of synaptic plasticity (Cellerino et al., 1992). We performed immunofluorescent histochemistry and quantified anti-PV reactivity in the mouse visual cortex following *early exposure* to oil or low-dose BPA. PV-reactive cells were distributed in all cortical layers in both oil and BPA treated animals (**Figures 2A,B**). We found no statistically significant difference in PV cell density in binocular visual cortex between the two conditions (**Figure 2C**). Since cortical thickness can affect cell packing density and contribute to attenuation or inflation in cell counts, and BPA may affect overall brain development, we next sought to determine if cortical thickness was altered in BPA-treated mice. Comparable rostro-caudal regions of the visual cortex were measured in both the Oil-treated and BPA-treated mice. We found no significant differences in cortical thickness between the two groups (**Figure 2D**).

Myelin basic protein (MBP) is a compact myelin marker which is developmentally up-regulated in a layer specific manner. MBP up-regulation is thought to contribute to the closure (inhibition) of critical period plasticity in the rodent cortex (McGee et al., 2005). To determine whether MBP expression was regulated by early exposure to BPA, oil and BPA-exposed brain tissue was immunohistochemically stained with an antibody against MBP. Low magnification images showed dense myelin fiber staining in layer 6 of the visual cortex, which gradually declined in superficial layers in both experimental conditions (**Figure 3A**, oil-treated; **Figure 3B**, BPA-treated). Lamina-specific analysis of MBP immuno-reactivity showed no significant difference between experimental conditions across layers (**Figure 3C**; Oil-treated, open circles; BPA-treated, filled circles). As expected, MBP immunoreactivity was significantly denser in infragranular layers within experimental conditions, showing significantly more reactivity in Layers 4, 5, and 6 in both oil and BPA-treated animals. When all layers were pooled, we found no significant difference in anti-MBP immunoreactivity following BPA exposure (**Figure 3D**).

LOW-DOSE BPA EXPOSURE AFFECTS DENDRITIC SPINE DENSITY

Functional synaptic changes during plasticity are accompanied by structural changes at the level of the dendritic spine. We wondered whether low dose BPA exposure early in development affected the maturation of dendritic spines which could affect the implementation of later synaptic changes. To investigate the effects of low-dose BPA exposure on dendritic spine morphology, we used confocal microscopy to analyze fixed sections of somatosensory cortex from GFP-M animals which express GFP in subsets of cortical neurons (**Figures 4A–D**). Animals were treated with a low-dose of BPA from postnatal day 5 (P5) to P21 and sacrificed between P35 and P39 for microscopy analysis (**Figure 4E**). Primary apical dendritic branches of layer 5 cortical neurons residing in layer 2/3 were imaged at high magnification and dendritic spines were counted. Quantitative analysis

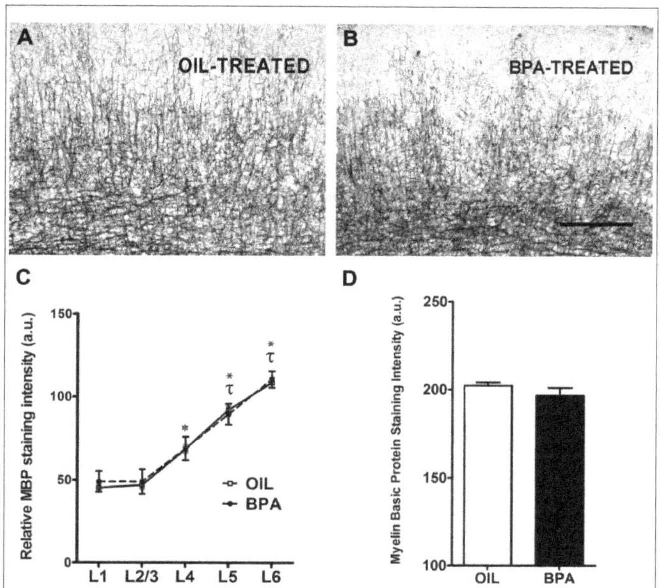

FIGURE 3 | Myelin basic protein expression is unchanged in BPA exposed mice. Representative examples of anti-myelin basic protein immunoreactivity in the binocular visual cortex of mice treated with oil **(A)** or low-dose BPA **(B)**. **(C)** Quantification of relative MBP staining intensity across cortical layers shows no significant differences across treatment conditions (Oil-treated, open circles; BPA-treated, closed circles). Asterisk denotes significance across layers *within* the oil-treated group. Specifically, layers 4–6 in the oil-treated groups were significantly different from their neighboring layers as well as from layers 1–3. Tau denotes significance across layers *within* the BPA-treated groups, where only layers 5–6 were significantly different from other layers. **(D)** Quantitative analysis of myelin basic protein immuno-staining intensity throughout all cortical layers. No significant differences were observed between BPA and oil treated animals. Scale bar = 100 μm.

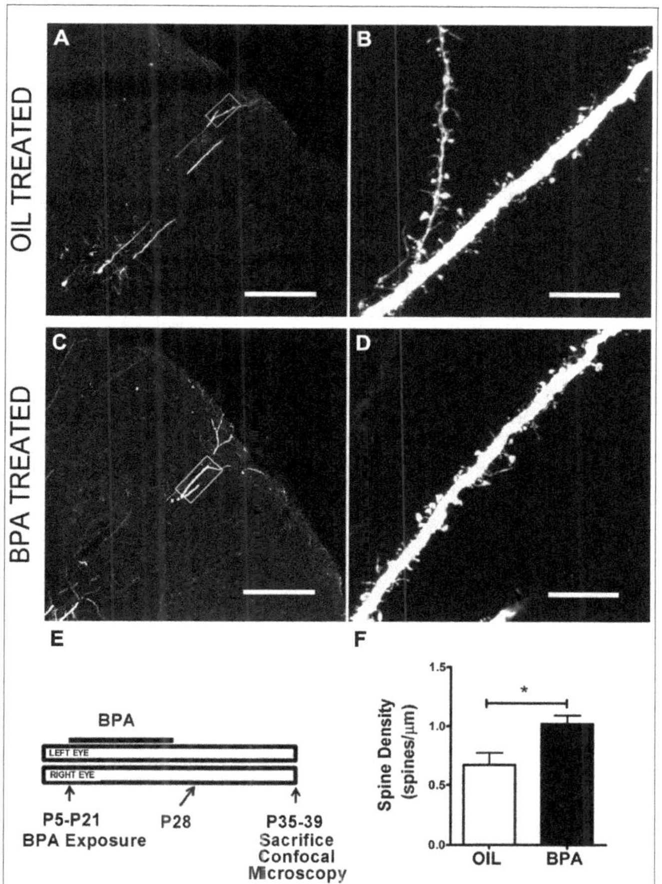

FIGURE 4 | Dendritic spine density is increased in BPA exposed mice. Confocal images showing representative examples of apical dendrites of layer 5 neurons in somatosensory cortex at low magnification following oil **(A)** and BPA treatment **(C)**. High magnification images of boxed regions in **(A)** and **(C)** showing distribution and qualitative appearance of dendritic spines in oil **(B)** and BPA treated animals **(D)**. **(E)** Schematic showing exposure parameters for BPA treatment. **(F)** Quantitative analysis showing that BPA exposure during the early postnatal period increases dendritic spine density on apical dendrites of layer 5 neurons (solid bar) relative to oil control (clear bar). $^*p < 0.05$. Scale bars: **A,C** = 200 μm; **B,D** = 10 μm.

showed a significant increase in dendritic spine density in animals treated with BPA, as compared to mice treated with oil (**Figure 4F**, oil = 0.667 spines/μm; BPA = 1.022 spines/μm; $p < 0.05$; Student's *t*-test).

Next, we sought to determine if BPA induced morphological changes in dendritic spines (**Figure 5A**). No significant differences in spine head diameter, spine length or relative neck diameter were found between oil and BPA-treated animals (**Figure 5B**). Comparison of spine morphological parameters can be used to determine the developmental profile of dendritic spines. For example, a high head:neck ratio would indicate a mushroom headed (mature) spine, while a low spine head:neck and spine length:head diameter might indicate a more immature phenotype. For both oil and BPA-treated animals, spines appeared to exist as a morphological continuum rather than fall into distinct morphological classes. Furthermore, the distribution of spine morphological parameters overlapped extensively between the two conditions, suggesting that the morphological distribution of dendritic spines in BPA-exposed animals is similar to that in controls (**Figure 5C**).

Increased dendritic spine density in BPA treated mice could result from increased formation of dendritic spines or a defect in spine elimination which is prominent during adolescence (Zuo et al., 2005). To determine whether the dynamics of spines were altered we imaged dendritic spines chronically in somatosensory cortex *in vivo* using two photon microscopy (**Figures 6A,B**). We found no change in either formation or elimination rates of dendritic spines over a period of 4 days at P28 (**Figure 6C**), suggesting that increased spine density in BPA-treated animals is established earlier in development and that early BPA treatment affects activity-dependent plasticity without affecting the basal dynamic turnover of dendritic spines during adolescence.

MICROGLIAL DENSITY IS NOT AFFECTED BY EARLY BPA EXPOSURE

Given the changes we observed in dendritic spine density, we sought to investigate the potential effects on microglia distribution following low-dose BPA exposure. Microglia are the

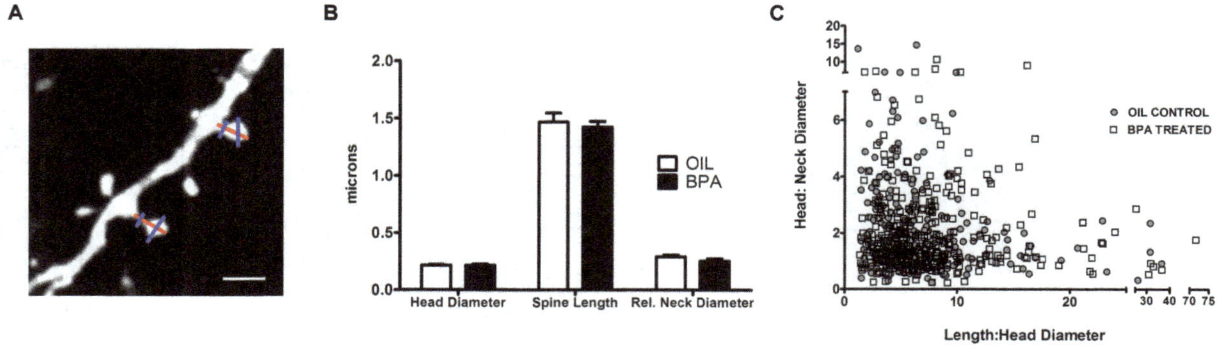

FIGURE 5 | Quantitative analysis of dendritic spine morphological changes in BPA exposed mice. (A) A representative high magnification confocal image of dendritic spines on apical dendrites of layer 5 neurons. Lines indicated measurements of dendritic spine parameters. Spine Length measurements (tip of the spine to its base at the dendrite, red line); Spine head diameter (measured at the widest point of spine, blue line) and relative neck width (blue line across neck). Scale bar = 2.5 μm. **(B)** Morphological measurements of dendritic spines, including spine head diameter, spine length and relative neck diameter, were similar for oil treated (clear bar) vs. BPA treated (solid bar) mice. **(C)** Spines can be loosely classified into morphological "types" by comparing their relative head, neck, and length dimensions. The complete overlap of spines from the two conditions indicates that BPA exposure does not elicit a change in spine type distribution (oil = filled in circle, BPA = open square).

resident immune cells of the brain and have been implicated in synaptic regulation (Trapp et al., 2007; Perry and O'Connor, 2010; Kettenmann et al., 2013). Previous reports show an effect of low-dose BPA or bisphenol AF (BPAF) exposure on glia, specifically GFAP-positive astrocytes (Yamaguchi et al., 2006; Kunz et al., 2011; Iwasaki et al., 2013) and microglia (Lee et al., 2013). Following low-dose BPA (or oil) exposure, brain tissue was stained with anti-Iba-1, an antibody that specifically labels microglia. Low mag images were collected (**Figures 7A,B**) showing densely labeled cell bodies and fine microglial processes. Quantitative analysis of microglial density was performed in the primary visual cortex. We found no significant difference in microglial density between animals treated with low-dose BPA and animals treated with oil (**Figure 7C**).

While both oil and BPA-exposed mice exhibited microglia that appeared to have a resting, ramified morphology, we wanted to determine whether BPA-exposure results in long lasting microglial activation. Using double-immunofluorescent reactivity, we tested the expression pattern of several microglial activation-state markers, including: the cell-surface activation molecule, MHC-II (major histocompatibility complex, type II), and CD68 (a glycoprotein involved in phagocytosis; ED-1). All of these markers were expressed in tissue from animals that had received intracranial injections of LPS, especially around the injection site, where these markers co-localized with Iba-1 (**Figures 8A–D**). In contrast, none of the markers were expressed in oil or BPA-treated tissue (**Figures 8E–L**) suggesting that early BPA exposure does not result in long lasting microglial activation.

DISCUSSION

The goal of our study was to investigate the consequences of chronic low-dose BPA exposure (one half of the U.S. EPA's rodent reference dose) during postnatal development (Richter et al., 2007), a critical period when the brain is highly plastic and is thus extremely vulnerable to environmental insults. Exposure during this period has not been well studied despite the fact that childhood is typically the period when human exposures are greatest (Mielke and Gundert-Remy, 2009; Groff, 2010; von Goetz et al., 2010) and also when cortical circuitry is undergoing its greatest experience-dependent refinement. To address this issue, we used MD, a model of neuronal plasticity, which shares many common mechanisms with learning and memory. For binocular mammals reared in a normal visual environment, the majority of neurons in binocular visual cortex respond to stimulation of either eye. If, however, one eye is temporarily deprived of visual input, there is a loss in binocularity and a decrease in the number of cortical neurons in binocular visual cortex responding to vision through that eye. The resulting *OD shift* toward the non-deprived eye has been well documented (Wiesel and Hubel, 1963a,b; Gordon and Stryker, 1996) and is coincident with structural events underlying experience-dependent circuit refinement; including reorganization of cortical circuitry, cell and structural changes, and regulation of important subsets of proteins that regulate synaptic strength (Hensch, 2005). We have shown that mice exposed to low-dose BPA early in development have impaired ODP during the visual critical period when compared to control animals. This effect is not driven by developmental regulation of PV-expressing neurons or MBP levels by BPA exposure and may instead be mediated by altered development of excitatory synapses. The attenuation in ODP was not seen in animals treated within the critical window of visual development (*late exposure*), suggesting that BPA's effects on cortical plasticity may be limited to a specific period of early development.

LONG TERM EFFECTS OF DEVELOPMENTAL BPA EXPOSURE

Experience dependent plasticity of cortical synapses is critically important for functional development and for the remodeling of neuronal networks throughout life. Our finding that BPA exposure can reduce the activity-dependent shift in OD

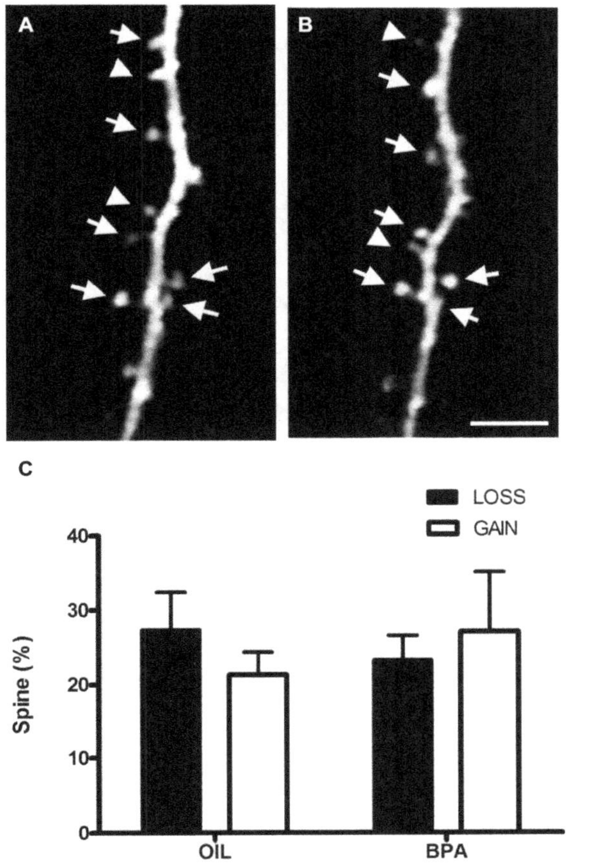

FIGURE 6 | Bisphenol-A exposure does not alter dendritic spine dynamics. *In vivo* two-photon images of the same dendritic section taken 4 days apart [Day 0 **(A)**; Day 4 **(B)**] in the somatosensory cortex of a BPA treated mouse. Stable spines are marked with arrows. Arrowheads at Day 0 mark spines that will be eliminated and at Day 4 they mark newly formed spines. **(C)** Quantitative analysis of spine formation and elimination in oil and BPA-treated animals. No significant differences between conditions were observed. Scale bar = 5 μm.

during the visual critical period suggests that BPA can have profound effects on plastic processes within the brain. All the more importantly, ODP plasticity was not induced until 7 days after BPA exposure was discontinued, suggesting that short exposure to BPA during a specific developmental period can have long-lasting effects on the brain. While ODP is a sensory-induced plasticity, similar underlying mechanisms govern learning and memory storage throughout the brain and throughout life (Tropea et al., 2009b; Sur et al., 2013). Additionally, ODP is affected in mouse models of neurodevelopmental disorders (Dolen et al., 2007; Tropea et al., 2009a) suggesting that deficits in ODP may reflect more generalized defects in activity-dependent brain rewiring.

One possible explanation for the effects of BPA on ODP is that BPA may delay or accelerate the development of cortical circuits, making them unable to undergo activity-dependent remodeling during the normal visual critical period (Hensch, 2005) To examine this possibility we investigated two prominent features of cortical development that are known to play an important role in regulating the plastic state of visual cortical circuits.

Inhibition is critical in regulating cortical activity and the excitatory to inhibitory balance is carefully adjusted throughout development and adulthood (Desai et al., 2002). Inhibitory connections generally mature later than their excitatory counterparts (Long et al., 2005), and a specific level of inhibition is permissive for plasticity and opens the critical period for ODP. Conversely, as inhibition continues to mature during the visual critical period, its higher levels inhibit plasticity and close the critical period (Hensch, 2005). Inhibitory neurons, however, are remarkably diverse and show stereotyped and specific connectivity within the cortex. It is becoming clear that PV-expressing neurons are particularly important in opening and closing the visual critical period (Sugiyama et al., 2008; Tropea et al., 2009b). We did not observe a change in PV neuron density in the binocular visual cortex after BPA treatment suggesting that PV cells develop normally and that this pathway is not responsible for the reduction in plasticity elicited by BPA.

Another important determinant of cortical maturity that is inhibitory for plasticity is myelination. Myelination matures during the visual critical period, in a layer specific manner, and limits plasticity by signaling through its receptors which are highly distributed throughout the cortex (McGee et al., 2005). This is analogous to myelin's role in inhibiting recovery after damage in the CNS (Bregman et al., 1995). However, we also found no evidence of a change in MBP distribution in the visual cortex after BPA treatment, suggesting that myelination is not a target of BPA and does not contribute to deficits in ODP after early BPA treatment.

THE EFFECT OF BPA ON DENDRITIC SPINES

The lack of changes in important regulators of ODP and cortical maturity, led us to examine the excitatory connections between cortical neurons. Dendritic spines are synaptic compartments whose dynamic behavior is tightly linked to circuit plasticity (Mataga et al., 2004). They receive the synaptic inputs from efferent axons, experience rapid and dramatic changes in density and morphological dynamics during the induction of longer term potentiation and depression (Dunaevsky et al., 1999; Bhatt et al., 2009), as well as during ODP (Hofer et al., 2009). BPA has been found to affect spines, although in a complex manner. Some studies report that administration of BPA alone results in increased spine numbers in the hippocampal CA1 field (Ogiue-Ikeda et al., 2008) while co-administration of BPA and estrogen attenuates increased spine density in rat hippocampus (MacLusky et al., 2005) and prefrontal cortex (Leranth et al., 2008). BPA's effects on spine density are dependent on timing of exposure (Elsworth et al., 2013) and other studies report decreases in spine density after BPA treatment (Eilam-Stock et al., 2012; Elsworth et al., 2013; Bowman et al., 2014). Our results support the idea that BPA affects dendritic spine morphogenesis, as we observed increased dendritic spine density in the somatosensory cortex of BPA-exposed mice. While we were not able to assess dendritic spines in visual cortex due to the low expression of GFP in this brain area at these

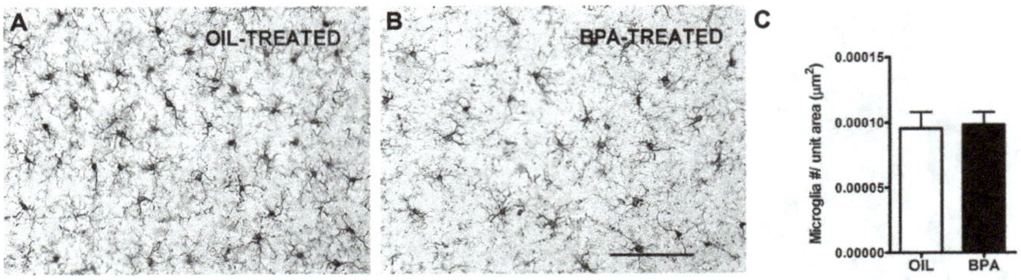

FIGURE 7 | Microglial density is unchanged in BPA exposed mice. Representative images showing microglia labeled using Anti-Iba1 immunoreactivity in mice treated with oil **(A)** or low-dose BPA **(B)**. **(C)** Quantitative analysis of Iba1-labeled cell density throughout the cortical layers of visual cortex demonstrates no change in microglial density following BPA exposure. Scale bar = 100 μm.

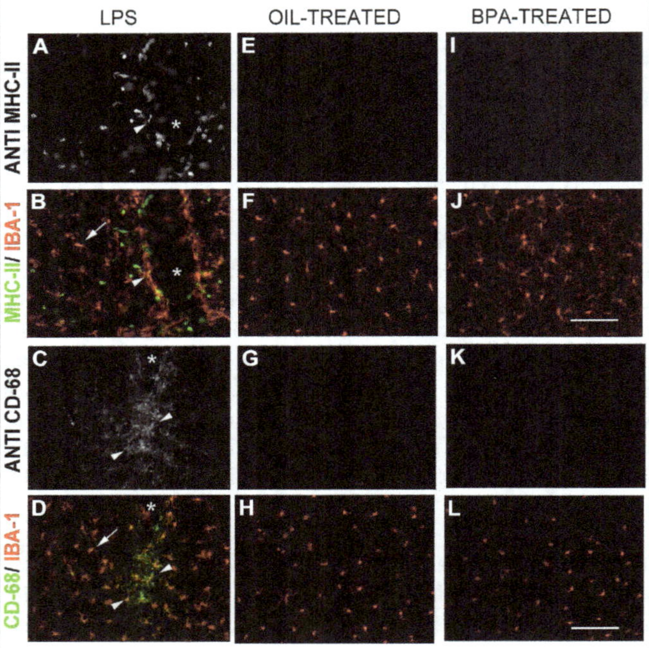

FIGURE 8 | Bisphenol-A exposure does not result in long lasting microglial activation. Immunofluorescent reactivity of microglial activation state markers following intracranial LPS injections **(A–D)**, Oil **(E–H)**, and BPA treatment **(I–L)**. Notice that MHC II **(A,B)** and CD68 **(I–L)** are robustly expressed around the injection site in LPS treated tissue and show some co-localization with Iba-1. These markers are absent in oil and BPA-treated tissue. Arrows denote ramified microglia; arrowheads denote co-labeled (activated) microglia. Scale bar = 100 μm.

early ages, developmental timelines of spinogenesis are similar across primary sensory areas (Elston and Fujita, 2014). The fact that increased spine density after BPA treatment has been reported in different brain areas and different neuronal classes (MacLusky et al., 2005; Xu et al., 2010, 2013b; Eilam-Stock et al., 2012), also suggests that BPA has a widespread effect on the development of brain circuitry. If initial circuit development is altered during the time of BPA exposure, this may affect future plastic processes by altering the excitatory/inhibitory ratio or by altering the flow of information throughout the brain. Additionally, BPA may differentially regulate different periods of dendritic spine and circuit development. Dendritic spine density is known to increase during development during early periods of spinogenesis. Excess and inappropriate connections are then pruned, although the extent of pruning differs between cortical area and between species (Elston et al., 2009, 2010, 2011; Bianchi et al., 2013; Elston and Fujita, 2014). Whether BPA affects synaptogenesis by inducing the outgrowth of inappropriate synapses, or whether it interferes with normal pruning processes that occur during this period of development remains to be explored, although our experiments indicate that BPA does not have a lasting effect on basal spine dynamics.

Increased density of dendritic spines after BPA treatment may reflect altered neuronal activity during cortical development. Early studies showed that visual deprivation decreases spine density in visual cortex and delays the maturation of circuits (Valverde, 1967, 1968). Similar changes occur in the adult somatosensory cortex after deprivation (Kossut, 1998). Thus BPA may alter firing patterns or developmental maturation of cortical pyramidal neurons. It is important to note that we did not observe changes in dendritic spine morphology after BPA treatment. Synaptic morphology is tightly linked with synaptic strength and function (Arellano et al., 2007), suggesting that BPA increases cortical interconnectivity without affecting the maturation and strength of individual synapses. This agrees with our data on PV and MBP expression in the visual cortex and further supports the conclusion that BPA does not delay or accelerate cortical maturation. However, synaptic strength on single neurons is usually tightly regulated by homeostatic processes, whereby if more synapses are made, all synapses are weakened to ensure an optimal level of activity in single neurons (Turrigiano and Nelson, 2004). An increase in synaptic density without a concomitant decrease in synaptic strength may indicate a dysregulation of homeostatic processes by BPA (Xu et al., 2013a,b, 2014). As a caveat, it should be noted that in our study we did not attempt to quantify changes in the complexity of the dendritic tree of pyramidal neurons after BPA treatment, because of the difficulty of getting complete dendritic arbors in thin fixed sections (Elston et al., 2001). Dendritic development is also complex and the way dendritic tree size and branching change with age varies widely between brain areas and species (Benavides-Piccione et al., 2006; Elston et al., 2009, 2010, 2011; Bianchi et al., 2013; Elston and Fujita, 2014). If BPA alters the timing or extent of dendritic outgrowth or pruning, this could greatly change the total number of spines and synapses on each individual neuron in a way that is not directly related to dendritic spine density, and may also have profound effects on the response properties of these neurons (Elston and Fujita, 2014). In fact, BPA has been shown to promote dendritic outgrowth in culture (Xu et al., 2010, 2014). Further studies exploring how BPA affects dendritic arbor development in cortical neurons *in vivo* will be needed to get a full picture of how BPA affects synaptic development in sensory cortices.

BPA EXPOSURE AND HUMAN HEALTH

Bisphenol-A exposure in humans is generally considered to be lifelong, low and constant, coming mostly from food and beverages but also from the handling of paper receipts, and dust (Vandenberg et al., 2007; Biedermann et al., 2010; Lakind and Naiman, 2011). However, many toxicants are multipotent and can have different effects depending on when they are administered. In this study we attempted to tease out the effects of BPA in a specific developmental period – a time that spans the third trimester and the first years of human life (P5–P21 in mice). This is a period of particular growth in the brain, when neural connections are rapidly made and remodeled. It is also a time when children are at particular risk for BPA exposure through baby bottles and many objects they put in their mouth. We reasoned that this could be a time of particular sensitivity to BPA exposure. Indeed we found a significant decrement in plasticity after BPA exposure during this time period but not acutely, if BPA was administered during the visual critical period when plasticity was assayed. Although it is important to note that the duration and route of exposure, as well as the dose were not uniform in these two experiments, our results may suggest that BPA exposure has its own "critical period" in terms of its long term effects on the activity-dependent remodeling of neuronal circuits, and that the period of late pregnancy and early childhood may be a period of increased sensitivity of the brain to BPA exposure.

The looming question remains of whether effects of BPA exposure observed in rodents can be generalized to humans. The consequences of BPA exposure on human health remain controversial (Vandenberg et al., 2007; Goodman et al., 2009; Beronius et al., 2010). While several studies have reported a negative health impact of exposure in rodents (Howdeshell et al., 1999; Vandenberg et al., 2007; Adewale et al., 2009; Cabaton et al., 2011) others have reported no effect at all (Howdeshell et al., 1999; Tyl et al., 2002, 2008; Ryan et al., 2010). Additionally, experimental variables for the exposure methods – dose, route of administration, diet are factors that widely vary across studies (Thigpen et al., 2007; Vandenberg et al., 2007; Goodman et al., 2009; Myers et al., 2009; Beronius et al., 2010) further challenging extrapolation of rodent studies to human health. It is important to note that in the early exposure paradigm in our study pups received BPA lactationally as only the dams were treated with BPA. The pups therefore received a very small daily amount of BPA because the dams ingested one half of the U.S. EPA's rodent reference dose, and lactational transfer is limited (Doerge et al., 2010). A number of studies have now suggested that BPA's effects on the body are non-linear with low doses having disproportionally large effects (Beausoleil et al., 2013; Liang et al., 2014). This further complicates our understanding of how BPA may affect human health but underscores the need to understand the effects of doses smaller than those deemed safe by the EPA.

In this study, we set out to look at the question of whether childhood exposure to daily, low levels of BPA could interfere with normal development of neuronal connectivity. What we found suggests that, in fact, it can; in a profound way; even after exposure has ended. More work is needed to determine the mechanisms by which BPA effects brain development.

ACKNOWLEDGMENTS

We are particularly grateful to Cynthia Rittenhouse for project planning, data collection, analysis, intellectual contribution and manuscript preparation. We thank Jenny Mosier, Manpreet Brar, Cassandra Lamantia, Nicole Zwald and Kristiana Lachiusa for their assistance in animal treatment, data collection and analysis. We thank Jianhua Cang for sharing Matlab code for OD analysis. This work was supported by the National Institutes of Health (NIH) grants EY019277 (Ania K. Majewska), T32 ES 7026-34 and EY013319 (Emily A. Kelly), and P30 ES001247 (pilot award to Ania K. Majewska and Lisa A. Opanashuk).

REFERENCES

Adewale, H. B., Jefferson, W. N., Newbold, R. R., and Patisaul, H. B. (2009). Neonatal bisphenol-a exposure alters rat reproductive development and ovarian morphology without impairing activation of gonadotropin-releasing hormone neurons. *Biol. Reprod.* 81, 690–699. doi: 10.1095/biolreprod.109.078261

Arellano, J. I., Benavides-Piccione, R., Defelipe, J., and Yuste, R. (2007). Ultrastructure of dendritic spines: correlation between synaptic and spine morphologies. *Front. Neurosci.* 1:131–143. doi: 10.3389/neuro.01.1.1.010.2007

Beausoleil, C., Ormsby, J. N., Gies, A., Hass, U., Heindel, J. J., Holmer, M. L., et al. (2013). Low dose effects and non-monotonic dose responses for endocrine active chemicals: science to practice workshop: workshop summary. *Chemosphere* 93, 847–856. doi: 10.1016/j.chemosphere.2013.06.043

Benavides-Piccione, R., Hamzei-Sichani, F., Ballesteros-Yanez, I., Defelipe, J., and Yuste, R. (2006). Dendritic size of pyramidal neurons differs among mouse cortical regions. *Cereb. Cortex* 16, 990–1001. doi: 10.1093/cercor/bhj041

Beronius, A., Ruden, C., Hakansson, H., and Hanberg, A. (2010). Risk to all or none? A comparative analysis of controversies in the health risk assessment of Bisphenol A. *Reprod. Toxicol.* 29, 132–146. doi: 10.1016/j.reprotox.2009.11.007

Bhatt, D. H., Zhang, S., and Gan, W. B. (2009). Dendritic spine dynamics. *Annu. Rev. Physiol.* 71, 261–282. doi: 10.1146/annurev.physiol.010908.163140

Bianchi, S., Stimpson, C. D., Duka, T., Larsen, M. D., Janssen, W. G., Collins, Z., et al. (2013). Synaptogenesis and development of pyramidal neuron dendritic morphology in the chimpanzee neocortex resembles humans. *Proc. Natl. Acad. Sci. U.S.A.* 110(Suppl. 2), 10395–10401. doi: 10.1073/pnas.1301224110

Biedermann, S., Tschudin, P., and Grob, K. (2010). Transfer of bisphenol A from thermal printer paper to the skin. *Anal. Bioanal. Chem.* 398, 571–576. doi: 10.1007/s00216-010-3936-9

Bogart, L. J., Levy, A. D., Gladstone, M., Allen, P. D., Zettel, M., Ison, J. R., et al. (2011). Loss of prestin does not alter the development of auditory cortical dendritic spines. *Neural Plast.* 2011, 305621. doi: 10.1155/2011/305621

Bowman, R. E., Luine, V., Khandaker, H., Villafane, J. J., and Frankfurt, M. (2014). Adolescent bisphenol-A exposure decreases dendritic spine density: role of sex and age. *Synapse* 68, 498–507. doi: 10.1002/syn.21758

Brede, C., Fjeldal, P., Skjevrak, I., and Herikstad, H. (2003). Increased migration levels of bisphenol A from polycarbonate baby bottles after dishwashing, boiling and brushing. *Food Addit. Contam.* 20, 684–689. doi: 10.1080/0265203031000119061

Bregman, B. S., Kunkel-Bagden, E., Schnell, L., Dai, H. N., Gao, D., and Schwab, M. E. (1995). Recovery from spinal cord injury mediated by antibodies to neurite growth inhibitors. *Nature* 378, 498–501. doi: 10.1038/378498a0

Cabaton, N. J., Wadia, P. R., Rubin, B. S., Zalko, D., Schaeberle, C. M., Askenase, M. H., et al. (2011). Perinatal exposure to environmentally relevant levels of bisphenol A decreases fertility and fecundity in CD-1 mice. *Environ. Health Perspect.* 119, 547–552. doi: 10.1289/ehp.1002559

Celio, M. R. (1986). Parvalbumin in most gamma-aminobutyric acid-containing neurons of the rat cerebral cortex. *Science* 231, 995–997. doi: 10.1126/science.3945815

Cellerino, A., Siciliano, R., Domenici, L., and Maffei, L. (1992). Parvalbumin immunoreactivity: a reliable marker for the effects of monocular deprivation in the rat visual cortex. *Neuroscience* 51, 749–753. doi: 10.1016/0306-4522(92)90514-3

Chugh, D., Nilsson, P., Afjei, S. A., Bakochi, A., and Ekdahl, C. T. (2013). Brain inflammation induces post-synaptic changes during early synapse formation in adult-born hippocampal neurons. *Exp. Neurol.* 250, 176–188. doi: 10.1016/j.expneurol.2013.09.005

Desai, N. S., Cudmore, R. H., Nelson, S. B., and Turrigiano, G. G. (2002). Critical periods for experience-dependent synaptic scaling in visual cortex. *Nat. Neurosci.* 5, 783–789. doi: 10.1038/nn878

Doerge, D. R., Twaddle, N. C., Vanlandingham, M., and Fisher, J. W. (2010). Pharmacokinetics of bisphenol A in neonatal and adult Sprague-Dawley rats. *Toxicol. Appl. Pharmacol.* 247, 158–165. doi: 10.1016/j.taap.2010.06.008

Dolen, G., Osterweil, E., Rao, B. S., Smith, G. B., Auerbach, B. D., Chattarji, S., et al. (2007). Correction of fragile X syndrome in mice. *Neuron* 56, 955–962. doi: 10.1016/j.neuron.2007.12.001

Dunaevsky, A., Tashiro, A., Majewska, A., Mason, C., and Yuste, R. (1999). Developmental regulation of spine motility in the mammalian central nervous system. *Proc. Natl. Acad. Sci. U.S.A.* 96, 13438–13443. doi: 10.1073/pnas.96.23.13438

Eilam-Stock, T., Serrano, P., Frankfurt, M., and Luine, V. (2012). Bisphenol-A impairs memory and reduces dendritic spine density in adult male rats. *Behav. Neurosci.* 126, 175–185. doi: 10.1037/a0025959

Elston, G. N., Benavides-Piccione, R., and Defelipe, J. (2001). The pyramidal cell in cognition: a comparative study in human and monkey. *J. Neurosci.* 21, RC163.

Elston, G. N., and Fujita, I. (2014). Pyramidal cell development: postnatal spinogenesis, dendritic growth, axon growth, and electrophysiology. *Front. Neuroanat.* 8:78. doi: 10.3389/fnana.2014.00078

Elston, G. N., Oga, T., and Fujita, I. (2009). Spinogenesis and pruning scales across functional hierarchies. *J. Neurosci.* 29, 3271–3275. doi: 10.1523/JNEUROSCI.5216-08.2009

Elston, G. N., Oga, T., Okamoto, T., and Fujita, I. (2011). Spinogenesis and pruning in the anterior ventral inferotemporal cortex of the macaque monkey: an intracellular injection study of layer III pyramidal cells. *Front. Neuroanat.* 5:42. doi: 10.3389/fnana.2011.00042

Elston, G. N., Okamoto, T., Oga, T., Dornan, D., and Fujita, I. (2010). Spinogenesis and pruning in the primary auditory cortex of the macaque monkey (*Macaca fascicularis*): an intracellular injection study of layer III pyramidal cells. *Brain Res.* 1316, 35–42. doi: 10.1016/j.brainres.2009.12.056

Elsworth, J. D., Jentsch, J. D., Vandevoort, C. A., Roth, R. H., Redmond, D. E. Jr., and Leranth, C. (2013). Prenatal exposure to bisphenol A impacts midbrain dopamine neurons and hippocampal spine synapses in non-human primates. *Neurotoxicology* 35, 113–120. doi: 10.1016/j.neuro.2013.01.001

Feng, G., Mellor, R. H., Bernstein, M., Keller-Peck, C., Nguyen, Q. T., Wallace, M., et al. (2000). Imaging neuronal subsets in transgenic mice expressing multiple spectral variants of GFP. *Neuron* 28, 41–51. doi: 10.1016/S0896-6273(00)00084-2

Goodman, J. E., Witorsch, R. J., Mcconnell, E. E., Sipes, I. G., Slayton, T. M., Yu, C. J., et al. (2009). Weight-of-evidence evaluation of reproductive and developmental effects of low doses of bisphenol A. *Crit. Rev. Toxicol.* 39, 1–75. doi: 10.3109/10408440903279946

Gordon, J. A., and Stryker, M. P. (1996). Experience-dependent plasticity of binocular responses in the primary visual cortex of the mouse. *J. Neurosci.* 16, 3274–3286. doi: 10.1016/j.cell.2008.05.054

Groff, T. (2010). Bisphenol A: invisible pollution. *Curr. Opin. Pediatr.* 22, 524–529. doi: 10.1097/MOP.0b013e32833b03f8

Hajszan, T., and Leranth, C. (2010). Bisphenol A interferes with synaptic remodeling. *Front. Neuroendocrinol.* 31:519–530. doi: 10.1016/j.yfrne.2010.06.004

Hensch, T. K. (2005). Critical period mechanisms in developing visual cortex. *Curr. Top. Dev. Biol.* 69, 215–237. doi: 10.1016/S0070-2153(05)69008-4

Hofer, S. B., Mrsic-Flogel, T. D., Bonhoeffer, T., and Hubener, M. (2009). Experience leaves a lasting structural trace in cortical circuits. *Nature* 457, 313–317. doi: 10.1038/nature07487

Howdeshell, K. L., Hotchkiss, A. K., Thayer, K. A., Vandenbergh, J. G., and Vom Saal, F. S. (1999). Exposure to bisphenol A advances puberty. *Nature* 401, 763–764. doi: 10.1038/44517

Howdeshell, K. L., Peterman, P. H., Judy, B. M., Taylor, J. A., Orazio, C. E., Ruhlen, R. L., et al. (2003). Bisphenol A is released from used polycarbonate animal cages into water at room temperature. *Environ. Health Perspect.* 111, 1180–1187. doi: 10.1289/ehp.5993

Hubel, D. H., and Wiesel, T. N. (1970). The period of susceptibility to the physiological effects of unilateral eye closure in kittens. *J. Physiol.* 206, 419–436.

Imai, Y., Ibata, I., Ito, D., Ohsawa, K., and Kohsaka, S. (1996). A novel gene iba1 in the major histocompatibility complex class III region encoding an EF hand protein expressed in a monocytic lineage. *Biochem. Biophys. Res. Commun.* 224, 855–862. doi: 10.1006/bbrc.1996.1112

Itoh, K., Yaoi, T., and Fushiki, S. (2012). Bisphenol A, an endocrine-disrupting chemical, and brain development. *Neuropathology* 32, 447–457. doi: 10.1111/j.1440-1789.2011.01287.x

Iwasaki, R., Matsuura, Y., Ohtori, S., Suzuki, T., Kuniyoshi, K., and Takahashi, K. (2013). Activation of astrocytes and microglia in the C3-T4 dorsal horn by lower trunk avulsion in a rat model of neuropathic pain. *J. Hand Surg. Am.* 38, 841–846. doi: 10.1016/j.jhsa.2013.01.034

Joskow, R., Barr, D. B., Barr, J. R., Calafat, A. M., Needham, L. L., and Rubin, C. (2006). Exposure to bisphenol A from bis-glycidyl dimethacrylate-based dental sealants. *J. Am. Dent. Assoc.* 137, 353–362. doi: 10.14219/jada.archive.2006.0185

Kalatsky, V. A., and Stryker, M. P. (2003). New paradigm for optical imaging: temporally encoded maps of intrinsic signal. *Neuron* 38, 529–545. doi: 10.1016/S0896-6273(03)00286-1

Kang, J. H., Kito, K., and Kondo, F. (2003). Factors influencing the migration of bisphenol A from cans. *J. Food Prot.* 66, 1444–1447.

Kettenmann, H., Kirchhoff, F., and Verkhratsky, A. (2013). Microglia: new roles for the synaptic stripper. *Neuron* 77, 10–18. doi: 10.1016/j.neuron.2012.12.023

Kossut, M. (1998). Experience-dependent changes in function and anatomy of adult barrel cortex. *Exp. Brain Res.* 123, 110–116. doi: 10.1007/s002210050551

Kunz, N., Camm, E. J., Somm, E., Lodygensky, G., Darbre, S., Aubert, M. L., et al. (2011). Developmental and metabolic brain alterations in rats exposed to bisphenol A during gestation and lactation. *Int. J. Dev. Neurosci.* 29, 37–43. doi: 10.1016/j.ijdevneu.2010.09.009

Lakind, J. S., and Naiman, D. Q. (2011). Daily intake of bisphenol A and potential sources of exposure: 2005-2006 national health and nutrition examination survey. *J. Expo. Sci. Environ. Epidemiol.* 21, 272–279. doi: 10.1038/jes.2010.9

Lee, S., Kim, Y. K., Shin, T. Y., and Kim, S. H. (2013). Neurotoxic effects of bisphenol AF on calcium-induced ROS and MAPKs. *Neurotox. Res.* 23, 249–259. doi: 10.1007/s12640-012-9353-4

Leranth, C., Szigeti-Buck, K., Maclusky, N. J., and Hajszan, T. (2008). Bisphenol A prevents the synaptogenic response to testosterone in the brain of adult male rats. *Endocrinology* 149, 988–994. doi: 10.1210/en.2007-1053

Liang, Q., Gao, X., Chen, Y., Hong, K., and Wang, H. S. (2014). Cellular mechanism of the nonmonotonic dose response of bisphenol a in rat cardiac myocytes. *Environ. Health Perspect.* doi: 10.1289/ehp.1307491

Long, M. A., Cruikshank, S. J., Jutras, M. J., and Connors, B. W. (2005). Abrupt maturation of a spike-synchronizing mechanism in neocortex. *J. Neurosci.* 25, 7309–7316. doi: 10.1523/JNEUROSCI.0375-05.2005

MacLusky, N. J., Hajszan, T., and Leranth, C. (2005). The environmental estrogen bisphenol a inhibits estradiol-induced hippocampal synaptogenesis. *Environ. Health Perspect.* 113, 675–679. doi: 10.1289/ehp.7633

Majewska, A., Yiu, G., and Yuste, R. (2000). A custom-made two-photon microscope and deconvolution system. *Pflugers. Arch.* 441, 398–408. doi: 10.1007/s004240000435

Majewska, A. K., Newton, J. R., and Sur, M. (2006). Remodeling of synaptic structure in sensory cortical areas *in vivo*. *J. Neurosci.* 26, 3021–3029. doi: 10.1523/JNEUROSCI.4454-05.2006

Mataga, N., Mizuguchi, Y., and Hensch, T. K. (2004). Experience-dependent pruning of dendritic spines in visual cortex by tissue plasminogen activator. *Neuron* 44, 1031–1041. doi: 10.1016/j.neuron.2004.11.028

McGee, A. W., Yang, Y., Fischer, Q. S., Daw, N. W., and Strittmatter, S. M. (2005). Experience-driven plasticity of visual cortex limited by myelin and Nogo receptor. *Science* 309, 2222–2226. doi: 10.1126/science.1114362

Mielke, H., and Gundert-Remy, U. (2009). Bisphenol A levels in blood depend on age and exposure. *Toxicol. Lett.* 190, 32–40. doi: 10.1016/j.toxlet.2009.06.861

Myers, J. P., Zoeller, R. T., and Vom Saal, F. S. (2009). A clash of old and new scientific concepts in toxicity, with important implications for public health. *Environ. Health Perspect.* 117, 1652–1655. doi: 10.1289/ehp.0900887

Ogiue-Ikeda, M., Tanabe, N., Mukai, H., Hojo, Y., Murakami, G., Tsurugizawa, T., et al. (2008). Rapid modulation of synaptic plasticity by estrogens as well as endocrine disrupters in hippocampal neurons. *Brain Res. Rev.* 57, 363–375. doi: 10.1016/j.brainresrev.2007.06.010

Perry, V. H., and O'Connor, V. (2010). The role of microglia in synaptic stripping and synaptic degeneration: a revised perspective. *ASN Neuro* 2, e00047. doi: 10.1042/AN20100024

Richter, C. A., Birnbaum, L. S., Farabollini, F., Newbold, R. R., Rubin, B. S., Talsness, C. E., et al. (2007). *In vivo* effects of bisphenol A in laboratory rodent studies. *Reprod. Toxicol.* 24, 199–224. doi: 10.1016/j.reprotox.2007.06.004

Rochester, J. R. (2013). Bisphenol A and human health: a review of the literature. *Reprod. Toxicol.* 42, 132–155. doi: 10.1016/j.reprotox.2013.08.008

Ryan, B. C., Hotchkiss, A. K., Crofton, K. M., and Gray, L. E. Jr. (2010). *In utero* and lactational exposure to bisphenol A, in contrast to ethinyl estradiol, does not alter sexually dimorphic behavior, puberty, fertility, and anatomy of female LE rats. *Toxicol. Sci.* 114, 133–148. doi: 10.1093/toxsci/kfp266

Sugiyama, S., Di Nardo, A. A., Aizawa, S., Matsuo, I., Volovitch, M., Prochiantz, A., et al. (2008). Experience-dependent transfer of Otx2 homeoprotein into the visual cortex activates postnatal plasticity. *Cell* 134, 508–520. doi: 10.1016/j.cell.2008.05.054

Sur, M., Nagakura, I., Chen, N., and Sugihara, H. (2013). Mechanisms of plasticity in the developing and adult visual cortex. *Prog. Brain Res.* 207, 243–254. doi: 10.1016/B978-0-444-63327-9.00002-3

Suzuki, K., Ishikawa, K., Sugiyama, K., Furuta, H., and Nishimura, F. (2000). Content and release of bisphenol A from polycarbonate dental products. *Dent. Mater. J.* 19, 389–395. doi: 10.4012/dmj.19.389

Szychowski, K. A., and Wojtowicz, A. K. (2013). Components of plastic disrupt the function of the nervous system. *Postepy. Hig. Med. Dosw. (Online)* 67, 499–506. doi: 10.5604/17322693.1051001

Thigpen, J. E., Setchell, K. D., Padilla-Banks, E., Haseman, J. K., Saunders, H. E., Caviness, G. F., et al. (2007). Variations in phytoestrogen content between different mill dates of the same diet produces significant differences in the time of vaginal opening in CD-1 mice and F344 rats but not in CD Sprague-Dawley rats. *Environ. Health Perspect.* 115, 1717–1726. doi: 10.1289/ehp.10165

Trapp, B. D., Wujek, J. R., Criste, G. A., Jalabi, W., Yin, X., Kidd, G. J., et al. (2007). Evidence for synaptic stripping by cortical microglia. *Glia* 55, 360–368. doi: 10.1002/glia.20462

Tropea, D., Giacometti, E., Wilson, N. R., Beard, C., Mccurry, C., Fu, D. D., et al. (2009a). Partial reversal of Rett Syndrome-like symptoms in MeCP2 mutant mice. *Proc. Natl. Acad. Sci. U.S.A.* 106, 2029–2034. doi: 10.1073/pnas.0812394106

Tropea, D., Van Wart, A., and Sur, M. (2009b). Molecular mechanisms of experience-dependent plasticity in visual cortex. *Philos. Trans. R. Soc. Lond. B Biol. Sci.* 364, 341–355. doi: 10.1098/rstb.2008.0269

Tropea, D., Majewska, A. K., Garcia, R., and Sur, M. (2010). Structural dynamics of synapses *in vivo* correlate with functional changes during experience-dependent plasticity in visual cortex. *J. Neurosci.* 30, 11086–11095. doi: 10.1523/JNEUROSCI.1661-10.2010

Turrigiano, G. G., and Nelson, S. B. (2004). Homeostatic plasticity in the developing nervous system. *Nat. Rev. Neurosci.* 5, 97–107. doi: 10.1038/nrn1327

Tyl, R. W., Myers, C. B., Marr, M. C., Sloan, C. S., Castillo, N. P., Veselica, M. M., et al. (2008). Two-generation reproductive toxicity study of dietary bisphenol A in CD-1 (Swiss) mice. *Toxicol. Sci.* 104, 362–384. doi: 10.1093/toxsci/kfn084

Tyl, R. W., Myers, C. B., Marr, M. C., Thomas, B. F., Keimowitz, A. R., Brine, D. R., et al. (2002). Three-generation reproductive toxicity study of dietary bisphenol A in CD Sprague-Dawley rats. *Toxicol. Sci.* 68, 121–146. doi: 10.1093/toxsci/68.1.121

U.S. Food and Drug Administration. (2010). *Update on Bisphenol A for Use in Food Contract Applications.* Available at: http://www.fda.gov/NewsEvents/PublicHealthFocus/ucm197739.htm [accessed May 4, 2010].

Valverde, F. (1967). Apical dendritic spines of the visual cortex and light deprivation in the mouse. *Exp. Brain Res.* 3, 337–352. doi: 10.1007/BF00237559

Valverde, F. (1968). Structural changes in the area striata of the mouse after enucleation. *Exp. Brain Res.* 5, 274–292. doi: 10.1007/BF00235903

Vandenberg, L. N., Hauser, R., Marcus, M., Olea, N., and Welshons, W. V. (2007). Human exposure to bisphenol A (BPA). *Reprod. Toxicol.* 24, 139–177. doi: 10.1016/j.reprotox.2007.07.010

von Goetz, N., Wormuth, M., Scheringer, M., and Hungerbuhler, K. (2010). Bisphenol a: how the most relevant exposure sources contribute to total consumer exposure. *Risk Anal.* 30, 473–487. doi: 10.1111/j.1539-6924.2009.01345.x

Wiesel, T. N., and Hubel, D. H. (1963a). Effects of visual deprivation on morphology and physiology of cells in the cats lateral geniculate body. *J. Neurophysiol.* 26, 978–993.

Wiesel, T. N., and Hubel, D. H. (1963b). Single-cell responses in striate cortex of kittens deprived of vision in one eye. *J. Neurophysiol.* 26, 1003–1017.

Xu, X., Liu, X., Zhang, Q., Zhang, G., Lu, Y., Ruan, Q., et al. (2013a). Sex-specific effects of bisphenol-A on memory and synaptic structural modification in hippocampus of adult mice. *Horm. Behav.* 63, 766–775. doi: 10.1016/j.yhbeh.2013.03.004

Xu, X., Xie, L., Hong, X., Ruan, Q., Lu, H., Zhang, Q., et al. (2013b). Perinatal exposure to bisphenol-A inhibits synaptogenesis and affects the synaptic morphological development in offspring male mice. *Chemosphere* 91, 1073–1081. doi: 10.1016/j.chemosphere.2012.12.065

Xu, X., Lu, Y., Zhang, G., Chen, L., Tian, D., Shen, X., et al. (2014). Bisphenol A promotes dendritic morphogenesis of hippocampal neurons through estrogen receptor-mediated ERK1/2 signal pathway. *Chemosphere* 96, 129–137. doi: 10.1016/j.chemosphere.2013.09.063

Xu, X., Ye, Y., Li, T., Chen, L., Tian, D., Luo, Q., et al. (2010). Bisphenol-A rapidly promotes dynamic changes in hippocampal dendritic morphology through estrogen receptor-mediated pathway by concomitant phosphorylation of NMDA receptor subunit NR2B. *Toxicol. Appl. Pharmacol.* 249, 188–196. doi: 10.1016/j.taap.2010.09.007

Yamaguchi, H., Zhu, J., Yu, T., Sasaki, K., Umetsu, H., Kidachi, Y., et al. (2006). Low-level bisphenol A increases production of glial fibrillary acidic protein in differentiating astrocyte progenitor cells through excessive STAT3 and Smad1 activation. *Toxicology* 226, 131–142. doi: 10.1016/j.tox.2006.06.011

Zuo, Y., Yang, G., Kwon, E., and Gan, W. B. (2005). Long-term sensory deprivation prevents dendritic spine loss in primary somatosensory cortex. *Nature* 436, 261–265. doi: 10.1038/nature03715

8

Super-resolution 2-photon microscopy reveals that the morphology of each dendritic spine correlates with diffusive but not synaptic properties

Kevin Takasaki and Bernardo L. Sabatini *

Department of Neurobiology, Harvard Medical School, Howard Hughes Medical Institute, Boston, MA, USA

***Correspondence:**
Bernardo L. Sabatini, Department of Neurobiology, Harvard Medical School, Howard Hughes Medical Institute, 220 Longwood Ave., Boston, MA 02115, USA
e-mail: bsabatini@hms.harvard.edu

The structure of dendritic spines suggests a specialized function in compartmentalizing synaptic signals near active synapses. Indeed, theoretical and experimental analyses indicate that the diffusive resistance of the spine neck is sufficient to effectively compartmentalize some signaling molecules in a spine for the duration of their activated lifetime. Here we describe the application of 2-photon microscopy combined with stimulated emission depletion (STED-2P) to the biophysical study of the relationship between synaptic signals and spine morphology, demonstrating the utility of combining STED-2P with modern optical and electrophysiological techniques. Morphological determinants of fluorescence recovery time were identified and evaluated within the context of a simple compartmental model describing diffusive transfer between spine and dendrite. Correlations between the neck geometry and the amplitude of synaptic potentials and calcium transients evoked by 2-photon glutamate uncaging were also investigated.

Keywords: dendritic spine, 2-photon microscopy, stimulated emission microscopy, super resolution microscopy, synaptic transmission

INTRODUCTION

Dendritic spines are small, subcellular structures that house the post-synaptic machinery associated with glutamatergic synapses, typically consisting of a bulbous head joined to the parent dendrite by a channel-like neck (Harris and Stevens, 1989; Alvarez and Sabatini, 2007). The special morphology of dendritic spines suggests that they biochemically compartmentalize diffusible signaling cascades by restricting the transfer of molecules between the spine head and dendrite. Indeed, the rapid kinetics of calcium (Ca) signaling in the spine head compared to the slowed mixing of Ca across the neck under physiological conditions ensures independent signaling in each compartment for this second messenger (Sabatini et al., 2002). Such compartmentalization presumably permits the highly spatially specific induction of Ca dependent plasticity at one synapse without affecting its neighbors (Yuste and Denk, 1995; Matsuzaki et al., 2004; Harvey and Svoboda, 2007). Nevertheless, not all intracellular signals are functionally compartmentalized, and during plasticity induction, certain signaling molecules activated in the spine head are able to escape and influence neighboring synapses (Harvey and Svoboda, 2007; Harvey et al., 2008; Murakoshi et al., 2011). Thus, the ability of a biochemical signal to spread beyond the spine depends on the molecular properties of the messengers involved, mechanisms of retention and inactivation, and passive constraints imposed by the geometry of the spine and dendrite (Yasuda and Murakoshi, 2011).

In addition to biochemical signaling cascades, the excitatory synapses of dendritic spines support electrical signaling via post-synaptic potentials. It has long been hypothesized that the morphology of dendritic spines might play a role in regulating the spread of electrical signals. The opening of ion channels located in the spine, local capacitive charging of the spine head, and the electrical resistance of the neck could potentially shape the amplitude, time course, and spatial spread of synaptic potentials. However, in contrast to clear confirmation of the compartmentalization of certain biochemical signals, whether spine morphology regulates synaptically evoked electrical activity has been controversial (Tsay and Yuste, 2004). Numerous studies have examined whether the geometry of spines has, or in theory could have, a measurable impact on electrical signaling by affecting the generation and propagation of membrane potentials during synaptic transmission; the results of these studies have provided evidence supporting (Bloodgood and Sabatini, 2005; Araya et al., 2006; Bloodgood et al., 2009; Harnett et al., 2012) and rejecting (Harris and Stevens, 1989; Koch and Zador, 1993; Svoboda et al., 1996; Palmer and Stuart, 2009) a role of spine geometry in regulating the electrical function of synapses. Nevertheless, functional studies that are independent of accurate measurements of spine dimensions reveal significant drops in potential across the spine neck that alter voltage-dependent processes, such as the activation of voltage-gated ion channels and relief of the Mg block of NMDA-type glutamate receptors (Bloodgood et al., 2009; Harnett et al., 2012). Furthermore, computational models support additional potential functions of the spine morphology in normalizing synaptic potentials (for example rendering their amplitude insensitive to the morphology of the parent dendrite; Gulledge et al., 2012) and correlative structure-function studies have found that the amplitude of synaptic potentials falls for longer spines (Araya et al., 2006).

A challenge in establishing an understanding of the structure-function relationship of dendritic spines has been an inability to obtain high-resolution structural information in an experimental context that permits functional analysis. The diffraction limited resolution of 2-photon laser scanning microscopy (2PLSM), the standard method of imaging dendritic spines in living tissue, is too coarse (~400 nm) to accurately measure the dimensions of the spine neck, which can be less than 100 nm in diameter, or fine features of the head, which can have non-spherical morphology.

We and others have implemented in-tissue superresolution 2PLSM realized via stimulated emission depletion (STED) (Ding et al., 2009; Bethge et al., 2013; Takasaki et al., 2013). STED-2P permits fluorescence imaging of neurons in brain tissue to a resolution of ~50 nm, sufficient for accurate reconstruction of spine morphology. We use this approach, coupled with electrophysiological analysis, fluorescence recovery after photo-bleaching (FRAP), and two-photon laser glutamate uncaging, to determine what features of synaptic signaling are predicted by the morphology of the spine. To preserve the highest imaging resolution, analysis was limited to spines near the surface of acute brain slices. This analysis demonstrates a clear structure-function relationship for diffusional transfer of a small molecule, such that the physical dimensions of each spine, with rare exceptions, predict the time course of diffusional equilibration across the neck. On the other hand, we find no correlation between morphology and the sizes of uncaging evoked synaptic potentials (uEPSPs) and associated Ca transients (ΔCa_{uEPSP}). This latter result, given the previously established impact of spine neck resistance on synaptic signaling, suggests the possibility of counter-balanced regulation of synaptically-activated ion channels, such as glutamate receptors and voltage-gated ion channels, that normalize synaptic signals in the face of variable spine morphology.

MATERIALS AND METHODS

Experiments were performed with a custom microscope that combines 2PLSM and STED microscopy utilizing electronically synchronized Ti:Sapphire pulsed lasers (Takasaki et al., 2013). In order to achieve sufficient depletion without inducing multiphoton excitation, the depletion beam is temporally stretched to several hundred picoseconds, precluding its use for two-photon mediated photo-release of glutamate from MNI-glutamate. Therefore, in order to uncage glutamate, a third Ti:Sapphire pulsed laser was incorporated that delivered femtosecond pulses of 720 nm light (**Figure 1**).

ELECTROPHYSIOLOGY, GLUTAMATE UNCAGING, AND Ca IMAGING

All animal handling and procedures were performed in accordance with protocols approved by the Harvard IACUC and in accordance with federal guidelines. Acute brain slices were prepared from the hippocampus of young mice (C57BL6, ages p15–p18) as described previously (Bloodgood and Sabatini, 2007). After recovery, slices were transferred to the recording chamber in the microscope and bathed in ACSF recirculating with a small volume, closed system (10 ml). Three mM methoxy-nitroindolinyl-caged glutamate (MNI-glutamate) was added in photolysis experiments with 10 μM D-serine to prevent glutamate receptor desensitization. All physiological experiments were performed at 34°C. Whole-cell patch pipettes were filled with a $KMeSO_4$-based internal solution containing 300 μM Alexa Fluor 594 and 300 μM Fluo-5F, a moderate affinity calcium indicator. Cells were allowed to dye fill for 15–20 min after break-in before beginning the experiment. Photobleaching of Alexa 594 was accomplished with 2 ms pulses, whereas glutamate uncaging utilized 0.5 ms pulses. Uncaging evoked Ca transients in the spine head (ΔCa_{uEPSP}) are expressed as a fraction of saturating green fluorescence obtained in the presence of 1 mM [Ca], as described

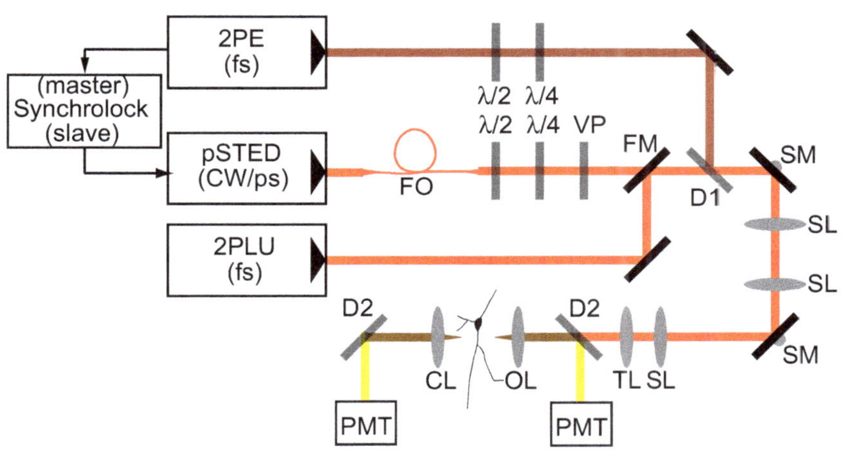

FIGURE 1 | Schematic of microscope. Laser pulses from a femtosecond-pulsed Ti-Sapph laser tuned to 810 nm for two-photon excitation (2PE) are synchronized by an electronic feedback circuit (Synchrolock) with those of a picosecond-pulsed Ti-Sapph laser (pSTED) tuned to 736 nm for stimulated emission. The STED laser can be exchanged by a flip mirror (FM) with the beam from a femtosecond-pulsed Ti-Sapph laser tuned to 720 nm for two-photon laser-induced uncaging (2PLU) of caged compounds, such as caged glutamate. STED pulses are stretched to ~200 ps by dispersion through a 120 m single-mode polarization-maintaining fiber optic (FO) and phase patterned to achieve a helical wavefront by a vortex phase plate (VP). The 2PE and STED lasers are combined by a dichroic (D1). Fluorescence is separated from excitation and depletion light by a dichroic (D2) and collected by photomultiplier tubes (PMT). λ/2 and λ/4 are half- and quarter-waveplates used to adjust the polarization. SL, Scan lens; TL, Tube lens; SM, Scanning mirror; OL, Objective lens; CL, Condenser lens.

previously (Bloodgood and Sabatini, 2007). This method allows comparison of Ca transient amplitudes across microscopes and laboratories since it is independent of photon collection and detection efficiency.

MODELING OF DIFFUSIVE COMPARTMENTALIZATION IN DENDRITIC SPINES

The morphology of dendritic spines imposes geometric constraints on the diffusion of biochemical materials within the spine and between the spine and its parent dendrite. A simple model describing transfer of freely diffusing substances between the spine head and dendrite can be obtained by approximating the spine head and dendrite as compartments of homogeneous concentration separated by a passive barrier imposed by the spine neck (Svoboda et al., 1996). The only time varying quantity in this model is the concentration in the spine head, $C_H(t)$, while the constant parameters are the cytoplasmic diffusion coefficient, D, the volume of the spine head, V_H, the concentration in the dendrite, C_d, which functions as a particle reservoir and can be set to 0, and the geometric resistance of the spine neck, W_N, which relates the dimensions of the neck to a resistance to diffusive transfer across it. The equation governing the time course of C_H is then

$$\frac{dC_H}{dt} = -\frac{D}{V_H W_N} C_H \tag{1}$$

This behavior is directly analogous to capacitive discharge in an electrical RC circuit, and there is an analogous correspondence of the geometry of a resistor and its resistance to the diffusive resistance of the spine neck. That is,

$$W_N = \frac{l_N}{a_N} \tag{2}$$

where l_N is the neck length, and a_N is its cross-sectional area. Given a step change in concentration, equations (1) and (2) predict exponential relaxation with a recovery time given by

$$\tau = \frac{V_H l_N}{D a_N}. \tag{3}$$

RESULTS

MORPHOLOGICAL DETERMINANTS OF DIFFUSIONAL TRANSFER IN DENDRITIC SPINES

In order to determine if the structure of each dendritic spine determines the time-course of passive diffusional equilibration across the spine neck, we utilized a custom-built STED-2P microscope equipped with a third pulse Ti-Sapphire laser (**Figure 1**; see Materials and Methods). To observe diffusional transfer across the spine neck, we performed FRAP and measured the relaxation of a step perturbation to concentration of fluorescent dye in the spine head. Spine heads were visualized under STED-2P for morphological analysis (**Figure 2A**), and fluorescence from the spine head was measured over time by line scanning with conventional 2PLSM (**Figure 2B**). During the line scan, the spine head was exposed to 2 ms illumination with laser pulses centered on 720 nm from a third mode-locked Ti:sapphire laser (Chameleon XR), producing a rapid reduction in head fluorescence attributable to photobleaching which was followed by a recovery period driven by diffusional transfer across the neck (**Figure 2C**).

FRAP recovery times, determined as the time constant of an exponential fit to the fluorescence, showed strong linear correlation with neck length ($r = 0.75$, $p < 0.0001$, $n = 38$) (**Figure 2D**), but no significant correlation with head volume ($r = -0.19$, $p = 0.26$, $n = 38$) (**Figure 2E**). The dependence of recovery time on neck diameter appeared non-linear and was fit by a power function, $f(x) = a + bx^n$, with $n = -3.28 \pm 1.79$ which is consistent with the value of -2 expected from modeling as a resistor (**Figure 2F**). The data was also fit by the same function with the exponent, n, fixed to -2 with a 1% increase in the residual sum of squares compared with the unconstrained fit.

To examine the validity of the simple model leading to equation (3), we compared recovery times against a parameter defined as a combination of morphological parameters, $\zeta = \frac{V_H l_N}{d_N^2}$, so that equation (3) becomes

$$\tau = \frac{4}{\pi D} \zeta. \tag{4}$$

Comparison of recovery time constant against ζ showed strong linear correlation ($r = 0.76$, $p < 0.0001$, $n = 38$) and was well fit by a line with a slope of 44 ± 7 (**Figure 3A**). Given equation (4), this slope value yields an estimate for the diffusion coefficient, $D = 29\,\mu m^2/s$. The inverse and linear correlations of **Figures 2B**, **3A**, respectively, are consistent with accurate measurement of the morphological parameters that determine the time course of diffusional equilibration across the spine neck. Nevertheless, some dendritic spines deviate strongly from the predicted behavior, exhibiting equilibration time inconsistent with that predicted by the model. For example, the spine shown in **Figure 3B** and indicated in **Figure 3A** has a head that is similar in size and width to the neck, rendering invalid the discretized capacitor and resistor model described above. For these spines, more complex geometric models that incorporate the non-zero volume of the neck, which adds a non-zero transit time and introduces a significant reservoir of molecules, may be required.

IMPACT OF SPINE STRUCTURE ON SYNAPTIC POTENTIALS AND Ca TRANSIENTS

Measurement of the subthreshold membrane potential within a dendritic spine is technically challenging due to poor electrophysiological access and the lack of optical voltage indicators with sufficient sensitivity to measure small depolarizations in individual spines. Ca influx through endogenous voltage-dependent sources, such as voltage-gated Ca channels (VGCCs) and the NMDA-type glutamate receptor (NMDAR), can be used as an indirect measurement of spine voltage. As a first step toward exploring the relationship between spine morphology and electrical compartmentalization, we combined two-photon photolysis of caged glutamate, whole-cell electrophysiology, and Ca imaging with STED-2P for morphological imaging.

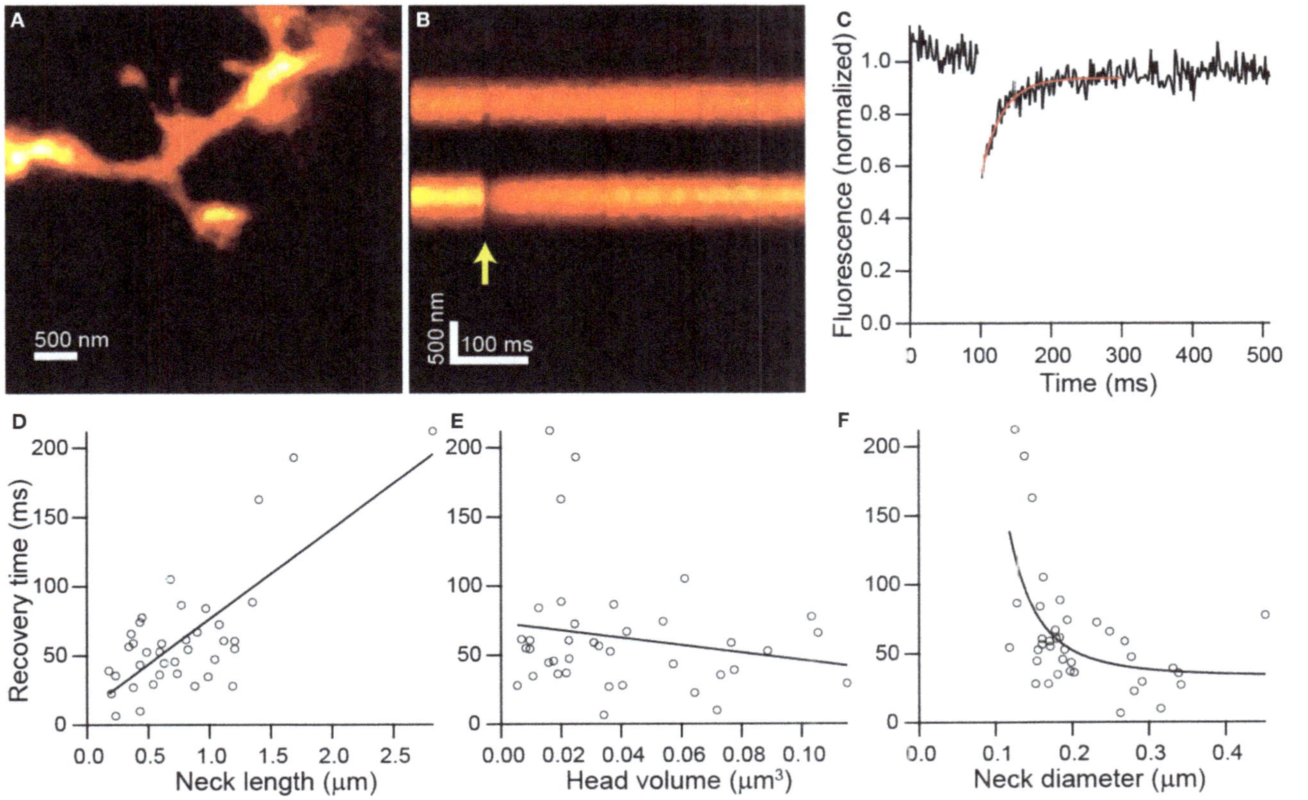

FIGURE 2 | Combined FRAP and STED-2P analysis. (A) STED-2P image of a dendritic spine on the apical dendrite of a CA1 hippocampal neurons filled with Alexa Fluor 594 through a somatic whole-cell recording pipette. **(B)** 2PLSM linescan taken through the spine and dendrite in **(A)**. The photobleaching pulse was delivered on the spine head after a 100 ms delay (*yellow arrow*). **(C)** Fluorescence in the spine head over time quantified from **(B)**. Recovery was fit with a decaying exponential (*red line*) to obtain the recovery time constant. **(D–F)** Recovery time constants plotted against neck length **(D)**, head volume **(E)**, and neck diameter **(F)**.

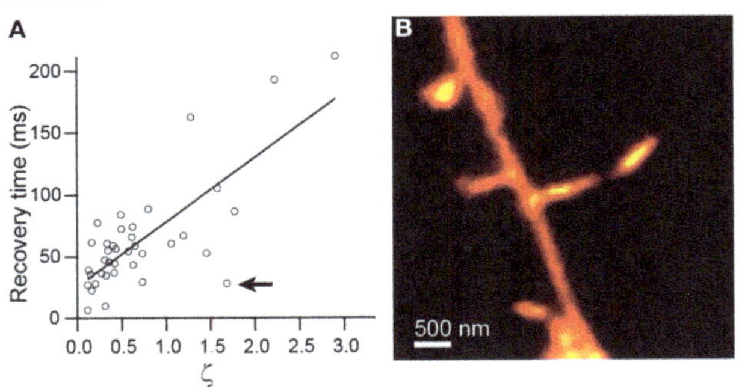

FIGURE 3 | Modeling of diffusive transfer across the spine neck. (A) Recovery times from **Figure 2** plotted against ζ. **(B)** STED-2P image of the spine producing the outlying point marked by the arrow in **(A)**.

Dendritic spines were visualized by 2PLSM and STED-2P (**Figure 4A**) using the microscope described above. In this set of experiments, the third laser was used for the photolytic release (uncaging) of glutamate from MNI-glutamate. No shifts in holding current or increases in green fluorescence from the Ca sensitive fluorophore were observed during STED-2P imaging, likely due to the relatively low two-photon cross-section of MNI-glutamate (0.06 GM) which prevents significant uncaging by the dispersed STED pulse. Before uncaging, the amplifier was switched into current clamp mode with current injection to maintain a resting potential near −60 mV. While line scanning over the dendrite and spine, delivery of 0.5 ms illumination with laser pulses centered on 720 nm from a third mode-locked Ti:sapphire laser (Chameleon XR) generated transient increases in green fluorescence selectively in the spine head, as well as small depolarizations measured at the soma (**Figures 4B–D**). Green fluorescence from Ca-bound Fluo-5F was baseline subtracted and then normalized to red fluorescence from Alexa Fluor 594 ($\Delta G/R$) to account for volume variation of the intracellular space. This metric was then normalized to the saturated G/R ratio (G/R_{sat}) corresponding to the fully bound indicator as described in Bloodgood and Sabatini (2007) to obtain a measurement of Ca influx ($\Delta G/G_{sat}$) comparable across microscopes with varying collection efficiencies.

To investigate potential correlations between the amplitude of uncaging-evoked excitatory post-synaptic potentials (uEPSPs) and peak changes in green fluorescence ($\Delta G/G_{sat}$) with spine morphology, we compared these measurements against measurements of spine neck diameter and length (**Figure 5**).

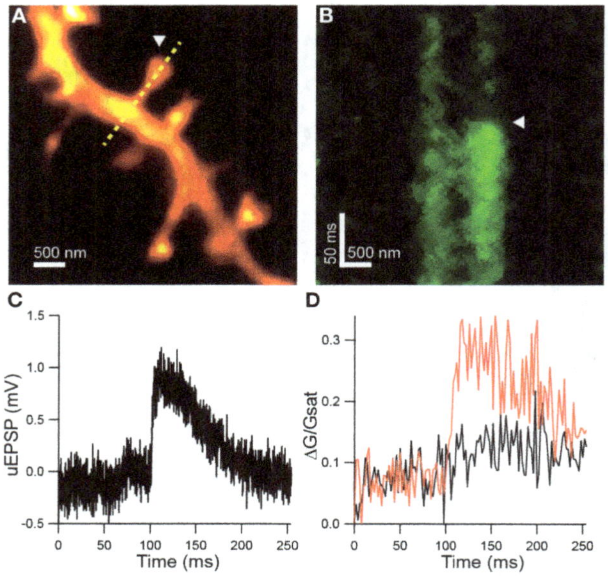

FIGURE 4 | Functional analysis of STED-2P resolved dendritic spines. **(A)** STED-2P image of dendritic spines. MNI-glutamate was uncaged at a point located near a target spine (*white arrowhead*) while line scanning over the spine and dendrite (*yellow dashed line*). **(B)** Green fluorescence, indicative of Ca-bound Fluo 5F, measured in line scan. MNI-glutamate uncaging following a 100 ms delay (*white arrowhead*) produced a transient increase in green fluorescence. **(C)** Somatic membrane potential recording of the uEPSP elicited from the synapse in **(A)**. **(D)** Quantification of Fluo 5F fluorescence in the spine head (*red*) and in the dendrite (*black*) as imaged in **(B)**.

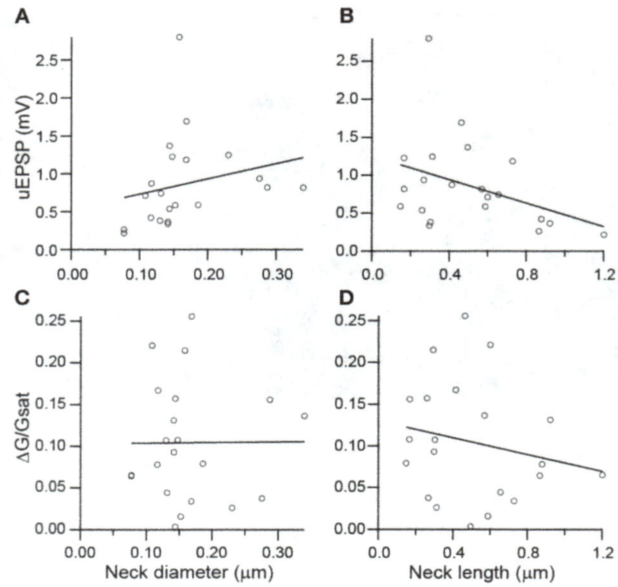

FIGURE 5 | Lack of correlations between spine dimensions, synaptic potentials, and associated Ca transients. **(A,B)** uEPSP amplitude plotted against spine neck diameter **(A)** and length **(B)**. **(C,D)** Amplitude of uncaging evoked Ca transient plotted against neck diameter **(C)** and length **(D)**.

No significant correlations were observed between uEPSP amplitude and neck diameter ($r = 0.23$, $p = 0.32$, $n = 21$; **Figure 5A**), peak calcium and neck diameter ($r = 0.23$, $p = 0.98$, $n = 21$; **Figure 5C**), or peak calcium and neck length ($r = -0.20$, $p = 0.38$, $n = 21$; **Figure 5D**). A weak negative correlation was observed between uEPSP amplitude and neck length ($r = -0.38$, $p = 0.09$, $n = 21$; **Figure 5B**).

DISCUSSION

DIFFUSIVE PROPERTIES OF DENDRITIC SPINES

Experiments performed by various groups have investigated correlations between diffusive transfer of calcium, small molecules, and proteins with neck morphological parameters, and modulation of diffusive transfer in response to perturbations. Notably, activity-dependent plasticity of diffusive transfer of both small molecules and proteins has been observed (Bloodgood and Sabatini, 2005; Grunditz et al., 2008). In the Bloodgood study, synaptic activity paired with back-propagating dendritic action potentials induced changes in diffusive transfer that could not be fully explained by observed changes in spine head volume and neck length according to equation (3), thus highlighting the possible involvement of activity-induced remodeling of spine neck width. However, experiments performed with conventional fluorescence microscopy have been unable to measure sub-resolution features, such as the diameters of many spine necks, and have not been able to fully address the role of spine neck morphology in diffusive transfer. Indeed, studies have used diffusive measurements, such as the spread of synaptic Ca (Noguchi et al., 2005) or FRAP (Grunditz et al., 2008), as indirect measurements of spine neck geometry.

Our findings indicate that for a large fraction of spines, incorporation of accurate morphological measurements into a simple biophysical model predicts the passive diffusion behavior of a small molecule across the spine neck. Conversely, utilizing this model and accurate measurements of the spine neck allows for an estimate of diffusion coefficients of small fluorophores in the spine. Such analysis reveals $D = 29\,\mu m^2/s$ for Alexa Fluor 594, a value nearly 10-fold smaller than that obtained from analysis of diffusion in Xenopus oocytes (Nitsche et al., 2004). This discrepancy may be the result of differences in methodology (FRAP vs. dye spreading) or in the local cytoplasmic environment. In support of the latter possibility, measurement of the diffusion coefficients of small molecule fluorophores in the dendrites of cerebellar stellate cells also demonstrates a near 10-fold slowing, perhaps attributable to special properties of the dendroplasm (Soler-Llavina and Sabatini, 2006).

There is a small fraction of dendritic spines for which the simple biophysical model fails to predict diffusive behavior. Recent theoretical work has clarified the approximations and limits of the biophysical model underlying equation (3) (Holcman and Schuss, 2011), and has further explored the role that subtle morphological features might play in the regulation of biochemical compartmentalization and signaling in spines. More sophisticated analysis is likely necessary to explain the diffusive properties of spines with non-canonical shapes.

CORRELATION OF MORPHOLOGY AND SYNAPTIC SIGNALS

Our studies failed to find a significant correlation between the dimensions of the spine head and neck and uncaging-evoked synaptic potentials and Ca transients. Previous studies have demonstrated that many factors, including spine geometry and NMDAR subunit composition (Sobczyk and Svoboda, 2007) determine the amplitude and time course of synaptic Ca signals. In contrast, Araya et al. demonstrated that synaptic potentials were strongly inversely correlated with spine length (Araya et al., 2006) although it was not possible to determine the number of AMPA-type glutamate receptors in each spine. Our data might support the lack of a functional impact of spine shape on electrical or Ca signaling. Conversely, it may indicate the existence of counter-balancing regulatory mechanisms that adjust synaptically activated ion channels to negate the effects of spine morphology. The large variability present in the uEPSP and Ca measurements likely requires studies with very large N or more sensitive techniques to reveal significant interactions by correlative population approaches.

CONCLUSION

The experiments described here demonstrate the use of STED-2P for structure-function studies in combination with experimental methods such as FRAP, whole-cell electrophysiology, caged neurotransmitter photolysis, and calcium imaging. Various theoretical and experimental findings have addressed the question of how spine morphology influences synaptic function, and the ability to probe biochemical and electrical function at an individual spine with simultaneous high-resolution measurement of morphology enables quantitative studies of such biophysical questions.

These methods could be extended to new experimental conditions or other biological systems in which nanoscale structure is of interest. For example, similar studies could be performed on dendritic spines of other cell types, such as spiny projection neurons of the striatum or Purkinje cells of the cerebellum, or on spines with perturbed structure and function in models of disease, such as tuberous sclerosis complex (Tavazoie et al., 2005) or Alzheimer's disease (Shankar et al., 2008). Alternatively, biophysical studies of dendritic spines with STED-2P could be improved upon with the application of novel experimental techniques. For example, the study of electrical compartmentalization and the role of spine geometry in regulating electrical signaling would benefit from methods able to directly measure membrane potential by an optical signal (Kralj et al., 2011; Jin et al., 2012).

REFERENCES

Alvarez, V. A., and Sabatini, B. L. (2007). Anatomical and physiological plasticity of dendritic spines. *Annu. Rev. Neurosci.* 30, 79–97. doi: 10.1146/annurev.neuro.30.051606.094222

Araya, R., Jiang, J., Eisenthal, K. B., and Yuste, R. (2006). The spine neck filters membrane potentials. *Proc. Natl. Acad. Sci. U.S.A.* 103, 17961–17966. doi: 10.1073/pnas.0608755103

Bethge, P., Chereau, R., Avignone, E., Marsicano, G., and Nagerl, U. V. (2013). Two-photon excitation STED microscopy in two colors in acute brain slices. *Biophys. J.* 104, 778–785. doi: 10.1016/j.bpj.2012.12.054

Bloodgood, B. L., Giessel, A. J., and Sabatini, B. L. (2009). Biphasic synaptic Ca influx arising from compartmentalized electrical signals in dendritic spines. *PLoS Biol.* 7:e1000190. doi: 10.1371/journal.pbio.1000190

Bloodgood, B. L., and Sabatini, B. L. (2005). Neuronal activity regulates diffusion across the neck of dendritic spines. *Science* 310, 866–869. doi: 10.1126/science.1114816

Bloodgood, B. L., and Sabatini, B. L. (2007). Nonlinear regulation of unitary synaptic signals by CaV(2.3) voltage-sensitive calcium channels located in dendritic spines. *Neuron* 53, 249–260. doi: 10.1016/j.neuron.2006.12.017

Ding, J. B., Takasaki, K. T., and Sabatini, B. L. (2009). Supraresolution imaging in brain slices using stimulated-emission depletion two-photon laser scanning microscopy. *Neuron* 63, 429–437. doi: 10.1016/j.neuron.2009.07.011

Grunditz, A., Holbro, N., Tian, L., Zuo, Y., and Oertner, T. G. (2008). Spine neck plasticity controls postsynaptic calcium signals through electrical compartmentalization. *J. Neurosci.* 28, 13457–13466. doi: 10.1523/JNEUROSCI.2702-08.2008

Gulledge, A. T., Carnevale, N. T., and Stuart, G. J. (2012). Electrical advantages of dendritic spines. *PLoS ONE* 7:e36007. doi: 10.1371/journal.pone.0036007

Harnett, M. T., Makara, J. K., Spruston, N., Kath, W. L., and Magee, J. C. (2012). Synaptic amplification by dendritic spines enhances input cooperativity. *Nature* 491, 599–602. doi: 10.1038/nature11554

Harris, K. M., and Stevens, J. K. (1989). Dendritic spines of CA 1 pyramidal cells in the rat hippocampus: serial electron microscopy with reference to their biophysical characteristics. *J. Neurosci.* 9, 2982–2997.

Harvey, C. D., and Svoboda, K. (2007). Locally dynamic synaptic learning rules in pyramidal neuron dendrites. *Nature* 450, 1195–1200. doi: 10.1038/nature06416

Harvey, C. D., Yasuda, R., Zhong, H., and Svoboda, K. (2008). The spread of Ras activity triggered by activation of a single dendritic spine. *Science* 321, 136–140. doi: 10.1126/science.1159675

Holcman, D., and Schuss, Z. (2011). Diffusion laws in dendritic spines. *J. Math. Neurosci.* 1:10. doi: 10.1186/2190-8567-1-10

Jin, L., Han, Z., Platisa, J., Wooltorton, J. R., Cohen, L. B., and Pieribone, V. A. (2012). Single action potentials and subthreshold electrical events imaged in neurons with a fluorescent protein voltage probe. *Neuron* 75, 779–785. doi: 10.1016/j.neuron.2012.06.040

Koch, C., and Zador, A. (1993). The function of dendritic spines: devices subserving biochemical rather than electrical compartmentalization. *J. Neurosci.* 13, 413–422.

Kralj, J. M., Douglass, A. D., Hochbaum, D. R., Maclaurin, D., and Cohen, A. E. (2011). Optical recording of action potentials in mammalian neurons using a microbial rhodopsin. *Nat. Methods* 9, 90–95. doi: 10.1038/nmeth.1782

Matsuzaki, M., Honkura, N., Ellis-Davies, G. C., and Kasai, H. (2004). Structural basis of long-term potentiation in single dendritic spines. *Nature* 429, 761–766. doi: 10.1038/nature02617

Murakoshi, H., Wang, H., and Yasuda, R. (2011). Local, persistent activation of Rho GTPases during plasticity of single dendritic spines. *Nature* 472, 100–104. doi: 10.1038/nature09823

Nitsche, J. M., Chang, H. C., Weber, P. A., and Nicholson, B. J. (2004). A transient diffusion model yields unitary gap junctional permeabilities from images of cell-to-cell fluorescent dye transfer between Xenopus oocytes. *Biophys. J.* 86, 2058–2077. doi: 10.1016/S0006-3495(04)74267-8

Noguchi, J., Matsuzaki, M., Ellis-Davies, G. C., and Kasai, H. (2005). Spine-neck geometry determines NMDA receptor-dependent Ca2+ signaling in dendrites. *Neuron* 46, 609–622. doi: 10.1016/j.neuron.2005.03.015

Palmer, L. M., and Stuart, G. J. (2009). Membrane potential changes in dendritic spines during action potentials and synaptic input. *J. Neurosci.* 29, 6897–6903. doi: 10.1523/JNEUROSCI.5847-08.2009

Sabatini, B. L., Oertner, T. G., and Svoboda, K. (2002). The life cycle of Ca(2+) ions in dendritic spines. *Neuron* 33, 439–452. doi: 10.1016/S0896-6273(02)00573-1

Shankar, G. M., Li, S., Mehta, T. H., Garcia-Munoz, A., Shepardson, N. E., Smith, I., et al. (2008). Amyloid-beta protein dimers isolated directly from Alzheimer's brains impair synaptic plasticity and memory. *Nat. Med.* 14, 837–842. doi: 10.1038/nm1782

Sobczyk, A., and Svoboda, K. (2007). Activity-dependent plasticity of the NMDA-receptor fractional Ca2+ current. *Neuron* 53, 17–24. doi: 10.1016/j.neuron.2006.11.016

Soler-Llavina, G. J., and Sabatini, B. L. (2006). Synapse-specific plasticity and compartmentalized signaling in cerebellar stellate cells. *Nat. Neurosci.* 9, 798–806. doi: 10.1038/nn1698

Svoboda, K., Tank, D. W., and Denk, W. (1996). Direct measurement of coupling between dendritic spines and shafts. *Science* 272, 716–719. doi: 10.1126/science.272.5262.716

Takasaki, K. T., Ding, J. B., and Sabatini, B. L. (2013). Live-cell superresolution imaging by pulsed STED two-photon excitation microscopy. *Biophys. J.* 104, 770–777. doi: 10.1016/j.bpj.2012.12.053

Tavazoie, S. F., Alvarez, V. A., Ridenour, D. A., Kwiatkowski, D. J., and Sabatini, B. L. (2005). Regulation of neuronal morphology and function by the tumor suppressors Tsc1 and Tsc2. *Nat. Neurosci.* 8, 1727–1734. doi: 10.1038/nn1566

Tsay, D., and Yuste, R. (2004). On the electrical function of dendritic spines. *Trends Neurosci.* 27, 77–83. doi: 10.1016/j.tins.2003.11.008

Yasuda, R., and Murakoshi, H. (2011). The mechanisms underlying the spatial spreading of signaling activity. *Curr. Opin. Neurobiol.* 21, 313–321. doi: 10.1016/j.conb.2011.02.008

Yuste, R., and Denk, W. (1995). Dendritic spines as basic functional units of neuronal integration. *Nature* 375, 682–684. doi: 10.1038/375682a0

9

Fine structure of synapses on dendritic spines

Michael Frotscher[1]*, Daniel Studer[2], Werner Graber[2], Xuejun Chai[1], Sigrun Nestel[3] and Shanting Zhao[1]

[1] Institute for Structural Neurobiology, Center for Molecular Neurobiology Hamburg, University Medical Center Hamburg-Eppendorf, Hamburg, Germany
[2] Institute of Anatomy, University of Bern, Bern, Switzerland
[3] Institute of Anatomy and Cell Biology, University of Freiburg, Freiburg, Germany

***Correspondence:**
Michael Frotscher, Institute for Structural Neurobiology, Center for Molecular Neurobiology Hamburg, University Medical Center Hamburg-Eppendorf, Falkenried 94, 20251 Hamburg, Germany
e-mail: michael.frotscher@zmnh.uni-hamburg.de

Camillo Golgi's "Reazione Nera" led to the discovery of dendritic spines, small appendages originating from dendritic shafts. With the advent of electron microscopy (EM) they were identified as sites of synaptic contact. Later it was found that changes in synaptic strength were associated with changes in the shape of dendritic spines. While live-cell imaging was advantageous in monitoring the time course of such changes in spine structure, EM is still the best method for the simultaneous visualization of all cellular components, including actual synaptic contacts, at high resolution. Immunogold labeling for EM reveals the precise localization of molecules in relation to synaptic structures. Previous EM studies of spines and synapses were performed in tissue subjected to aldehyde fixation and dehydration in ethanol, which is associated with protein denaturation and tissue shrinkage. It has remained an issue to what extent fine structural details are preserved when subjecting the tissue to these procedures. In the present review we report recent studies on the fine structure of spines and synapses using high-pressure freezing (HPF), which avoids protein denaturation by aldehydes and results in an excellent preservation of ultrastructural detail. In these studies, HPF was used to monitor subtle fine-structural changes in spine shape associated with chemically induced long-term potentiation (cLTP) at identified hippocampal mossy fiber synapses. Changes in spine shape result from reorganization of the actin cytoskeleton. We report that cLTP was associated with decreased immunogold labeling for phosphorylated cofilin (p-cofilin), an actin-depolymerizing protein. Phosphorylation of cofilin renders it unable to depolymerize F-actin, which stabilizes the actin cytoskeleton. Decreased levels of p-cofilin, in turn, suggest increased actin turnover, possibly underlying the changes in spine shape associated with cLTP. The findings reviewed here establish HPF as an appropriate method for studying the fine structure and molecular composition of synapses on dendritic spines.

Keywords: dendritic spine, cofilin, actin cytoskeleton, immunogold labeling, electron microscopy, high-pressure freezing

INTRODUCTION

Early studies by Ramón y Cajal (1911) and his contemporaries already indicated that dendritic spines are not artifacts of the silver impregnation technique introduced by Camillo Golgi (Golgi, 1873). Querton (1898) observed changes in dendritic spines during hibernation, suggesting that dendritic spines are plastic structural elements that are subject to modification in an activity-dependent manner. By means of electron microscopy (EM) Gray (1959) showed that spines are postsynaptic elements, indicating that changes in spine number reflect changes in the connectivity pattern of the neuronal network. While studying network plasticity, many authors reported that afferent denervation affected the number of dendritic spines on postsynaptic cells. Thus, enucleation or dark rearing was found to result in a loss of dendritic spines in Golgi-impregnated neurons of the visual cortex (e.g., Valverde, 1967, 1968; Fifková, 1970). In contrast, the stimulation of an animal increased the number of dendritic spines and synapses (see Shapiro and Vukovic, 1970; Frotscher et al., 1975; Greenough et al., 1985). As far as the complex spines postsynaptic to hippocampal mossy fiber boutons (MFB) are concerned, we showed some time ago that removal of the entorhinal cortex during development results in *trans*-synaptic malformation of these spines (Frotscher et al., 1977). Collectively, these findings pointed to an inductive role of afferent fibers in the formation of their postsynaptic elements (Hámori, 1973). These observations in fixed tissue were supported by real-time microscopy studies showing *de novo* formation of dendritic spines following long-term potentiation (LTP) induction (Engert and Bonhoeffer, 1999). Recent studies further revealed that the structure of individual spines is not static but subject to change. Thin, long spines were assumed to be nascent spines, compared to the large mushroom-shaped spines that were associated with memory traces (Matsuzaki et al., 2004). Thus, the different spine categories, thin, stubby, and mushroom-shaped (Peters and Kaiserman-Abramof, 1970), appeared to represent different functional states. Theoretical considerations, as well as experimental data, led to the conclusion that dendritic spines are small devices that subserve chemical compartmentalization by amplifying and isolating synaptically induced second messengers such as calcium (Koch et al., 1992).

Changes in spine structure were accompanied by changes in the actin cytoskeleton and shifts in the equilibrium between F-actin and G-actin (Okamoto et al., 2004) by virtue of actin-depolymerizing proteins such as cofilin. The severing activity of cofilin is terminated by phosphorylation of the protein (Arber et al., 1998; Yang et al., 1998), and increased spine size in LTP was found to be associated with increased phosphorylation of cofilin (Chen et al., 2007; Rex et al., 2009), indicating stabilization of the spine cytoskeleton.

Several groups have reported on the changes in synaptic ultrastructure following LTP induction (Desmond and Levy, 1988; Buchs and Muller, 1996; Toni et al., 1999; Geinisman, 2000; Harris et al., 2003). Collectively, these studies indicated restructuring of synapses following LTP induction, ranging from synapse enlargement to the formation of spine-like protrusions.

With the present review article we pursue the following aims: first, we briefly summarize the literature on the fine structure of synapses on dendritic spines. Naturally, such a survey can only highlight some subjectively selected papers and remains incomplete. Second, we address the issue of tissue preservation for EM. We summarize recent studies in which high-pressure freezing (HPF) was used as an alternative method to conventional aldehyde fixation of neural tissue. Third, we report on the use of HPF in EM immunogold labeling studies. Without fixation in aldehyde solution, antigenicity to phosphorylated cofilin (p-cofilin) was found to be much better preserved than after conventional fixation for EM (Studer et al., 2014). Thus, this review summarizes our knowledge on spine synapses as well summarizing recent attempts to improve the preservation of their fine structure and molecular composition.

FINE STRUCTURE OF SYNAPSES ON DENDRITIC SPINES

Palade and Palay (1954) and Palay (1956, 1958) were the first to describe synapses by using electron microscopic methods. However, it was Gray (1959) who clearly showed that the heads of dendritic spines were postsynaptic elements of asymmetric synapses. He called them "asymmetric" because their postsynaptic density was thicker than the presynaptic membrane specialization. He differentiated them from the "symmetric" synapses often found on cell bodies. Today, we know that the presynaptic boutons of asymmetric synapses on spines contain the excitatory neurotransmitter glutamate, whereas the symmetric contacts formed on cell bodies are GABAergic inhibitory synapses. Harris and Weinberg (2012) have recently provided a comprehensive survey of the ultrastructure of synapses in the mammalian brain.

George Gray also discovered the spine apparatus, an enigmatic organelle consisting of sacs of endoplasmic reticulum intervened by electron dense bars (Gray, 1959). A spine apparatus is found in many, but not all, spines of forebrain neurons. It is absent in spines of cerebellar Purkinje cells (Peters et al., 1991). More recent studies have provided evidence that the spine apparatus is involved in synaptic plasticity and learning and memory. Thus, mouse mutants deficient in synaptopodin, a protein present in renal podocytes and dendritic spines (Mundel et al., 1997; Deller et al., 2000), do not form this organelle and are impaired in LTP and spatial learning (Deller et al., 2003).

Spine counts roughly reveal the number of excitatory synapses on dendritic spines, but there is no one-to-one relationship. In addition to the synapse on the spine head, there may be contacts on the spine neck (Peters and Kaiserman-Abramof, 1970), and the presynaptic bouton of this second synapse may contain a different neurotransmitter, for instance acetylcholine (Frotscher and Léránth, 1986).

In addition to their asymmetric membrane specializations and the presynaptic vesicle-filled bouton, synapses on spines are recognizable by a widening of the extracellular space at the site of the contact, i.e., the synaptic cleft. Synaptic contact zones or release sites may be perforated by a small protrusion of the spine, the spinule (Westrum and Blackstad, 1962; Tarrant and Routtenberg, 1977; Sorra et al., 1998), assumed to be involved in *trans*-endocytosis (Spacek and Harris, 2004). As first described by Steward and Levy (1982), ribosomes are often found at the base of spines or near synaptic contacts, suggesting local protein synthesis.

The fine structural characteristics of spine synapses briefly described here were observed in sections of a thickness of about 50 nm. The heads of large dendritic spines have a diameter of up to 1 μm and are thus much larger. This implies that conventional thin sections only show a small fraction of the spine, its synapses and organelles – unless three-dimensional reconstructions from complete series of thin sections were performed. This is relevant for conclusions regarding the regular occurrence of organelles in a spine or the frequency of synaptic contacts, and one should therefore rather talk of spine profiles when looking at single sections. Moreover, with the exception of some structurally unique synapses, in single sections we hardly know what the presynaptic and postsynaptic partners are. We do not know the functional history of a given spine or spine profile, nor do we know its age. Finally, we cannot be sure that all structures we see represent their native state in the living animal, which needs to be anesthetized and fixed with aldehyde solutions for subsequent EM. Given all these obstacles, it is remarkable that thorough EM analyses provided reliable data on structural changes at spine synapses associated with functional synaptic plasticity such as LTP. Intuitively, one would assume that synaptic strengthening is not only associated with a *de novo* formation of dendritic spines (Engert and Bonhoeffer, 1999) but also with an increase in the number of synaptic contacts. Remarkably, most investigators using conventional fixation and embedding procedures found neither an increase in synapse number (Geinisman, 2000) nor splitting of spines (Harris et al., 2003), but modification of preexisting contacts. For instance, Desmond and Levy (1988) reported an increase of synaptic interface surface area in LTP, and Geinisman (2000) showed an increase in the number of perforated synapses at the expense of non-perforated synapses. Harris et al. (2003) provided evidence of the formation of small spine-like protrusions that encountered presynaptic boutons already synapsing with neighboring spines. Toni et al. (1999) used calcium accumulation to determine activated synapses and observed an increase in the proportion of axon terminals contacting two or more dendritic spines.

A couple of questions arise at this point: How can we reliably identify potentiated synapses in a volume of tissue? How can we reliably identify the presynaptic and the postsynaptic neuron of a given synaptic contact? Can we optimize tissue fixation and dehydration to minimize protein denaturation and shrinkage?

HIGH-PRESSURE FREEZING AS AN ALTERNATIVE TO CONVENTIONAL ALDEHYDE FIXATION FOR EM

In conventional EM the tissue is subjected to chemical fixation using aldehyde solutions and is dehydrated in ascending series of ethanol. These steps are associated with protein denaturation and tissue shrinkage, respectively, depending on the water content of the various tissue components. Little information is available in the literature on how quickly the tissue is fixed upon exposition to the aldehyde solution. In addition, perfusion of an animal with fixation solution requires anesthesia, opening of the chest, and rinsing of the circulatory system with a rinsing solution before the fixative is administered. It is unknown to what extent these manipulations interfere with the preservation of fine-structural detail, in particular with the preservation of subtle structural changes induced by a preceding stimulation experiment. As far as dendritic spines are concerned, it has been previously shown, using real-time microscopy, that they undergo structural changes upon stimulation (Matsuzaki et al., 2004), but we do not know whether subtle stimulation-induced ultrastructural changes in spine shape, in synaptic structure, and in the molecular composition of spine synapses are preserved by conventional fixation and dehydration procedures.

One way to avoid conventional fixation and dehydration is by shock-freezing the tissue under high pressure, followed by cryosubstitution of the tissue water. HPF immobilizes the tissue in less than a second, resulting in tissue vitrification and excellent preservation of ultrastructural detail (Studer et al., 2001, 2014). Following HPF, the samples are collected in liquid nitrogen and then transferred to the freeze-substitution device. There, the tissue water is substituted by acetone and the sample osmicated for embedding in Epon. For EM immunogold labeling, the water is substituted by methanol (without osmication) and the sample embedded in Lowicryl HM20 (for details see Studer et al., 2014).

High-pressure freezing has been developed since rapid freezing without pressure only preserved the very surface of the tissue, whereas more remote portions showed ice crystal formation damaging cells and organelles. Shock-freezing of the tissue surface was pioneered by Van Harreveld et al. (1965), who studied the extracellular space in central nervous tissue. Heuser et al. (1979) dropped the tissue on a cooled metal block to capture synaptic vesicle fusion. Freezing under high pressure, however, lowers the freezing point of water and increases vitrification depth 10-fold (Sartori et al., 1993). Although HPF thus seems to be a clear improvement when compared to chemical fixation using aldehydes, we do not want to conceal the problems associated with this approach. First, tissue samples need to be small and easily accessible to be rapidly frozen. This may turn out to be critical when the sample needs to be transferred from the recording chamber to the high-pressure freezer, which causes a time delay. Moreover, in order to fit into the cavity of the specimen carrier, the region of interest might have to be punched out from a larger tissue sample. Ice crystal formation may occur when the samples or the instruments to handle them during further preparation are not properly cooled. Finally, warming up in an organic solvent prior to polymerization may lead to a reorganization and loss of some proteins (see Studer et al., 2014, for critical steps of the HPF procedure). Taken together, HPF is an alternative to conventional aldehyde fixation, but application of this complex method makes it necessary to carefully select the questions to be addressed.

Brain biopsies and acute brain slices have successfully been subjected to HPF (Studer et al., 2014). Optimal results were obtained with slice cultures (Zhao et al., 2012a,b; Studer et al., 2014). In contrast to acute slices, in which numerous neurons and their processes are acutely damaged by slice preparation, the tissue is allowed to recover and reorganize in slice cultures during incubation *in vitro*, and tissue debris is removed, thus resulting in flattening of the slice. When prepared, slice cultures are about 300 μm in thickness and flatten to about 200 μm during an incubation period of 1–2 weeks. Slice cultures are thus optimal for HPF since they are sufficiently thin to be completely frozen without the formation of ice crystals. Moreover, tissue-specific characteristics are nicely preserved in this culture model ("organotypic" slice cultures), even after extended periods of incubation *in vitro*. We recognized all known tissue components and good fine-structural preservation of *stratum lucidum* of the hippocampal region CA3 in slice cultures subjected to HPF. The unmyelinated mossy fiber axons, their giant expansions, and their postsynaptic complex spines (*excrescences*) originating from proximal dendrites of CA3 pyramidal neurons, were clearly discernible under these conditions (Zhao et al., 2012a,b; Studer et al., 2014; **Figure 1**). With regard to dendritic spines, we noticed an excellent preservation of their synaptic contacts and prominent asymmetric membrane specializations, the characteristic widening of the extracellular space at active zones (synaptic cleft), and organelles such as ribosomes and the spine apparatus (**Figure 2**). Moreover, we were able to monitor subtle changes in spine fine structure associated with the induction of chemical LTP (cLTP) by using slice cultures that were immediately subjected to HPF following the experiment (Zhao et al., 2012a). Other investigators that applied HPF to the study of the nervous system observed filamentous projections from the postsynaptic membrane specialization, linking the postsynaptic density to the actin cytoskeleton (Rostaing et al., 2006), and they studied the three-dimensional architecture of the presynaptic terminal matrix (Siksou et al., 2007).

cLTP-INDUCED FORMATION OF SMALL SPINES AT HIPPOCAMPAL MOSSY FIBER SYNAPSES

Long-term potentiation can be induced in various ways. Chemical LTP is advantageous when using HPF since the tissue can be incubated in the drug for a certain period of time and then be shock-frozen without any additional manipulation. In contrast, electrical stimulation requires the removal of the tissue

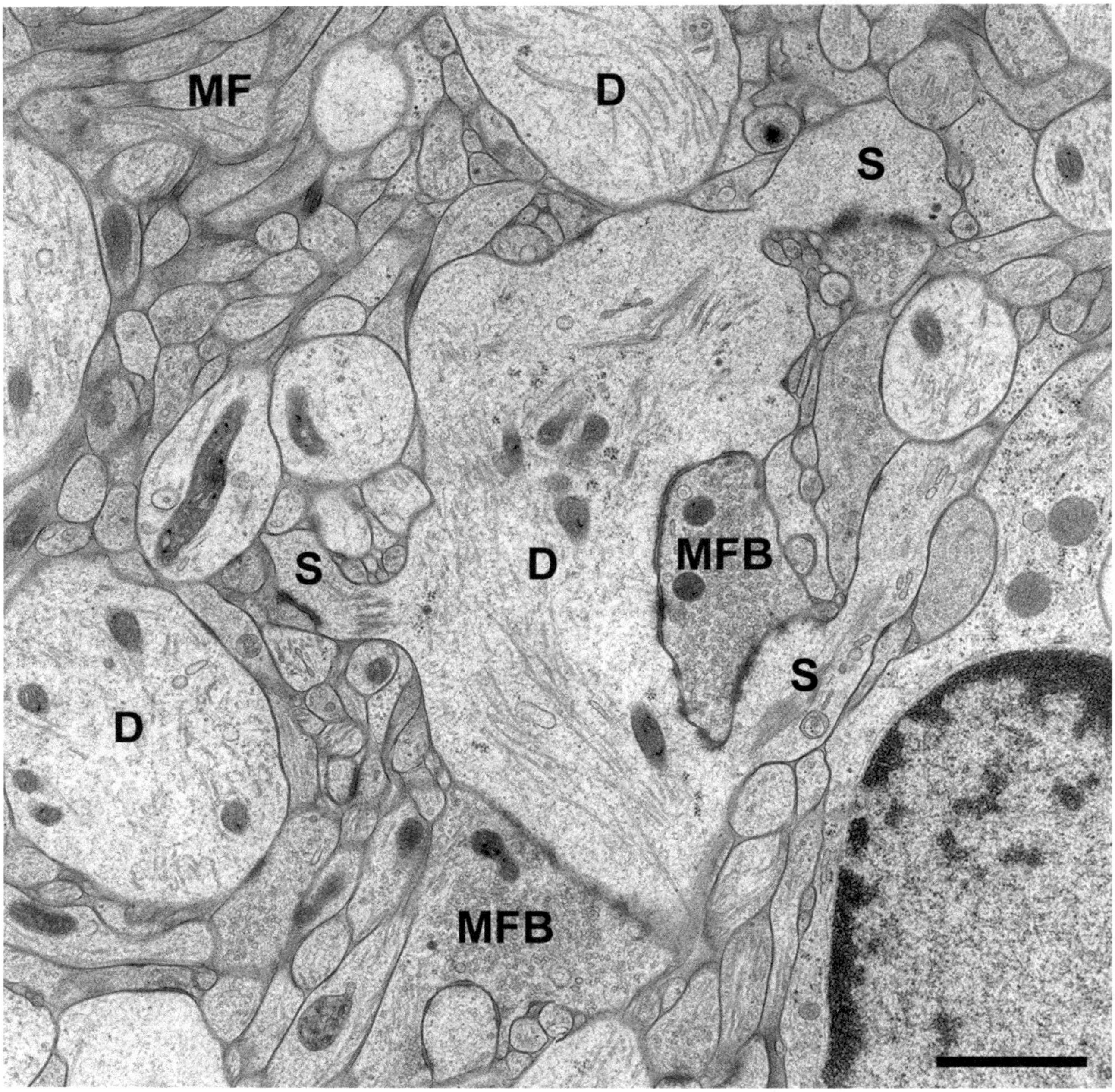

FIGURE 1 | CA3 region of Hippocampus in a slice culture incubated for 2 weeks *in vitro* (DIV). The tissue was high-pressure frozen in the absence of chemical fixatives, subjected to freeze substitution, osmicated, and finally embedded in Epon (see Studer et al., 2014, for details on the method). Note that all tissue components of *stratum lucidum* are well preserved after the incubation period and subsequent freezing procedure. As known from many studies in perfusion-fixed material, the *stratum lucidum* mainly contains the thin unmyelinated axons of the mossy fibers (MF) and their giant boutons (mossy fiber bouton, MFB). The postsynaptic elements, the proximal dendrites (D) of CA3 pyramidal cells, are located in between the bundles of mossy fibers and give rise to large complex spines (S) for the contact with MFBs. Scale bar: 1 μm.

from the recording chamber and transfer to the high-pressure freezer, which includes a time delay. Moreover, electrical stimulation affects an indeterminate number of synapses, whereas a large fraction of synapses are stimulated when using cLTP (Hosokawa et al., 1995). In the studies reported on here, we induced cLTP by exposing the tissue, organotypic slice cultures of hippocampus, to 25 mM tetraethylammonium (TEA) for 10 min. Control tissue was exposed to the control medium during that period of time. Whole-cell patch-clamp recordings from TEA-exposed CA3 pyramidal neurons, the target cells of hippocampal mossy fibers (MF), did indeed show strong potentiation of excitatory postsynaptic potentials (EPSPs) when

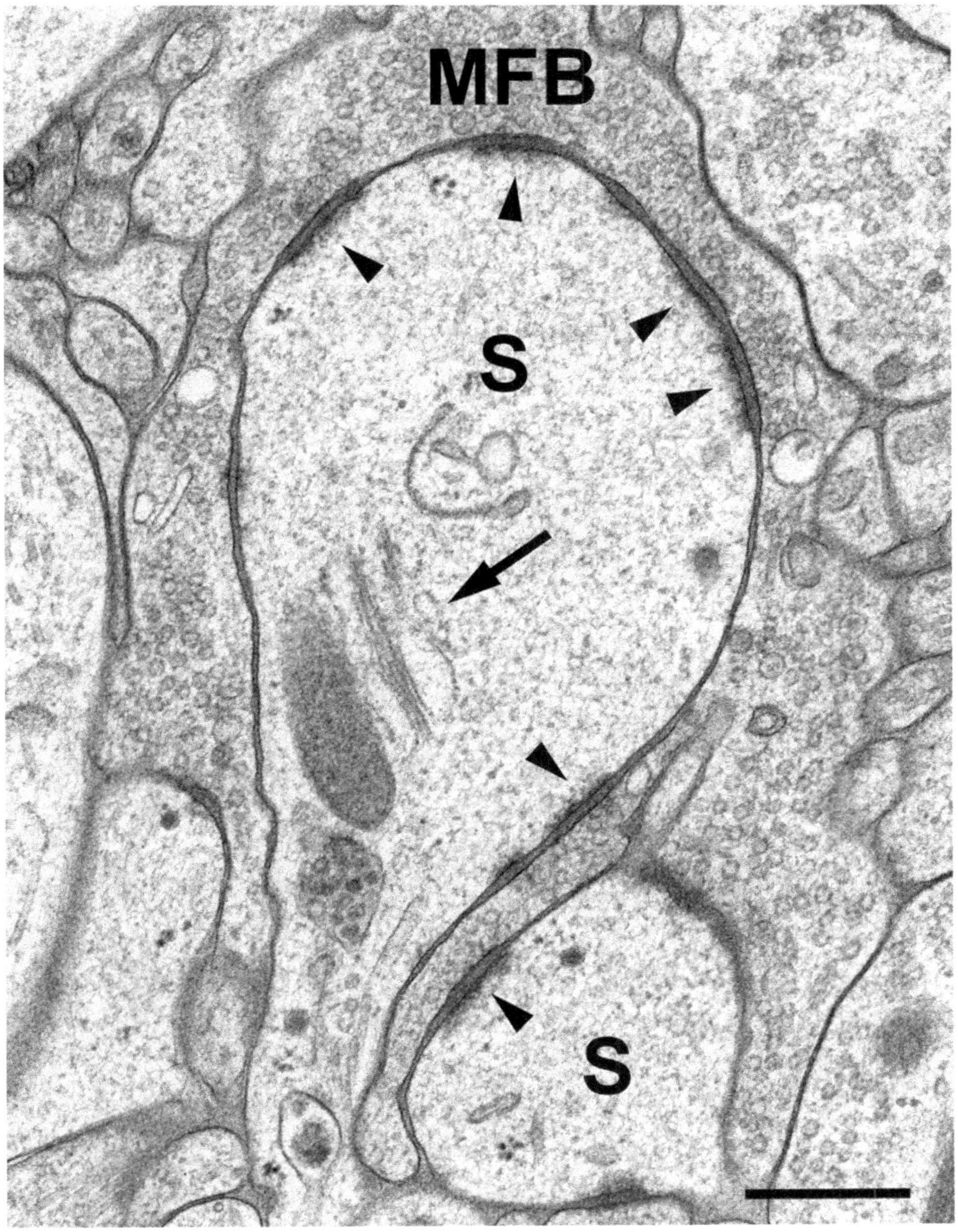

FIGURE 2 | High-pressure frozen slice culture after 2 weeks of incubation *in vitro*. Freeze substitution, osmication, and embedding in Epon. Large complex spines (S) of a CA3 pyramidal cell dendrite, engulfed by a large MFB. The arrow points to a spine apparatus with sacs of smooth endoplasmic reticulum and electron-dense bars. Arrowheads indicate active zones. Note the widening of the extracellular space at synaptic sites and prominent postsynaptic densities that extend fine filiform protrusions into the spine cytoplasm. Occasionally, ribosomes are seen near active zones. Scale bar: 200 nm.

compared to recording under control conditions (Zhao et al., 2012a,b). Following TEA treatment and incubation in control medium, respectively, the tissue was immediately shock-frozen using an EM PACT2 high-pressure freezer from Leica Microsystems (Vienna). The material was then subjected to cryosubstitution and embedding in Epon or Lowicryl HM20 (Zhao et al., 2012a,b; Studer et al., 2014). Epon embedding was used for studies on structural changes at spine synapses, whereas Lowicryl embedding was preferred in immunogold labeling experiments.

In our analysis, we focused on the easily identifiable mossy fiber synapse in the hippocampus formed between axons of dentate granule cells and large complex spines on proximal dendrites of CA3 pyramidal neurons (Blackstad and Kjaerheim, 1961;

Hamlyn, 1962). When studying TEA-exposed tissue and control tissue in the electron microscope, several observations were made. First, we noticed small omega-shaped invaginations of the presynaptic membrane of MFBs following TEA treatment. Most likely, these membrane invaginations represent vesicle fusions with the presynaptic membrane as a result of the strong TEA-induced stimulation. In fact, quantitative assessment of the number of vesicles in stimulated and non-stimulated tissue revealed a significant decrease in the number of vesicles in MFBs of TEA-treated cultures when compared to control cultures (Zhao et al., 2012a). We interpreted this decrease in synaptic vesicles, together with an increased number of fusion events, as resulting from stimulation, and expected to see an increase in the length of the presynaptic MFB membrane. Indeed, while there was no difference in the area of MFB profiles, there was an increase in the ratio of mossy fiber perimeter/mossy fiber area, indicating a more labyrinthine course of the presynaptic membrane in stimulated mossy fiber synapses. On the postsynaptic side, we observed an increase in the complexity of the large spines or *excrescences* in contact with MFBs. In particular, we observed the formation of small, filopodia-like protrusions originating from the large complex spines (Zhao et al., 2012a,b). Thus, the more labyrinthine course of the presynaptic membrane was accompanied by a more convoluted appearance of the postsynaptic spine surface. These results confirmed and extended previous work on experience-dependent growth of mossy fiber synapses observed in light microscopic studies (Galimberti et al., 2006, 2010). The formation of these filopodia-like protrusions was accompanied by an increase in the number of synaptic contacts. Collectively, these findings indicated growth of mossy fiber synapses in response to intense stimulation. Moreover, the results showed that HPF combined with EM is a suitable method of capturing such activity-induced changes at spine synapses with high resolution. The reader is referred to our original paper (Zhao et al., 2012a) for the complete data set and to our protocol for details on the methods (Studer et al., 2014).

Appropriate controls are an important issue in studies on synaptic plasticity. As mentioned, TEA-stimulated slice cultures of hippocampus were compared to non-stimulated cultures. In addition, we used slice cultures from Munc13-1 mouse mutants that are impaired with respect to vesicle priming and docking (Augustin et al., 1999). Indeed, when we compared TEA-stimulated Munc13-1 slice cultures with non-stimulated cultures from these mutants,

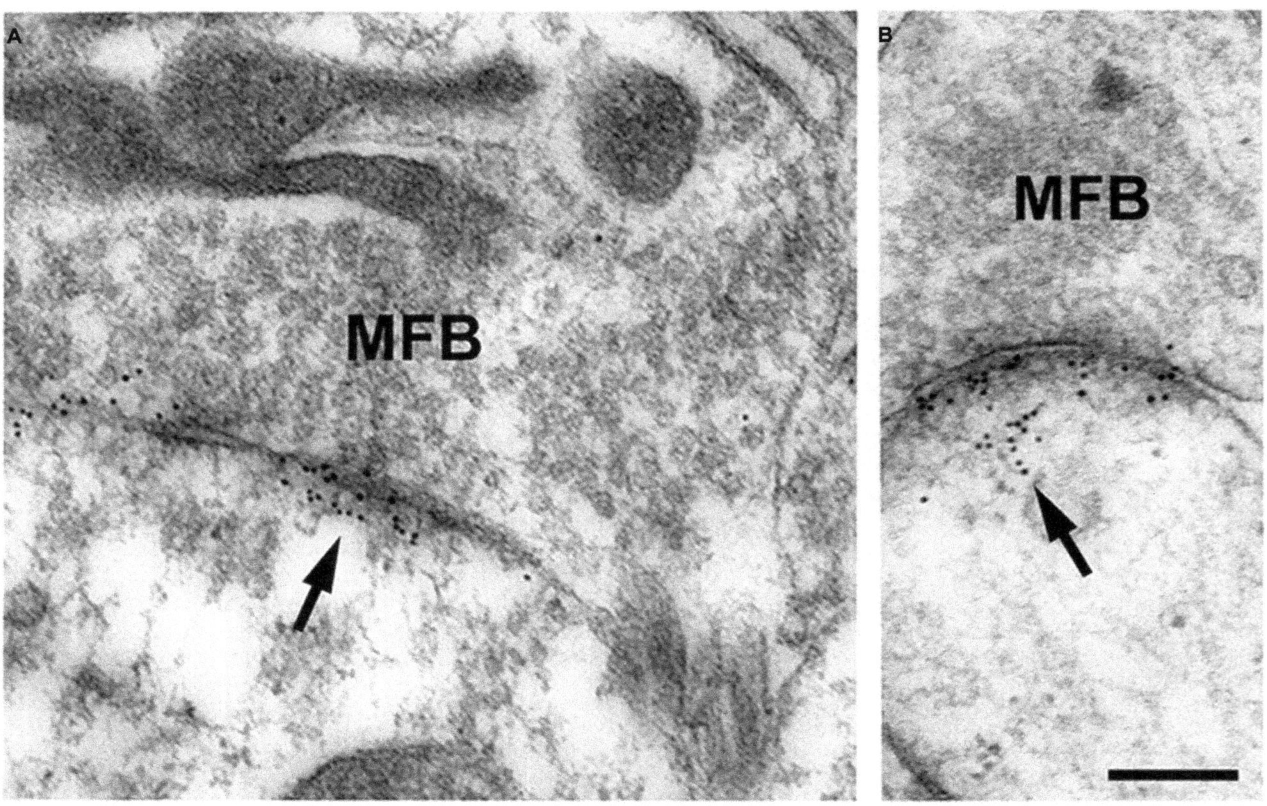

FIGURE 3 | (A,B) High-pressure frozen slice culture of hippocampus incubated *in vitro* for 2 weeks. Freeze substitution, embedding of the tissue in Lowicryl HM20 (no osmication), and postembedding immunogold labeling for p-cofilin in thin sections of the CA3 region. Note the specific accumulations of gold grains (arrows) at synaptic sites of MFB. Only occasionally are gold grains seen at other locations. Thin sections were incubated in rabbit anti-p-cofilin (ser3; 1:100; Santa Cruz Biotechnology, Heidelberg, Germany); secondary antibodies were gold-labeled (goat-anti-rabbit, 10 nm gold grains; British Biocell, Cardiff, UK). Sections were post-stained with uranyl acetate and lead citrate. For control, the primary antibody was omitted; no specific staining was seen under these conditions. Scale bar: 200 nm.

no differences were observed with respect to the formation of the filopodia-like spine protrusions and number of synaptic contacts (Zhao et al., 2012a). Also, there was no difference in the number of synaptic vesicles and the perimeter of the presynaptic bouton membrane between stimulated and non-stimulated cultures of Munc13-1 mutant mice.

CHANGES IN COFILIN PHOSPHORYLATION INDUCED BY cLTP

Tetraethylammonium-induced stimulation resulted in the formation of small spines and new synaptic contacts. However, when measuring the length of these synaptic contacts, we noticed that they were shorter than in controls (Zhao et al., 2012a). We regarded this as a hint that the spine-like protrusions and their synaptic contacts were still in the process of growth after the 10-min TEA stimulation. Restructuring of spines requires remodeling of the actin cytoskeleton, which is particularly enriched in dendritic spines (Fischer et al., 1998, 2000; Matus, 2000; Star et al., 2002; Fukazawa et al., 2003; Okamoto et al., 2004; Hotulainen et al., 2009; Hotulainen and Hoogenraad, 2010). Remodeling of the actin cytoskeleton involves active, actin-depolymerizing (non-phosphorylated) cofilin to build new actin filaments and change spine shape. Accordingly, levels of p-cofilin might be decreased in early phases of LTP induction and may be associated with spine restructuring.

In our studies on structural synaptic plasticity of mossy fiber synapses we used HPF and postembedding immunogold labeling for p-cofilin following cLTP induction by TEA. Consistent with previous EM immunogold studies for cofilin (Racz and Weinberg, 2006), we noticed accumulations of gold grains at synaptic contacts (**Figure 3**; Studer et al., 2014). Interestingly enough, we found a statistically significant decrease in the number of gold grains at mossy fiber synapses of TEA-stimulated slice cultures when compared to non-stimulated cultures (**Figure 4**). In TEA-stimulated cultures the number of gold grains at active zones of mossy fiber synapses, up to a distance of 100 nm from the membrane specialization, amounted to 3.7 ± 2.7 SD compared to 5.6 ± 3.0 SD in the control cultures. This result suggested a relative increase in non-p-cofilin and hence active cytoskeletal reorganization at the time point of immobilization by HPF. Remarkably, this decrease in p-cofilin immunoreactivity was not observed in TEA-stimulated slice cultures from Munc13-1 mutant mice (TEA: 4.5 ± 2.8 SD; control: 4.6 ± 3.3 SD; **Figure 4**), consistent with the lack of TEA-induced structural changes at spines in slice cultures from these mutants (Zhao et al., 2012a). Our results are in line with other studies pointing to an involvement of cofilin in changes in spine structure and reorganization of the actin cytoskeleton associated with LTP (Fukazawa et al., 2003; Lisman, 2003; Zhou et al., 2004; Chen et al., 2007; Rex et al., 2009). In mutants deficient in LIM kinase-1 (LIMK-1), the kinase that phosphorylates cofilin, LTP is enhanced associated with changes in spine morphology and a reduced length of the postsynaptic density (Meng et al., 2002).

An interesting side effect of the immunogold labeling studies was that, in general, the number of gold grains indicating p-cofilin immunoreactivity was much larger in slice cultures subjected to HPF, compared to cultures conventionally fixed using aldehyde solutions. It is of note that this was not due to increased background staining (Studer et al., 2014). These observations point

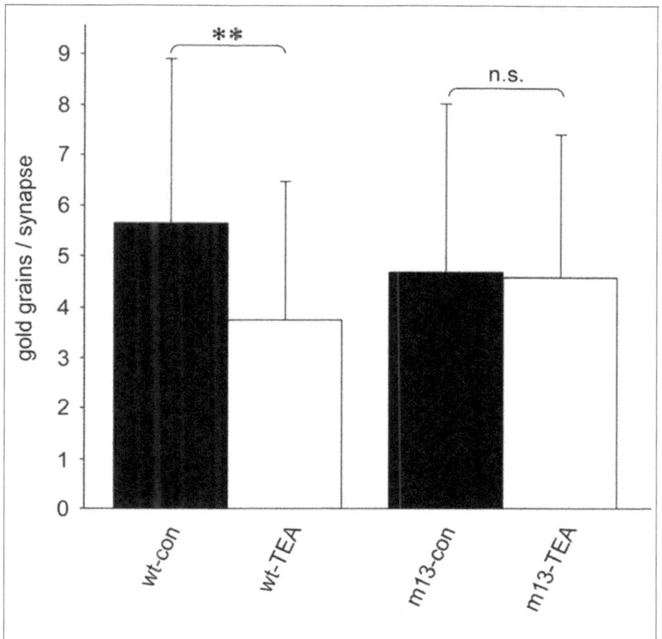

FIGURE 4 | Quantitative estimation of the number of gold grains per active zone at mossy fiber synapses in *stratum lucidum* of CA3 in hippocampal slice cultures subjected to HPF, freeze substitution, embedding in Lowicryl HM20 (no osmication), thin-sectioning, and immunogold labeling for p-cofilin. The number of gold grains at mossy fiber synapses is significantly higher in wild-type control cultures (wt-con) compared to wt cultures treated with TEA (wt-TEA; mean ± SD; $^{**}p < 0.01$). This difference between control tissue and TEA-treated tissue was not observed in cultures from Munc13-1 mutants (m13-con and m13-TEA, respectively). n.s., not significant. All gold grains within 100 nm of the postsynaptic density were regarded as specific labeling and were counted (60 active zones per experimental group; two-sided Student's *t*-test; $\alpha = 0.05$). See Studer et al. (2014) for details on the method.

to an increased signal-to-noise ratio of immunolabeling following freezing, freeze substitution, and embedding in Lowicryl, as similarly described in previous studies (e.g., Moreira et al., 1998). This is likely because protein denaturation by aldehydes and robust dehydration in ethanol are avoided. Thus, HPF combined with freeze substitution and Lowicryl embedding may be a useful alternative to conventional EM immunocytochemical methods.

MOSSY FIBER BOUTONS AND THEIR POSTSYNAPTIC SPINES ARE RESTRUCTURED IN AN ACTIVITY-DEPENDENT MANNER

Numerous studies, including those on the famous patient H.M., have indicated that the hippocampal formation plays an important role in learning and memory processes. What does this mean at the level of cells, projections, and synapses? Sensory perception of novel, probably dangerous changes in the environment will require behavioral adjustment to cope with the new situation. In higher centers, such as the cerebral cortex and hippocampus, behavioral adjustment involves associations and recall of previous, similar situations. It is generally assumed that this "learning" about a novel environment is achieved by modification of the neuronal circuit. Information about the environment is fed into the hippocampus via the entorhinal cortex, which receives input from a large variety of sensory centers. Circuit modification is then assumed to take place in the hippocampus, particularly in the synapses of the trisynaptic pathway (Andersen et al., 1971), involving the synapses of entorhinal fibers with dentate granule cells, granule cell synapses (mossy fiber synapses) with CA3 pyramidal neurons and mossy cells, and CA3 pyramidal cell projections (Schaffer collaterals) to CA1 pyramidal neurons. Plasticity of transmission at hippocampal synapses, including changes in the structure of spines and synaptic contacts as seen in LTP or LTD (long-term depression), has accordingly become a widely studied cellular model of learning and memory processes.

Potentiation or depression of synaptic transmission is associated with molecular and structural changes at synapses. In this review, we report on the formation of finger-shaped protrusions emerging from the complex spines of mossy fiber synapses and *de novo* formation of active zones in response to cLTP induction. These structural changes were associated with decreased phosphorylation of cofilin, suggesting active remodeling of the actin cytoskeleton in the complex spines. It is most likely that these fine-structural and molecular changes underlie the experience-dependent increase in complexity of mossy fiber synapses observed in light microscopic studies (Galimberti et al., 2006, 2010).

ACKNOWLEDGMENTS

The authors thank Professor Nils Brose (Max Planck Institute for Experimental Medicine, Göttingen, Germany) for providing the Munc13-1 mouse mutants and Mrs. Liz Grundy for reading the manuscript. The work reviewed in this article was supported by grants from the Deutsche Forschungsgemeinschaft (grant number: FR 620/12-1; SFB 780: project A4) and the Swiss National Foundation (grant number: 3100AO_118394). Michael Frotscher is Senior Research Professor of the Hertie Foundation.

REFERENCES

Andersen, P., Bliss, T. V. P., and Skrede, K. K. (1971). Lamellar organization of hippocampal excitatory pathways. *Exp. Brain Res.* 13, 222–238. doi: 10.1007/BF00234087

Arber, S., Barbayannis, F. A., Hanser, H., Schneider, C., Stanyon, C. A., Bernard, O., et al. (1998). Regulation of actin dynamics through phosphorylation of cofilin by LIM-kinase. *Nature* 393, 805–809. doi: 10.1038/31729

Augustin, I., Rosenmund, C., Südhof, T. C., and Brose, N. (1999). Munc13-1 is essential for fusion competence of glutamatergic synaptic vesicles. *Nature* 400, 457–461. doi: 10.1038/22768

Blackstad, T. W., and Kjaerheim, A. (1961). Special axo-dendritic synapses in the hippocampal cortex: electron and light microscopic studies on the layer of mossy fibers. *J. Comp. Neurol.* 117, 133–159. doi: 10.1002/cne.901170202

Buchs, P. A., and Muller, D. (1996). Induction of long-term potentiation is associated with major ultrastructural changes of activated synapses. *Proc. Natl. Acad. Sci. U.S.A.* 93, 8040–8045. doi: 10.1073/pnas.93.15.8040

Chen, L. Y., Rex, C. S., Casale, M. S., Gall, C. M., and Lynch, G. (2007). Changes in synaptic morphology accompany actin signaling during LTP. *J. Neurosci.* 27, 5363–5372. doi: 10.1523/JNEUROSCI.0164-07.2007

Deller, T., Korte, M., Chabanis, S., Drakew, A., Schwegler, H., Stefani, G. G., et al. (2003). Synaptopodin-deficient mice lack a spine apparatus and show deficits in synaptic plasticity. *Proc. Natl. Acad. Sci. U.S.A.* 100, 10494–10499. doi: 10.1073/pnas.1832384100

Deller, T., Merten, T., Roth, S. U., Mundel, P., and Frotscher, M. (2000). Actin-associated protein synaptopodin in the rat hippocampal formation: localization in the spine neck and close association with the spine apparatus of principal neurons. *J. Comp. Neurol.* 418, 164–181. doi: 10.1002/(SICI)1096-9861(20000306)418:2<164::AID-CNE4>3.0.CO;2-0

Desmond, N. L., and Levy, W. B. (1988). Synaptic interface surface area increases with long-term potentiation in the hippocampal dentate gyrus. *Brain Res.* 453, 308–314. doi: 10.1016/0006-8993(88)90171-0

Engert, F., and Bonhoeffer, T. (1999). Dendritic spine changes associated with hippocampal long-term synaptic plasticity. *Nature* 399, 66–70. doi: 10.1038/19978

Fifková, E. (1970). The effect of unilateral deprivation on visual centers in rats. *J. Comp. Neurol.* 140, 431–438. doi: 10.1002/cne.901400404

Fischer, M., Kaech, S., Knutti, D., and Matus, A. (1998). Rapid actin-based plasticity in dendritic spines. *Neuron* 20, 847–854. doi: 10.1016/S0896-6273(00)80467-5

Fischer, M., Kaech, S., Wagner, U., Brinkhaus, H., and Matus, A. (2000). Glutamate receptors regulate actin-based plasticity in dendritic spines. *Nat. Neurosci.* 3, 887–894. doi: 10.1038/78791

Frotscher, M., Hámori, J., and Wenzel, J. (1977). Transneuronal effects of entorhinal lesions in the early postnatal period on synaptogenesis in the hippocampus of the rat. *Exp. Brain Res.* 30, 549–560. doi: 10.1007/BF00237644

Frotscher, M., and Léránth, C. (1986). The cholinergic innervation of the rat fascia dentata: identification of target structures on granule cells by combining choline acetyltransferase immunocytochemistry and Golgi impregnation. *J. Comp. Neurol.* 243, 58–70. doi: 10.1002/cne.902430106

Frotscher, M., Mannsfeld, B., and Wenzel, J. (1975). Umweltabhängige Differenzierung der Dendritenspines an Pyramidenneuronen des Hippocampus (CA1) der Ratte. *J. Hirnforsch.* 16, 443–450.

Fukazawa, Y., Saitoh, Y., Ozawa, F., Ohta, Y., Mizuno, K., and Inokuchi, K. (2003). Hippocampal LTP is accompanied by enhanced F-actin content within the dendritic spine that is essential for late LTP maintenance in vivo. *Neuron* 38, 447–460. doi: 10.1016/S0896-6273(03)00206-X

Galimberti, I., Bednarek, E., Donato, F., and Caroni, P. (2010). EphA4 signaling in juveniles establishes topographic specificity of structural plasticity in the hippocampus. *Neuron* 65, 627–642. doi: 10.1016/j.neuron.2010.02.016

Galimberti, I., Gogolla, N., Alberi, S., Santos, A. F., Muller, D., and Caroni, P. (2006). Long-term rearrangements of hippocampal mossy fiber terminal connectivity in the adult regulated by experience. *Neuron* 50, 749–763. doi: 10.1016/j.neuron.2006.04.026

Geinisman, Y. (2000). Structural synaptic modifications associated with hippocampal LTP and behavioral learning. *Cereb. Cortex* 10, 952–962. doi: 10.1093/cercor/10.10.952

Golgi, C. (1873). Sulla struttura della sostanza grigia della cervello. *Gazz. Med. Ital. Lombardia* 6, 244–246.

Gray, E. G. (1959). Axo-somatic and axodendritic synapses of the cerebral cortex: an electron microscope study. *J. Anat. (London)* 93, 420–433.

Greenough, W. T., Hwang, H.-M. F., and Gorman, C. (1985). Evidence for active synapse formation or altered postsynaptic metabolism in visual cortex of rats reared in complex environments. *Proc. Natl. Acad. Sci. U.S.A.* 82, 4549–4552. doi: 10.1073/pnas.82.13.4549

Hamlyn, L. H. (1962). The fine structure of the mossy fibre endings in the hippocampus of the rabbit. *J. Anat.* 96, 112–120. doi: 10.1007/BF00455273

Hámori, J. (1973). The inductive role of presynaptic axons in the development of postsynaptic spines. *Brain Res.* 62, 337–344. doi: 10.1016/0006-8993(73)90694-X

Harris, K. M., Fiala, J. C., and Ostroff, L. (2003). Structural changes at dendritic spine synapses during long-term potentiation. *Philos. Trans. R. Soc. Lond. Biol. Sci.* 358, 745–748. doi: 10.1098/rstb.2002.1254

Harris, K. M., and Weinberg, R. J. (2012). Ultrastructure of synapses in the mammalian brain. *Cold Spring Harb. Perspect. Biol.* 4:a005587. doi: 10.1101/cshperspect.a 005587

Heuser, J. E., Reese, T. S., Dennis, M. J., Jan, Y., Jan, L., and Evans, L. (1979). Synaptic vesicle exocytosis captured by quick freezing and correlated with quantal transmitter release. *J. Cell Biol.* 81, 275–300. doi: 10.1083/jcb.81.2.275

Hosokawa, T., Rusakov, D. A., Bliss, T. V., and Fine, A. (1995). Repeated confocal imaging of individual dendritic spines in the living hippocampal slice: evidence for changes in length and orientation associated with chemically induced LTP. *J. Neurosci.* 15, 5560–5573. doi: 10.1038/19978

Hotulainen, P., and Hoogenraad, C. C. (2010). Actin in dendritic spines: connecting dynamics to function. *J. Cell Biol.* 189, 619–629. doi: 10.1083/jcb.201003008

Hotulainen, P., Llano, O., Smirnov, S., Tanhuanpää, K., Faix, J., and Rivera, C., et al. (2009). Defining mechanisms of actin polymerization and depolymerization during dendritic spine morphogenesis. *J. Cell. Biol.* 185, 323–339. doi: 10.1083/jcb.200809046

Koch, C., Zador, A., and Brown, T. H. (1992). Dendritic spines: convergence of theory and experiment. *Science* 256, 973–974. doi: 10.1126/science.1589781

Lisman, J. (2003). Actin's actions in LTP-induced synapse growth. *Neuron* 38, 361–365. doi: 10.1016/S0896-6273(03)00257-5

Matsuzaki, M., Honkura, N., Ellis-Davies, G. C. R., and Kasai, H. (2004). Structural basis of long-term potentiation in single dendritic spines. *Nature* 429, 761–766. doi: 10.1038/nature02617

Matus, A. (2000). Actin-based plasticity in dendritic spines. *Science* 290, 754–758. doi: 10.1126/science.290.5492.754

Meng, Y., Zhang, Y., Tregoubov, V., Janus, C., Cruz, L., Jackson, M., et al. (2002). Abnormal spine morphology and enhanced LTP in LIMK-1 knockout mice. *Neuron* 35, 121–133. doi: 10.1016/S0896-6273(02)00758-4

Moreira, J. E., Dodane, V., and Reese, T. S. (1998). Immunoelectronmicroscopy of soluable and membrane proteins with a sensitive postembedding method. *J. Histochem. Cytochem.* 46, 847–854. doi: 10.1177/002215549804600708

Mundel, P., Heid, H. W., Mundel, T. M., Krüger, M., Reiser, J., and Kriz, W. (1997). Synaptopodin: an actin-associated protein in telencephalic dendrites and renal podocytes. *J. Cell Biol.* 139, 193–204. doi: 10.1083/jcb.139.1.193

Okamoto, K. I., Nagai, T., Miyawaki, A., and Hayashi, Y. (2004). Rapid and persistent modulation of actin dynamics regulates postsynaptic reorganization underlying bidirectional plasticity. *Nat. Neurosci.* 7, 1104–1112. doi: 10.1038/nn1311

Palade, G. E., and Palay, S. L. (1954). Electron microscope observations of interneuronal and neuromuscular synapses. *Anat. Rec.* 118, 335–336.

Palay, S. L. (1956). Synapses in the central nervous system. *J. Biophys. Biochem. Cytol.* 2, 193–206. doi: 10.1083/jcb.2.4.193

Palay, S. L. (1958). The morphology of synapses of the central nervous system. *Exp. Cell Res.* 5, 275–293.

Peters, A., and Kaiserman-Abramof, I. R. (1970). The small pyramidal neuron of the rat cerebral cortex. The perikaryon, dendrites and spines. *J. Anat.* 127, 321–356. doi: 10.1002/aja.1001270402

Peters, A., Palay, S. L., and Webster, H. F. (1991). *The Fine Structure of the Nervous System.* New York: Oxford University Press. 9

Querton, L. (1898). Le sommeil hibernal et les modifications des neurones cerebraux. *Ann. Soc. Roy. Sci. Med. Nat. (de Bruxelles)* 7, 147–204.

Racz, B., and Weinberg, R. J. (2006). Spatial organization of cofilin in dendritic spines. *Neuroscience* 138, 447–456. doi: 10.1016/j.neuroscience.2005.11.025

Ramón y Cajal, S. R. (1911). *Histologie du Système Nerveux de lhomme et des Vertébrés,* Vol. 2. Paris: Maloine.

Rex, C. S., Chen, L. Y., Sharma, A., Liu, J., Babayan, A. H., Gall, C. M., et al. (2009). Different Rho GTPase-dependent signaling pathways initiate sequential steps in the consolidation of long-term potentiation. *J. Cell Biol.* 186, 85–97. doi: 10.1083/jcb.200901084

Rostaing, P., Real, E., Siksou, L., Lechaire, J. P., Boudier, P., Boeckers, T. M., et al. (2006). Analysis of synaptic ultrastructure without fixative using high-pressure freezing and tomography. *J. Neurosci.* 24, 3463–3474. doi: 10.1111/j.1460-9568.2006.05234.x

Sartori, N., Richter, K., and Dubochet, J. (1993). Vitrification depth can be increased more than 10-fold by high-pressure freezing. *J. Microsc.* 172, 55–61. doi: 10.1111/j.1365-2818.1993.tb03393.x

Shapiro, S., and Vukovic, K. R. (1970). Early experience upon cortical dendrites: A proposed model for development. *Science* 167, 292–294. doi: 10.1126/science.167.3916.292

Siksou, L., Rostaing, P., Lechaire, J. P., Boudier, P., Ohtsuka, T., Fejtova, A., et al. (2007). Three-dimensional architecture of presynaptic terminal cytomatrix. *J. Neurosci.* 27, 6868–6877. doi: 10.1523/JNEUROSCI.1773-07.2007

Sorra, K. E., Fiala, J. C., and Harris, K. M. (1998). Critical assessment of the involvement of perforations, spinules, and spine branching in hippocampal synapse formation. *J. Comp. Neurol.* 398, 225–240. doi: 10.1002/(SICI)1096-9861(19980824)398:2<225::AID-CNE5>3.0.CO;2-2

Spacek, J., and Harris, K. M. (2004). Trans-endocytosis via spinules in adult rat hippocampus. *J. Neurosci.* 24, 4233–4241. doi: 10.1523/JNEUROSCI.0287-04.2004

Star, E. N., Kwiatkowski, D. J., and Murthy, V. N. (2002). Rapid turnover of actin in dendritic spines and its regulation by activity. *Nat. Neurosci.* 5, 239–246. doi: 10.1038/nn811

Steward, O., and Levy, W. B. (1982). Preferential localization of polyribosomes under the base of dendritic spines in granule cells of the dentate gyrus. *J. Neurosci.* 2, 284–291.

Studer, D., Graber, W., Al-Amoudi, A., and Eggli, P. A. (2001). A new approach for cryofixation by high-pressure freezing. *J. Microsc.* 203, 285–294. doi: 10.1046/j.1365-2818.2001.00919.x

Studer, D., Zhao, S., Chai, X., Jonas, P., Graber, W., Nestel, S., et al. (2014). Capture of activity-induced ultrastructural changes at synapses by high-pressure freezing of brain tissue. *Nat. Protoc.* 9, 1480–1495. doi: 10.1038/nprot.2014.099

Tarrant, S. B., and Routtenberg, A. (1977). The synaptic spinule in the dendritic spine: electron microscopic study of the hippocampal dentate gyrus. *Tissue Cell* 9, 461–473. doi: 10.1016/0040-8166(77)90006-4

Toni, N., Buchs, P. A., Nikonenko, I., Bron, C. R., and Muller, D. (1999). LTP promotes formation of multiple spine synapses between a single axon terminal and a dendrite. *Nature* 402, 421–425. doi: 10.1038/46574

Valverde, F. (1967). Apical dendritic spines and light deprivation in the mouse. *Exp. Brain Res.* 3, 337–352. doi: 10.1007/BF00237559

Valverde, F. (1968). Structural changes in the area striata of the mouse after enucleation. *Exp. Brain Res.* 5, 274–292. doi: 10.1007/BF00235903

Van Harreveld, A., Crowell, J., and Malhotra, S. K. (1965). A study of extracellular space in central nervous tissue by freeze-substitution. *J. Cell Biol.* 25, 117–137. doi: 10.1083/jcb.25.1.117

Westrum, L. E., and Blackstad, T. (1962). An electron microscopic study of the stratum radiatum of the rat hippocampus (regio superior, CA1) with particular emphasis on synaptology. *J. Comp. Neurol.* 119, 281–309. doi: 10.1002/cne.901190303

Yang, N., Higuchi, O., Ohashi, K., Nagata, K., Wada, A., Kangawa, K., et al. (1998). Cofilin phosphorylation by LIM-kinase 1 and its role in Rac-mediated actin reorganization. *Nature* 393, 809–812. doi: 10.1038/31735

Studer, D., Chai, X., Graber, W., Brose, N., Nestel, S., et al. (2012a). Structural plasticity of hippocampal mossy fiber synapses as revealed by high-pressure freezing. *J. Comp. Neurol.* 520, 2340-2351. doi: 10.1002/cne.23040

Zhao, S., Studer, D., Chai, X. Graber, W., Brose, N., Nestel, S., et al. (2012b). Structural plasticity of spines at giant mossy fiber synapses. *Front. Neural Circuits* 6:103. doi: 103389/fncir.2012.00103

Zhou, Q., Homma, K. J., and Poo, M. (2004). Shrinkage of dendritic spines associated with long-term depression of hippocampal synapses. *Neuron* 44, 749–757. doi: 10.1016/j.neuron.2004.11.011

10

Fluorescent labeling of dendritic spines in cell cultures with the carbocyanine dye "DiI"

Connie Cheng, Olivia Trzcinski and Laurie C. Doering*

Department of Pathology and Molecular Medicine, McMaster University, Hamilton, ON, Canada

Correspondence:
Laurie C. Doering, Department of Pathology and Molecular Medicine, McMaster University, 1280 Main Street West, Hamilton, ON L8S 4K1, Canada
e-mail: doering@mcmaster.ca

Analyzing cell morphology is a key component to understand neuronal function. Several staining techniques have been developed to facilitate the morphological analysis of neurons, including the use of fluorescent markers, such as DiI (1,1′-dioctadecyl-3,3,3′,3′-tetramethylindocarbocyanine perchlorate). DiI is a carbocyanine membrane dye that exhibits enhanced fluorescence upon insertion of its lipophilic hydrocarbon chains into the lipid membrane of cells. The high photostability and prominent fluorescence of the dye serves as an effective means of illuminating cellular architecture in individual neurons, including detailed dendritic arborizations and spines in cell culture and tissue sections. Here, we specifically optimized a simple and reliable method to fluorescently label and visualize dissociated hippocampal neurons using DiI and high-resolution confocal microscopic imaging. With high efficacy, this method accurately labels neuronal and synaptic morphology to permit quantitative analysis of dendritic spines. Accurate imaging techniques of these fine neuronal specializations are vital to the study of their morphology and can help delineate structure-function relationships in the central nervous system.

Keywords: DiI, carbocyanine dye, dendritic spine, morphology, confocal microscopy, paraformaldehyde, neuronal function

INTRODUCTION

Dendritic spines are small protrusions from the dendritic shaft of various types of neurons that act as the postsynaptic compartments of most excitatory synapses in the central nervous system (CNS). They are known to play a significant role in neuronal plasticity and synaptic integration through their ability to undergo structural rearrangements during development (Rochefort and Konnerth, 2012). Morphological features of spines, such as size, shape, and density, have been shown to reflect important synaptic functional attributes and the potential for plasticity. Spine morphology is highly variable and has been classified into several different types based on their structure: filopodia, long-thin, stubby, and mushroom-shaped (Yuste, 2011; **Figure 1**). On the same dendrite, a continuum of shapes can be observed and the morphology can change rapidly through activity-dependent and -independent mechanisms (Penzes and Rafalovich, 2012). The density of spines can be understood in terms of the levels of connectivity within the neuronal network, as well as the integrative capabilities of the neuron. As such, abnormalities in the shape and density of spines can often signify an aspect of disease (Fiala et al., 2002). Therefore, structural classifications of spines with accurate labeling and imaging techniques can spawn vital information on neuronal function, and in turn offer insight into the etiology of neurological diseases (Lin and Koleske, 2010; Penzes et al., 2011).

For over a century, the Golgi staining technique has been the classical method for neuronal labeling and dendritic spine analysis (Neely et al., 2009). Although Golgi staining has played a crucial role in the advancement of anatomical neurobiology, a major drawback of this technique is that the tissue fixation used for Golgi is often incompatible with other methods to study morphology, such as immunocytochemistry. Furthermore, the Golgi method provides inconsistent, low frequency staining, which results in the insecurity of a selection bias (Staffend and Meisel, 2011b). In addition, long periods of time (often weeks) are required to reach the final product. Due to the lack of specificity and reproducibility, researchers have decreasingly relied on this technique (Ranjan and Mallick, 2010). A variety of methods have been developed to circumvent some of the limitations of the Golgi staining, most notably through the use of fluorescent markers. In fact, labeling cells and tissues with fluorescent markers is one of the most widely used methods of cellular examination employed to date (Colello et al., 2012). Fluorescence immunolabeling is a highly specific method that is commonly used to visualize cell structure, facilitate protein localization, and study cell interactions at the light microscopic level. Some of these other methods used to evaluate cellular morphology include various commercially available dyes, fluorochrome labeled antibodies, and genetically encoded fluorescent proteins, such as green fluorescent protein (GFP; Staffend and Meisel, 2011a). Specifically with GFP, transgenic animals and cultured cells can be designed to drive fluorescent expression under specific promoters (Malinow et al., 2010). However, although GFP-labeling provides great specificity of fluorescent expression, a similar end result can be accomplished in a much shorter time frame and with far fewer supplies/materials by employing lipophilic DiI labeling.

The fluorescent lipophilic dye dialkylcarbocyanine, also called "DiI" [1,1′-dioctadecyl-3,3,3′,3′-tetramethylindocarbocyanine perchlorate; DiIC$_{18}$(3)], has traditionally been used for anterograde

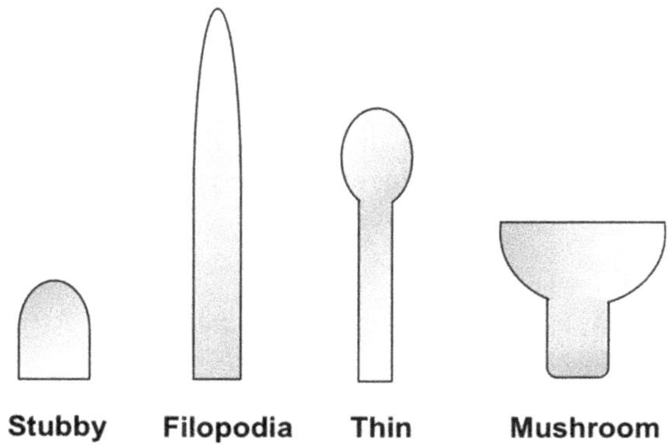

FIGURE 1 | Schematic representation of spine morphologies. Spines display a wide diversity of morphologies. They are commonly classified into four different categories (as illustrated from left to right): stubby, filopodia, thin, and mushroom-shaped. Stubby spines are devoid of a neck and are particularly prominent during postnatal development. Thin spines are most common and have a thin, long neck and a small bulbous head, whereas mushroom spines are those with a large head. Lastly, dendritic filopodia are typically longer, normally have no clear head, and often represent immature spines.

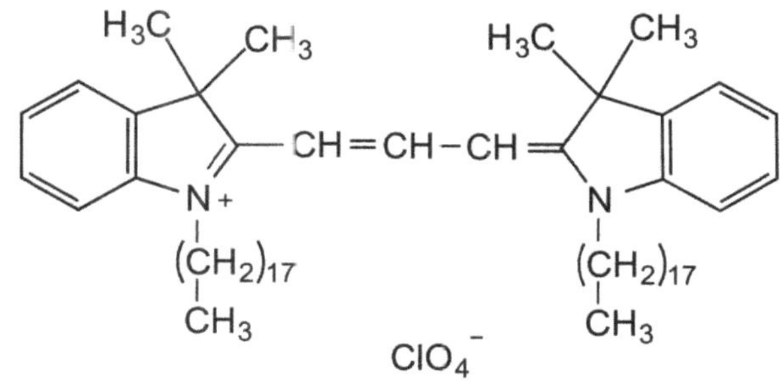

FIGURE 2 | Chemical structure of carbocyanine dye DiI. The fluorescent lipophilic dye "DiI" [1,1′-dioctadecyl-3,3,3′,3′ tetramethylindocarbocyanine perchlorate; DiIC18(3)] is commonly used as an anterograde and retrograde neuronal tracer. DiI labels cell membranes by inserting its two long (C_{18} carbon) hydrocarbon chains into the lipid bilayers.

and retrograde neuronal tracing (Honig and Hume, 1989). Structurally, the molecule consists of a hydrophilic head that lies above the plasma cell membrane and two lipophilic hydrocarbon side chains that insert into the hydrophobic plasma membrane (Bruce et al., 1997; **Figure 2**). The orange-red fluorescent dye is weakly fluorescent until it is incorporated into the membrane. DiI partitions and diffuses through the cell membrane to sufficiently highlight dendrites and their spinous protrusions, providing a well-defined outline of neuronal processes (Sherazee and Alvarez, 2013). The fluorescence provided by the carbocyanine dye is very strong and robust and withstands illumination, e.g., in a confocal laser scanning microscope (Gan et al., 1999; Lanciego and Wouterlood, 2011). Typical applications of this technique include the study of neuronal morphology during development and altered development in neurological disorders (Bruce et al., 1997; Braun and Segal, 2000; Smith et al., 2009; Li et al., 2010). This dye can be applied to a variety of cell types, live or fixed tissue (Terasaki et al., 1994), as well as diverse species such as rodents, primates, and zebrafish (Gan et al., 2000; O'Brien and Lummis, 2006; Seabold et al., 2010; Arsenault and O'Brien, 2013). In slice preparations, DiI labeling is commonly known as "DiOlistic labeling," in which beads coated with the lipophilic dye are "ballistically" ejected with a gene gun on to brain tissue (Lo et al., 1994). This technique has been developed as a useful and simple means to label neurons and glia in their entirety, unveiling even the most detailed structures, such as dendritic spines (Haber et al., 2006). To date, very few procedures are available that allow the direct application of DiI to cultured cells. Our protocol described here results in high quality staining and imaging of dissociated cell cultures with lipophilic DiI labeling and confocal microscopy. This visualization approach enables a detailed analysis of dendritic spine morphology, density, topographical distribution, and connectivity.

MATERIALS AND METHODS

ANIMALS

An in-house mouse breeding colony was used to generate primary cell cultures of hippocampal neurons for DiI labeling. The mice were housed and bred at the McMaster University Central Animal Facility. All experiments complied with the guidelines set out by the Canadian Council on Animal Care and were approved by the McMaster Animal Research Ethics Board.

CELL CULTURE PREPARATION

Primary hippocampal neurons were generated as previously described by our laboratory with minor modifications (Jacobs and Doering, 2010). Briefly, four embryonic day 15–17, E15–17 (day of sperm plug counted as E1) pups were randomly removed from the pregnant dam. Hippocampi were dissected in calcium and magnesium-free Hank's buffered salt solution (CMF-HBSS) and tissues were digested with 2.5% trypsin for 15 min in a 37°C water bath. The supernatant was removed, rinsed with three successive washes of CMF-HBSS and re-suspended in neural growth media (NGM) containing 1X Neurobasal (Life Technologies), 0.5 mM GlutaMAX (Life Technologies), and 2.0% B-27 Supplement (Invitrogen). Cells were subsequently plated on 12 mm glass coverslips (Bellco) in 24 multi-well plates, pre-treated with 1 mg/mL poly-L-lysine (Sigma) and 10 μg/ml laminin (Life Technologies), immediately after dissociation at a density of 16,000 cells per well. Neurons were subsequently incubated at 37°C with 5% CO_2 and remained in culture for 17 days *in vitro* (*DIV*) to allow for the development and maturation of dendritic spines. Every 3–4 days, the neurons were fed by replacing one half of the media with fresh NGM.

DiI LABELING PROCEDURE

Dendritic spines were identified using the well-characterized fluorescent marker DiI. Application of the dye was adapted from established protocols (Westmark et al., 2011). The neurons were fixed with freshly prepared 2.0% paraformaldehyde (PFA) for 15 min. Each well was gently washed with Dulbecco's phosphate-buffered saline (DPBS, Invitrogen). For the staining, the wells were aspirated and sprinkled with solid DiI crystals (Life Technologies-Molecular Probes, Cat. #D-3911). Approximately 2–3 crystals were added using a pair of fine forceps to each well. To prevent dehydration of the cells, a small amount of DPBS was dispensed to the edge of the wells. Special care was taken to deliver the smallest crystals to prevent clumping of the dye. The neurons were exposed to the crystals for 10 min on an orbital shaker set at a low speed. The shaker motion ensured that the crystals were adequately distributed to augment complete staining across the surface of the coverslip. The plate was then removed from the shaker and the wells were copiously washed with DPBS to remove all crystals. This procedure was repeated until no crystals were visible. The cells were incubated with DPBS in the dark overnight at room temperature to allow for the diffusion of the dye. The following day, the coverslips were rinsed three times with dH_20 for 5–10 min each. The coverslips were removed, completely air-dried, and mounted on slides with prolong gold antifade (Life Technologies – Molecular Probes). Coverslips cured for a minimum of 24 h to allow the liquid mountant to form a semi-rigid gel. Cells were visualized after 72 h from the time of the initial staining to allow the dye to fully migrate across neuronal membranes and diffuse throughout the neurons to highlight spine structures. All images were taken within 7–10 days after coverslipping to minimize fading.

CONFOCAL IMAGING

Visual imaging of the dendritic spines was acquired using a Zeiss 510 confocal laser-scanning microscope (LSM 510). All images were taken using a $63\times/1.2$ water immersion lens. A 543 nm Hene-1 Rhodamine laser was utilized to visualize the fluorescence emitted by DiI. To view the specimen with reflected fluorescent light, the reflector turret was programmed to position F set 15 in correlation to the Rhodamine laser, and the single-track configuration was chosen. We used 1024×1024 pixels for image size and set the scan speed at a setting of 4. Scan direction and line averaging were also adjusted to a setting of 4. The pinhole diameter was configured to 1 Airy unit (124 μm). Series stacks were collected from the bottom to the top covering all dendrites and protrusions, with an optical slice thickness of 0.5–1 μm. The resulting images (4–6) were then reconstructed to identify hidden protrusions according to Z-stack projections of the maximum intensity.

DENDRITIC SPINE ANALYSIS

ImageJ software (http://rsbweb.nih.gov/ij/) was used for viewing the confocal images and for spine quantification. In order to increase the magnification for a better view of the spines without loss of image quality, the resolution of the stack image was increased by a factor of 5 in the X and Y directions with the plug-in Transform J Scale (Pop et al., 2012). The length of a spine was obtained by drawing a line from its emerging point on the dendrite to the tip of its head. Approximately, 8–10 neurons selected at random were analyzed per condition across two coverslips. Density and morphology of spines were scored in dendritic segments 10 μm in length. Spines were classified into one of the four morphological subtypes: filopodial, thin, stubby, and mushroom-shaped.

STATISTICAL ANALYSIS

Spine density was determined by summing the total number of spines per dendritic segment length and then calculating the average number of spines per 10 μm. These values were then averaged to yield the number of spines per 10 μm for each animal. Statistics were performed using GraphPad Prism. Differences were detected with a one-way analysis of variance. Following one-way ANOVA, *post hoc* differences were resolved using the Tukey's multiple comparison test. A p-value of <0.05 was considered significant. All values are expressed as mean $\pm$ SEM.

RESULTS

LABORATORY PREPARED VERSUS COMMERCIAL GRADE PARAFORMALDEHYDE FIXATION

To determine an optimized protocol for the fluorescent visualization of dendritic spines with the carbocyanine dye in dissociated cultures, we explored patterns of DiI labeling in neurons fixed with laboratory prepared paraformaldehyde (PFA) in PBS or commercial grade formalin at 2.0%. When the cells were prepared with either fixative, the DiI crystals diffused efficiently along the neuronal membranes to permit the effective visualization of the somas and dendritic processes studded with delicate spinous protrusions. However, the laboratory prepared PFA samples facilitated enhanced staining and clarity for the crisp visualization of spines compared to formalin. Commercial grade formalin which typically contains $\sim$10–15% methanol prevents polymerization in storage. Given that DiI is soluble in organic solvents, the use of methanol or acetone fixation is highly discouraged. Taking this into consideration, we investigated whether neurons fixed with acetone would be ineffectively labeled with DiI. We were able to confirm that cells had adhered to the coverslip (as visualized by DAPI) when fixed with acetone, but as expected, the dye unsuccessfully permeated throughout the dendritic segments (results not shown). Additionally, it is important to note that the use of any fixative stored for extended periods of time may risk decomposition and in turn yield poor fixation of samples.

VARIATIONS IN PARAFORMALDEHYDE CONCENTRATION ALTER CLARITY

Labeling neurons with the fluorescent marker DiI provides a well-defined outline of neuronal cell bodies, dendritic arbors (**Figure 3**), and spine subtypes (**Figure 4**). To determine the most effective conditions for optimal DiI diffusion along dendritic segments, we tested varying concentrations of laboratory PFA fixative at 1.5, 2.0, and 4.0%. Qualitative analysis revealed that the structural integrity of dendrites could not be maintained with a higher concentration of fixation. Namely, the extent of dendritic branching visualized by the dye in cells fixed with 4.0% PFA was hindered compared to cells fixed using 1.5 or 2.0% PFA (**Figure 5A**). In some cases, dye diffusion was limited to where the dye was applied, such that distal dendrites and spines on the same neuron were often not stained, including other neighboring neurons. Swelling of the dendrites (varicosities) were also apparent often hindering accurate measurements of the spines (**Figure 5B**). For instance, the dye would aggregate along the dendrites at spines, causing them to appear "stubby" in shape. However, this often yielded a false morphological classification, as the shape or appearance of spines was attributed to the dye's inability to completely diffuse throughout the neuronal processes. Furthermore, higher concentrations

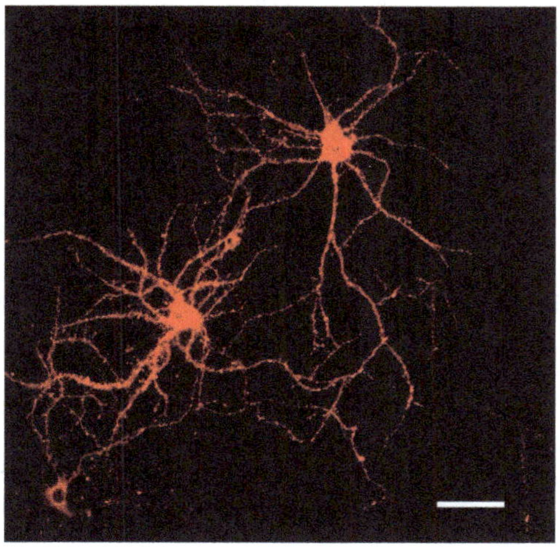

FIGURE 3 | Representative images of DiI labeled neurons. DiI highlighting the dendritic complexity and topographical connectivity of neurons. Dendritic arbors and spines are sufficiently filled and visualized in their entirety with the fluorescent dye. Scale bar = 50 μm.

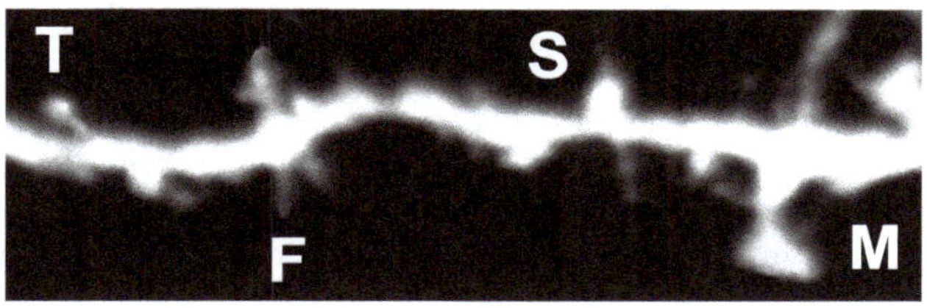

FIGURE 4 | Representative image of DiI labeled spines. Filopodia-like (F), long-thin (T), stubby (S), and mushroom (M) spines are identified based on structural measures.

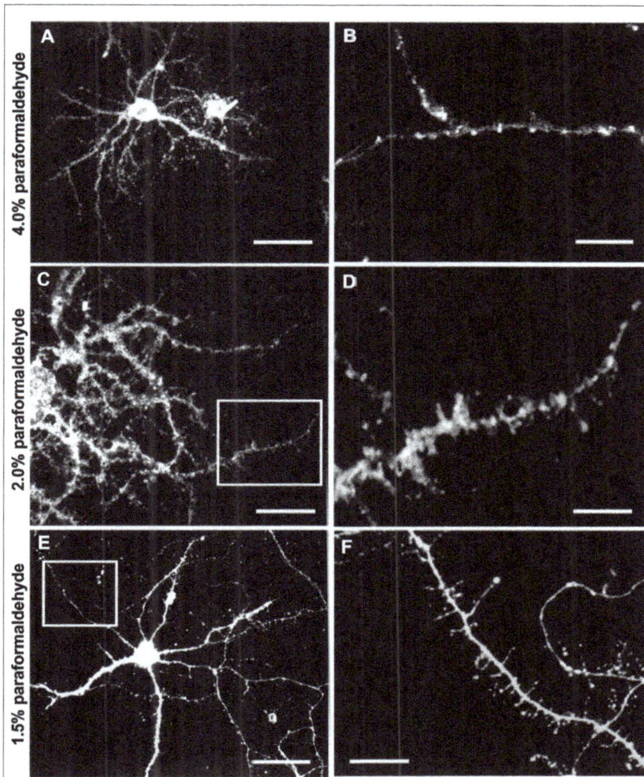

FIGURE 5 | DiI labeled neurons fixed with varying concentrations of paraformaldehyde (PFA). Application of DiI crystals on fixed cells produces a very high degree of detail. **(A)** Cell fixed with 4.0% PFA. **(B)** The use of 4.0% PFA fixative significantly compromises DiI diffusion through the dendrites. Multiple varicosities are highlighted along the dendrite and spines are poorly resolved. **(C)** Cell fixed with 2.0 % PFA. **(D)** The use of 2.0% PFA generates high quality DiI labeling of spines. Various subtypes of spines are evident along the dendritic segment. **(E)** Cell fixed with 1.5% PFA. **(F)** The use of 1.5% PFA yields comparable results to the use of 2.0% fixative. Fine, thin filopodial projections are resolved. Scale bar **(A,C,E)** = 50 μm; Scale bar **(B,D,F)** = 5 μm.

of PFA typically yielded autofluorescence, which may explain the diffuse background fluorescence coupled with reduced illumination of the spines evident in **Figure 5B**. Ultimately, we discovered that laboratory prepared PFA utilized at lower concentrations was most effective, as it encouraged complete filling of the dendritic segments and finer processes through rapid dye diffusion. Specifically, the images obtained with 1.5–2.0% PFA delineated fine dendritic spines in comparable detail to the traditional Golgi staining method (**Figures 5C–F**). Hence, optimal fixation can greatly improve the quality of DiI neuronal labeling.

QUANTITATIVE ANALYSIS OF SPINE DENSITY AND MORPHOLOGY

Spine density and morphology were assessed in DiI labeled neurons fixed with varying concentrations of PFA (1.5, 2.0, and 4.0%) to investigate dye permeability. No significant differences in spine density were observed in neurons fixed with either 1.5 or 2.0% PFA (**Figure 6**). Alternatively, neurons fixed with 2.0% PFA yielded significantly higher spine densities when compared to neurons fixed with 4.0% PFA ($^{*}p = 0.012$), potentially as a result of increased DiI labeling. These findings suggest and reinforce our observation that the use of a stronger fixative hinders the dye's ability to completely diffuse and fill fine processes, like spines. Notably, despite the appearance of an increased proportion of "stubby" spines in neurons fixed with a higher concentration of fixative (**Figure 5B**), no significant differences resulted in any of the comparisons made in the composition of spine morphologies with varying concentrations of fixative (results not shown). Still, our recommendation holds that initial fixation with milder concentrations of PFA fixative at 1.5–2.0% generates the most consistent and superior results.

SUMMARY OF FINDINGS

The results obtained through this protocol demonstrated that DiI staining in cells prepared with a lower percentage of fixative yielded the highest quality of images. The detailed images generated by this protocol allow us to perform an accurate quantitative analysis of spine structures and spine density. Stubby and mushroom shaped dendritic spines were most evident by their prominent "pinhead" fluorescence directly on the dendritic spine when positioned perpendicularly to the plane of focus on the microscope slide, or as thick protrusions off the dendrite. Filopodial dendritic spines

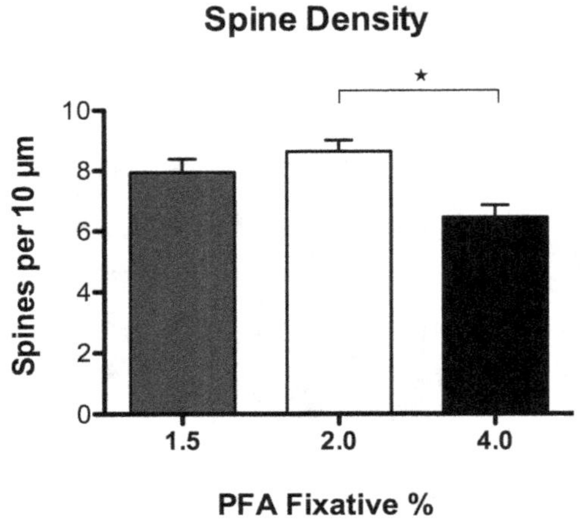

FIGURE 6 | Spine density analysis of DiI labeled neurons fixed with varying concentrations of paraformaldehyde (PFA). No significant differences in spine density were observed in neurons fixed with 1.5% or 2.0% PFA. Neurons fixed with 2.0% PFA yielded significantly higher spine densities when compared to neurons fixed with 4.0% PFA (* $p < 0.05$).

were most visible when their characteristic long and thin protrusions extended upward/downward from the dendritic branch. The high-resolution images that can be obtained using this technique allow us to delineate spine morphologies to provide insight into the areas of synapse formation, development, and remodeling in the CNS.

DISCUSSION

Several methods to study neuronal structure include histological stains, immunocytochemistry, electroporation of fluorescent dyes, transfection of fluorescent constructs, and the Golgi technique. Although the Golgi technique offers valuable results, this method is time consuming and often lacks reliability. DiI fluorescence labeling has gained popularity, but optimization of the method is essential to accurately quantitate and evaluate fine neuronal structures such as dendritic spines. In lieu of the DiOlistic literature, reported protocols differ vastly for cell/tissue fixation, dye delivery, and diffusion times, with no report on the impact that these different conditions have on the quality of labeling. Here, we outlined a procedure that allows the direct application of DiI to cells in culture; a method that has not been thoroughly explored. The present protocol sought to define the optimal conditions for the fluorescent illumination of individual neurons, including the soma, dendritic arborizations, and spines in cell culture through the use of confocal microscopy. Confocal microscopic analysis of fluorescently labeled neurons has improved resolution of dendritic morphology and has been suggested to provide a more accurate measurement of spines (Lee et al., 2009; Schmitz et al., 2011). Among the most important parameters of this procedure, fixation properties impacted the success of labeling most profoundly.

OPTIMIZATION OF CELL FIXATION

Amid the DiOlistic literature, a variety of fixation conditions have been reported that produce acceptable levels of DiI labeling. The use of 4.0% PFA is most commonly reported by standard immunohistochemical and immunocytochemical protocols, while many DiI labeling protocols indicate the use of both 1.5 or 4.0% PFA (i.e., Kim et al., 2007; Staffend and Meisel, 2011b; Westmark et al., 2011). To explore this range, we compared the image quality of neurons obtained from 1.5, 2.0, and 4.0% concentrations of fixative. The use of 4.0% PFA fixative significantly compromised DiI diffusion through the dendritic processes (**Figure 5B**). This was apparent by reduced image quality due to increased background fluorescence and inconsistent labeling. However, fixation with both 1.5 and 2.0% PFA yielded similar results with superior diffusion of the lipophilic dye DiI along the neuronal membranes (**Figures 5C–F**). We determined this to be a significant finding since 4.0% PFA has been reported to yield successful results in both tissue slices and cell culture labeling. We discovered that a milder concentration of PFA fixative increased the extent of DiI diffusion, resulting in complete visualization of dendrites and spines. A higher concentration of fixative may interfere and prevent the dye from penetrating the membrane. We strived to further augment our cell fixation technique through a direct comparison of the effectiveness of using freshly prepared laboratory PFA versus commercially produced formalin. Utilization of 1.5–2.0% laboratory PFA produced images with higher clarity and less background fluorescence. The use of commercially -produced formalin (containing methanol) may have adversely impacted the labeling. When evaluating spine density, we found that milder fixation conditions with 2.0% PFA more effectively incorporated DiI into the spines than their 4.0% PFA counterpart. With the use of a weaker fix, more spines were resolved and identified, resulting in an increase in spine density. Together, our results suggest the use of 1.5–2.0% freshly prepared buffered PFA as the superior fixative. As a precaution, utilizing 2.0% (rather than 1.5%) PFA fixative ensures that the cells are effectively fixed and adhered to the coverslip.

DENDRITIC ORDER OF ANALYSIS

To quantitatively analyze the dendritic spines, we utilized confocal imaging of the cells. The resolution obtained with the confocal microscope permitted the study of individual spines. However, Z stack images with a step interval of 0.5–1 μm supplemented each XY image for accurate spine quantification. The sides of the dendrite were meticulously examined for vertical protrusions stretching upward and downward off the dendrite in addition to the spines extending upward toward the observer. At higher magnification, we were able to morphologically classify some of the dendritic protrusions. However, the spines that extended vertically toward the observer were difficult to morphologically classify from an aerial perspective. Additionally, extra care was taken while examining possible protrusions positioned on the dendritic trunk that extended vertically upward toward the observer; filopodia and thin shaped spines were likely to exhibit less fluorescence in comparison to stubby and mushroom-shaped counterparts, due to less absorption of the dye with reduced surface volume. This point was particularly significant in accurately deciphering the morphology of spines. Moreover, the aggregation of overlapping dendritic processes and complex branching/arborization at times hindered the accurate evaluation of spines. For instance, the areas of the dendritic trunk located closer to the soma-exhibited extreme intertwining with numerous surrounding dendrites that complicated the isolation and differentiation of spines. Additionally, swellings of the dendritic trunk tended to conceal the presence of shorter spines even with a detailed analysis using a series of Z stack images.

Providing that spine density may vary across different order dendrites (primary, secondary, tertiary, etc.), systematic sampling of dendritic order is necessary when analyzing spine density and morphology. Branch ordering schemes are frequently used, wherein the dendrites emerging from the cell soma are primary, their first branches are secondary and so on, with increasing order until the tips are reached. Branches may also vary in diameter. The total number of images collected will depend on the experimental requirements and the degree of variability within a neuron, and across neurons and animals (Ruszczycki et al., 2012). For the purpose of this study, image collection was restricted to the three-dimensional structure of secondary and tertiary dendrites. These parameters were consciously considered to improve accuracy in conducting spine measurements (Rosenzweig and Wojtowicz, 2011). Differences in spine measurements on different order dendrites could potentially draw further insight on neural connectivity in the brain.

OPTIMIZATION OF DiI DELIVERY

Less than optimal cellular DiI labeling can be attributed to a variety of sources. For troubleshooting purposes, the most common problems, probable causes, and solutions are outlined in **Table 1**.

POSSIBLE LIMITATIONS OF THIS METHOD

Although this approach has proven to be effective, it is important to address some of the limitations to the technique. For instance, DiI labeling can be highly variable, because dye crystal size, density, and penetration are all very difficult factors to control. Despite the majority of cells being labeled, the application of extracellular solid DiI crystals often restricted complete staining of all neurons in its entirety within a culture well. Dye diffusion was constrained to neurons that were in close proximity to the crystals, whereas more distal neurons or terminal branches were not prominently stained or filled in. As such, this method is most appropriate for the structural analysis of dendritic spines rather than a comprehensive analysis of dendritic arborization. While these methods produce an accurate analysis on a single-cell resolution, extrapolating the acquired data to a larger neuronal population might prove inaccurate if the staining technique selectively labels only subsets of neurons. Additional selection bias might also occur in these cases if the researcher chooses to measure "convenient" cells, which are visualized more clearly and without overlap with other neurons. Therefore, it is of the utmost importance to ensure that cultures are grown at a sufficient density that limits overlapping processes and permits the isolation of single entities (spines). By using the appropriate concentration of fixative, this can ensure that most neuronal processes are appropriately filled in. Additionally, ensuring that the solid dye is thoroughly distributed during the staining procedure will highlight a larger proportion of cells per sample in a well.

As the morphology of dendritic spines is highly variable, a sufficient sampling size is essential for statistical analysis. With light or epifluorescent microscopy, the dendrite may obscure spines that lie above or below the visual plane, such that only spines extending laterally can be accurately counted. However, this problem cannot be completely remedied by three-dimensional confocal microscopy. To compensate, some studies have applied correction factors for hidden spines (Bannister and Larkman, 1995).

It is also desirable to combine DiI labeling with immunofluorescent staining, with which detailed co-localization can be analyzed using confocal microscopy. The two techniques, however, are often incompatible because Triton X-100, a conventional detergent or permeabilization reagent commonly used to enhance antibody penetration into tissues or cells, causes diffusion of DiI from the labeled structures (Neely et al., 2009). Since Triton X-100 solubilizes lipid molecules almost indiscriminately, it is most likely that Triton X-100 compromises the retention of DiI in the cellular membrane. As a result, the dye potentially leaks out of the membrane, causing the label to disappear after immunocytochemical procedures (Matsubayashi et al., 2008). The ability to perform a dual staining would better allow investigators to phenotypically characterize DiI labeled cells. In future studies, it may be valuable to couple DiI labeling with other fluorescent markers and/or antibodies to immunocytochemically identify other target proteins of interest within a neuron. Investigating appropriate fluorescent immunocytochemical protocols compatible with DiI neuronal tracing would serve as a useful tool in advancing current labeling techniques.

ADVANTAGES OF THIS METHOD

The methods outlined above using DiI labeling offer a reproducible protocol that have several advantages for the analysis of dendritic spine structures using photostable fluorescence. This protocol offers the opportunity to systematically analyze a large quantity of dendritic spines in high detail, which cannot be achieved through other neuronal identification methods. Furthermore, fluorescent staining and imaging by confocal microscopy yields a series of Z stack images. Many densely compacted segments and spine protrusions often do not lie favorably in the plane of focus and thus cannot be reliably counted. Confocal imaging with DiI labeling permits the sensitive detection of spines by allowing a three-dimensional analysis of spines and dendrites to avoid over and undersaturated pixels. This is particularly vital for the identification of spinous protrusions on the dendritic trunk and most proximal to the soma, and in other cases where there is frequent overlap of the dendrites. Finally, our described methods are simple and do not increase the costs or effort, and more importantly do not compromise the integrity of the neurons or the quality of the staining and data acquired. Taken together, these characteristics make DiI a powerful technique for identifying and studying early events in neuronal development and brain connectivity with significant implications for neurological disease.

CONCLUSION

Given the literature, a variety of labeling and diffusion conditions can produce acceptable levels of fluorescent DiI labeling. Our goal was to explicitly compare specific methodological components to determine a DiI protocol that produces reproducible staining

Table 1 | Troubleshooting guide for optimal DiI labeling.

Problems	Potential causes/corrective measures
High background is visible.	Residual crystals will result in high background. Avoid adding a surplus of DiI crystals. An excess of crystals will yield high autofluorescence and debris in the cultures. Ensure that coverslips are rinsed well with dH_2O until no DiI crystals are visible to the naked eye. Lastly, it is desirable to limit the duration of exposure of the sample to the laser to minimize the degree of phototoxic damage to the ultrastructure and any non-specific signal.
Dye bleeds upon exposure to light.	Glycerol-based mounting media (i.e., Prolong Gold, Vectashield, etc.) can extract membrane-bound dyes upon exposure to light. DiI is light sensitive and long-term exposure will cause fluorescence to fade. Higher magnification objectives (i.e., 63×) are necessary to produce better image resolution and enhance sensitivity of spine detection; however, samples are subject to increased light exposure. High intensity light renders the dye to photobleaching. Minimize duration of light exposure if possible.
Slides are fading.	Ensure that images are captured as soon as possible after mounting. Illumination with light will cause fluorescence to diminish. Slides can be used at least 6 months to a year if stored in the dark at 4°C.
Coverslips appear cloudy.	Ensure that coverslips are rinsed well with dH_2O or salt residue/film will accumulate clouding the coverslip. Apply more washes if necessary.
Bubbles are apparent after mounting.	Avoid the formation of air bubbles. Ensure that coverslips are completely dry before mounting. Do not apply an excess of mounting medium. Apply a small amount using a dropper to the coverslip and gently pick up the coverslip using the slide. As the coverslip pulls against the slide, allow the mountant to gradually permeate without applying additional pressure.
Absence or lack of cells present.	Fixation of cells may have been unsuccessful. Higher concentration of fixative may be required if cells are not adhering to the coverslip. Always use freshly prepared fixative. Avoid rigorous washes that may cause cells to lift.
Low frequency staining of neurons.	Due to the dye's indiscriminate nature, this technique often generates sparse fluorescent labeling. During the application, DiI crystals must be thoroughly dispersed to maximize the staining of cells. High concentration of fixative may also obstruct dye diffusion. Do not extend the duration of fix, as it will affect labeling. Overfixation will disrupt the cell membrane integrity causing DiI to leak out of the cell.
Streaking across coverslips.	Scratching of the coverslip with the glass pipette during extraction of solutions from the well impacts image quality. Since this procedure involves numerous washes, it is important to slowly add or remove solutions from the wells to prevent lifting of the cells. One can practice gentle pipetting techniques using the sides of the wells to allow solutions to slowly cover the cells. Extract solutions from the side of the well to avoid contact with coverslip and prevent scratching.
Difficulty isolating single neuronal processes for analysis.	Overlapping of cells and processes may be caused by high density. Reduce plating density.
Dendritic spines are poorly resolved.	Confocal imaging parameters may not be optimal for assessing spine morphology. For high-resolution images obtained at high magnification, slower image acquisition should be used. Adjust settings for detector gain, line averaging, and speed of scanning to improve image quality. The same imaging parameters should be used throughout the study.

of dendritic spines in dissociated cultures. Dendritic spines are significant structural substrates for synaptic plasticity and in turn are vital to the proper functioning of the CNS. Spines serve as a functional integrative unit whose morphology is tightly correlated with its function. An accurate neuronal visualization method provides valuable insight into the neuronal organization of various areas of the brain. Importantly, our technique provides an alternative method to fluorescently label neurons and dendritic spines in a convenient and cost-effective manner. Our technique further enables the analysis of dendritic spine topographical distribution, quantitative measurement, and morphological assessment. Such findings would be highly applicable to the investigation of the etiology of various disorders in which spine pathology has been implicated. As a result, this accurate, efficient, and economical staining technique has a wide array of applicability to the study of CNS neurobiology in normal and disease states.

ACKNOWLEDGMENTS

This work has been supported by NSERC (National Sciences and Engineering Research Council of Canada) and the Fondation Jérôme LeJeune (Paris).

REFERENCES

Arsenault, J., and O'Brien, J. A. (2013). Optimized heterologous transfection of viable adult organotypic brain slices using an enhanced gene gun. *BMC Res. Notes* 6:544. doi: 10.1186/1756-0500-6-544

Bannister, N. J., and Larkman, A. U. (1995). Dendritic morphology of CA1 pyramidal neurones from the rat hippocampus: II. Spine distributions. *J. Comp. Neurol.* 360, 161–171. doi: 10.1002/cne.903600112

Braun, K., and Segal, M. (2000). FMRP involvement in formation of synapses among cultured hippocampal neurons. *Cereb. Cortex* 10, 1045–1052. doi: 10.1093/cercor/10.10.1045

Bruce, L. L., Christensen, M. A., and Fritzsch, B. (1997). Electron microscopic differentiation of directly and transneuronally transported DiI and applications for studies of synaptogenesis. *J. Neurosci. Methods* 73, 107–112. doi: 10.1016/S0165-0270(96)02218-2

Colello, R. J., Tozer, J., and Henderson, S. C. (2012). Confocal laser scanning microscopic photoconversion: a new method to stabilize fluorescently labeled cellular elements for electron microscopic analysis. *Curr. Protoc. Neurosci.* Chap. 2, Unit 2.15. doi: 10.1002/0471142301.ns0215s58

Fiala, J. C., Spacek, J., and Harris, K. M. (2002). Dendritic spine pathology: cause or consequence of neurological disorders? *Brain Res. Rev.* 39, 29–54. doi: 10.1016/S0165-0173(02)00158-3

Gan, W. B., Bishop, D. L., Turney, S. G., and Lichtman, J. W. (1999). Vital imaging and ultrastructural analysis of individual axon terminals labeled by iontophoretic application of lipophilic dye. *J. Neurosci. Methods* 93, 13–20. doi: 10.1016/S0165-0270(99)00096-5

Gan, W. B., Grutzendler, J., Wong, W. T., Wong, R. O., and Lichtman, J. W. (2000). Multicolor "DiOlistic" labeling of the nervous system using lipophilic dye combinations. *Neuron* 27, 219–225. doi: 10.1016/S0896-6273(00)00031-3

Haber, M., Zhou, L., and Murai, K. K. (2006). Cooperative astrocyte and dendritic spine dynamics at hippocampal excitatory synapses. *J. Neurosci.* 26, 8881–8891. doi: 10.1523/JNEUROSCI.1302-06.2006

Honig, M. G., and Hume, R. I. (1989). DiI and diO: versatile fluorescent dyes for neuronal labelling and pathway tracing. *Trends Neurosci.* 12, 333–341. doi: 10.1016/0166-2236(89)90040-4

Jacobs, S., and Doering, L. C. (2010). "Primary dissociated astrocyte and neuron co-culture," in *Protocols for Neural Cell Culture*, 4th Edn, ed. L. C. Doering (Berlin: Springer), 269–283.

Kim, B. G., Dai, H. N., McAtee, M., Vicini, S., and Bregman, B. S. (2007). Labeling of dendritic spines with the carbocyanine dye DiI for confocal microscopic imaging in lightly fixed cortical slices. *J. Neurosci. Methods* 162, 237–243. doi:10.1016/j.jneumeth.2007.01.016

Lanciego, J. L., and Wouterlood, F. G. (2011). A half century of experimental neuroanatomical tracing. *J. Chem. Neuroanat.* 42, 157–183. doi: 10.1016/j.jchemneu.2011.07.001

Lee, P.-C., Chang, H.-M., Lin, C.-Y., Chiang, A.-S., and Ching, Y.-T. (2009). Constructing neuronal structure from 3D confocal microscopic images. *J. Med. Biol. Eng.* 29, 1–6.

Li, M., Cui, Z., Niu, Y., Liu, B., Fan, W., Yu, D., et al. (2010). Synaptogenesis in the developing mouse visual cortex. *Brain Res. Bull.* 81, 107–113. doi: 10.1016/j.brainresbull.2009.08.028

Lin, Y.-C., and Koleske, A. J. (2010). Mechanisms of synapse and dendrite maintenance and their disruption in psychiatric and neurodegenerative disorders. *Annu. Rev. Neurosci.* 33, 349–378. doi: 10.1146/annurev-neuro-060909-153204

Lo, D. C., McAllister, A. K., and Katz, L. C. (1994). Neuronal transfection in brain slices using particle-mediated gene transfer. *Neuron* 13, 1263–1268. doi: 10.1186/1756-0500-6-544

Malinow, R., Hayashi, Y., Maletic-Savatic, M., Zaman, S. H., Poncer, J.-C., Shi, S.-H., et al. (2010). Introduction of green fluorescent protein (GFP) into hippocampal neurons through viral infection. *Cold Spring Harb. Protoc.* 2010:pdb.prot5406. doi: 10.1101/pdb.prot5406

Matsubayashi, Y., Iwai, L., and Kawasaki, H. (2008). Fluorescent double-labeling with carbocyanine neuronal tracing and immunohistochemistry using a cholesterol-specific detergent digitonin. *J. Neurosci. Methods* 174, 71–81. doi: 10.1016/j.jneumeth.2008.07.003

Neely, M. D., Stanwood, G. D., and Deutch, A. Y. (2009). Combination of diOlistic labeling with retrograde tract tracing and immunohistochemistry. *J. Neurosci. Methods* 184, 332–336. doi: 10.1016/j.jneumeth.2009.08.016

O'Brien, J. A., and Lummis, S. C. R. (2006). Diolistic labeling of neuronal cultures and intact tissue using a hand-held gene gun. *Nat. Protoc.* 1, 1517–1521. doi: 10.1038/nprot.2006.258

Penzes, P., Cahill, M. E., Jones, K. A., VanLeeuwen, J.-E., and Woolfrey, K. M. (2011). Dendritic spine pathology in neuropsychiatric disorders. *Nat. Neurosci.* 14, 285–293. doi: 10.1038/nn.2741

Penzes, P., and Rafalovich, I. (2012). Regulation of the actin cytoskeleton in dendritic spines. *Adv. Exp. Med. Biol.* 970, 81–95. doi: 10.1007/978-3-7091-0932-8_4

Pop, A. S., Levenga, J., Esch, C. E. F., Buijsen, R. A. M., Nieuwenhuizen, I. M., Li, T., et al. (2012). Rescue of dendritic spine phenotype in Fmr1 KO mice with the mGluR5 antagonist AFQ056/Mavoglurant. *Psychopharmacology* doi: 10.1007/s00213-012-2947-y

Ranjan, A., and Mallick, B. N. (2010). A modified method for consistent and reliable Golgi-cox staining in significantly reduced time. *Front. Neurol.* 1:157. doi: 10.3389/fneur.2010.00157

Rochefort, N. L., and Konnerth, A. (2012). Dendritic spines: from structure to *in vivo* function. *EMBO Rep.* 13, 699–708. doi: 10.1038/embor.2012.102

Rosenzweig, S., and Wojtowicz, J. M. (2011). Analyzing dendritic growth in a population of immature neurons in the adult dentate gyrus using laminar quantification of disjointed dendrites. *Front. Neurosci.* 5:34. doi: 10.3389/fnins.2011.00034

Ruszczycki, B., Szepesi, Z., Wilczynski, G. M., Bijata, M., Kalita, K., Kaczmarek, L., et al. (2012). Sampling issues in quantitative analysis of dendritic spines morphology. *BMC Bioinformatics* 13:213. doi: 10.1186/1471-2105-13-213

Schmitz, S. K., Hjorth, J. J., Joemai, R. M. S., Wijntjes, R., Eijgenraam, S., de Bruijn, P., et al. (2011). Automated analysis of neuronal morphology, synapse number and synaptic recruitment. *J. Neurosci. Methods* 195, 185–193. doi: 10.1016/j.jneumeth.2010.12.011

Seabold, G. K., Daunais, J. B., Rau, A., Grant, K. A., and Alvarez, V. A. (2010). DiOLISTIC labeling of neurons from rodent and non-human primate brain slices. *J. Vis. Exp.* 6:pii 2081. doi: 10.3791/2081

Sherazee, N., and Alvarez, V. A. (2013). DiOlistics: delivery of fluorescent dyes into cells. *Methods Mol. Biol.* 940, 391–400. doi: 10.1007/978-1-62703-110-3_28

Smith, D. L., Pozueta, J., Gong, B., Arancio, O., and Shelanski, M. (2009). Reversal of long-term dendritic spine alterations in Alzheimer disease models. *Proc. Natl. Acad. Sci. U.S.A.* 106, 16877–16882. doi: 10.1073/pnas.0908706106

Staffend, N. A., and Meisel, R. L. (2011a). DiOlistic labeling in fixed brain slices: phenotype, morphology, and dendritic spines. *Curr. Protoc. Neurosci.* Chap. 2, Unit 2.13. doi: 10.1002/0471142301.ns0213s55

Staffend, N. A., and Meisel, R. L. (2011b). DiOlistic labeling of neurons in tissue slices: a qualitative and quantitative analysis of methodological variations. *Front. Neuroanat.* 5:14. doi: 10.3389/fnana.2011.00014

Terasaki, M., Slater, N. T., Fein, A., Schmidek, A., and Reese, T. S. (1994). Continuous network of endoplasmic reticulum in cerebellar Purkinje neurons. *Proc. Natl. Acad. Sci. U.S.A.* 91, 7510–7514.

Westmark, C. J., Westmark, P. R., O'Riordan, K. J., Ray, B. C., Hervey, C. M., Salamat, M. S., et al. (2011). Reversal of fragile X phenotypes by manipulation of AβPP/Aβ levels in Fmr1KO mice. *PLoS ONE* 6:e26549. doi: 10.1371/journal.pone.0026549

Yuste, R. (2011). Dendritic spines and distributed circuits. *Neuron* 71, 772–781. doi: 10.1016/j.neuron.2011.07.024

11

Integration of multiscale dendritic spine structure and function data into systems biology models

James J. Mancuso[1,2], Jie Cheng[1,2], Zheng Yin[1,2], Jared C. Gilliam[1,2], Xiaofeng Xia[1,2], Xuping Li[1,2] and Stephen T. C. Wong[1,2]*

[1] *Department of Systems Medicine and Bioengineering, Houston Methodist Research Institute, Houston, TX, USA*
[2] *TT and WF Chao Center for Bioinformatics Research and Imaging for Neurosciences, Houston Methodist Research Institute, Houston, TX, USA*

Correspondence:
Stephen T. C. Wong, Department of Systems Medicine and Bioengineering, Houston Methodist Research Institute, 6670 Bertner St., Houston, TX 77030, USA
e-mail: stwong@houstonmethodist.org

Comprising 10^{11} neurons with 10^{14} synaptic connections the human brain is the ultimate systems biology puzzle. An increasing body of evidence highlights the observation that changes in brain function, both normal and pathological, consistently correlate with dynamic changes in neuronal anatomy. Anatomical changes occur on a full range of scales from the trafficking of individual proteins, to alterations in synaptic morphology both individually and on a systems level, to reductions in long distance connectivity and brain volume. The major sites of contact for synapsing neurons are dendritic spines, which provide an excellent metric for the number and strength of signaling connections between elements of functional neuronal circuits. A comprehensive model of anatomical changes and their functional consequences would be a holy grail for the field of systems neuroscience but its realization appears far on the horizon. Various imaging technologies have advanced to allow for multi-scale visualization of brain plasticity and pathology, but computational analysis of the big data sets involved forms the bottleneck toward the creation of multiscale models of brain structure and function. While a full accounting of techniques and progress toward a comprehensive model of brain anatomy and function is beyond the scope of this or any other single paper, this review serves to highlight the opportunities for analysis of neuronal spine anatomy and function provided by new imaging technologies and the high-throughput application of older technologies while surveying the strengths and weaknesses of currently available computational analytical tools and room for future improvement.

Keywords: dendritic spines, microscopy, image analysis, systems biology, modeling and simulations, big data

SYSTEMS BIOLOGY

The nervous system is so complex that studies have had to focus on individual or small numbers of components at a single level of organization. Such a reductionist approach has helped reveal many processes that govern neuronal and brain function and has led the foundation of the field of neuroscience. Translating the logic of this reductionist approach to modern neuroscience results in a framework that is rooted in the scientific method and premised on biological discovery and understanding of disease mechanisms. Although the logic remains compelling, the traditional reductionist framework often leads to the study of individual proteins, subcellular structures, or neurons in isolation and can neglect the dynamic interaction of all components and how their interaction can lead to a more comprehensive understanding of neuronal function and dysfunction. Owing to recent advances in biotechnologies and computational sciences, biologists are now gaining the capability to go beyond the interactions of components within a single level of biological organization and the study of one or a few components at a time. The application of engineering precepts to biological systems has spawned the field of systems biology. Biologists are increasingly able to integrate information and form networks of interacting components across many organisms, from multiple levels of biological organization, such as cells, organs, and populations, and about entire systems, such as all the genes in a genome, to obtain new knowledge that incorporates more of the complexity that characterizes biological systems (see **Figure 1**).

Recent advances in imaging approaches have provided investigators with the means to acquire not only quantitative information about fine neuronal structures, including dendritic spines, *in vivo* or *in vitro* but also to examine their complete biological context including interactions with neighboring cells, connectivity, and chemical and protein composition. To date, comprehensive approaches to integrate these large data sets from fluorescence microscopy, electron microscopy (EM), and various imaging modalities, such as coherent anti-Stokes Raman spectroscopy (CARS), second harmonic generation (SHG), and autofluorescence imaging, that take advantage of intrinsic signals in living biological samples have been slowed by signal to noise issues and the lack of automated analysis algorithms. This has hindered their full use in a

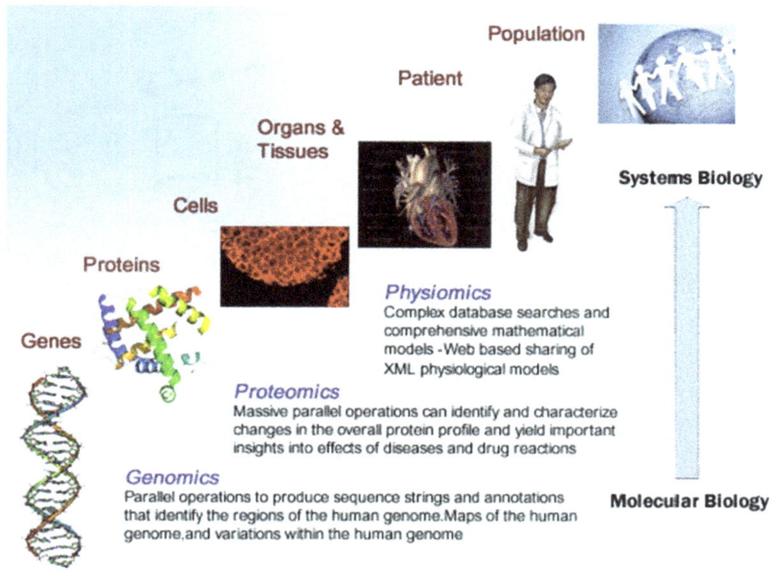

FIGURE 1 | Illustrates the principles of the systems medicine approach. Multi-scale data from a range of sources is integrated to provide a more comprehensive understanding of a disease state.

comprehensive systems biology analysis of dendritic spine pathology, and relegated their use to experimental paradigms that address biomedical questions from a traditional, reductionist standpoint.

The principle steps guiding the development of systems medicine models from brain imaging data are as follows: (1) generation and collection of large volumes of relevant imaging data; (2) systematic analysis and quantification of imaging data; (3) integration of analyzed imaging data with other data sources to create a systems level model of disease. This review primarily focuses on progress made to date on the first two steps as well as room for future improvement, while touching briefly on the promise of the third step (**Figure 2**).

NEURONAL ANATOMY (INCLUDING DENDRITIC SPINES)

Elements of the central nervous system are well known to exhibit strong correlations between anatomy and function on a number of different scales (Lee et al., 2012; Wang et al., 2013). Various subpopulations of neurons show variations in morphology which often underlie fundamental differences in signal integration and transmission properties of the individual subpopulations; the integration of these many diverse neuronal subtypes forms the foundation for basic and higher order brain processes. Throughout the nervous system various processes, both normal, such as development and aging, and pathological, such as neurodegeneration and drug addiction, manifest as changes in neuronal anatomy (Elston and Rosa, 1997, 1998; Engert and Bonhoeffer, 1999; Maletic-Savatic et al., 1999; Elston, 2000; Jacobs et al., 2001; Elston et al., 2011a; Bosch and Hayashi, 2012). While the study of neuronal anatomy alone may not be sufficient to ascertain a full understanding of neuronal circuit and brain disease pathology, the large data sets that are readily obtained from high resolution systematic imaging of brain regions provide an excellent resource for integration into comprehensive, big data models of neuronal function and pathology (Jacobs et al., 1997; Elston et al., 2009, 2010a,b, 2011b; Sasaki et al., 2014). Full understanding is far off due to the sheer complexity of the nervous system; there are approximately 10^{11} neurons making approximately 10^{14} synaptic connections (Williams and Herrup, 1988; Nimchinsky et al., 2004). A comprehensive evaluation of neuronal morphology and connectivity far exceeds the limits of our abilities to gather and analyze data at this time.

Among the most notable and plastic neuronal structures, dendritic spines are post-synaptic protuberances found primarily at non-symmetrical excitatory synapses directly opposed to a presynaptic bouton as illustrated by the high resolution of EM (Jones, 1968). Normally composed of a round spine head with a volume ranging from 0.015 to 0.77 μm^3 (DeFelipe et al., 1988; Petralia et al., 1994a,b,c; Knott et al., 2006; Arellano et al., 2007) and a thinner spine neck, dendritic spines serve as the point of contact between two neurons highly enriched in postsynaptic signaling components such as GluR (De Paola et al., 2006). They provide isolated sites for local integration and molecular compartmentalization of second messenger pathways such as calcium essential for normal synaptic scaling and learning and memory (Shepherd, 1996; Yuste et al., 2000; Yuste and Bonhoeffer, 2001; Alvarez and Sabatini, 2007). A rich literature exists of comparative studies among brain regions and species, allowing us to discover correlations between brain and neuronal anatomy, particularly in dendritic spines, and cognitive differences in healthy animals (Benavides-Piccione et al., 2002; Ballesteros-Yáñez et al., 2006).

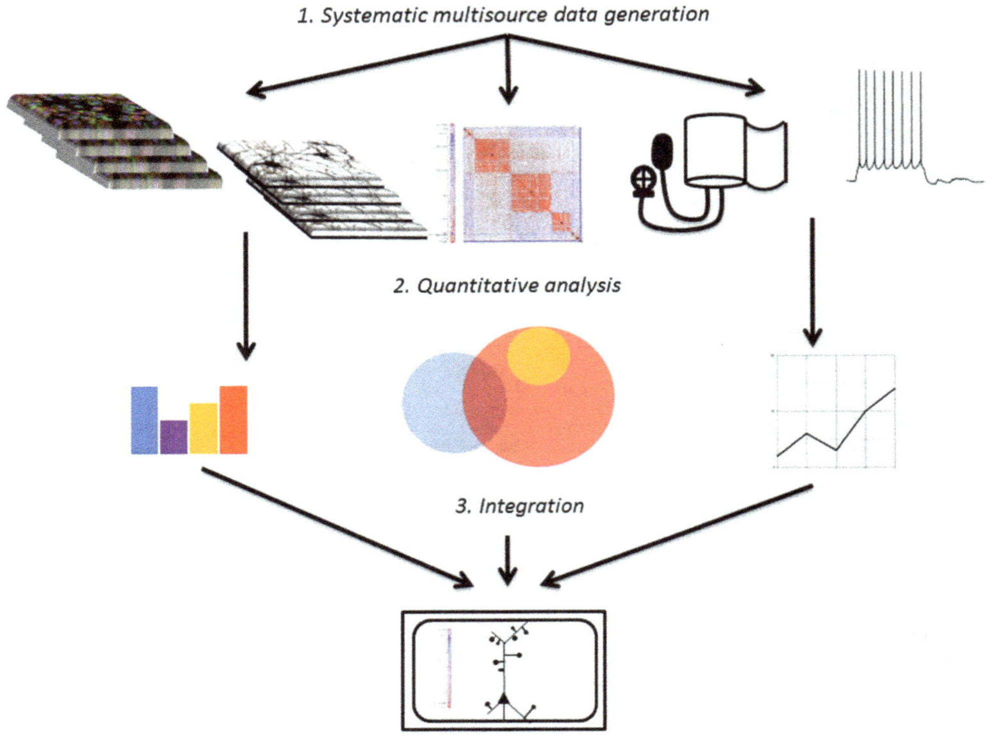

FIGURE 2 | Overall workflow schematic. Systematic raw data sets from diverse sources are collected (or extracted from public databases) and analyzed to provide manageable input for modeling. Data sets are then integrated to create models of function and disease that can be used to predict physiology and therapy.

DENDRITIC SPINE ABNORMALITIES AND COGNITIVE IMPAIRMENT

It has long been recognized that neurodegenerative disease and other neurological pathology often manifests as an alteration in neuronal anatomy and in particular in the number, shape, and distribution of dendritic spines (Goldman-Rakic, 1996; DeFelipe, 2004; Alonso-Nanclares et al., 2005; Glausier and Lewis, 2013; He and Portera-Cailliau, 2013; Licznerski and Duman, 2013; Pozueta et al., 2013; Smith and Villalba, 2013; Villalba and Smith, 2013; Wong and Guo, 2013), most likely correlating with alterations in neuronal signaling and axonal and neuronal death. Additionally, treatments that reduce the cognitive symptoms of neurodegenerative disease also reverse spine pathology (Smith et al., 2009). Unfortunately for patients and clinicians, these alterations can only be observed in small amount of tissues sampled from specific brain areas via biopsy, or post-mortem tissue received from deceased patients. The accumulation of senile plaques and tau bundles are the most well-known anatomical hallmarks of Alzheimer's disease, but it is synapse loss, exemplified by a reduction in dendritic spine density in the cerebral cortex and hippocampus, that best correlates with disease progression (Moolman et al., 2004). A decrease in length and complexity of the dendritic arbor as well as a significant reduction in spine density in medium spiny neurons of the dopamine receiving areas of the brain have long been observed as pathological hallmarks of Parkinson's disease (Stephens et al., 2005). Rett syndrome patients display a prominent reduction in dendritic arbor complexity, dendritic spine density, total number of neurons, and total brain volume which appears within the first year of the patient's life (Belichenko and Dahlström, 1995a,b; Armstrong, 2005). That these anatomical abnormalities are recapitulated in animal models (Smrt et al., 2007; Belichenko et al., 2009) of the disease reveals that Rett Syndrome is a disorder of neuronal development and reconfirms the correlation between dendritic spine anatomy and neuronal function or dysfunction.

Epilepsy is a neurological disorder resulting from network hyperactivity in neuronal circuits that causes chronic seizures (Bromfield et al., 2006). The principle hyperactive neurons in epilepsy are found in the medial temporal lobe and are characterized by dense excitatory synaptic inputs through dendritic spines. As one might expect, the chronic hyperactivity found in epilepsy correlates with significant changes in spine density, but it is unclear whether spine loss is a cause of epilepsy or a compensatory change in response to it (Wong and Guo, 2013). Further complicating the issue anatomical, and functional changes in the brain coincide with gene transcriptional chances, but a cause on effect relationship has not been established in either direction (Arion et al., 2006). This situation is not the exception but the rule for post mortem studies of diseased human tissue.

Here animal models of human disease are extremely useful for elucidating the causes and mechanisms of synaptic dysfunction. Not only do they offer the lack of confounding genetic and environmental factors found in human patients, but they offer investigators the potential to study disease progression at defined time points. Still, the use of imperfect animal models of human disease yields an understanding of these diseases and disease mechanisms that is overly simplistic (Chesselet and Carmichael, 2012) and the validity of these models in accurately predicting human disease is highly variable. Only comprehensive integration and iteration of clinical studies and mechanistic studies in animal models (under constant evaluation) can provide an accurate vision of the causes and mechanisms of complex neurodegenerative diseases.

Directed anatomical studies of neurons and populations of neurons along with protein expression and electrophysiological studies have been instrumental in the development of models that predict how the electrical properties of neurons vary with changes in cell shape; these works have contributed to a large number of popular software packages that model neuronal activity under various conditions (Hines and Carnevale, 2001; Bower and Beeman, 2007). The field of systems and computational neuroscience is mature and continues to flourish. In addition, a wide range of complementary knowledge can be gained by systematic analysis of available data sets and the acquisition of new high throughput data sets; chief among these are image data sets on multiple scales and from a variety of modalities which to data remain largely underutilized.

MULTISCALE IMAGING APPROACHES (FROM BIG TO SMALL)

Clinical imaging approaches such as CT, PET, and MRI have successfully illustrated pathological hallmarks of neurodegenerative disease such as loss of brain mass (Thompson et al., 2007; Schuff et al., 2009), alterations in long range connectivity (Daianu et al., 2013), and toxic protein accumulations such a senile plaques (Cohen et al., 2012; Johnson et al., 2012). These approaches, fMRI in particular, provide functional information regarding systems-level neuronal signaling and pathology, but lack the resolution for imaging individual synapses or subcellular components such as dendritic spines. Still, they provide another valuable resource for integration into systems biology models of brain function and pathology and excellent work, including the Alzheimer's Disease Neuroimaging Initiative (ADNI) and related projects (Mueller et al., 2005; Bradshaw et al., 2013; Daianu et al., 2013) is already taking advantage of it. A full account of the uses of these clinical imaging approaches or their limitations is beyond the scope of this review.

Determination of the number, morphology, and dynamics of synapses in populations of neurons is a well-accepted metric for neuronal health, development, and function that can provide investigators with information about specific brain regions and neuronal subtypes. To date, optical microscopy provides one of the most attractive tools for mechanistic studies of synaptic health and dysfunction applicable to both neurodegenerative disease patients (post-mortem tissues) and animal models of human disease. Dating back over 100 years, Golgi staining and brightfield microscopy of brain tissue sections has long been the workhorse for studies of neuronal anatomy. Invented by Camillo Golgi in his kitchen, the Golgi stain is elegant in its simplicity. It is based on the precipitation of silver or mercury chromate granules along the membranes of neurons in fixed tissue. These dense black particles clearly and stably stain neurons, leaving their anatomy including fine structures visible to bright field microscopy with high signal to noise (Pannese, 1999). It is particularly worth noting that the Golgi method randomly and sparsely labels cells throughout a field of view, allowing differentiation of the fine processes of a cell of interest from the dense background of connected circuitry (**Figure 3**). Santiago Ramon y Cajal took advantage of this fantastic approach to painstakingly document the anatomy of cells throughout the nervous system. For this combination the two men shared the Nobel Prize in Physiology or Medicine in 1906 (Grant, 2007).

Since that time these approaches have been widely modified and modernized and cell filling and stereology have been the workhorses in gathering data that have led to a systematic understanding of neuronal structure down to the synapse level (Elston, 2003; Elston and Fujita, 2014). Standard tissue preparation, staining, and bright field microscopy, while an extremely effective approach in the identification, characterization, and quantification of dendritic spines from specific regions of the brain, does have its limitations. Principle among these is the fact that tissues used in these approaches are by their very nature taken post-mortem and processed. Additionally, because bright field microscopy achieves no separation between photons originating at the focal plane and those arising above or below, 3-dimensional resolution is lacking; a considerable amount of neuronal structure is lost, simply because the nervous system does not exist entirely in two dimensions. For instance, the number of dendritic spines as measured by bright-field microscopy is greatly underestimated due to the exclusion spines that only protrude from the parent dendrite in the z-plane (Harris and Stevens, 1988). Slices also must be cut extremely thin, which eliminates most long range synaptic connectivity. Finally, the two-dimensional resolution limits observation of changes in structures below the micron range, which is appropriate for changes in dendritic spines but nothing smaller including structures in the spine such as post-synaptic density.

EX VIVO AND *IN VIVO* IMAGING

All fixed tissue imaging approaches by design face that limitation that they provide only a snapshot of neuronal anatomy at a given time. Only imaging of live cells, tissues, or organisms allow for the observation of dynamic processes. The widespread genetic introduction of fluorescent indicator dyes and recombinant fluorescent proteins derived from jellyfish has revolutionized live cell imaging including the imaging of neurons. Using transgenic animal models or viral transduction, fluorescent proteins such as GFP have been introduced into specific, genetically defined populations of neurons and other neural cells (Feng et al., 2000; Gong et al., 2003). Random insertion of transgenes leads to mouse models with neurons labeled sparsely enough to allow for high resolution imaging of fine anatomical structures such

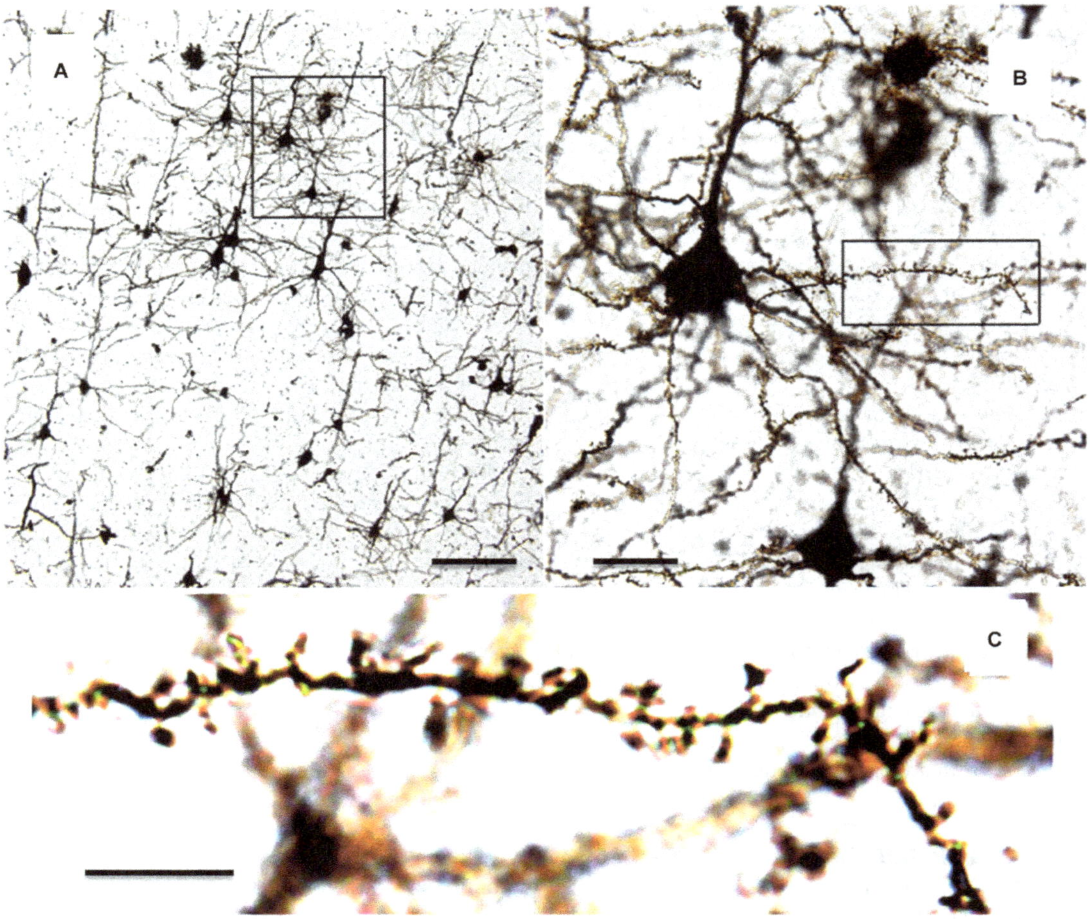

FIGURE 3 | Photomicrographs of Golgi-stained mouse cortical neurons from slices. **(A)** Neurons in brain slices are randomly and sporadically labeled allowing visualization of individual neurons. Scale = 50 μm. **(B)** Enlargement of boxed area in **(A)** showing dendrites and spines belonging to individual neurons. Scale = 10 μm. **(C)** Enlargement of boxed area in **(B)** showing individual dendritic spines which can be counted and analyzed. Scale = 5 μm. (adapted from Mancuso et al., 2013).

as dendritic spines (Feng et al., 2000). The combination of fluorescent labels with confocal microscopy, which uses a pinhole to discard those photons arising outside of the focal plane, allows these processes to be imaged at near diffraction resolution in three-dimension (3D). Due to their electrical excitability, electrophysiological recording is of course the standard method to observe and manipulate the function of neurons or populations of neurons. Still, confocal microscopy is limited by the scattering of excitation and emission photons to imaging structures 50 μm below the surface due to photodamage that occurs with the higher laser powers necessary with increasing imaging depth.

By reducing light scattering in the excitation path and restricting fluorescence activation to a tiny focal volume, allowing for 100% collection of emission signal, non-linear, multiphoton imaging with near infrared wavelengths, has enabled researchers to image neuronal structures as far as 1 micron deep (Theer et al., 2003) and over extended periods without significant light-induced tissue damage. Live tissue imaging coupled with physiological studies provides the capability to correlate changes in neuronal anatomy with functional measurements and manipulations in the same neuron or neurons (Kasai et al., 2010). Indeed such studies have led to our understanding of the mechanisms of synaptic plasticity at the single synapse level (Zhou et al., 2004; Yang et al., 2008) as well as the entry, diffusion, and intracellular release of calcium caused by synaptic activation and downstream signaling events and the role of dendritic spine morphology (Denk et al., 1995; Yuste et al., 1999; Holthoff et al., 2002; Araya et al., 2014).

The convergence of advances in microscopy and genetic tools for neuronal labeling has led to the advent of high resolution *in vivo* imaging of neuronal function and anatomy including imaging of the dendritic spine dynamics in awake, moving animals (Dombeck et al., 2009; Scott et al., 2013). This allows investigators to look at changes in dendritic spine density and anatomy and how they relate to the response of an animal to normal environmental stimuli (Jung and Herms, 2014). A number of studies have combined anatomical imaging and stereological analysis of neuronal structure including dendritic spines with electrophysiology by filling cells with fluorescent dye through the recording pipette and other imaging modalities in order to paint a picture of the elaborate changes that occur in models of disease (Day et al., 2006).

Formation and pruning of spines as well as changes in spine size and shape are a part of normal development, essential for the function of neuronal circuits (Calabrese, 2006). While more than one mechanism of synapse formation exists, in the most common model of neuronal development a postsynaptic neuron projects numerous small, thin filapodia which receive random inputs from neighboring synaptic terminals (Bhatt et al., 2009). The filipodia that receive sufficient inputs of the proper timing, mature into full dendritic spines and form a specific synapse, while those that do not are eliminated. While in adulthood most dendritic spines are stable over a long period of time, a proportion appear and disappear in any given period according to their inputs and it is thought that these changes highlight experience-dependent remodeling of neuronal circuits (Knott and Holtmaat, 2008). More specifically, it has been demonstrated in adult neurons that changes in the size and shape of dendritic spines correlate with plasticity at individual synapses (Matsuzaki et al., 2004).

All cellular level biological processes and synapse dynamics specifically are extremely dependent on the context of their cell-cell interactions and general environment (Hu and Wang, 2010; Petzold and Murthy, 2011; Van Beek and Claassen, 2011; Dallérac et al., 2013), which is a fundamental facet of systems medicine. It should be noted that the aforementioned fluorescence techniques based on protein expression or dye labeling only show labeled structures and neglect surrounding tissue. Label-free imaging approaches, while exhibiting much lower signal to noise, are then essential for placing labeled structures in the proper biological context. Among these, two photon autofluorescence (TPEAF) imaging, taking advantage of autofluorescent metabolic intermediates such as NADH, has long been used to image cells and distinguish among populations of cells based on metabolic rate (Williams et al., 1994; Piston et al., 1995; Monici, 2005). Second harmonic generation is another valuable non-linear, label-free imaging approach often used to visualize ordered arrays of proteins as are seen in structures such as cytoskeleton (Vanzi et al., 2012). More recently CARS imaging and its various subtypes have emerged as valuable tools for measuring chemical diversity in biological samples with high spatial resolution and is now used to distinguish cells based on the distribution of specific biological moieties, particularly various species of lipid molecules (Evans and Xie, 2008). Recently, the Wong lab developed a novel multimodal imaging approach combining TPAEF, SHG, and CARS in order to differentiate lung cancerous tissue from normal and desmoplastic edge (Xu et al., 2013). Lipid droplets and cell nuclei were well characterized in CARS images, and elastin and collagen fibers were illustrated by TPEAF and SHG modalities, respectively. A major obstacle to using these modalities as a component for systems levels models of neuronal function and dysfunction has been the development of appropriate computational tools for the systematic and quantitative analysis of such multimodal data. In this case the signal to noise issues that plague label-free approaches were improved by employing Sternberg's rolling ball method (Sternberg, 1983) to adaptively estimate background followed by denoising. Images were then processed using the eigenvalues of a Hessian matrix to find "tube-like" structures and a Robust Automatic Threshold Selection (RATS) to complete the segmentation (Wilkinson and Schut, 1998). With any such multimodal approach no one size fits all image analysis paradigm exists due to heterogeneity in signals and in anatomy, as such, specific approaches are necessary for each.

SUPER-RESOLUTION AND ELECTRON MICROSCOPY

Spine size, shape, and number alone do not give a complete portrayal of synaptic changes, both normal and pathological. Modulation of normal synapse physiology and function is accompanied by architectural rearrangements of intra-terminal ultrastructures that occur on timescales ranging from milliseconds to minutes. Macromolecular fluctuations of this magnitude are difficult to study using conventional imaging and biochemical methods as these methods lack the blend of resolution, cellular context, stability, and sensitivity needed to study native cellular processes. Neurological diseases are caused by genetic mutations affecting these native processes. Many of these mutations are also suspected of altering the ultrastructural architectures within neurons at the nanometer level.

Traditionally, EM has been employed to examine these nanoscopic subcellular changes (Kuwajima et al., 2013). Originally it was Gray (1959a,b) who used EM to conclusively demonstrate that the dendritic spines of pyramidal neurons are in fact the sites of synaptic contact. The postsynaptic density (PSD), the electron dense region of synaptic contact located on the distal tip of dendritic spines, has been a highly effective target of EM and its anatomy well-characterized in various brain regions (Cohen et al., 2012). In addition the application of proteomics approaches such as matrix-laser desorption/ionization-time-of-flight (MALDI-TOF) mass spectrometry (MS) have enabled researchers to gain a quantitative working knowledge of the protein composition of PSDs from a variety of brain regions in a number of neuronal subtypes under number of different conditions. While these results continue to suffer from some degree of false negatives and positives due to the nature of the detergent solubilization protocols used to isolate PSD proteins (Sheng and Hoogenraad, 2007), further refinement of data generation approaches for PSD proteomics will make data gained an excellent candidate for incorporation into our modeling approach.

Work from the Reid lab (Bock et al., 2011) provides an excellent example of integration of a large scale reconstruction of brain connectivity from EM data with *in vivo* functional data. Using intravital microscopy of a fluorescent calcium indicator in order to elucidate a single visual functional trait, orientation selectivity of a group of neurons, the group then correlated that activity with synaptic connectivity terminating in dendritic spines as determined by EM. It should be noted that the data acquired by this study at the lowest resolution necessary to carry out these goals on a single area of the visual cortex was upwards of 35 TB and characterization of this huge data set was entirely manual and constituted a herculean effort. Systematic application of this type of approach in normal and diseased tissue on a scale necessary to formulate models about function and dysfunction in synaptic circuitry certainly awaits a more rapid, less labor intensive analytical approach.

More recently, superresolution light microscopy approaches have arisen that allow for the examination of dendritic spine processes on a nanometer scale (Bethge et al., 2013; Loew and Hell, 2013; Takasaki et al., 2013). Taking advantage of the intrinsic properties of fluorophores or fluorescent proteins, these approaches, such as STED, STORM, and PALM, circumvent the normal diffraction barrier, allowing for light microscopy at nanometer resolution. Because they do not require special processing of the tissues involved, these approaches are compatible with live cell imaging. The combination of superresolution light microscopy with two photon excitation enabled researchers to resolve structures as small as the dendritic spine neck in thin slices and leaves open the possibility of accomplishing the same task *in vivo*. A recent study from the Rizzoli lab (Wilhelm et al., 2014) provides an excellent example of an approach to incorporate superresolution imaging of the synapse with omics data, in this case proteomic data, in order to construct a comprehensive model of the presynaptic bouton with the potential to expand our understanding of vesicle release and synaptic signaling. While this particular biological preparation, due to its simplicity, lends itself beautifully to such a comprehensive approach, a modified approach could certainly be applied to a number of other more complex preparations.

Cryo-electron tomography (cryo-ET) has emerged as a powerful technique, well-suited to imaging normal and abnormal macromolecular assemblies while preserving their native cellular contexts. Cryo-electron tomography is a 3D imaging technique that is increasingly being utilized to study the close relationship between neuron function and subcellular organization (Harapin et al., 2013; Lučič et al., 2013). The strength of cryo-ET centers on its use of isotonic cellular preservation, which captures fragile cellular structures in their native, near-physiological state. Cryopreserved specimens are imaged on an electron microscope while being tilted from −70° to +70° during the imaging process. The observed cellular features are imaged as a collection of 2D micrographs that are computationally combined into a single 3D tomogram, which is a nanometer-scale map of the original cell (Milne et al., 2013). The high-quality spacial information contained within these tomograms has revealed detailed views of eukaryotic cells that, if applied toward neurological disease, hold the potential to further the understanding of neurodegeneration.

Synapses are comprised of the necessary pre- and postsynaptic biological components for sending, receiving, and responding physiologically to neuromodulatory signals. These components include biosynthetic organelles such as endoplasmic reticula and mitochondria, various lipid-based cellular membranes, membrane delineated ion channels and protein complexes, cytoskeletal assemblies and their associated cellular trafficking machinery, and lipid vesicles bearing chemical neurotransmitters. Changes in one synaptic component, inevitably lead to compensatory changes in other related components. Fluctuations in the presynaptic membrane potential are known to modulate the rate of synaptic vesicle fusion with the plasma membrane and the release of chemical neurotransmitter into the synaptic cleft. Previous cryo-ET studies have shed light on the arrangements of presynaptic cytoskeletal structures (Fernández-Busnadiego et al., 2010), such as actin filaments and microtubules, as well as the number of transmitter-containing vesicles and their distributions in conventional (Fernández-Busnadiego et al., 2013; Harlow et al., 2013) and ribbon-type active zones (Lenzi et al., 1999). Similar methods could conceivably be used to extend the current understanding of vesicle numbers and fusion (Bharat et al., 2014) in diseased neurons as a proxy for measuring neurotransmitter release kinetics in diseases, such as Alzheimer's or Parkinson's, known to affect cognitive function. Similarly, cryo-ET could be applied to human diseases to investigate macromolecular structures downstream of transmitter release at the synaptic cleft (Lucić et al., 2005) and postsynaptic nerve terminals located on dendritic spines (Swulius et al., 2012). Because spine density is affected in neural pathologies, there is a clear link to the critical nature of synaptic junctions and dendritic spines in normal neuron function. Currently, spine count is primarily used as an indicator of neural distress, but little is known about the early morphological changes that occur within the synapse that contribute to the numerical decline of dendritic spines. By elucidating ultrastructures on either side of the synapse, depth of understanding could be gained regarding the changes occurring within neurons affected during Alzheimer's or Parkinson's, and also whether changes in spine density follows a unified progression or whether each affected spine holds clues to further understanding of disease.

Mitochondria play a critical role in supporting the energy demands of neurons, and dysfunctional mitochondrial metabolism has been implicated in the pathogenesis of a number of neurodegenerative diseases (Itoh et al., 2013; Maresca et al., 2013). Mitochondria are present along the axon length and within pre- and postsynaptic termini. Within or near dendritic spines, mitochondria are thought to generate sufficient energy for ATP-intensive processes including kinesin-based protein and vesicular transport, endocytosis and recycling of neurotransmitter receptors, as well as biosynthetic responses resulting from presynaptic stimuli. In addition, mitochondria are a major source of reactive oxygen species (ROS) within eukaryotic cells, which are thought to contribute to oxidative damage in neurons. Cryo-electron tomography has been used to study mitochondrial morphologies in photoreceptor synaptic termini (Perkins et al., 2012) and the Calyx of Held (Perkins et al., 2010), and protocols have been designed that would allow mitochondrial studies in axons as well (Shahmoradian et al., 2014). In addition, previous tomographic studies that measured neuronal membrane systems (Nickell et al., 2007; Gilliam et al., 2012) and intracellular transport systems (Gilliam et al., 2012) demonstrate the feasibility of using these approaches to investigate mitochondria as well. Future cryo-ET investigations correlating mitochondrial size and cristae surface area (a function of ATP synthesis levels) and the statistical analysis of axonal vesicles numbers could provide critical clues to understanding how defects in axonal transport promote dendritic spine loss and neurodegeneration.

The normal cycle of eukaryotic biosynthetic processes includes lysosomal degradation of lipid membranes and proteins. Abnormal accumulation of this cellular debris lies behind disease progression in lysosomal storage disorders and may play a similar role in other diseases associated with cellular accumulations. Protein misfolding and aggregation results in accumulations of α-synuclein found in Parkinson's Disease (Lee et al., 2014) as well as accumulations of tau and amyloid-beta polypeptides responsible for the hallmark neuritic plaques and neurofibrillary tangles associated with Alzheimer's Disease (Bloom, 2014). It is not presently clear whether synaptic peptide accumulations are strictly extracellular or whether accumulations occur within spines as well. However, synapses are armed with machinery for both exocytosis and endocytosis as it pertains to vesicle fusion, vesicle retrieval, and membrane recycling. Alterations in these processes within dendritic spines may lead to intraterminal protein accumulations that would be visible by cryo-ET. While few tomographic studies have focused on transgenic models of neurodegenerative disease (Frank et al., 2010; Gilliam et al., 2012), recent studies point to the value of cryo-ET as a critical tool for evaluating neurotoxic protein aggregation (Nicoll et al., 2013; Shahmoradian et al., 2013) as a means of evaluating such diseases. Future application of cryo-ET towards neurological dysfunction will likely reveal clues to understanding abnormal protein aggregation allowing that data to be integrated into models of disease pathogenesis.

All EM work and cryo-ET in particular still requires a great deal of manual intervention from human operators, despite great advances in analytical tools. Most large scale studies employ sparse reconstruction strategies whose resolution is limited by the sampling method employed in order to make data acquisition and analysis feasible (Harris et al., 2006). Dense reconstruction awaits improvements in the computational tools required to analyze the large data sets involved, including: (1) automatic alignment and segmentation of sections; and (2) generation of 3D reconstructions. While cryo-ET data appears to face some of the greatest hurdles in its potential integration into larger scale models of synaptic function and dysfunction, it also offers some of the greatest promise toward a larger understanding of mechanisms of signaling beyond simple connectivity.

COMPUTATIONAL TOOLS FOR AUTOMATED SPINE ANALYSIS

As current high-resolution imaging techniques allow for the collection of the massive amounts of 3D anatomical data or data series needed to feed systems level models, the bottleneck in these studies has become accurate quantification and classification of anatomical structures. Manual spine analysis is very time consuming and it is not feasible especially for the analysis of a large set of 3D and 4D images. Besides, the results are hard to reproduce due to investigator subjectivity and variability. Programs which can automatically and rapidly detect and measure spines of large datasets of 3D neuronal images with little human intervention are much needed to study the mechanisms regulating spine morphology. In this section we will first describe the general pipeline for automatic spine detection. Then, some existing popular tools for automated detection and quantitative analysis of spines will be presented, as well as their pros and cons. Major challenges and some new desired functions of the software will be briefly discussed at the end.

A general pipeline for spine detection is composed of image preprocessing, segmentation, spine labeling and post-processing. The purpose of preprocessing is to increase the signal-to-noise ratio of the image so that it can be better segmented. Two most commonly used preprocessing techniques are denoising and deconvolution. Noise can be caused by the microscope or a detector such as a charge-coupled device (CCD) camera or photomultiplier tube (PMT). Low pass filters such as Gaussian filter or median filter are usually used to remove the speckle noise. Deconvolution is applied to revise the optical distortion that takes place during microscopic imaging. Depending on whether the point spread function (PSF) is known, there are two types of deconvolution methods available. Blind deconvolution is widely used in fluorescence microscopic image restoration which has two different approaches. The Richardson–Lucy deconvolution algorithm is the most commonly used iterative algorithm, while the Wiener deconvolution is the most common non-iterative algorithms for blind deconvolution.

The purpose of segmentation is to distinguish the foreground objects (e.g., dendrites and spines) from the background of the image. Many segmentation methods have been proposed for spine identification. The segmentation based on a global threshold can be easily applied (Koh et al., 2002); however, it is difficult to segment faint or thin spines without distorting the spine shapes with a single global threshold. Adaptive thresholding, which computes local thresholds, can partially solve the problem by calculating local thresholds at different regions (Cheng et al., 2007; Rodriguez et al., 2008). Many more sophisticated methods such as level set and Bayesian segmentation are also used (Fan et al., 2009; Oriented Markov Random Field Based Dendritic Spine Segmentation for Fluorescence Microscopy Images by Cheng). In many cases, these kinds of methods have superior segmentation results than the threshold based methods. However, the results can also be largely degraded because of the poor image quality, e.g., image with low SNR (signal to noise ratio).

To detect each single object, labeling is performed after segmentation. A major challenge toward automated spine detection and classification is laying out the criteria that define dendritic spines. This makes automated detection difficult to surpass manual detection. A common approach is based on the medial axis of dendrites which can be obtained by skeletonization. The spines are detected as the small protrusions along the boundaries of the dendrites. Usually diameter estimation is performed after skeletonization for dendritic morphometry. One simple way is to assume that the branch cross-section at any node is approximated as circular, which, however, will introduce quantization errors for small structures such as thin dendrites and spines. Rayburst sampling algorithm has been proposed to solve the problem. It is capable of continuous

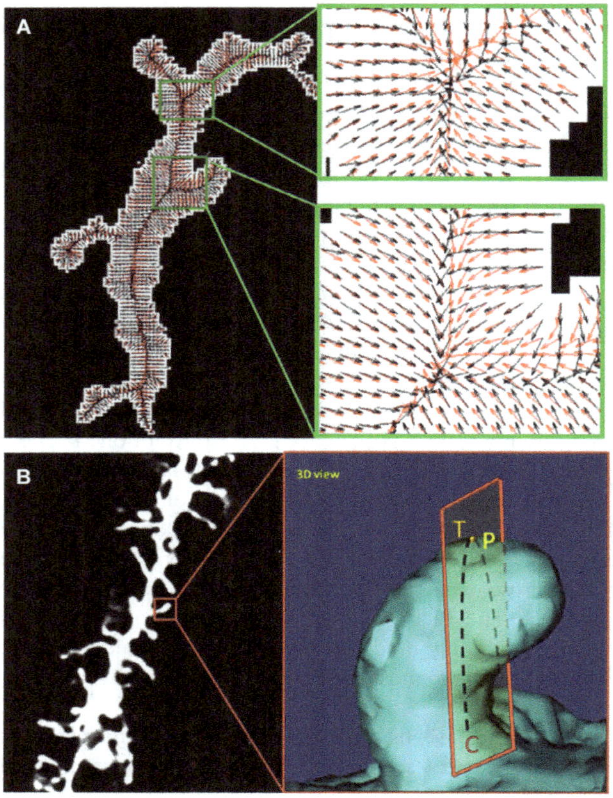

FIGURE 4 | Comparison of two alternative spine detection algorithms. **(A)** Gradient vector field (GVF) analyses for centerline extraction (reprinted from Zhang et al., 2010). **(B)** Detection of Spine Tip Area Using Minimal Cross-Sectional Curvature (reprinted from He et al., 2012).

and more accurate radius estimation by using the original grayscale data instead of the segmented images. (Rodriguez et al., 2006).

After labeling, postprocessing is performed to refine the final results. For example, to separate two attached spines, or to remove the false spines, the detection of which can be caused by nearby axon pieces. If necessary, manual editing is also performed at this stage.

During the past decade, several software tools have been developed for automatic dendritic spine analysis. NeuronIQ was developed by Dr. Stephen Wong's lab (**Figure 4**) with two versions designed for 2D and 3D analysis respectively (Cheng et al., 2007; Zhang et al., 2007, 2010). The 2D version is based on the maximal intensity projection (MIP) of image stacks and has much less computational complexity compared with the 3D versions. The 3D version provides 3D rendering and visualization. For both versions, measurement results can be exported to files using standard formats for further processing, modeling and statistical analysis. NeuronStudio was developed by Rodriguez et al. (2006) for automatic tracing and reconstruction of neuron structures from confocal image stacks. Rendering and 3D visualization are also provided. Imaris is a commercial software which can be used for dendritic spine analysis (Swanger et al., 2011). The Filament Tracer module provides the functioning of automatic spine detection and is capable of processing a large dataset of time-lapse images. Neurolucida is a powerful tool for neuron reconstructions and quantitative analysis from microscopy images (Aguiar et al., 2013). AutoSpine can be used for automatic detection and quantitication of dendritic spines based on the tracing results from Neurolucida. Some popular bioimage informatics platforms such as ImageJ have also been used for automated spine analysis. For example, Orlowski and Bjarkam (2012) proposed a simple method of spine counting based on the binarization and skeletonization functions provided by ImageJ.

All of the above mentioned software tools are capable of the fast, accurate, and automated quantification of dendritic spines, however with relative strengths and weaknesses. NeuronIQ and NeuronStudio are in house developed tools which are specially designed for dendritic spine analysis. They are standalone tools which are the easiest to be used nevertheless with the least flexibility, i.e., it is hard for the users to check the codes and introduce some new functionality by themselves. FilamentTracer and AutoSpine are modules of another software package and cannot be used alone. For example, FilamentTracer depends on Imaris for visualization, analysis and segmentation; while AutoSpine analyze the dendritic spines based on the images of dendritic branches obtained from Neurolucida and AutoNeuron. No doubt it is more complex for the users. However, with the support of other modules, FilamentTracer and AutoSpine are more powerful in visualization and data analysis. ImageJ has the highest flexibility and is the most powerful tool for users with some programming knowledge. The users can design their own approaches for dendritic spine analysis, with the help of the ever increasing plugins pool. The users can also change the plugins by themselves according to some specific requirements of the projects, since all the plugins' source codes are publicly available.

One of the major challenges still faced for automated spine detection is the poor performance when processing images with complex backgrounds (e.g., with complex patterns of crossing neuronal projections) or when spine density is very high. Another challenge is to deal with the partial volume effects or a large spacing between neighboring slices. Additionally, the existing tools only focus on the structural and morphological analysis of dendritic spines. For a comprehensive integration of the many varied types of spine imaging data available, it is necessary to develop methods for analysis and incorporation of spine functional data. For example, to include trafficking of specific macromolecules into spines, or correlate the trafficking of synaptic molecules with morphological parameters by investigating the fluorescence intensity of dendritic spine heads. Additionally, the aforementioned tools are designed to process data sets of images of high contrast labeled neurons. While signal to noise issues in these samples is not trivial, it pales in comparison to the issues faced when attempting to analyze data from the label-free imaging modalities highlighted earlier. The generation of a whole new arsenal of new computational tools to process, analyze, and quantify these types of imaging data forms a major obstacle to their potential

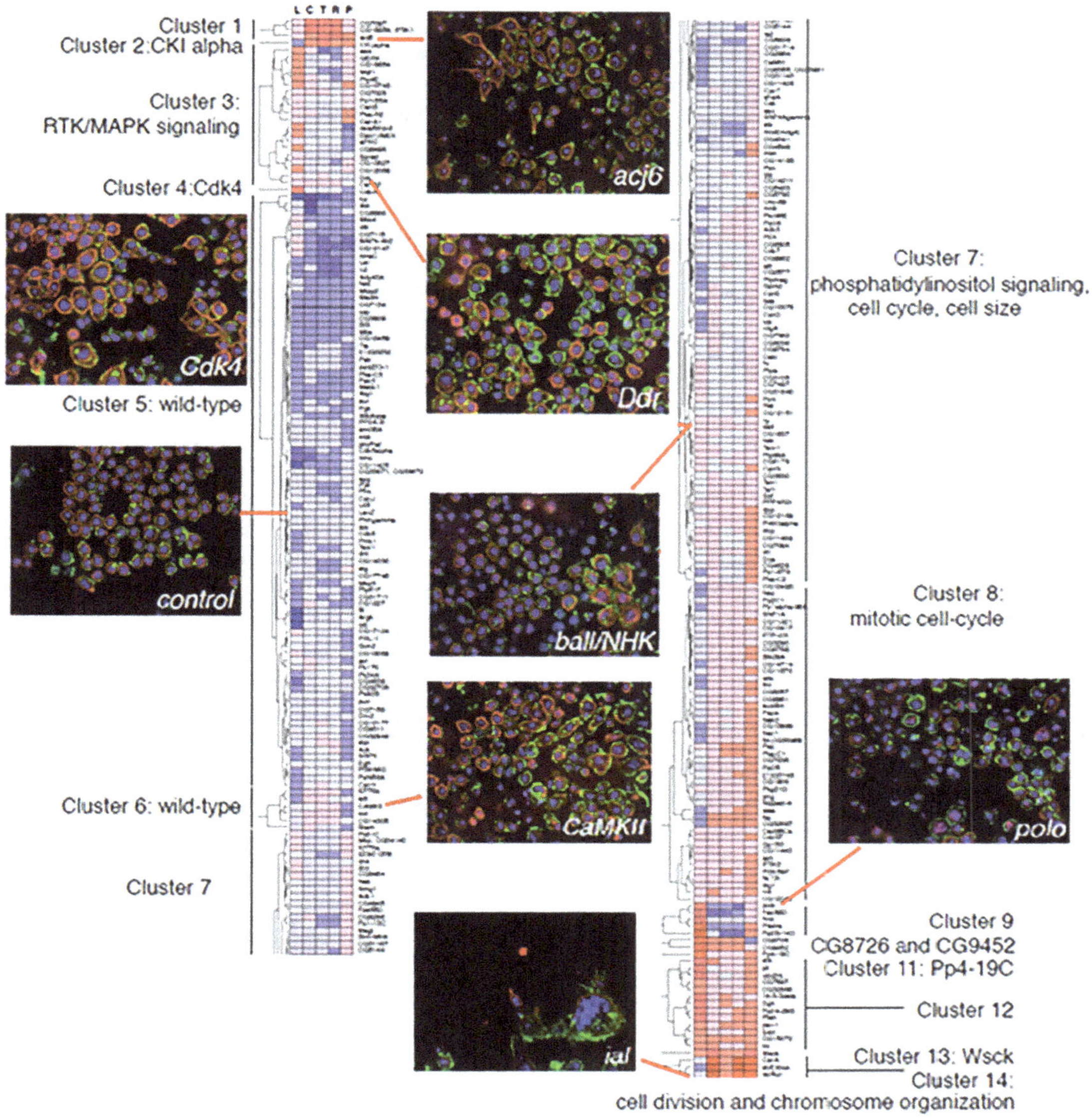

FIGURE 5 | Example of raw cell morphology imaging data of cells with gene-specific knockdowns and the corresponding gene expression profiling. Data gathered reveals clusters of co-expressed genes that correlate with transitions to specific morphological states.

integration into models for the prediction of neuronal function and dysfunction.

TYING IT ALL TOGETHER: CORRELATIONS BETWEEN CHANGES IN CELL SHAPE AND CHANGES IN GENE NETWORKS

A prototype for incorporating anatomical changes into systems level models of cell biology activity serves as a blueprint for our third step, the integration of analyzed neuronal imaging data into a comprehensive systems model of brain function. Recently, Yin et al., building on previous work by Bakal et al., employed one of the first systems level approaches to correlating cell morphological complexity to gene function (Bakal et al., 2007; Yin et al., 2013, 2014). After light microscopic imaging of populations of individual cells in culture, *Drosophila* KC-167 cells were classified into five distinct groups based on morphology. A Quantitative Morphological Signature (QMS) was established and used to quantify cell shape changes by comparing to each of these groups. Gene signaling networks were then altered using RNAi (**Figure 5**) and the effects of these gene network alterations on population complexity properties, including cell number and distribution of cell shapes within a population, were analyzed. Work was performed in insect cells as well as mouse and human metastatic melanoma cells and showed that cells exhibit discrete changes in morphology correlating to low energy regions in shape space in response to changes in gene function. Based on the morphological profile generated by their alteration, genes then separate themselves into groups. This work showed that classes of genes conserved across species induce similar changes in cell morphology and that many of these mechanisms are likely conserved among cell types. This suggests that gene networks have evolved to tightly control the topology of a cell's space shape in response to external and internal stimuli.

Previous work has successfully used this approach on cells which adopt a neuron-like morphology (Bakal et al., 2007) and despite the increasing levels of complexity involved, this concept likely applies to the morphology of adult neurons and their individual subcellular structures in the context of normal and pathological stimuli, allowing the correlation of genetic, developmental, and environmental changes to alterations in the balance of populations of structures. Dendritic spines, in particular provide an excellent substrate into which to expand this approach due to their abundance and well-documented variation in size, shape, and location. Investigators attempting to perform similar studies on neurons are faced with variations in the synaptic inputs received as well as neuronal subtype heterogeneity. Still, the major hurdle in realizing neuronal morphology correlation with gene and -omic data on a systems level is the need for population-level automated analysis of dendritic spines.

DISCUSSION

As the days of studying individual biological processes on the level of single entities operating in a vacuum give way to a more comprehensive approach that acknowledges the complex interplay between the many participants in a biological system, new data that can enrich systems models are at a premium. The correlation between the anatomy and function of neurons is well documented and many changes to normal neuronal anatomy are known to occur in various neurological disease states. One of the most prominent anatomical features of excitatory and other types of neurons, dendritic spines, which are the postsynaptic terminus of glutamatergic neurons, have long served as one of the most common anatomical indicators of neuronal function and dysfunction, including development, synaptic plasticity, and aging as well as schizophrenia, epilepsy, and Alzheimer's disease. While helpful in directed spine counting experiments aimed at exploring the mechanism and severity of diseases, the large-scale, systematic imaging data of populations of neurons forms a largely untapped resource for integration with other data sources, such as proteomics or gene expression profiling, into comprehensive, systems medicine models of brain function and dysfunction. The old adage that a picture is worth a thousand words certainly applies in this case, as the potential imaging sets involved hold huge potential as big data sources. The exploitation of that resource faces many non-trivial obstacles in the acquisition, analysis, and modeling of imaging data, which we point out in this review.

Advances in microscopy technologies coupled with the exploding field of genetically encoded indicator proteins and their directed expression has given investigators the tools to gather very specific, high resolution imaging data in a number of contexts including in live, awake animals. The principle hurdle in incorporating such data sets into systems models is the development of algorithms that can convert large amounts of irregular imaging data into categorized quantitative data appropriate for those models. Large strides have been made in the development of automated or semi-automated software tools that detect and characterize dendritic spines from labeled neurons, but work does still remain in order to achieve accurate, fully automated spine detection, particularly from high density or low signal-to-noise images. These shortcomings are greatly magnified when dealing with more complex, yet more information rich images such as those attained from label-free imaging. While it is unlikely that any one size fits all solution exists, constant improvement in the accuracy of automated dendritic spine detection and characterization from images acquired from a variety of imaging modalities is already underway. Label-free multi-modal imaging of specific aspects of the surrounding tissues offers an excellent prospective method to place high resolution dendritic spine imaging in the proper biological context. The integration of characterized dendritic spine imaging with multimodal imaging of the surrounding environment and the wealth of currently available omics and brain functional data is the next step in the evolution of modeling brain function and dysfunction.

ACKNOWLEDGMENTS

The authors would like to acknowledge generous funding from: R01 AG028928, TT & WF Chao Foundation, John S. Dunn Research Foundation to Stephen T. C. Wong and R21 AG042585 to Xiaofeng Xia.

REFERENCES

Aguiar, P., Sousa, M., and Szucs, P. (2013). Versatile morphometric analysis and visualization of the three-dimensional structure of neurons. *Neuroinformatics* 11, 393–403. doi: 10.1007/s12021-013-9188-z

Alonso-Nanclares, L., Garbelli, R., Sola, R. G., Pastor, J., Tassi, L., Spreafico, R., et al. (2005). Microanatomy of the dysplastic neocortex from epileptic patients. *Brain J. Neurol.* 128, 158–173. doi: 10.1093/brain/awh331

Alvarez, V. A., and Sabatini, B. L. (2007). Anatomical and physiological plasticity of dendritic spines. *Annu. Rev. Neurosci.* 30, 79–97. doi: 10.1146/annurev.neuro.30.051606.094222

Araya, R., Vogels, T. P., and Yuste, R. (2014). Activity-dependent dendritic spine neck changes are correlated with synaptic strength. *Proc. Natl. Acad. Sci. U S A* 111, E2895–E2904. doi: 10.1073/pnas.1321869111

Arellano, J. I., Espinosa, A., Fairén, A., Yuste, R., and DeFelipe, J. (2007). Non-synaptic dendritic spines in neocortex. *Neuroscience* 145, 464–469. doi: 10.1016/j.neuroscience.2006.12.015

Arion, D., Sabatini, M., Unger, T., Pastor, J., Alonso-Nanclares, L., Ballesteros-Yáñez, I., et al. (2006). Correlation of transcriptome profile with electrical activity in temporal lobe epilepsy. *Neurobiol. Dis.* 22, 374–387. doi: 10.1016/j.nbd.2005.12.012

Armstrong, D. D. (2005). Neuropathology of rett syndrome. *J. Child Neurol.* 20, 747–753. doi: 10.1177/08830738050200090901

Bakal, C., Aach, J., Church, G., and Perrimon, N. (2007). Quantitative morphological signatures define local signaling networks regulating cell morphology. *Science* 316, 1753–1756. doi: 10.1126/science.1140324

Ballesteros-Yáñez, I., Benavides-Piccione, R., Elston, G. N., Yuste, R., and DeFelipe, J. (2006). Density and morphology of dendritic spines in mouse neocortex. *Neuroscience* 138, 403–409. doi: 10.1016/j.neuroscience.2005.11.038

Belichenko, N. P., Belichenko, P. V., and Mobley, W. C. (2009). Evidence for both neuronal cell autonomous and nonautonomous effects of methyl-CpG-binding protein 2 in the cerebral cortex of female mice with Mecp2 mutation. *Neurobiol. Dis.* 34, 71–77. doi: 10.1016/j.nbd.2008.12.016

Belichenko, P. V., and Dahlström, A. (1995a). Confocal laser scanning microscopy and 3-D reconstructions of neuronal structures in human brain cortex. *NeuroImage* 2, 201–207. doi: 10.1006/nimg.1995.1026

Belichenko, P. V., and Dahlström, A. (1995b). Studies on the 3-dimensional architecture of dendritic spines and varicosities in human cortex by confocal laser scanning microscopy and Lucifer yellow microinjections. *J. Neurosci. Methods* 57, 55–61. doi: 10.1016/0165-0270(94)00125-z

Benavides-Piccione, R., Ballesteros-Yáñez, I., DeFelipe, J., and Yuste, R. (2002). Cortical area and species differences in dendritic spine morphology. *J. Neurocytol.* 31, 337–346. doi: 10.1023/A:1024134312173

Bethge, P., Chéreau, R., Avignone, E., Marsicano, G., and Nägerl, U. V. (2013). Two-photon excitation STED microscopy in two colors in acute brain slices. *Biophys. J.* 104, 778–785. doi: 10.1016/j.bpj.2012.12.054

Bharat, T. A. M., Malsam, J., Hagen, W. J. H., Scheutzow, A., Söllner, T. H., and Briggs, J. A. G. (2014). SNARE and regulatory proteins induce local membrane protrusions to prime docked vesicles for fast calcium-triggered fusion. *EMBO Rep.* 15, 308–314. doi: 10.1002/embr.201337807

Bhatt, D. H., Zhang, S., and Gan, W.-B. (2009). Dendritic spine dynamics. *Annu. Rev. Physiol.* 71, 261–282. doi: 10.1146/annurev.physiol.010908.163140

Bloom, G. S. (2014). Amyloid-β and tau: the trigger and bullet in Alzheimer disease pathogenesis. *JAMA Neurol.* 71, 505–508. doi: 10.1001/jamaneurol.2013.5847

Bock, D. D., Lee, W.-C. A., Kerlin, A. M., Andermann, M. L., Hood, G., Wetzel, A. W., et al. (2011). Network anatomy and in vivo physiology of visual cortical neurons. *Nature* 471, 177–182. doi: 10.1038/nature09802

Bosch, M., and Hayashi, Y. (2012). Structural plasticity of dendritic spines. *Curr. Opin. Neurobiol.* 22, 383–388. doi: 10.1016/j.conb.2011.09.002

Bower, J. M., and Beeman, D. (2007). Constructing realistic neural simulations with GENESIS. *Methods Mol. Biol.* 401, 103–125. doi: 10.1007/978-1-59745-520-6_7

Bradshaw, E. M., Chibnik, L. B., Keenan, B. T., Ottoboni, L., Raj, T., Tang, A., et al. (2013). CD33 Alzheimer's disease locus: altered monocyte function and amyloid biology. *Nat. Neurosci.* 16, 848–850. doi: 10.1038/nn.3435

Bromfield, E. B., Cavazos, J. E., and Sirven, J. I. (2006). Basic mechanisms underlying seizures and epilepsy [WWW document]. Available online at: http://www.ncbi.nlm.nih.gov/books/NBK2510/. Accessed on July 7 2014.

Calabrese, B. (2006). Development and regulation of dendritic spine synapses. *Physiology* 21, 38–47. doi: 10.1152/physiol.00042.2005

Cheng, J., Zhou, X., Miller, E., Witt, R. M., Zhu, J., Sabatini, B. L., et al. (2007). A novel computational approach for automatic dendrite spines detection in two-photon laser scan microscopy. *J. Neurosci. Methods* 165, 122–134. doi: 10.1016/j.jneumeth.2007.05.020

Chesselet, M.-F., and Carmichael, S. T. (2012). Animal models of neurological disorders. *Neurotherapeutics* 9, 241–244. doi: 10.1007/s13311-012-0118-9

Cohen, A. D., Rabinovici, G. D., Mathis, C. A., Jagust, W. J., Klunk, W. E., and Ikonomovic, M. D. (2012). Using pittsburgh compound B for in vivo PET imaging of fibrillar amyloid-beta. *Adv. Pharmacol.* 64, 27–81. doi: 10.1016/b978-0-12-394816-8.00002-7

Daianu, M., Jahanshad, N., Nir, T. M., Toga, A. W., Jack, C. R. Jr., Weiner, M. W., et al. (2013). Breakdown of brain connectivity between normal aging and Alzheimer's disease: a structural k-core network analysis. *Brain Connect.* 3, 407–422. doi: 10.1089/brain.2012.0137

Dallérac, G., Chever, O., and Rouach, N. (2013). How do astrocytes shape synaptic transmission? Insights from electrophysiology. *Front. Cell. Neurosci.* 7:159. doi: 10.3389/fncel.2013.00159

Day, M., Wang, Z., Ding, J., An, X., Ingham, C. A., Shering, A. F., et al. (2006). Selective elimination of glutamatergic synapses on striatopallidal neurons in Parkinson disease models. *Nat. Neurosci.* 9, 251–259. doi: 10.1038/nn1632

DeFelipe, J. (2004). Cortical microanatomy and human brain disorders: epilepsy. *Cortex* 40, 232–233. doi: 10.1016/s0010-9452(08)70962-6

DeFelipe, J., Conti, F., Van Eyck, S. L., and Manzoni, T. (1988). Demonstration of glutamate-positive axon terminals forming asymmetric synapses in cat neocortex. *Brain Res.* 455, 162–165. doi: 10.1016/0006-8993(88)90127-8

Denk, W., Sugimori, M., and Llinás, R. (1995). Two types of calcium response limited to single spines in cerebellar Purkinje cells. *Proc. Natl. Acad. Sci. U S A* 92, 8279–8282. doi: 10.1073/pnas.92.18.8279

De Paola, V., Holtmaat, A., Knott, G., Song, S., Wilbrecht, L., Caroni, P., et al. (2006). Cell type-specific structural plasticity of axonal branches and boutons in the adult neocortex. *Neuron* 49, 861–875. doi: 10.1016/j.neuron.2006.02.017

Dombeck, D. A., Graziano, M. S., and Tank, D. W. (2009). Functional clustering of neurons in motor cortex determined by cellular resolution imaging in awake behaving mice. *J. Neurosci.* 29, 13751–13760. doi: 10.1523/jneurosci.2985-09.2009

Elston, G. N. (2000). Pyramidal cells of the frontal lobe: all the more spinous to think with. *J. Neurosci.* 20, RC95. doi: 10.1007/springerreference_223714

Elston, G. N. (2003). Cortex, cognition and the cell: new insights into the pyramidal neuron and prefrontal function. *Cereb. Cortex* 13, 1124–1138. doi: 10.1093/cercor/bhg093

Elston, G. N., Benavides-Piccione, R., Elston, A., Manger, P. R., and DeFelipe, J. (2011a). Pyramidal cells in prefrontal cortex of primates: marked differences in neuronal structure among species. *Front. Neuroanat.* 5:2. doi: 10.3389/fnana.2011.00002

Elston, G. N., and Fujita, I. (2014). Pyramidal cell development: postnatal spinogenesis, dendritic growth, axon growth and electrophysiology. *Front. Neuroanat.* 8:78. doi: 10.3389/fnana.2014.00078

Elston, G. N., Oga, T., and Fujita, I. (2009). Spinogenesis and pruning scales across functional hierarchies. *J. Neurosci.* 29, 3271–3275. doi: 10.1523/jneurosci.5216-08.2009

Elston, G. N., Oga, T., Okamoto, T., and Fujita, I. (2010a). Spinogenesis and pruning from early visual onset to adulthood: an intracellular injection study of layer III pyramidal cells in the ventral visual cortical pathway of the macaque monkey. *Cereb. Cortex* 20, 1398–1408. doi: 10.1093/cercor/bhp203

Elston, G. N., Oga, T., Okamoto, T., and Fujita, I. (2011b). Spinogenesis and pruning in the anterior ventral inferotemporal cortex of the macaque monkey: an intracellular injection study of layer III pyramidal cells. *Front. Neuroanat.* 5:42. doi: 10.3389/fnana.2011.00042

Elston, G. N., Okamoto, T., Oga, T., Dornan, D., and Fujita, I. (2010b). Spinogenesis and pruning in the primary auditory cortex of the macaque monkey (*Macaca fascicularis*): an intracellular injection study of layer III pyramidal cells. *Brain Res.* 1316, 35–42. doi: 10.1016/j.brainres.2009.12.056

Elston, G. N., and Rosa, M. G. (1997). The occipitoparietal pathway of the macaque monkey: comparison of pyramidal cell morphology in layer III of functionally related cortical visual areas. *Cereb. Cortex* 7, 432–452. doi: 10.1093/cercor/7.5.432

Elston, G. N., and Rosa, M. G. (1998). Morphological variation of layer III pyramidal neurones in the occipitotemporal pathway of the macaque monkey visual cortex. *Cereb. Cortex* 8, 278–294. doi: 10.1093/cercor/8.3.278

Engert, F., and Bonhoeffer, T. (1999). Dendritic spine changes associated with hippocampal long-term synaptic plasticity. *Nature* 399, 66–70.

Evans, C. L., and Xie, X. S. (2008). Coherent anti-stokes raman scattering microscopy: chemical imaging for biology and medicine. *Annu. Rev. Anal. Chem. (Palo Alto Calif)* 1, 883–909. doi: 10.1146/annurev.anchem.1.031207.112754

Fan, J., Zhou, X., Dy, J. G., Zhang, Y., and Wong, S. T. C. (2009). An automated pipeline for dendrite spine detection and tracking of 3D optical microscopy neuron images of in vivo mouse models. *Neuroinformatics* 7, 113–130. doi: 10.1007/s12021-009-9047-0

Feng, G., Mellor, R. H., Bernstein, M., Keller-Peck, C., Nguyen, Q. T., Wallace, M., et al. (2000). Imaging neuronal subsets in transgenic mice expressing multiple spectral variants of GFP. *Neuron* 28, 41–51. doi: 10.1016/s0896-6273(00)00084-2

Fernández-Busnadiego, R., Asano, S., Oprisoreanu, A.-M., Sakata, E., Doengi, M., Kochovski, Z., et al. (2013). Cryo-electron tomography reveals a critical role of RIM1α in synaptic vesicle tethering. *J. Cell Biol.* 201, 725–740. doi: 10.1083/jcb.201206063

Fernández-Busnadiego, R., Zuber, B., Maurer, U. E., Cyrklaff, M., Baumeister, W., and Lucic, V. (2010). Quantitative analysis of the native presynaptic cytomatrix by cryoelectron tomography. *J. Cell Biol.* 188, 145–156. doi: 10.1083/jcb.200908082

Frank, T., Rutherford, M. A., Strenzke, N., Neef, A., Pangršič, T., Khimich, D., et al. (2010). Bassoon and the synaptic ribbon organize $Ca^{2}+$ channels and vesicles to add release sites and promote refilling. *Neuron* 68, 724–738. doi: 10.1016/j.neuron.2010.10.027

Gilliam, J. C., Chang, J. T., Sandoval, I. M., Zhang, Y., Li, T., Pittler, S. J., et al. (2012). Three-Dimensional architecture of the rod sensory cilium and its disruption in retinal neurodegeneration. *Cell* 151, 1029–1041. doi: 10.1016/j.cell.2012.10.038

Glausier, J. R., and Lewis, D. A. (2013). Dendritic spine pathology in schizophrenia. *Neuroscience* 251, 90–107. doi: 10.1016/j.neuroscience.2012.04.044

Goldman-Rakic, P. S. (1996). The prefrontal landscape: implications of functional architecture for understanding human mentation and the central executive.

Philos. Trans. R. Soc. Lond. B Biol. Sci. 351, 1445–1453. doi: 10.1098/rstb.1996.0129

Gong, S., Zheng, C., Doughty, M. L., Losos, K., Didkovsky, N., Schambra, U. B., et al. (2003). A gene expression atlas of the central nervous system based on bacterial artificial chromosomes. *Nature* 425, 917–925. doi: 10.1038/nature02033

Grant, G. (2007). How the 1906 nobel prize in physiology or medicine was shared between golgi and cajal. *Brain Res. Rev.* 55, 490–498. doi: 10.1016/j.brainresrev.2006.11.004

Gray, E. G. (1959a). Axo-somatic and axo-dendritic synapses of the cerebral cortex: an electron microscope study. *J. Anat.* 93, 420–433.

Gray, E. G. (1959b). Electron microscopy of synaptic contacts on dendrite spines of the cerebral cortex. *Nature* 183, 1592–1593. doi: 10.1038/1831592a0

Harapin, J., Eibauer, M., and Medalia, O. (2013). Structural analysis of supramolecular assemblies by cryo-electron tomography. *Structure* 21, 1522–1530. doi: 10.1016/j.str.2013.08.003

Harlow, M. L., Szule, J. A., Xu, J., Jung, J. H., Marshall, R. M., and McMahan, U. J. (2013). Alignment of synaptic vesicle macromolecules with the macromolecules in active zone material that direct vesicle docking. *PloS One* 8:e69410. doi: 10.1371/journal.pone.0069410

Harris, K. M., Perry, E., Bourne, J., Feinberg, M., Ostroff, L., and Hurlburt, J. (2006). Uniform serial sectioning for transmission electron microscopy. *J. Neurosci.* 26, 12101–12103. doi: 10.1523/jneurosci.3994-06.2006

Harris, K. M., and Stevens, J. K. (1988). Dendritic spines of rat cerebellar Purkinje cells: serial electron microscopy with reference to their biophysical characteristics. *J. Neurosci.* 8, 4455–4469.

He, C. X., and Portera-Cailliau, C. (2013). The trouble with spines in fragile X syndrome: density, maturity and plasticity. *Neuroscience* 251, 120–128. doi: 10.1016/j.neuroscience.2012.03.049

He, T., Xue, Z., Kim, Y., and Wong, S. T. (2012). "Three-dimensional dendritic spine detection based on minimal cross-sectional curvature," in *2012 9th IEEE International Symposium on Biomedical Imaging (ISBI). Presented at the 2012 9th IEEE International Symposium on Biomedical Imaging (ISBI)*, 1639–1642. doi: 10.1109/ISBI.2012.6235891

Hines, M. L., and Carnevale, N. T. (2001). NEURON: a tool for neuroscientists. *Neuroscientist* 7, 123–135. doi: 10.1177/107385840100700207

Holthoff, K., Tsay, D., and Yuste, R. (2002). Calcium dynamics of spines depend on their dendritic location. *Neuron* 33, 425–437. doi: 10.1016/s0896-6273(02)00576-7

Hu, S., and Wang, L. V. (2010). Photoacoustic imaging and characterization of the microvasculature. *J. Biomed. Opt.* 15:011101. doi: 10.1117/1.3281673

Itoh, K., Nakamura, K., Iijima, M., and Sesaki, H. (2013). Mitochondrial dynamics in neurodegeneration. *Trends Cell Biol.* 23, 64–71. doi: 10.1016/j.tcb.2012.10.006

Jacobs, B., Driscoll, L., and Schall, M. (1997). Life-span dendritic and spine changes in areas 10 and 18 of human cortex: a quantitative Golgi study. *J. Comp. Neurol.* 386, 661–680. doi: 10.1002/(sici)1096-9861(19971006)386:4<661::aid-cne11>3.0.co;2-n

Jacobs, B., Schall, M., Prather, M., Kapler, E., Driscoll, L., Baca, S., et al. (2001). Regional dendritic and spine variation in human cerebral cortex: a quantitative golgi study. *Cereb. Cortex* 11, 558–571. doi: 10.1093/cercor/11.6.558

Johnson, K. A., Fox, N. C., Sperling, R. A., and Klunk, W. E. (2012). Brain imaging in Alzheimer disease. *Cold Spring Harb. Perspect. Med.* 2:a006213. doi: 10.1101/cshperspect.a006213

Jones, E. G. (1968). An electron microscopic study of the terminations of afferent fiber systems onto the somatic sensory cortex of the cat. *J. Anat.* 103, 595–597.

Jung, C. K. E., and Herms, J. (2014). Structural dynamics of dendritic spines are influenced by an environmental enrichment: an in vivo imaging study. *Cereb. Cortex* 24, 377–384. doi: 10.1093/cercor/bhs317

Kasai, H., Fukuda, M., Watanabe, S., Hayashi-Takagi, A., and Noguchi, J. (2010). Structural dynamics of dendritic spines in memory and cognition. *Trends Neurosci.* 33, 121–129. doi: 10.1016/j.tins.2010.01.001

Knott, G., and Holtmaat, A. (2008). Dendritic spine plasticity—Current understanding from in vivo studies. *Brain Res. Rev.* 58, 282–289. doi: 10.1016/j.brainresrev.2008.01.002

Knott, G. W., Holtmaat, A., Wilbrecht, L., Welker, E., and Svoboda, K. (2006). Spine growth precedes synapse formation in the adult neocortex in vivo. *Nat. Neurosci.* 9, 1117–1124. doi: 10.1038/nn1747

Koh, I. Y. Y., Lindquist, W. B., Zito, K., Nimchinsky, E. A., and Svoboda, K. (2002). An image analysis algorithm for dendritic spines. *Neural Comput.* 14, 1283–1310. doi: 10.1162/089976602753712945

Kuwajima, M., Spacek, J., and Harris, K. M. (2013). Beyond counts and shapes: studying pathology of dendritic spines in the context of the surrounding neuropil through serial section electron microscopy. *Neuroscience* 251, 75–89. doi: 10.1016/j.neuroscience.2012.04.061

Lee, H.-J., Bae, E.-J., and Lee, S.-J. (2014). Extracellular α–synuclein-a novel and crucial factor in Lewy body diseases. *Nat. Rev. Neurol.* 10, 92–98. doi: 10.1038/nrneurol.2013.275

Lee, K. F. H., Soares, C., and Beique, J.-C. (2012). Examining form and function of dendritic spines. *Neural Plast.* 2012:704103. doi: 10.1155/2012/704103

Lenzi, D., Runyeon, J. W., Crum, J., Ellisman, M. H., and Roberts, W. M. (1999). Synaptic vesicle populations in saccular hair cells reconstructed by electron tomography. *J. Neurosci.* 19, 119–132.

Licznerski, P., and Duman, R. S. (2013). Remodeling of axo-spinous synapses in the pathophysiology and treatment of depression. *Neuroscience* 251, 33–50. doi: 10.1016/j.neuroscience.2012.09.057

Loew, L. M., and Hell, S. W. (2013). Superresolving dendritic spines. *Biophys. J.* 104, 741–743. doi: 10.1016/j.bpj.2013.01.011

Lučič, V., Rigort, A., and Baumeister, W. (2013). Cryo-electron tomography: the challenge of doing structural biology in situ. *J. Cell Biol.* 202, 407–419. doi: 10.1083/jcb.201304193

Lucić, V., Yang, T., Schweikert, G., Förster, F., and Baumeister, W. (2005). Morphological characterization of molecular complexes present in the synaptic cleft. *Structure* 13, 423–434. doi: 10.1016/j.str.2005.02.005

Maletic-Savatic, M., Malinow, R., and Svoboda, K. (1999). Rapid dendritic morphogenesis in CA1 hippocampal dendrites induced by synaptic activity. *Science* 283, 1923–1927. doi: 10.1126/science.283.5409.1923

Mancuso, J. J., Chen, Y., Li, X., Xue, Z., and Wong, S. T. C. (2013). Methods of dendritic spine detection: from Golgi to high-resolution optical imaging. *Neuroscience* 251, 129–140. doi: 10.1016/j.neuroscience.2012.04.010

Maresca, A., la Morgia, C., Caporali, L., Valentino, M. L., and Carelli, V. (2013). The optic nerve: a "mito-window" on mitochondrial neurodegeneration. *Mol. Cell. Neurosci.* 55, 62–76. doi: 10.1016/j.mcn.2012.08.004

Matsuzaki, M., Honkura, N., Ellis-Davies, G. C. R., and Kasai, H. (2004). Structural basis of long-term potentiation in single dendritic spines. *Nature* 429, 761–766. doi: 10.1038/nature02617

Milne, J. L. S., Borgnia, M. J., Bartesaghi, A., Tran, E. E. H., Earl, L. A., Schauder, D. M., et al. (2013). Cryo-electron microscopy–a primer for the non-microscopist. *FEBS J.* 280, 28–45. doi: 10.1111/febs.12078

Monici, M. (2005). Cell and tissue autofluorescence research and diagnostic applications. *Biotechnol. Annu. Rev.* 11, 227–256. doi: 10.1016/s1387-2656(05)11007-2

Moolman, D. L., Vitolo, O. V., Vonsattel, J.-P. G., and Shelanski, M. L. (2004). Dendrite and dendritic spine alterations in Alzheimer models. *J. Neurocytol.* 33, 377–387. doi: 10.1023/b:neur.0000044197.83514.64

Mueller, S. G., Weiner, M. W., Thal, L. J., Petersen, R. C., Jack, C., Jagust, W., et al. (2005). The Alzheimer's disease neuroimaging initiative. *Neuroimaging Clin. N. Am.* 15, 869–877. doi: 10.1007/springerreference_34009

Nickell, S., Park, P. S.-H., Baumeister, W., and Palczewski, K. (2007). Three-dimensional architecture of murine rod outer segments determined by cryoelectron tomography. *J. Cell Biol.* 177, 917–925. doi: 10.1083/jcb.200612010

Nicoll, A. J., Panico, S., Freir, D. B., Wright, D., Terry, C., Risse, E., et al. (2013). Amyloid-β nanotubes are associated with prion protein-dependent synaptotoxicity. *Nat. Commun.* 4:2416. doi: 10.1038/ncomms3416

Nimchinsky, E. A., Yasuda, R., Oertner, T. G., and Svoboda, K. (2004). The number of glutamate receptors opened by synaptic stimulation in single hippocampal spines. *J. Neurosci.* 24, 2054–2064. doi: 10.1523/jneurosci.5066-03.2004

Orlowski, D., and Bjarkam, C. R. (2012). A simple reproducible and time saving method of semi-automatic dendrite spine density estimation compared to manual spine counting. *J. Neurosci. Methods* 208, 128–133. doi: 10.1016/j.jneumeth.2012.05.009

Pannese, E. (1999). The golgi stain: invention, diffusion and impact on neurosciences. *J. Hist. Neurosci.* 8, 132–140. doi: 10.1076/jhin.8.2.132.1847

Perkins, G. A., Scott, R., Perez, A., Ellisman, M. H., Johnson, J. E., and Fox, D. A. (2012). Bcl-xL-mediated remodeling of rod and cone synaptic mitochondria after postnatal lead exposure: electron microscopy, tomography and oxygen consumption. *Mol. Vis.* 18, 3029–3048.

Perkins, G. A., Tjong, J., Brown, J. M., Poquiz, P. H., Scott, R. T., Kolson, D. R., et al. (2010). The micro-architecture of mitochondria at active zones: electron tomography reveals novel anchoring scaffolds and cristae structured for high-rate metabolism. *J. Neurosci.* 30, 1015–1026. doi: 10.1523/jneurosci.1517-09.2010

Petralia, R. S., Wang, Y. X., and Wenthold, R. J. (1994a). Histological and ultrastructural localization of the kainate receptor subunits, KA2 and GluR6/7, in the rat nervous system using selective antipeptide antibodies. *J. Comp. Neurol.* 349, 85–110. doi: 10.1002/cne.903490107

Petralia, R. S., Wang, Y. X., and Wenthold, R. J. (1994b). The NMDA receptor subunits NR2A and NR2B show histological and ultrastructural localization patterns similar to those of NR (1). *J. Neurosci.* 14, 6102–6120.

Petralia, R. S., Yokotani, N., and Wenthold, R. J. (1994c). Light and electron microscope distribution of the NMDA receptor subunit NMDAR1 in the rat nervous system using a selective anti-peptide antibody. *J. Neurosci.* 14, 667–696.

Petzold, G. C., and Murthy, V. N. (2011). Role of astrocytes in neurovascular coupling. *Neuron* 71, 782–797. doi: 10.1016/j.neuron.2011.08.009

Piston, D. W., Masters, B. R., and Webb, W. W. (1995). Three-dimensionally resolved NAD(P)H cellular metabolic redox imaging of the in situ cornea with two-photon excitation laser scanning microscopy. *J. Microsc.* 178, 20–27. doi: 10.1111/j.1365-2818.1995.tb03576.x

Pozueta, J., Lefort, R., and Shelanski, M. L. (2013). Synaptic changes in Alzheimer's disease and its models. *Neuroscience* 251, 51–65. doi: 10.1016/j.neuroscience.2012.05.050

Rodriguez, A., Ehlenberger, D. B., Dickstein, D. L., Hof, P. R., and Wearne, S. L. (2008). Automated three-dimensional detection and shape classification of dendritic spines from fluorescence microscopy images. *PLoS One* 3:e1997. doi: 10.1371/journal.pone.0001997

Rodriguez, A., Ehlenberger, D. B., Hof, P. R., and Wearne, S. L. (2006). Rayburst sampling, an algorithm for automated three-dimensional shape analysis from laser scanning microscopy images. *Nat. Protoc.* 1, 2152–2161. doi: 10.1038/nprot.2006.313

Sasaki, T., Aoi, H., Oga, T., Fujita, I., and Ichinohe, N. (2014). Postnatal development of dendritic structure of layer III pyramidal neurons in the medial prefrontal cortex of marmoset. *Brain Struct. Funct.* doi: 10.1007/s00429-014-0853-2. [Epub ahead of print].

Schuff, N., Woerner, N., Boreta, L., Kornfield, T., Shaw, L. M., Trojanowski, J. Q., et al. (2009). MRI of hippocampal volume loss in early Alzheimer's disease in relation to ApoE genotype and biomarkers. *Brain* 132, 1067–1077. doi: 10.1093/brain/awp007

Scott, B. B., Brody, C. D., and Tank, D. W. (2013). Cellular resolution functional imaging in behaving rats using voluntary head restraint. *Neuron* 80, 371–384. doi: 10.1016/j.neuron.2013.08.002

Shahmoradian, S. H., Galaz-Montoya, J. G., Schmid, M. F., Cong, Y., Ma, B., Spiess, C., et al. (2013). TRiC's tricks inhibit huntingtin aggregation. *Elife* 2:e00710. doi: 10.7554/eLife.00710

Shahmoradian, S. H., Galiano, M. R., Wu, C., Chen, S., Rasband, M. N., Mobley, W. C., et al. (2014). Preparation of primary neurons for visualizing neurites in a frozen-hydrated state using cryo-electron tomography. *J. Vis. Exp.* 84:e50783. doi: 10.3791/50783

Sheng, M., and Hoogenraad, C. C. (2007). The postsynaptic architecture of excitatory synapses: a more quantitative view. *Annu. Rev. Biochem.* 76, 823–847. doi: 10.1146/annurev.biochem.76.060805.160029

Shepherd, G. M. (1996). The dendritic spine: a multifunctional integrative unit. *J. Neurophysiol.* 75, 2197–2210.

Smith, D. L., Pozueta, J., Gong, B., Arancio, O., and Shelanski, M. (2009). Reversal of long-term dendritic spine alterations in Alzheimer disease models. *Proc. Natl. Acad. Sci. U S A* 106, 16877–16882. doi: 10.1073/pnas.0908706106

Smith, Y., and Villalba, R. M. (2013). Dendrite spines plasticity in brain disorders. *Neuroscience* 251, 1. doi: 10.1016/j.neuroscience.2013.08.045

Smrt, R. D., Eaves-Egenes, J., Barkho, B. Z., Santistevan, N. J., Zhao, C., Aimone, J. B., et al. (2007). Mecp2 deficiency leads to delayed maturation and altered gene expression in hippocampal neurons. *Neurobiol. Dis.* 27, 77–89. doi: 10.1016/j.nbd.2007.04.005

Stephens, B., Mueller, A. J., Shering, A. F., Hood, S. H., Taggart, P., Arbuthnott, G. W., et al. (2005). Evidence of a breakdown of corticostriatal connections in Parkinson's disease. *Neuroscience* 132, 741–754. doi: 10.1016/j.neuroscience.2005.01.007

Sternberg, S. R. (1983). Biomedical image processing. *Computer* 16, 22–34.

Swanger, S. A., Yao, X., Gross, C., and Bassell, G. J. (2011). Automated 4D analysis of dendritic spine morphology: applications to stimulus-induced spine remodeling and pharmacological rescue in a disease model. *Mol. Brain* 4:38. doi: 10.1186/1756-6606-4-38

Swulius, M. T., Farley, M. M., Bryant, M. A., and Waxham, M. N. (2012). Electron cryotomography of postsynaptic densities during development reveals a mechanism of assembly. *Neuroscience* 212, 19–29. doi: 10.1016/j.neuroscience.2012.03.042

Takasaki, K. T., Ding, J. B., and Sabatini, B. L. (2013). Live-cell superresolution imaging by pulsed STED two-photon excitation microscopy. *Biophys. J.* 104, 770–777. doi: 10.1016/j.bpj.2012.12.053

Theer, P., Hasan, M. T., and Denk, W. (2003). Two-photon imaging to a depth of 1000 microm in living brains by use of a Ti:Al2O3 regenerative amplifier. *Opt. Lett.* 28, 1022–1024. doi: 10.1364/ol.28.001022

Thompson, P. M., Hayashi, K. M., Dutton, R. A., Chiang, M.-C., Leow, A. D., Sowell, E. R., et al. (2007). Tracking Alzheimer's disease. *Ann. N Y Acad. Sci.* 1097, 183–214. doi: 10.1196/annals.1379.017

Van Beek, A. H. E. A., and Claassen, J. A. H. R. (2011). The cerebrovascular role of the cholinergic neural system in Alzheimer's disease. *Behav. Brain Res.* 221, 537–542. doi: 10.1016/j.bbr.2009.12.047

Vanzi, F., Sacconi, L., Cicchi, R., and Pavone, F. S. (2012). Protein conformation and molecular order probed by second-harmonic-generation microscopy. *J. Biomed. Opt.* 17:060901. doi: 10.1117/1.jbo.17.6 060901

Villalba, R. M., and Smith, Y. (2013). Differential striatal spine pathology in Parkinson's disease and cocaine addiction: a key role of dopamine? *Neuroscience* 251, 2–20. doi: 10.1016/j.neuroscience.2013.07.011

Wang, Z., Chen, L. M., Negyessy, L., Friedman, R. M., Mishra, A., Gore, J. C., et al. (2013). The relationship of anatomical and functional connectivity to resting state connectivity in primate somatosensory cortex. *Neuron* 78, 1116–1126. doi: 10.1016/j.neuron.2013.04.023

Wilhelm, B. G., Mandad, S., Truckenbrodt, S., Kröhnert, K., Schäfer, C., Rammner, B., et al. (2014). Composition of isolated synaptic boutons reveals the amounts of vesicle trafficking proteins. *Science* 344, 1023–1028. doi: 10.1126/science.1252884

Wilkinson, M. H. F., and Schut, F. (1998). *Digital Image Analysis of Microbes: Imaging, Morphometry, Fluorometry and Motility Techniques and Applications.* Chichester, UK: John Wiley and Sons.

Williams, R. W., and Herrup, K. (1988). The control of neuron number. *Annu. Rev. Neurosci.* 11, 423–453. doi: 10.1146/annurev.neuro.11.1.423

Williams, R. M., Piston, D. W., and Webb, W. W. (1994). Two-photon molecular excitation provides intrinsic 3-dimensional resolution for laser-based microscopy and microphotochemistry. *FASEB J.* 8, 804–813.

Wong, M., and Guo, D. (2013). Dendritic spine pathology in epilepsy: cause or consequence? *Neuroscience* 251, 141–150. doi: 10.1016/j.neuroscience.2012.03.048

Xu, X., Cheng, J., Thrall, M. J., Liu, Z., Wang, X., and Wong, S. T. C. (2013). Multimodal non-linear optical imaging for label-free differentiation of lung cancerous lesions from normal and desmoplastic tissues. *Biomed. Opt. Express* 4, 2855–2868. doi: 10.1364/boe.4.002855

Yang, Y., Wang, X., Frerking, M., and Zhou, Q. (2008). Spine expansion and stabilization associated with long-term potentiation. *J. Neurosci.* 28, 5740–5751. doi: 10.1523/jneurosci.3998-07.2008

Yin, Z., Sadok, A., Sailem, H., McCarthy, A., Xia, X., Li, F., et al. (2013). A screen for morphological complexity identifies regulators of switch-like transitions between discrete cell shapes. *Nat. Cell Biol.* 15, 860–871. doi: 10.1038/ncb2764

Yin, Z., Sailem, H., Sero, J., Ardy, R., Wong, S. T. C., and Bakal, C. (2014). How cells explore shape space: a quantitative statistical perspective of cellular morphogenesis. *Bioessays* doi: 10.1002/bies.201400011. [Epub ahead of print].

Yuste, R., and Bonhoeffer, T. (2001). Morphological changes in dendritic spines associated with long-term synaptic plasticity. *Annu. Rev. Neurosci.* 24, 1071–1089. doi: 10.1146/annurev.neuro.24.1.1071

Yuste, R., Majewska, A., Cash, S. S., and Denk, W. (1999). Mechanisms of calcium influx into hippocampal spines: heterogeneity among spines, coincidence detection by NMDA receptors and optical quantal analysis. *J. Neurosci.* 19, 1976–1987.

Yuste, R., Majewska, A., and Holthoff, K. (2000). From form to function: calcium compartmentalization in dendritic spines. *Nat. Neurosci.* 3, 653–659. doi: 10.1038/76609

Zhang, Y., Chen, K., Baron, M., Teylan, M. A., Kim, Y., Song, Z., et al. (2010). A neurocomputational method for fully automated 3D dendritic spine detection and segmentation of medium-sized spiny neurons. *NeuroImage* 50, 1472–1484. doi: 10.1016/j.neuroimage.2010.01.048

Zhang, Y., Zhou, X., Witt, R. M., Sabatini, B. L., Adjeroh, D., and Wong, S. T. C. (2007). Dendritic spine detection using curvilinear structure detector and LDA classifier. *NeuroImage* 36, 346–360. doi: 10.1016/j.neuroimage.2007.02.044

Zhou, Q., Homma, K. J., and Poo, M. (2004). Shrinkage of dendritic spines associated with long-term depression of hippocampal synapses. *Neuron* 44, 749–757. doi: 10.1016/j.neuron.2004.11.011

12

Extracellular matrix control of dendritic spine and synapse structure and plasticity in adulthood

Aaron D. Levy[1,2†], Mitchell H. Omar[1,2†] and Anthony J. Koleske[1,2,3*]

[1] Interdepartmental Neuroscience Program, Yale University, New Haven, CT, USA
[2] Department of Molecular Biophysics and Biochemistry, Yale University, New Haven, CT, USA
[3] Department of Neurobiology, Yale University, New Haven, CT, USA

Correspondence:
Anthony J. Koleske, Department of Molecular Biophysics and Biochemistry, Yale University, 333 Cedar Street, Sterling Hall of Medicine CE-33, New Haven, CT 06420-8024, USA
e-mail: anthony.koleske@yale.edu

Dendritic spines are the receptive contacts at most excitatory synapses in the central nervous system. Spines are dynamic in the developing brain, changing shape as they mature as well as appearing and disappearing as they make and break connections. Spines become much more stable in adulthood, and spine structure must be actively maintained to support established circuit function. At the same time, adult spines must retain some plasticity so their structure can be modified by activity and experience. As such, the regulation of spine stability and remodeling in the adult animal is critical for normal function, and disruption of these processes is associated with a variety of late onset diseases including schizophrenia and Alzheimer's disease. The extracellular matrix (ECM), composed of a meshwork of proteins and proteoglycans, is a critical regulator of spine and synapse stability and plasticity. While the role of ECM receptors in spine regulation has been extensively studied, considerably less research has focused directly on the role of specific ECM ligands. Here, we review the evidence for a role of several brain ECM ligands and remodeling proteases in the regulation of dendritic spine and synapse formation, plasticity, and stability in adults.

Keywords: extracellular matrix, dendritic spine, chondroitin sulfate proteoglycans, agrin, reelin, extracellular proteases, RGD peptide, integrins

DENDRITIC SPINES ARE HIGHLY STRUCTURED POSTSYNAPTIC SIGNALING COMPARTMENTS

Dendritic spines are protrusions from the dendrite shaft of neurons that comprise the receptive contact at most excitatory synapses in the brain (Gray, 1959a,b; Harris and Kater, 1994; Hering and Sheng, 2001). Ultrastructurally, dendritic spines are composed of a thin neck supported by unbranched filamentous actin (F-actin) and a bulbous head containing a network of branched F-actin (Korobova and Svitkina, 2010; Tønnesen et al., 2014). The spine head also contains the membrane-associated postsynaptic density (PSD), a highly organized network of neurotransmitter receptors, adhesion receptors, scaffolding proteins, and downstream signaling molecules (Harris and Stevens, 1989; Kennedy, 1994, 1997; Hunt et al., 1996; Walikonis et al., 2000; Sheng and Kim, 2011; Harris and Weinberg, 2012). Scaffolding proteins and cell adhesion molecules (CAMs) connect the PSD to the spine actin cytoskeleton. Adhesion molecules also connect to both the presynaptic partner and the extracellular matrix (ECM) in and around the synaptic cleft (**Figure 1A**). These and other dendritic spine proteins regulate actin filament formation, turnover, and stability, thereby controlling dendritic spine structure.

Spines have a unique structure that is intrinsic to their function. The thin spine neck, ~100–300 nm in diameter (Harris and Stevens, 1989; Tønnesen et al., 2014), restricts diffusion to compartmentalize biochemical and electrical postsynaptic signaling (Majewska et al., 2000; Yuste et al., 2000; Sabatini et al., 2002; Noguchi et al., 2005; Carter and Sabatini, 2008; Harvey et al., 2008; Higley and Sabatini, 2012; Takasaki and Sabatini, 2014; Tønnesen et al., 2014). This compartmentalization enables molecular modifications specific to individual spines and synapses, including changes in synaptic efficacy and spine shape and size. Overall spine head size varies considerably among spines, from ~200–1400 nm in diameter (Harris and Stevens, 1989; Tønnesen et al., 2014). Spine size correlates with synaptic strength and larger spines commonly contain larger PSDs with more AMPA-type glutamate receptors and appose axon terminals with larger readily-releasable pools of neurotransmitter (Harris and Stevens, 1988, 1989; Matsuzaki et al., 2001). Therefore, large spines are more likely to produce strong excitatory postsynaptic currents and have greater influence on neuronal firing and network signaling.

DENDRITIC SPINE STRUCTURE IS DYNAMIC AND REGULATED BY ACTIVITY AND DEVELOPMENT

Recent advances in imaging and single synapse stimulation techniques have revealed that the size and transmission properties of individual dendritic spines can be altered rapidly in response to synaptic activity. Use of glutamate uncaging at individual spines has shown that long-term activity-dependent synaptic strengthening or weakening, also known as long-term potentiation (LTP) and long-term depression (LTD), respectively, occur at

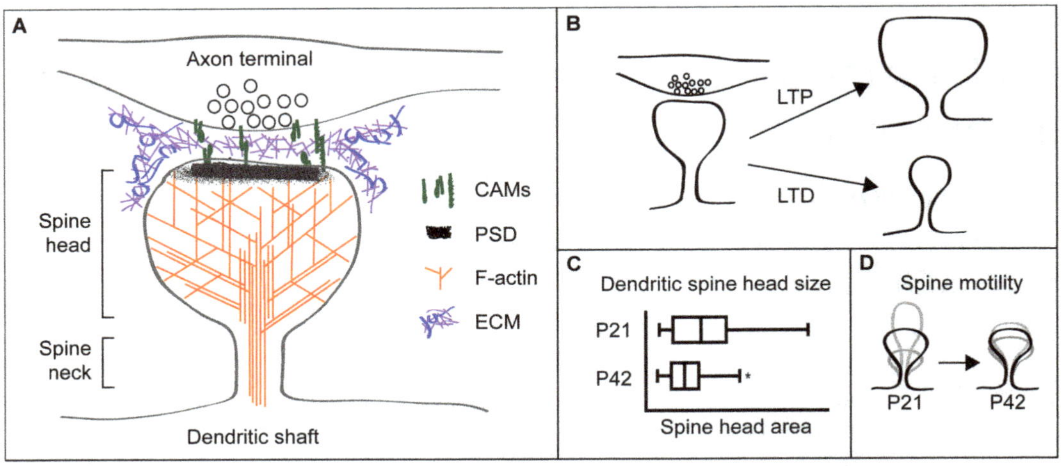

FIGURE 1 | Dendritic spines are highly structured and plastic synaptic specializations. (A) Schematic of a dendritic spine apposed to a presynaptic terminal. The spine head and neck are supported by a network of filamentous (F)-actin. Postsynaptic cell adhesion molecules (CAMs) connect to the postsynaptic density (PSD) and F-actin in the spine, and extend from the spine to associate with CAMs on the presynaptic terminal. Perisynapic and putative synaptic cleft extracellular matrix (ECM) may interact with multiple CAMs and other cell surface receptors. **(B)** Spine structural changes accompany synaptic plasticity, with long-term potentiation (LTP) increasing spine head size and long-term depression (LTD) decreasing head size. **(C)** Mouse hippocampal CA1 neuron spine head sizes were obtained from electron microscopy of the stratum radiatum. Spine head size and its variance decrease as animals mature from P21 (juvenile) to P42 (adult). Figure modified with permission from Kerrisk et al. (2013). **(D)** Spine motility, defined as changes in spine length over time, is high in juvenile animals. By contrast, spines from adult animals are relatively immotile.

discrete synapses and are associated with changes in spine size. High frequency synaptic stimulation that causes LTP promotes spine head enlargement, while low frequency stimulation that causes LTD results in spine head shrinkage (Matsuzaki et al., 2004; Nägerl et al., 2004; Zhou et al., 2004; Oh et al., 2013; **Figure 1B**). Furthermore, smaller spines are more likely to be lost following LTD-inducing stimulation paradigms (Bastrikova et al., 2008).

Experiments using longitudinal transcranial imaging of individual cortical spines support these *ex vivo* studies. Manipulating sensory input alters the likelihood that dendritic spines will or will not be lost (spine stability) over days, weeks, and months (Oray et al., 2004; Zuo et al., 2005a,b; Lai et al., 2012). Additionally, *in vivo* imaging experiments in mouse models show that stress and genetic abnormalities disrupt normal spine structural dynamics and stability (Pan et al., 2010; Liston et al., 2013). Excitingly, studies using imaging probes that report the activity of specific signaling pathways are beginning to elucidate the signaling events that underlie long-term changes in spine size and signaling properties (Murakoshi et al., 2011; Murakoshi and Yasuda, 2012; Lai and Ip, 2013; Oh et al., 2013; Zhai et al., 2013).

Spine structural plasticity is also heavily influenced by developmental stage. Juvenile animals have increased variance in spine head size (Sfakianos et al., 2007; Kerrisk et al., 2013; **Figure 1C**) and much more dynamic spine motility relative to spines in adult animals (Dunaevsky et al., 1999; Trachtenberg et al., 2002; Majewska and Sur, 2003; Holtmaat et al., 2005; **Figure 1D**). Furthermore, higher levels of spine formation and loss occur in adolescent mice vs. adults (Grutzendler et al., 2002).

While the age-dependent loss of spine plasticity has been reproducibly observed, the mechanisms that underlie this phenomenon are not well understood. Multiple synaptic proteins and signaling events differ between juvenile and adult animals as well as between wild type and disease-model animals, which might help to explain differences in spine stability (Scheetz and Constantine-Paton, 1994; Wu et al., 2009; Gundelfinger et al., 2010; Charrier et al., 2012; Akbik et al., 2013; Koleske, 2013). These observations do not, however, directly address whether or how specific pairing of pre- and post-synaptic compartments induces the machinery and mechanisms that confer increased synapse and dendritic spine stability. While it is a difficult experimental question to address, insights into this question are crucial to understanding neurological disorders and how we can gain control of synaptic flexibility.

BRAIN DISORDERS INVOLVE LOSS OF DENDRITIC SPINE STABILITY

Loss of dendritic spine stability in adulthood underlies several major neurological and psychiatric disorders, which are accompanied by perceptual, cognitive, memory, and behavioral deficits. For instance, cortical neurons in patients with Alzheimer's disease, Parkinson's disease, and other neurodegenerative disorders or dementia have decreased synapse and spine densities (Catalá et al., 1988; Katzman, 1989; Terry et al., 1991; Scheff and Price, 2003). Schizophrenia patients also have reduced cortical spine densities (Garey et al., 1998; Glantz and Lewis, 2000), and medium spiny neurons in Huntington's disease patients show spine densities that are increased earlier and reduced later in disease progression (Ferrante et al., 1991). Whether spine loss causes disease or results from other problems is unknown, but disrupted network connectivity via spine loss may underlie the cognitive deficits that occur in these patients. These observations demonstrate the importance of dendritic spine stability for normal brain function and suggest that a deeper comprehension of spine stabilization mechanisms could lead to a better understanding of these diseases and possibly new therapeutic approaches.

EXTRACELLULAR MATRIX RECEPTORS CONTROL DENDRITIC SPINE STABILITY AND REMODELING

Several studies demonstrate that specific ECM receptors can regulate dendritic spine stability and remodeling. Brain ECM is composed of secreted proteins and proteoglycans that assemble into cross-linked meshworks to provide structural support to the surrounding cells (Barros et al., 2011; Dansie and Ethell, 2011; Wlodarczyk et al., 2011; Soleman et al., 2013). The brain ECM forms a gel that surrounds neurons and glia, including the space adjacent to and between synapses (Nicholson and Syková, 1998). There, pre- and postsynaptic CAMs associate with one another and with the ECM to initiate and maintain synaptic contact (Bukalo and Dityatev, 2012; Missler et al., 2012). These transmembrane cell adhesion proteins connect to the intracellular dendritic spine actin network and influence the activities of actin regulatory molecules, thereby controlling spine shape (Huntley et al., 2002; Washbourne et al., 2004; Lin and Koleske, 2010; Benson and Huntley, 2012; Cheadle and Biederer, 2012; Sloniowski and Ethell, 2012; Koleske, 2013). Many adhesion molecules also influence synaptic transmission, a key regulator of spine structure (Chan et al., 2006, 2007; Huang et al., 2006; Shi and Ethell, 2006; Bukalo and Dityatev, 2012).

Integrin adhesion receptors are a major family of ECM receptors. Engagement of ECM by integrins triggers changes in cell morphology and motility powered by actin cytoskeletal rearrangements in diverse cell types (Horwitz et al., 1986; Tamkun et al., 1986; Otey and Burridge, 1990; Tawil et al., 1993; Wang et al., 1993; Chong et al., 1994; Gumbiner, 1996; Schwartz and Horwitz, 2006; Schwartz, 2010). Integrins are crucial in the brain as well, where they mediate processes such as migration, axonal outgrowth and pathfinding, and synaptic plasticity (DeFreitas et al., 1995; Chan et al., 2006, 2007; Shi and Ethell, 2006; Belvindrah et al., 2007a,b). Integrin signaling also modulates spine head size and stability during adolescence in mice (Warren et al., 2012; Kerrisk et al., 2013).

Other ECM receptors also function in the brain during adulthood, where they may stabilize spines. For example, dystroglycan, part of the dystrophin glycoprotein complex, plays important roles in axonal pathfinding (Wright et al., 2012) and synapse formation (Sato et al., 2008), but also associates with mature inhibitory synapses and modulates synaptic plasticity (Lévi et al., 2002; Satz et al., 2010; Pribiag et al., 2014). ApoER2, a receptor for the ECM protein reelin, is expressed from late embryonic periods through adulthood, where it is essential for proper migration of cortical neurons in development (Hack et al., 2007) but also plays roles in synapse maintenance and plasticity (Beffert et al., 2005, 2006; Trotter et al., 2011). These and other ECM receptor studies provide strong evidence that ECM regulates dendritic spine stability and remodeling.

STUDYING ECM-MEDIATED CONTROL OF SPINE STRUCTURE POSES UNIQUE DIFFICULTIES

Extracellular matrix molecules at synapses are likely candidates for regulators of synapse and dendritic spine stability. While studies have identified ECM receptors important for neuronal function and dendritic spine morphology, they often fail to identify the critical ECM ligands that drive these important processes. This failure may be partially due to the inherent difficulty of studying ECM components. Extracellular matrix molecules are secreted, so in the brain where many different cell types are intermingled, cell origin and site of function can be difficult to identify. The heterogenous cell population in the brain also complicates purification of ECM molecules from specific cell types. Additionally, many ECM molecules are large, such as laminins (800 kDa), and can have multiple interaction domains from the same molecule driving distinct pathways (Colognato and Yurchenco, 2000). Extracellular matrix biochemical activities are also altered by covalent modification and/or proteolytic processing, which can be triggered by synaptic activity (Nedivi et al., 1993; Qian et al., 1993; Sung et al., 1993; Szklarczyk et al., 2002; Chen et al., 2008; Horejs et al., 2014). Furthermore, it can be difficult to disentangle possible functions of ECM components in spine stabilization, e.g., providing extracellular rigidity, mediating spine-ECM adhesions, and/or inducing intracellular signaling cascades (**Figure 2**).

Regardless of the challenges posed by studying the roles of ECM in dendritic spine and synapse stability, emerging evidence indicates that specific ECM components are key regulators of dendritic spine and synapse structure, plasticity, and stability. Here, we review the evidence that specific ECM components and their interaction partners control dendritic spine and synapse structure and how remodeling of the ECM may contribute to dendritic spine plasticity and stability in adults.

ECM PROTEINS ARE KEY REGULATORS OF DENDRITIC SPINE AND SYNAPSE STABILITY AND REMODELING

CHONDROITIN SULFATE PROTEOGLYCANS RESTRICT FUNCTIONAL PLASTICITY AND STABILIZE SPINES

Chondroitin sulfate proteoglycans (CSPGs), including the lecticans (aggrecan, neurocan, versican and brevican), phosphacan, and leucine-rich CSPGs, are major components of the mature brain ECM. Each CSPG consists of a multi-domain protein core, important for interactions with other ECM molecules, as well as multiple glycosaminoglycan (GAG) side chains that can be degraded by the bacterial enzyme chondroitinaseABC (chABC). The GAG chains are critical for many CSPG functions (Galtrey and Fawcett, 2007), and the pattern of sulfation can define the specific response of the CSPG to signaling partners (Gama et al., 2006). Some CSPGs, notably brevican (Yamada et al., 1994), also exist in non-proteoglycan forms, and loss of CSPG protein core genes is associated with neurological disease (Cichon et al., 2011; Mühleisen et al., 2012). Many CSPGs assemble to form dense peri-neuronal nets (PNNs) around inhibitory neurons (Kwok et al., 2011), which can be identified by staining

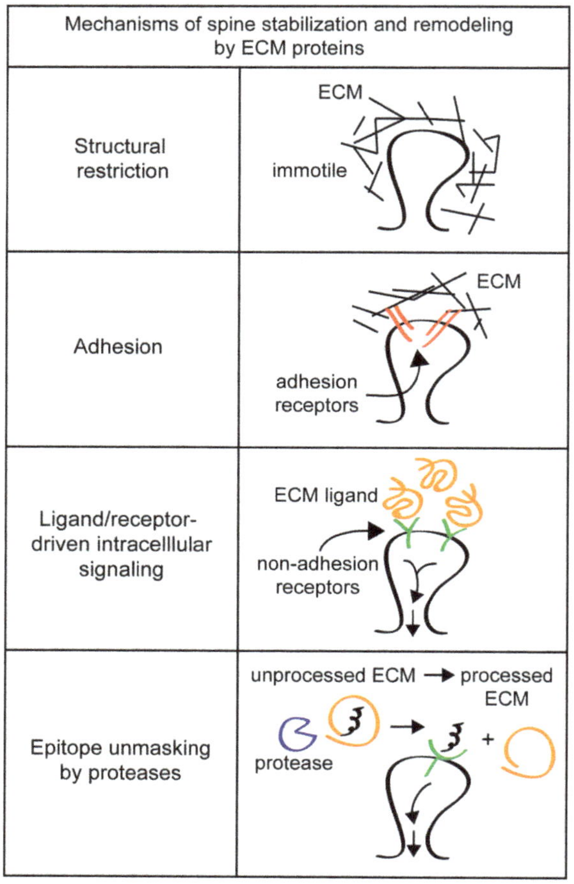

FIGURE 2 | Mechanisms of spine stabilization and remodeling by extracellular matrix (ECM) proteins. Extracellular matrix components can stabilize and remodel dendritic spines by a variety of different mechanisms. *Structural restriction*: ECM components such as chondroitin sulfate proteoglycans (CSPGs) can form a matrix around dendritic spines to provide extracellular rigidity and physically restrict spine motion. *Adhesion*: classical ECM proteins such as fibronectin and RGD-containing proteins can act as adhesion substrates and bind to integrin adhesion receptors to remodel spines. *Ligand/receptor-driven intracellular signaling*: ECM proteins like reelin function as ligands for non-adhesion receptors to drive intracellular signaling cascades that regulate spine remodeling and formation. *Epitope unmasking by proteases*: extracellular proteases such as tissue plasminogen activator (tPA) and the matrix metalloproteinase (MMPs) can cleave ECM proteins to reveal cryptic ligands that drive intracellular signaling to change spine morphology.

for GAG epitopes. In addition, a subset of excitatory neurons are also surrounded by more diffuse CSPGs (Wegner et al., 2003).

While the role of specific CSPG core proteins in dendritic spine structure and plasticity has not been extensively studied, a wealth of evidence indicates that the GAG chains of CSPGs restrict circuit plasticity *in vivo*, particularly in the visual system. In the primary visual cortex of rodents and other mammals, cells that receive geniculocortical inputs representing both eyes typically respond more strongly to stimulation of one eye, a phenomenon called ocular dominance (OD). Monocular deprivation (MD) enforced by closing one eye increases the proportion of cells that respond to stimulation of the open eye while reducing the proportion that respond to the closed eye, but only during a critical period for OD plasticity from P19-P35 (Wiesel and Hubel, 1963; Gordon and Stryker, 1996). Chondroitin sulfate proteoglycan expression in primary visual cortex increases through this critical period, and rearing mice in the dark, which delays critical period closure, also delays the developmental increase in CSPGs. This suggests that CSPG expression may be causally linked to the age-dependent loss of plasticity (Pizzorusso et al., 2002). Indeed, while MD normally cannot induce OD plasticity in adult rats after the critical period, MD can shift OD in adult rats that have had chABC injected directly into primary visual cortex (Pizzorusso et al., 2002). In a similar critical period plasticity paradigm, fear memories can be robustly erased by extinction training only during an early critical period, but chABC degradation of PNNs in the amygdala reinstates the ability to erase fear memories in adult rats (Gogolla et al., 2009). In addition, mice lacking the CSPGs neurocan or brevican have deficits in LTP maintenance without other apparent developmental defects, suggesting a role for CSPGs in adults (Zhou et al., 2001; Brakebusch et al., 2002). These results demonstrate that CSPGs are critical for the functional stability of neuronal circuits *in vivo*.

Chondroitin sulfate proteoglycans normally stabilize dendritic spines. The physiological changes induced by MD are associated with a reduction in spine density of layer II/III visual cortical neurons responsive to the deprived eye (Mataga et al., 2004; Pizzorusso et al., 2006). This loss of spines can be rescued by opening the deprived eye and closing the previously open eye, but only in juvenile animals. However, chABC treatment reinstates this plasticity in adult animals, demonstrating that CSPGs normally stabilize existing spines (Pizzorusso et al., 2006). Loss of CSPGs also enhances spine motility, measured as the magnitude of fluctuations in spine length over time (**Figure 1C**). Spine motility decreases with age (Majewska and Sur, 2003), but chABC treatment of adult visual cortex *in vivo* and of hippocampal organotypic slices *in vitro* enhances spine motility (Orlando et al., 2012; de Vivo et al., 2013), reverting spines to a more immature phenotype. This is similar to the effect of MD, which also increases spine motility (Oray et al., 2004). These results demonstrate that CSPGs stabilize dendritic spine structure and movement (**Figures 3A,B**).

Chondroitin sulfate proteoglycans interact with interneurons in PNNs and the development of inhibitory circuits is associated with closure of the critical period, suggesting the effects of chABC treatment on OD plasticity and spine stability may reflect alterations of inhibitory circuits (Pizzorusso et al., 2002). However, emerging evidence indicates that CSPGs can also act directly on spines, independently of PNNs and GABAergic neurons. Orlando et al. (2012) have shown that microinjection of chABC into the stratum radiatum of hippocampal slices, which lacks PNNs but has diffuse CSPG staining, increases CA1 pyramidal neuron spine motility and the number of spines with outgrowths from their heads, mimicking the effects of chABC bath application. This demonstrates that CSPGs normally stabilize spine structure and reduce spine head outgrowths independently of PNNs and inhibitory function (Orlando et al., 2012). These increases in

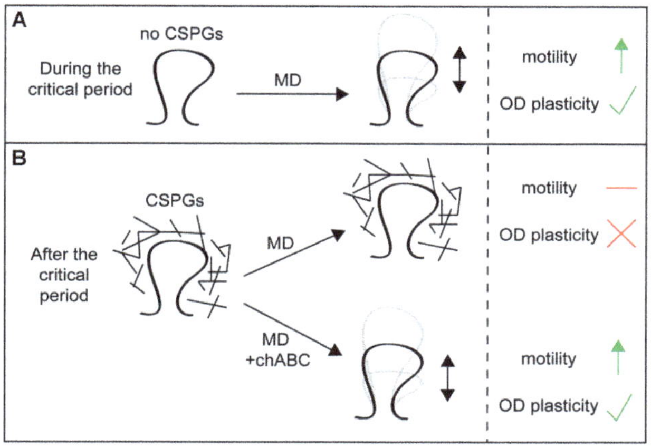

FIGURE 3 | Chondroitin sulfate proteoglycans around spines restrict spine dynamics and functional plasticity. (A) In juvenile animals during the critical period, CSPG expression is low and visual monocular deprivation (MD) can increase spine motility in primary visual cortex and drive changes in ocular dominance (OD) plasticity. **(B)** In adult animals after the critical period, CSPG expression is high and MD can no longer increase spine motility or drive OD plasticity. However, treatment with chondroitinaseABC (chABC) to degrade CSPG glycosaminoglycan (GAG) chains allows MD to once again increase spine motility and drive OD plasticity in adults, demonstrating that CSPGs restrict spine remodeling and functional plasticity in adult animals.

both motility and spine head outgrowth with chABC application require β1 integrin function, which has been shown to be involved in dendrite and spine stability (Warren et al., 2012). While CSPGs interact with and inhibit integrin function (Wu et al., 2002; Tan et al., 2011), whether these specific interactions regulate spine stability is unclear, and should be the target of future studies.

RGD PEPTIDES, AND POSSIBLY FIBRONECTIN, REGULATE DENDRITIC SPINE REMODELING

In the brain, there is little expression of most of the fibrous ECM proteins such as fibronectin, vitronectin, and the collagens that are major ECM components in other tissues (Ruoslahti, 1996a). Fibronectin mRNA and protein can be detected at low levels in discrete populations of neurons and astroglia, and its expression is increased in the hippocampus of adult animals by kainic acid treatment (Hoffman et al., 1998), but very little is known about the function of fibronectin in the brain. Instead, researchers have more commonly used synthetic peptides common to fibronectin and other matrix proteins that carry an arginine-glycine-aspartate (RGD) motif critical for binding to integrins and for adhesion (Ruoslahti and Pierschbacher, 1987; Ruoslahti, 1996b). RGD peptides have also been shown to evoke changes in synaptic plasticity and structural stability. For example, RGD peptides block the maintenance phase of LTP (Staubli et al., 1990; Bahr et al., 1997; Chun et al., 2001) and potentiate NMDA receptor (NMDAR) currents (Lin et al., 2003; Bernard-Trifilo et al., 2005), demonstrating that RGD-containing proteins may be involved in adult plasticity. RGD peptides also regulate structural stability in mature neurons, as treatment of 14 DIV cultured hippocampal neurons with RGD peptides induces an elongation of existing spines and causes filopodia formation. These changes can be blocked by NMDAR and CaMKII antagonists, suggesting that integrins regulate the stability of dendritic spines via NMDARs and CaMKII *in vitro* (Shi and Ethell, 2006). To be clear, studies using RGD peptides do not demonstrate that any specific RGD-containing ECM protein functions in the brain, as many extracellular proteins have RGD motifs, but they strongly suggest the involvement of integrin receptors in these diverse processes. In addition to traditional "outside-in" integrin activation described above, integrin adhesion can be activated by intracellular signaling partners in an "inside-out" mechanism (Calderwood, 2004; Moser et al., 2009). Inside-out signaling is active but has not been well studied in neurons, and may help explain changes in integrin-mediated ECM contact with changes in neuronal activity. For example, it has recently been shown that reelin signals through its receptors ApoER2 and VLDLR to promote integrin α5β1 adhesion to fibronectin by an inside-out mechanism to control neuronal positioning during cortical development (Sekine et al., 2012). More work needs to be done in the future to establish which RGD-containing brain proteins have effects on synaptic signaling, plasticity and spine structure, and how these signaling mechanisms interact with inside-out signaling pathways.

REELIN ENHANCES GLUTAMATERGIC TRANSMISSION AND PLASTICITY AND MAY STABILIZE SPINES

Reelin is a 385 kDa secreted ECM protein that is a key regulator of neuronal migration in development (Tissir and Goffinet, 2003; D'Arcangelo, 2014). However, even after neurons have reached their proper destination, reelin continues to modulate synaptic signaling pathways to control dendritic spine structure and synaptic plasticity. Reelin is expressed by layer I and II GABAergic interneurons, primarily Cajal-Retzius cells (Rodriguez et al., 2000), which project to other cortical layers where they secrete reelin into the ECM. Upon release, reelin surrounds and adheres to dendritic shafts and spines of cortical pyramidal cells (Rodriguez et al., 2000; Pappas et al., 2001), suggesting that it might regulate spine structure (Rodriguez et al., 2000). Indeed, younger (P21-P31) heterozygous *reelin+/–* mice, which have grossly normal neuron positioning but only half the level of reelin (Liu et al., 2001; Pappas et al., 2001), have significantly reduced dendritic spine density and altered spine morphology (Liu et al., 2001; Niu et al., 2008; Iafrati et al., 2014). Interestingly, by adulthood *reelin+/–* mice exhibit only minimal spine density loss compared to wild type, suggesting that compensatory mechanisms promote additional spine development when reelin levels are reduced (Ventruti et al., 2011).

In adult animals, reelin continues to promote synaptic function and regulate spine morphology. Adult *reelin+/–* mice have reduced levels of synaptic signaling molecules (Ventruti et al., 2011) as well as deficits in excitatory postsynaptic responses, LTP, and LTD (Qiu et al., 2006a), while addition of recombinant reelin to hippocampal slices or direct injection into the ventricles significantly enhances hippocampal LTP (Beffert et al., 2005; Pujadas et al., 2010; Rogers et al., 2011). Recombinant reelin also increases NMDA and AMPA currents in cultured hippocampal slices and primary hippocampal cultures (Chen et al., 2005; Qiu et al., 2006b; Groc et al., 2007; Qiu and Weeber, 2007). These results together demonstrate that reelin is both necessary and sufficient for adult plasticity and glutamatergic signaling. Reelin is also sufficient to promote spine remodeling, as postnatal overexpression of reelin in the mouse forebrain increases spine head size as well as the number of spines with multiple synaptic contacts, while leaving spine density unchanged. Turning off this reelin overexpression decreases spine size and density, indicating that in some cases reelin may also interact with spine stability mechanisms (Pujadas et al., 2010). In addition, injection of recombinant reelin into the ventricles of adult mice increases hippocampal CA1 spine density (Rogers et al., 2011), suggesting that reelin may also promote spine formation in adults. Interestingly, injection of reelin leads to an hours-long transient increase in reelin levels (Rogers et al., 2011), while genetic overexpression would cause a constant increase, suggesting the timing and duration of reelin expression may be important for its effect on spines. Together, these results indicate that in different contexts, reelin promotes synaptic transmission and plasticity and modulates spine dynamics and stability. Further work on stability would benefit from a conditional reelin knockout mouse that could be used to test the necessity of reelin for spine stability in adult animals.

Reelin levels also appear to affect disease pathology in humans. For example, reelin expression is reduced approximately 50% in patients with schizophrenia (Impagnatiello et al., 1998; Berretta, 2012) and *reelin* haploinsufficiency in mice causes increased neuron packing density, decreased GAD67 levels, reduced pre-pulse inhibition and loss of dendritic spines, all features associated with schizophrenia pathology (Tueting et al., 1999; Liu et al., 2001). Reelin may also be neuroprotective against Alzheimer's disease, as it has been shown to interact with soluble amyloid-β42, protect against amyloid-β42-induced spine loss and neuron death in cultured neurons, and reduce amyloid plaque development and memory loss in J20 Alzheimer's model mice (Pujadas et al., 2014). Together, these data show that reelin, which has important roles in neuron development and positioning, also plays critical roles in late onset diseases after development is complete.

AGRIN PROMOTES FILOPODIA AND DENDRITIC SPINE FORMATION

Agrin is best known for its prominent role in development of the vertebrate neuromuscular junction (NMJ) synapse, where it is deposited by motor neurons to induce acetylcholine receptor clustering in the muscle (Gautam et al., 1996; Glass et al., 1996; Sanes and Lichtman, 2001). Agrin is also widely expressed in the brain, with the highest levels of *agrin* expression coinciding with the peak period of synaptic development (O'Connor et al., 1994; Cohen et al., 1997). Indeed, antisense-mediated knockdown of agrin inhibits synapse development in cultured neurons (Ferreira, 1999; Bose et al., 2000). In contrast to knockdown systems, however, cultured *agrin–/–* neurons do not exhibit synaptic deficits (Li et al., 1999; Serpinskaya et al., 1999), suggesting that compensatory mechanisms may arise in the absence of endogenous agrin (Bose et al., 2000). Interestingly, knockdown of agrin in both mature (McCroskery et al., 2009) and immature (McCroskery et al., 2006) neuronal cultures reduces dendritic filopodia number, and agrin overexpression or clustering in immature cultured rat and mouse hippocampal neurons is sufficient to induce filopodia *in vitro* (Annies et al., 2006; McCroskery et al., 2006). As filopodia are precursors for dendritic spines (Ziv and Smith, 1996), these results support a role for agrin in promoting synapse and spine formation even in mature neurons. Indeed, *agrin–/–* mice in which perinatal lethality is rescued by muscle-specific agrin re-expression exhibit decreased cortical dendritic spine density (Ksiazek et al., 2007).

A role for agrin in spine and synapse stability is also supported by studies of neurotrypsin (also called motopsin or Prss12), an extracellular protease whose only known substrate is agrin (Gschwend et al., 1997; Molinari et al., 2002; Reif et al., 2007; Stephan et al., 2008). *neurotrypsin–/–* mice have reduced CA1 apical dendritic spine density (Mitsui et al., 2009). Neurotrypsin is released from presynaptic neurons in response to NMDAR-mediated activity and cleaves agrin at the synapse, suggesting that neurotrypsin might be involved in activity-dependent plasticity. Indeed, while neurons in hippocampal slices from adult *neurotrypsin–/–* mice have normal electrophysiological LTP, LTP-inducing stimuli fail to induce the formation of new filopodia in the knockouts, suggesting that neurotrypsin is required for some aspects of structural plasticity that accompany LTP in adult animals. Interestingly, a soluble cleavage fragment of agrin produced by neurotrypsin can rescue the loss of LTP-induced filopodia formation in *neurotrypsin–/–* mice (Matsumoto-Miyai et al., 2009; **Figure 4**). These results suggest a role for neurotrypsin and agrin in supporting new spine formation following LTP induction protocols in mature animals. Further work should address the molecular mechanisms downstream of agrin cleavage that promote filopodia formation and whether and how these new filopodia form functional dendritic spines and synapses.

TENASCINS ARE REQUIRED FOR SYNAPTIC PLASTICITY AND MAY INTERACT WITH SPINES

The tenascins are a family of ECM proteins that oligomerize through a tenascin association domain and interact with other ECM proteins and receptors through tenascin's EGF-like and fibronectin type III-repeats (Jones and Jones, 2000). Tenascin R (TNR) and tenascin C (TNC) are both expressed in the brain, TNR exclusively so, where they play roles in synaptic plasticity.

Tenascin R is required for normal plasticity, synaptic transmission, and behavior. Tenascin R knockout mice have impaired hippocampal LTP but normal LTD, increased basal synaptic transmission, and anxiety and motor deficits (Bukalo et al., 2001; Saghatelyan et al., 2001; Freitag et al., 2003; Gurevicius et al., 2004). Tenascin R is mainly associated with CSPGs in PNNs around inhibitory interneurons (Brückner et al., 2000), where it crosslinks some CSPG family members (Aspberg et al., 1997). Tenascin R's affect on LTP is due to it carrying the human natural killer-1 (HNK1) carbohydrate epitope (Kruse et al., 1985) which normally interferes with γ-aminobutyric acid type B $GABA_B$ receptor function. $GABA_B$ receptors block $GABA_A$ receptor-mediated inhibition by reducing presynaptic GABA release through a retrograde mechanism (Saghatelyan et al., 2001, 2003). Therefore the loss of HNK1 with *tenascin-R–/–* disinhibits $GABA_B$ receptors, allowing them to block $GABA_A$-mediated inhibition

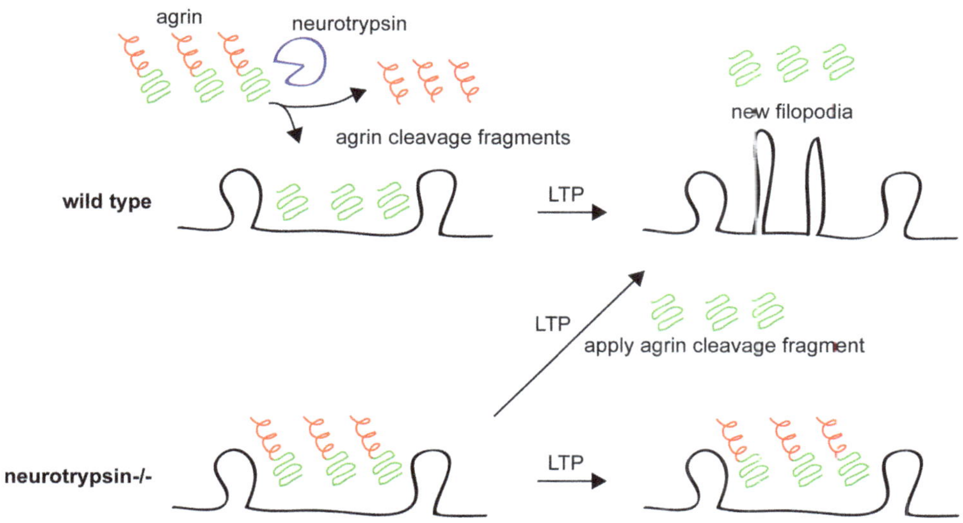

FIGURE 4 | Agrin cleavage by neurotrypsin plays an important role in filopodia formation following LTP. In wild type animals after an LTP stimulus, agrin is cleaved by neurotrypsin (top left) and the agrin fragment promotes growth of new dendritic filopodia (top right). In neurotrypsin knockout mice, agrin cannot be cleaved (bottom left) and new filopodia are not formed in response to an LTP-inducing stimulus (bottom right). However, application of a soluble recombinant neurotrypsin-dependent agrin cleavage fragment rescues this phenotype, promoting new filopodia growth after LTP even in neurotrypsin knockout hippocampal slices. See Matsumoto-Miyai et al. (2009).

and increase excitatory transmission (Saghatelyan et al., 2000, 2001; Nikonenko et al., 2003), raising the threshold for LTP induction (Bukalo et al., 2007).

A key role for TNR in spine stability has been described in the GABAergic granule cells of the olfactory bulb, which have non-conventional dendritic spines that serve both pre- and post-synaptic functions. Tenascin R is expressed and deposited in the olfactory bulb only in adults. Granule cells born in adult *tenascin-R–/–* mice have reduced spine density and reduced migration to the olfactory bulb, while granule cells born in juvenile animals are normal. The reduction in spine density is not secondary to migration defects, as interfering with TNR function after wild type adult-born granule cells have migrated to the olfactory bulb produces a similar reduction in spine density (David et al., 2013). These results demonstrate that TNR regulates the strength of inhibitory contacts onto excitatory neurons to alter adult synaptic plasticity and also regulates spine stability on a subset of inhibitory interneurons.

Tenascin C plays a role in modulating hippocampal plasticity. Tenascin C expression is high early in development but decreases through adolescence and is very low in adults (Ferhat et al., 1996). However, TNC expression can be transiently induced in adult animals by stimuli that cause LTP (Nakic et al., 1998), suggesting a role for TNC in plasticity. Indeed, *tenascin-C–/–* mice have reduced hippocampal CA1 LTP and lack CA1 LTD, though LTP in other regions of the hippocampus is normal (Evers et al., 2002; Strekalova et al., 2002). The specific role for TNC in neuron structure has been understudied, although one study suggests that TNC knockout causes redistribution of stubby dendritic spines in cortex away from primary dendrites and toward higher order dendrites (Irintchev et al., 2005). Further studies will undoubtedly reveal more detailed functions for TNC in spine formation, plasticity, and stability.

LAMININS ORGANIZE AND MAINTAIN SYNAPSES

Laminins are large, secreted, heterotrimeric glycoproteins made up of alpha (α), beta (β), and gamma (γ) subunits that interact with numerous transmembrane proteins, including integrin receptors, α-dystroglycan, and basal CAM/Lutheran (Horwitz et al., 1985; Buck and Horwitz, 1987; Smalheiser and Schwartz, 1987; Gehlsen et al., 1988; Ignatius and Reichardt, 1988; Gee et al., 1993; Henry and Campbell, 1996; El Nemer et al., 1998; Kikkawa et al., 2007; Aumailley, 2013; Yousif et al., 2013). Multiple α, β, and γ genes have been identified and they can combine to form over a dozen distinct heterotrimers (Aumailley et al., 2005; Aumailley, 2013). Each of the three subunits of laminin have an N-terminal short arm region, which mediates interactions with transmembrane receptors and other ECM molecules, and a coiled-coil domain, which mediates heterotrimerization. The α subunits also have a C-terminal globular domain that engages with cell surface receptors, including several integrins and α-dystroglycan (Colognato and Yurchenco, 2000; Aumailley, 2013).

Early experiments revealed that laminins can promote neurite growth from various cultured neuronal cells (Manthorpe et al., 1983; Liesi et al., 1984; Lander et al., 1985). Subsequently, Sanes and colleagues identified key roles for laminins at the NMJ where specific laminin subunits control development, maturation, and stability of the synapse (Sanes, 1982; Hunter et al., 1989a,b; Martin et al., 1995; Patton et al., 1997, 2001; Nishimune et al., 2008; Samuel et al., 2012). For example, β2 subunit-containing laminins are produced by the muscle and localize to the center of the synapse to direct acetylcholine receptor clustering (Martin et al., 1995). Additionally, an interaction between the β2 subunit and a presynaptic voltage-gated calcium channel maintains active zone organization (Nishimune et al., 2004). The α4 and α5 laminin subunits also play roles at the NMJ where they signal through the ECM receptor dystroglycan to promote postsynaptic maturation. The combined loss of laminins α4 and α5 results in smaller, much less elaborate synapses, and loss of α5 alone from the muscle causes a delay in synapse maturation (Nishimune et al., 2008). Interestingly, loss of laminin α4 also causes premature aging at the NMJ, accelerating age-related phenotypes by several months (Samuel et al., 2012). This work and additional evidence in the peripheral nervous system established laminins as major players in synapse formation and maintenance.

Recent evidence also supports roles for laminins in maintaining synapse structure and stability in the central nervous system. Mice lacking the laminin β2 subunit have disrupted hippocampal synapse structure, including misaligned pre- and postsynaptic partners and increased PSD length (Egles et al., 2007). Co-culturing experiments indicate that β2 laminin is produced by postsynaptic neurons in this system. In the hippocampus, kainic acid injection to induce excitotoxic injury degrades laminin γ1 and causes neuron death. These effects are absent in mice lacking the protease tissue plasminogen activator (tPA) and can be blocked with inhibitors of plasmin, an extracellular protease that is the substrate of tPA and degrades laminins. Importantly, adding a laminin antibody to disrupt laminin-neuron interactions can restore neuronal sensitivity to excitotoxic insult in tPA-deficient mice (Chen and Strickland, 1997). Furthermore, plasmin-mediated laminin degradation is associated with reduced LTP (Nakagami et al., 2000), although specific effects on dendritic spine size or stability have not been investigated.

The roles of laminins in the brain are not as well characterized as their roles in the peripheral nervous system. Nonetheless, these observations suggest that laminins function at synapses to maintain neuronal stability and synapse structure and function. More work is necessary to describe functions of specific laminin subunits in the brain as well as the receptors that mediate CNS laminin:neuronal interactions.

NETRIN:DCC SIGNALING REGULATES SPINE MORPHOLOGY AND LTP

Netrins are laminin-related proteins that play diverse conserved roles in neuronal morphogenesis and stability (Ishii et al., 1992; Serafini et al., 1994, 1996; Barallobre et al., 2000; Adler et al., 2006; Colón-Ramos et al., 2007; DeNardo et al., 2012; Smith et al., 2012). In mice and humans, the netrin family consists of three secreted molecules, netrins 1, 3, and 4, and two membrane-bound, GPI-anchored proteins, netrin G1 and G2. Receptors for secreted netrins include deleted in colorectal cancer (DCC), the UNC5 family of proteins, and specific integrin receptors (Chan et al., 1996; Keino-Masu et al., 1996; Leonardo et al., 1997; Yebra et al., 2003; Stanco et al., 2009). Interestingly, netrins share homology with the short arm regions of the β or γ subunits of laminin (Lai Wing Sun et al., 2011) and netrin 4 binds the short arm of laminin γ1 and γ3 subunits to form netrin:laminin complexes and disrupt laminin:laminin interactions (Schneiders et al., 2007).

Recent work suggests netrin:DCC interactions might regulate synapse structure and function in the brain. Loss of DCC after initial development causes smaller dendritic spine head size and impairs learning and LTP. Also, Netrin-1 and DCC co-fractionate from synapses of mature rats, and DCC is present at spines of CA1 pyramidal neurons in mature (60 DIV) cultured hippocampal slices (Horn et al., 2013). While this suggests that netrin can regulate both spine morphology and synaptic transmission in adulthood, further study is needed to understand the roles of netrins at synapses in the adult CNS.

ECM PROTEASES REGULATE SPINE AND SYNAPSE STABILITY AND REMODELING

TISSUE PLASMINOGEN ACTIVATOR CREATES A PERMISSIVE ENVIRONMENT FOR SPINE DESTABILIZATION

Tissue plasminogen activator (tPA) is a secreted extracellular serine protease best known for its role in cleaving and activating plasminogen into the active protease plasmin to prevent blood clots in the circulatory system (Collen, 1999). In the CNS, tPA is expressed and secreted widely (Sappino et al., 1993; Strickland, 2001), though its activity is located primarily in neurons of the hippocampus, amygdala, cerebellum and hypothalamus (Sappino et al., 1993; Baranes et al., 1998; Lochner et al., 2006). Tissue plasminogen activator was first identified as an activity-dependent immediate early gene strongly induced in rat hippocampus after seizures or LTP (Qian et al., 1993), suggesting a role for the protease in adult plasticity. Indeed, *tPA–/–* mice have deficits specifically in hippocampal LTP maintenance (Frey et al., 1996; Huang et al., 1996) with no problems in short term potentiation paradigms like pre-pulse facilitation or early-phase LTP. Tissue plasminogen activator is also sufficient to support late-phase LTP, as genetic overexpression of tPA enhances LTP proportional to the amount of gene overexpression (Madani et al., 1999). Tissue plasminogen activator can also regulate plasticity in other systems, including cerebellar motor learning (Seeds et al., 2003) and striatal LTD (Calabresi et al., 2000), and *tPA–/–* mice are resistant to chemically-induced synaptic potentiation (Huang et al., 1996; Baranes et al., 1998).

Tissue plasminogen activator is a key regulator of dendritic spine stability during plasticity, both in the visual system and in response to stress. Tissue plasminogen activator becomes activated in binocular primary visual cortex during MD, and tPA knockout blocks MD-induced OD plasticity shifts. Importantly, this loss of plasticity can be rescued by recombinant tPA (Mataga et al., 2002), demonstrating a critical role for tPA in OD plasticity. In addition, MD upregulates spine motility, and this effect can be mimicked by direct application of tPA or plasmin to visual cortex. Importantly, the increased motility induced by MD occludes that caused by plasmin application, suggesting that plasmin and MD function in the same pathway to permit MD-induced structural plasticity (Oray et al., 2004). In addition, while 4 days of MD causes spine pruning in visual cortex during the OD critical period, this spine loss is blocked in *tPA–/–* mice, indicating that tPA is also required for spine pruning in response to MD (Mataga et al., 2004). Chronic stress can also cause spine loss in the hippocampus and amygdala. Plasminogen is activated around dendritic spines by chronic stress, and knockout of tPA or plasminogen blocks stress-induced spine loss (Pawlak et al., 2005; Bennur et al., 2007). These results suggest that tPA negatively regulates spine stability and that its activation creates a permissive environment that destabilizes spines and promotes their loss.

One open question in the field is what substrates of tPA promote plasticity in each of these paradigms. Classically, tPA cleaves plasminogen to make the active protease plasmin, which can then degrade ECM targets. Indeed, plasmin can degrade laminin and the CSPG phosphacan to regulate LTP and hippocampal mossy fiber outgrowth (Nakagami et al., 2000; Wu et al., 2000). Plasmin also likely degrades ECM proteins in the MD paradigm, but its exact targets are unknown (Oray et al., 2004). However, it is important to note that tPA certainly has other non-ECM targets in the brain. For example, the loss of late LTP in tPA and plasminogen knockouts is mostly due to reduced proBDNF cleavage to create the mature form of BDNF (Pang et al., 2004). In addition, tPA can cleave the NR1 subunit of the NMDAR to potentiate NMDAR currents (Nicole et al., 2001). It is clear from these varied results that tPA and plasmin target a variety of ECM and non-ECM proteins to regulate synaptic and structural plasticity. It will be important to clearly identify the critical tPA targets in each experimental paradigm to better understand the role of tPA in dendritic spine regulation.

MATRIX METALLOPROTEINASES PLAY DIVERSE ROLES IN DENDRITIC SPINE REMODELING IN DISEASE, DEVELOPMENT, AND PLASTICITY

Matrix metalloproteinases (MMPs) are a large class of secreted and transmembrane proteases that can degrade many ECM proteins, transmembrane receptors, and other signaling proteins (Visse and Nagase, 2003). Matrix metalloproteinases were initially identified as critical for brain function because the mRNA for TIMP1, an endogenous inhibitor of MMPs, is upregulated in a kainic acid-induced epilepsy model, suggesting an activity-dependent role for MMPs in epilepsy (Nedivi et al., 1993; Rivera et al., 1997; Jaworski et al., 1999). In the kindling model of epilepsy (Morimoto et al., 2004), MMP9 knockout delays seizure onset while MMP9 overexpression speeds onset (Wilczynski et al., 2008). In addition, MMP2 and MMP9 are expressed in neurons and glia and are upregulated by kainate treatment (Szklarczyk et al., 2002), and other MMPs may also be expressed after injury or certain stimulations (Bilousova et al., 2006; Meighan et al., 2006). Importantly, kainate-induced seizures cause hippocampal spine loss that is blocked in *MMP9–/–* mice (Wilczynski et al., 2008).

MMP9 activity is also important in another pathophysiological condition, Fragile X syndrome (FXS). Mice with FXS have more long and thin spines than wild type mice, especially early in development. Treatment of FXS mice or hippocampal cultures derived from these mice with minocycline to inhibit MMP9 can normalize spine morphology (Bilousova et al., 2009), suggesting that hyperactive MMP9 in development prevents spine maturation. Indeed, MMP9 has recently been shown directly to be hyperactive in FXS mice, and disruption of the MMP9 gene in FXS mice normalizes the spine, behavioral, and signal transduction defects associated with FXS (Sidhu et al., 2014). These results demonstrate that pathophysiological activation of MMP9 can promote changes in dendritic spine morphology associated with disease (**Figure 5A**).

Matrix metalloproteinases also play roles in developmental processes such as spine protrusion and early maturation. For

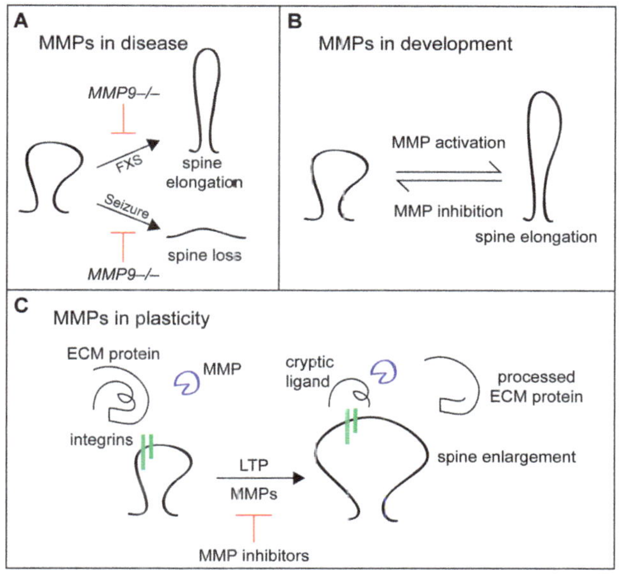

FIGURE 5 | Matrix metalloproteinases play diverse roles in dendritic spine remodeling in disease, development, and plasticity. **(A)** In Fragile X syndrome (FXS), MMP9 is hyperactive and dendritic spines are elongated early in development. MMP9 loss of function or inhibition with minocycline normalizes these spine defects. In epilepsy models, seizure-induced spine loss is blocked by inhibition of MMP activity. **(B)** In development, activation of MMPs, particularly MMP9, causes spine thinning and elongation, while MMP inhibition promotes the maturation of filopodia into mature, mushroom shaped spines. **(C)** Matrix metalloproteinases play a different role in adult plasticity, cleaving unknown ECM proteins to reveal cryptic integrin ligands that drive spine enlargement during LTP. In addition to changes in spine size, MMP activity is required for the maintenance phase of LTP.

example, bath application of activated MMP9 to young hippocampal cultures or organotypic slices and overexpression of activated MMP9 cause dendritic spines to become longer and thinner (Michaluk et al., 2011). Similarly, treatment of maturing hippocampal cultures with MMP7 causes spine elongation (Bilousova et al., 2006). By contrast, MMP inhibition of cultured neurons promotes maturation of thin filopodial spines into mature mushroom-shaped spines (Tian et al., 2007; Bilousova et al., 2009: **Figure 5B**). Matrix metalloproteinase activation promotes spine elongation at least in part through cleavage of intercellular cell adhesion molecule 5 (ICAM5). Full length ICAM5 is found in immature neurons and is cleaved by MMPs to release a soluble extracellular domain that promotes filopodial elongation (Tian et al., 2007). Soluble ICAM5 also increases AMPA receptor expression and cofilin phosphorylation, phenotypes that are associated with spine maturation and depend on β1 integrin (Conant et al., 2011; Lonskaya et al., 2013). Interestingly, ICAM5 localization in cortical neurons shifts during synapse development from predominately dendritic filopodia and spines to predominately the dendritic shaft, and this developmental shift is blocked in *MMP9–/–* mice (Kelly et al., 2014). These data indicate that ICAM5 is an important substrate of MMP9 during synaptogenesis. Together, these results show that MMPs have central roles in dendritic spine development and maturation.

Table 1 | Role(s) of ECM proteins in synaptic plasticity and/or regulation of spine structure.

ECM molecule	Role(s) in synaptic plasticity and/or regulation of spine structure	Evidence for role	References
CSPGs	Inhibit adult MD-induced OD plasticity	Degradation of CSPG GAG chains by treatment with chABC permits MD-induced OD plasticity after CP closure in adults.	Pizzorusso et al. (2002)
	Inhibit adult fear memory erasure	Treatment with chABC permits fear memory erasure after CP closure in adults.	Gogolla et al. (2009)
	Required for LTP maintenance	Adult neurocan and brevican knockouts have deficits in LTP maintenance.	Zhou et al. (2001), Brakebusch et al. (2002)
	Inhibit recovery of spine loss due to adult MD	Treatment with chABC allows spine density to recover in adults after MD when the opposite eyelid has been resutured.	Pizzorusso et al. (2006)
	Inhibit spine motility	Treatment with chABC increases spine motility.	Orlando et al. (2012), de Vivo et al. (2013)
RGD peptides	Inhibit LTP maintenance	RGD application to slices or cultured neurons inhibits the late phase of LTP.	Staubli et al. (1990), Bahr et al. (1997), Chun et al. (2001)
	Potentiate NMDA receptors	RGD application increases NMDAR-mediated currents.	Lin et al. (2003), Bernard-Trifilo et al. (2005)
	Increase spine length and promote filopodia formation	RGD application elongates existing spines and induces dendritic filopodia formation.	Shi and Ethell (2006)
Reelin	Enhances LTP	Recombinant reelin enhances LTP magnitude.	Beffert et al. (2005)
	Promotes glutamatergic transmission	Recombinant reelin increases NMDAR and AMPAR currents.	Chen et al. (2005), Qiu et al. (2006b), Groc et al. (2007), Qiu and Weeber (2007)
	Increases spine density	Spine density is reduced in *reelin+/–* mice and enhanced by recombinant reelin.	Liu et al. (2001), Niu et al. (2008), Rogers et al. (2011, 2013), Iafrati et al. (2014)
	Increases spine head size and promotes multi-synapse spines	Recombinant reelin drives these phenotypes.	Pujadas et al. (2010)
Agrin	Promotes filopodia formation	Filopodia formation is promoted by agrin clustering or overexpression and reduced by agrin knockdown.	Annies et al. (2006), McCroskery et al. (2006, 2009)
	Increases spine density	Spine density is reduced in *agrin–/–* and *neurotrypsin–/–* mice.	Ksiazek et al. (2007), Mitsui et al. (2009)
	Required for LTP-induced filopodia formation	LTP-induced filopodia formation is blocked in *neurotrypsin–/–* mice.	Matsumoto-Miyai et al. (2009)
Tenascins	TNR is required for LTP	LTP is impaired in *TNR–/–* mice.	Bukalo et al. (2001), Saghatelyan et al. (2001)
	TNR promotes basal transmission	Basal excitatory transmission is increased in *TNR–/–* mice.	Saghatelyan et al. (2001), Gurevicius et al. (2004)
	TNR required for olfactory bulb granule cell spine density	Spine density of newborn olfactory bulb granule cells is decreased in *TNR–/–* mice.	David et al. (2013)
	TNC is required for LTP and LTD	LTP and LTD are impaired in *TNC–/–* mice.	Evers et al. (2002), Strekalova et al. (2002)
	TNC is required for proper spine distribution along dendrites	Cortical dendritic spines are shifted toward higher order dendrites in *TNC–/–* mice.	Irintchev et al. (2005)
Laminin	Protects against excitotoxicty	Disrupting laminin resensitizes excitotoxic-insensitive neurons.	Chen and Strickland (1997)
	May stabilize LTP	Laminin degradation and loss of LTP are correlated.	Nakagami et al. (2000)
	May be required for synaptic structure	β2 laminin is required for synapse alignment and PSD length.	Egles et al. (2007)
Netrin	May be required for LTP	LTP is impaired in *DCC–/–* mice.	Horn et al. (2013)
	May inhibit spine growth	Spine heads are smaller in *DCC–/–* mice.	Horn et al. (2013)
tPA	Stabilizes LTP late phase	Late LTP is destabilized in *tPA–/–* mice and stabilized by recombinant tPA.	Huang et al. (1996), Frey et al. (1996), Baranes et al. (1998), Madani et al. (1999)
	Required for OD plasticity	OD plasticity is blocked in *tPA–/–* mice.	Mataga et al. (2002)

(Continued)

Table 1 | Continued

ECM molecule	Role(s) in synaptic plasticity and/or regulation of spine structure	Evidence for role	References
	Increases spine motility	Spine motility is upregulated by recombinant *tPA*.	Oray et al. (2004)
	Required for MD-induced spine pruning	Spine pruning caused by MD does not occur in *tPA–/–* mice.	Mataga et al. (2004)
	Require for stress-induced spine loss	Spine loss caused by stress is blocked in *tPA–/–* and *plasminogen–/–* mice.	Pawlak et al. (2005), Bennur et al. (2007)
MMPs	Required for kainate-induced spine loss	Spine loss is blocked in *MMP9–/–* mice.	Wilczynski et al. (2008)
	Required for FXS phenotypes	MMP9 inhibition or deletion rescues spine and behavioral phenotypes in FXS model mice	Bilousova et al. (2009), Sidhu et al. (2014)
	Promote spine elongation	Spine elongation is promoted by MMP activation and blocked by MMP inhibition in young systems.	Bilousova et al. (2006, 2009), Tian et al. (2007), Michaluk et al. (2011)
	Regulate ICAM5 cleavage and function	ICAM5 inhibits spine maturation, and MMPs are required for ICAM5 cleavage to promote spine elongation.	Tian et al. (2007), Conant et al. (2011), Lonskaya et al. (2013)
	Required for LTP late phase	LTP late phase is lost in *MMP9–/–* and *MMP2–/–* mice or when MMPs are inhibited.	Nagy et al. (2006), Wang et al. (2008)
	Required for spatial learning	Morris water maze acquisition is blocked by MMP inhibition.	Meighan et al. (2006)
	Promote LTP-induced spine volume increase	LTP-induced spine volume increase is blocked by MMP inhibition and promoted by local MMP application.	Wang et al. (2008), Szepesi et al. (2014)

Abbreviations: CSPG-chondroitin sulfate proteoglycans; GAG chains-glycosaminoglycan side chains; MD-monocular deprivation; OD-ocular dominance; LTP-long term potentiation; LTD-long term depression; chABC-chondroitinase ABC; CP-critical period; RGD peptide-Arginine-Glycine-Aspartate peptide; DCC-deleted in colorectal cancer (netrin receptor); tPA-tissue plasminogen activator; TNR/C-tenascin R or C; MMP-matrix metalloproteinase; FXS-Fragile X syndrome.

It is important to consider that the effects of MMPs on dendritic spines can differ greatly depending on the method of MMP manipulation and the maturity of the system. The MMP-dependent elongation of spines discussed above is dependent on manipulation of MMP activity in young or maturing systems or under pathophysiological conditions and requires general application of MMP-affecting drugs for long periods of time. In more mature systems and with local application of MMPs during plasticity events, MMP activity has the opposite effect. For example, local application of active MMP9 to dendritic spines in acute hippocampal slices is by itself sufficient to potentiate synapses and increase spine volume, the same changes that are caused by theta-burst pairing, which induces LTP. Notably, MMP9-induced potentiation and spine enlargement are occluded by prior theta-burst pairing, suggesting that MMP9 activation and LTP induction function in the same pathway to consolidate spine enlargement and LTP (Wang et al., 2008). Similarly, chemical LTP induction in mature cultured neurons increases spine head size of smaller spines in an MMP-dependent manner (Szepesi et al., 2014). In agreement with these findings, MMP9 is required for maintenance of LTP and LTP-induced spine volume increase in acute hippocampal slices from adult animals (Nagy et al., 2006; Wang et al., 2008), and inhibition of MMPs 3 and 9 blocks acquisition of spatial learning in adult animals (Meighan et al., 2006). Importantly, many of these acute phenotypes in mature systems depend on integrin β1 function (Nagy et al., 2006; Wang et al., 2008), suggesting that MMPs may reveal cryptic integrin ligands in the ECM that maintain spine structural plasticity in mature neurons (**Figure 5C**). Given the diverse effects of MMP targeting treatments on spine development, plasticity, and maintenance, further studies should address the molecular basis for the differential effects of MMP manipulation in both young and mature systems (Dziembowska and Wlodarczyk, 2012; Stawarski et al., 2014). In addition, the specific ECM molecules that signal through integrins are unknown, and future studies will hopefully link proteolysis of specific proteins by MMPs with specific changes in dendritic spines to understand the signaling mechanisms involved in MMP-mediated dendritic spine remodeling.

CONCLUSION

Precise regulation of dendritic spine and synapse formation, plasticity, and stability is essential for proper circuit and brain function. Emerging evidence indicates that ECM proteins, their receptors, and ECM proteases are major physiological regulators of spines and synapses (**Table 1**). Extracellular matrix molecules are potent regulators of the actin cytoskeleton, which dictates dendritic spine morphology and powers dynamic changes in dendritic spine shape. Moreover, the ECM surrounds neurons and its composition is influenced greatly by synaptic activity, making it an ideal substrate to influence spine and synapse structure and physiology.

Future studies in this field will be critical to identify the molecules that signal through ECM receptors such as integrins to control spine stability and plasticity. Elucidating these molecules and the mechanisms by which they function is essential to understand how differential stability and plasticity are achieved in adulthood vs. development, and in healthy individuals vs. those with neurodegenerative or late-onset psychiatric disease. Only then can we target these mechanisms therapeutically to gain control of synaptic flexibility and stability.

ACKNOWLEDGMENTS

The authors thank A. Scherer for his careful critiques and comments on this manuscript during its preparation.

REFERENCES

Adler, C. E., Fetter, R. D., and Bargmann, C. I. (2006). UNC-6/Netrin induces neuronal asymmetry and defines the site of axon formation. *Nat. Neurosci.* 9, 511–518. doi: 10.1038/nn1666

Akbik, F. V., Bhagat, S. M., Patel, P. R., Cafferty, W. B. J., and Strittmatter, S. M. (2013). Anatomical plasticity of adult brain is titrated by Nogo Receptor 1. *Neuron* 77, 859–866. doi: 10.1016/j.neuron.2012.12.027

Annies, M., Bittcher, G., Ramseger, R., Löschinger, J., Wöll, S., Porten, E., et al. (2006). Clustering transmembrane-agrin induces filopodia-like processes on axons and dendrites. *Mol. Cell. Neurosci.* 31, 515–524. doi: 10.1016/j.mcn.2005.11.005

Aspberg, A., Miura, R., Bourdoulous, S., Shimonaka, M., Heinegârd, D., Schachner, M., et al. (1997). The C-type lectin domains of lecticans, a family of aggregating chondroitin sulfate proteoglycans, bind tenascin-R by protein-protein interactions independent of carbohydrate moiety. *Proc. Natl. Acad. Sci. U S A* 94, 10116–10121. doi: 10.1073/pnas.94.19.10116

Aumailley, M. (2013). The laminin family. *Cell Adh. Migr.* 7, 48–55. doi: 10.4161/cam.22826

Aumailley, M., Bruckner-Tuderman, L., Carter, W. G., Deutzmann, R., Edgar, D., Ekblom, P., et al. (2005). A simplified laminin nomenclature. *Matrix Biol.* 24, 326–332. doi: 10.1016/j.matbio.2005.05.006

Bahr, B. A., Staubli, U., Xiao, P., Chun, D., Ji, Z. X., Esteban, E. T., et al. (1997). Arg-Gly-Asp-Ser-selective adhesion and the stabilization of long-term potentiation: pharmacological studies and the characterization of a candidate matrix receptor. *J. Neurosci.* 17, 1320–1329.

Barallobre, M. J., Del Rio, J. A., Alcantara, S., Borrell, V., Aguado, F., Ruiz, M., et al. (2000). Aberrant development of hippocampal circuits and altered neural activity in netrin 1-deficient mice. *Development* 127, 4797–4810.

Baranes, D., Lederfein, D., Huang, Y. Y., Chen, M., Bailey, C. H., and Kandel, E. R. (1998). Tissue plasminogen activator contributes to the late phase of LTP and to synaptic growth in the hippocampal mossy fiber pathway. *Neuron* 21, 813–825. doi: 10.1016/s0896-6273(00)80597-8

Barros, C. S., Franco, S. J., and Müller, U. (2011). Extracellular matrix: functions in the nervous system. *Cold Spring Harb. Perspect. Biol.* 3:a005108. doi: 10.1101/cshperspect.a005108

Bastrikova, N., Gardner, G. A., Reece, J. M., Jeromin, A., and Dudek, S. M. (2008). Synapse elimination accompanies functional plasticity in hippocampal neurons. *Proc. Natl. Acad. Sci. U S A* 105, 3123–3127. doi: 10.1073/pnas.0800027105

Beffert, U., Nematollah Farsian, F., Masiulis, I., Hammer, R. E., Yoon, S. O., Giehl, K. M., et al. (2006). ApoE receptor 2 controls neuronal survival in the adult brain. *Curr. Biol.* 16, 2446–2452. doi: 10.1016/j.cub.2006.10.029

Beffert, U., Weeber, E. J., Durudas, A., Qiu, S., Masiulis, I., Sweatt, J. D., et al. (2005). Modulation of synaptic plasticity and memory by Reelin involves differential splicing of the lipoprotein receptor Apoer2. *Neuron* 47, 567–579. doi: 10.1016/j.neuron.2005.07.007

Belvindrah, R., Graus-Porta, D., Goebbels, S., Nave, K. A., and Müller, U. (2007a). Beta1 integrins in radial glia but not in migrating neurons are essential for the formation of cell layers in the cerebral cortex. *J. Neurosci.* 27, 13854–13865. doi: 10.1523/JNEUROSCI.4494-07.2007

Belvindrah, R., Hankel, S., Walker, J., Patton, B. L., and Müller, U. (2007b). Beta1 integrins control the formation of cell chains in the adult rostral migratory stream. *J. Neurosci.* 27, 2704–2717. doi: 10.1523/jneurosci.2991-06.2007

Bennur, S., Shankaranarayana Rao, B. S., Pawlak, R., Strickland, S., McEwen, B. S., and Chattarji, S. (2007). Stress-induced spine loss in the medial amygdala is mediated by tissue-plasminogen activator. *Neuroscience* 144, 8–16. doi: 10.1016/j.neuroscience.2006.08.075

Benson, D. L., and Huntley, G. W. (2012). Synapse adhesion: a dynamic equilibrium conferring stability and flexibility. *Curr. Opin. Neurobiol.* 22, 397–404. doi: 10.1016/j.conb.2011.09.011

Bernard-Trifilo, J. A., Kramár, E. A., Torp, R., Lin, C.-Y., Pineda, E. A., Lynch, G., et al. (2005). Integrin signaling cascades are operational in adult hippocampal synapses and modulate NMDA receptor physiology. *J. Neurochem.* 93, 834–849. doi: 10.1111/j.1471-4159.2005.03062.x

Berretta, S. (2012). Extracellular matrix abnormalities in schizophrenia. *Neuropharmacology* 62, 1584–1597. doi: 10.1016/j.neuropharm.2011.08.010

Bilousova, T. V., Dansie, L., Ngo, M., Aye, J., Charles, J. R., Ethell, D. W., et al. (2009). Minocycline promotes dendritic spine maturation and improves behavioural performance in the fragile X mouse model. *J. Med. Genet.* 46, 94–102. doi: 10.1136/jmg.2008.061796

Bilousova, T. V., Rusakov, D. A., Ethell, D. W., and Ethell, I. M. (2006). Matrix metalloproteinase-7 disrupts dendritic spines in hippocampal neurons through NMDA receptor activation. *J. Neurochem.* 97, 44–56. doi: 10.1111/j.1471-4159.2006.03701.x

Bose, C. M., Qiu, D., Bergamaschi, A., Gravante, B., Bossi, M., Villa, A., et al. (2000). Agrin controls synaptic differentiation in hippocampal neurons. *J. Neurosci.* 20, 9086–9095.

Brakebusch, C., Seidenbecher, C. I., Asztely, F., Rauch, U., Matthies, H., Meyer, H., et al. (2002). Brevican-deficient mice display impaired hippocampal CA1 long-term potentiation but show no obvious deficits in learning and memory. *Mol. Cell. Biol.* 22, 7417–7427. doi: 10.1128/mcb.22.21.7417-7427.2002

Brückner, G., Grosche, J., Schmidt, S., Härtig, W., Margolis, R. U., Delpech, B., et al. (2000). Postnatal development of perineuronal nets in wild-type mice and in a mutant deficient in tenascin-R. *J. Comp. Neurol.* 428, 616–629. doi: 10.1002/1096-9861(20001225)428:4<616::aid-cne3>3.0.co;2-k

Buck, C. A., and Horwitz, A. F. (1987). Cell surface receptors for extracellular matrix molecules. *Annu. Rev. Cell Biol.* 3, 179–205. doi: 10.1146/annurev.cb.03.110187.001143

Bukalo, O., and Dityatev, A. (2012). Synaptic cell adhesion molecules. *Adv. Exp. Med. Biol.* 970, 97–128. doi: 10.1007/978-3-7091-0932-8_5

Bukalo, O., Schachner, M., and Dityatev, A. (2001). Modification of extracellular matrix by enzymatic removal of chondroitin sulfate and by lack of tenascin-R differentially affects several forms of synaptic plasticity in the hippocampus. *Neuroscience* 104, 359–369. doi: 10.1016/s0306-4522(01)00082-3

Bukalo, O., Schachner, M., and Dityatev, A. (2007). Hippocampal metaplasticity induced by deficiency in the extracellular matrix glycoprotein tenascin-R. *J. Neurosci.* 27, 6019–6028. doi: 10.1523/jneurosci.1022-07.2007

Calabresi, P., Napolitano, M., Centonze, D., Marfia, G. A., Gubellini, P., Teule, M. A., et al. (2000). Tissue plasminogen activator controls multiple forms of synaptic plasticity and memory. *Eur. J. Neurosci.* 12, 1002–1012. doi: 10.1046/j.1460-9568.2000.00991.x

Calderwood, D. A. (2004). Integrin activation. *J. Cell Sci.* 117, 657–666. doi: 10.1242/jcs.01014

Carter, A., and Sabatini, B. (2008). "Spine calcium signaling," in *Dendrites*, eds G. Stuart, N. Spruston and M. Hausser 2nd Edn. (New York: Oxford University Press), 287–308.

Catalá, I., Ferrer, I., Galofré, E., and Fábregues, I. (1988). Decreased numbers of dendritic spines on cortical pyramidal neurons in dementia. A quantitative Golgi study on biopsy samples. *Hum. Neurobiol.* 6, 255–259.

Chan, C.-S., Levenson, J. M., Mukhopadhyay, P. S., Zong, L., Bradley, A., Sweatt, J. D., et al. (2007). Alpha3-integrins are required for hippocampal long-term potentiation and working memory. *Learn. Mem.* 14, 606–615. doi: 10.1101/lm.648607

Chan, C.-S., Weeber, E. J., Zong, L., Fuchs, E., Sweatt, J. D., and Davis, R. L. (2006). Beta 1-integrins are required for hippocampal AMPA receptor-dependent synaptic transmission, synaptic plasticity and working memory. *J. Neurosci.* 26, 223–232. doi: 10.1523/jneurosci.4110-05.2006

Chan, S. S., Zheng, H., Su, M. W., Wilk, R., Killeen, M. T., Hedgecock, E. M., et al. (1996). UNC-40, a C. elegans homolog of DCC (Deleted in Colorectal Cancer), is required in motile cells responding to UNC-6 netrin cues. *Cell* 87, 187–195. doi: 10.1016/s0092-8674(00)81337-9

Charrier, C., Joshi, K., Coutinho-Budd, J., Kim, J.-E., Lambert, N., de Marchena, J., et al. (2012). Inhibition of SRGAP2 function by its human-specific paralogs induces neoteny during spine maturation. *Cell* 149, 923–935. doi: 10.1016/j.cell.2012.03.034

Cheadle, L., and Biederer, T. (2012). The novel synaptogenic protein Farp1 links postsynaptic cytoskeletal dynamics and transsynaptic organization. *J. Cell Biol.* 199, 985–1001. doi: 10.1083/jcb.201205041

Chen, Y., Beffert, U., Ertunc, M., Tang, T.-S., Kavalali, E. T., Bezprozvanny, I., et al. (2005). Reelin modulates NMDA receptor activity in cortical neurons. *J. Neurosci.* 25, 8209–8216. doi: 10.1523/jneurosci.1951-05.2005

Chen, Z. L., and Strickland, S. (1997). Neuronal death in the hippocampus is promoted by plasmin-catalyzed degradation of laminin. *Cell* 91, 917–925. doi: 10.1016/s0092-8674(00)80483-3

Chen, Z.-L., Yu, H., Yu, W.-M., Pawlak, R., and Strickland, S. (2008). Proteolytic fragments of laminin promote excitotoxic neurodegeneration by up-regulation of the KA1 subunit of the kainate receptor. *J. Cell Biol.* 183, 1299–1313. doi: 10.1083/jcb.200803107

Chong, L. D., Traynor-Kaplan, A., Bokoch, G. M., and Schwartz, M. A. (1994). The small GTP-binding protein Rho regulates a phosphatidylinositol 4-phosphate 5-kinase in mammalian cells. *Cell* 79, 507–513. doi: 10.1016/0092-8674(94)90259-3

Chun, D., Gall, C. M., Bi, X., and Lynch, G. (2001). Evidence that integrins contribute to multiple stages in the consolidation of long term potentiation in rat hippocampus. *Neuroscience* 105, 815–829. doi: 10.1016/s0306-4522(01)00173-7

Cichon, S., Mühleisen, T. W., Degenhardt, F. A., Mattheisen, M., Miró, X., Strohmaier, J., et al. (2011). Genome-wide association study identifies genetic variation in neurocan as a susceptibility factor for bipolar disorder. *Am. J. Hum. Genet.* 88, 372–381. doi: 10.1016/j.ajhg.2011.01.017

Cohen, N. A., Kaufmann, W. E., Worley, P. F., and Rupp, F. (1997). Expression of agrin in the developing and adult rat brain. *Neuroscience* 76, 581–596. doi: 10.1016/s0306-4522(96)00345-4

Collen, D. (1999). The plasminogen (fibrinolytic) system. *Thromb. Haemost.* 82, 259–270.

Colognato, H., and Yurchenco, P. D. (2000). Form and function: the laminin family of heterotrimers. *Dev. Dyn.* 218, 213–234. doi: 10.1002/(sici)1097-0177(200006)218:2<213::aid-dvdy1>3.0.co;2-r

Colón-Ramos, D. A., Margeta, M. A., and Shen, K. (2007). Glia promote local synaptogenesis through UNC-6 (netrin) signaling in *C. elegans*. *Science* 318, 103–106. doi: 10.1126/science.1143762

Conant, K., Lonskaya, I., Szklarczyk, A., Krall, C., Steiner, J., Maguire-Zeiss, K., et al. (2011). Methamphetamine-associated cleavage of the synaptic adhesion molecule intercellular adhesion molecule-5. *J. Neurochem.* 118, 521–532. doi: 10.1111/j.1471-4159.2010.07153.x

Dansie, L. E., and Ethell, I. M. (2011). Casting a net on dendritic spines: the extracellular matrix and its receptors. *Dev. Neurobiol.* 71, 956–981. doi: 10.1002/dneu.20963

D'Arcangelo, G. (2014). Reelin in the years: controlling neuronal migration and maturation in the Mammalian brain. *Adv. Neurosci.* 2014:19. doi: 10.1155/2014/597395

David, L. S., Schachner, M., and Saghatelyan, A. (2013). The extracellular matrix glycoprotein tenascin-R affects adult but not developmental neurogenesis in the olfactory bulb. *J. Neurosci.* 33, 10324–10339. doi: 10.1523/jneurosci.5728-12.2013

DeFreitas, M. F., Yoshida, C. K., Frazier, W. A., Mendrick, D. L., Kypta, R. M., and Reichardt, L. F. (1995). Identification of integrin alpha 3 beta 1 as a neuronal thrombospondin receptor mediating neurite outgrowth. *Neuron* 15, 333–343. doi: 10.1016/0896-6273(95)90038-1

DeNardo, L. A., de Wit, J., Otto-Hitt, S., and Ghosh, A. (2012). NGL-2 regulates input-specific synapse development in CA1 pyramidal neurons. *Neuron* 76, 762–775. doi: 10.1016/j.neuron.2012.10.013

de Vivo, L., Landi, S., Panniello, M., Baroncelli, L., Chierzi, S., Mariotti, L., et al. (2013). Extracellular matrix inhibits structural and functional plasticity of dendritic spines in the adult visual cortex. *Nat. Commun.* 4:1484. doi: 10.1038/ncomms2491

Dunaevsky, A., Tashiro, A., Majewska, A. K., Mason, C. A., and Yuste, R. (1999). Developmental regulation of spine motility in the mammalian central nervous system. *Proc. Natl. Acad. Sci. U S A* 96, 13438–13443. doi: 10.1073/pnas.96.23.13438

Dziembowska, M., and Wlodarczyk, J. (2012). MMP9: a novel function in synaptic plasticity. *Int. J. Biochem. Cell Biol.* 44, 709–713. doi: 10.1016/j.biocel.2012.01.023

Egles, C., Claudepierre, T., Manglapus, M. K., Champliaud, M.-F., Brunken, W. J., and Hunter, D. D. (2007). Laminins containing the beta2 chain modulate the precise organization of CNS synapses. *Mol. Cell. Neurosci.* 34, 288–298. doi: 10.1016/j.mcn.2006.11.004

El Nemer, W., Gane, P., Colin, Y., Bony, V., Rahuel, C., Galactéros, F., et al. (1998). The Lutheran blood group glycoproteins, the erythroid receptors for laminin, are adhesion molecules. *J. Biol. Chem.* 273, 16686–16693. doi: 10.1074/jbc.273.27.16686

Evers, M. R., Salmen, B., Bukalo O., Rollenhagen, A., Bösl, M. R., Morellini, F., et al. (2002). Impairment of L-type Ca2+ channel-dependent forms of hippocampal synaptic plasticity in mice deficient in the extracellular matrix glycoprotein tenascin-C. *J. Neurosci.* 22, 7177–7194.

Ferhat, L., Chevassus au Louis, N., Jorquera, I., Niquet, J., Khrestchatisky, M., Ben-Ari, Y., et al. (1996). Transient increase of tenascin-C in immature hippocampus: astroglial and neuronal expression. *J. Neurocytol.* 25, 53–66. doi: 10.1007/bf02284785

Ferrante, R. J., Kowall, N. W., and Richardson, E. P. (1991). Proliferative and degenerative changes in striatal spiny neurons in Huntington's disease: a combined study using the section-Golgi method and calbindin D28k immunocytochemistry. *J. Neurosci.* 11, 3877–3887.

Ferreira, A. (1999). Abnormal synapse formation in agrin-depleted hippocampal neurons. *J. Cell Sci.* 112(Pt. 24), 4729–4738.

Freitag, S., Schachner, M., and Morellini, F. (2003). Behavioral alterations in mice deficient for the extracellular matrix glycoprotein tenascin-R. *Behav. Brain Res.* 145, 189–207. doi: 10.1016/s0166-4328(03)00109-8

Frey, U., Muller, M., and Kuhl, D. (1996). A different form of long-lasting potentiation revealed in tissue plasminogen activator mutant mice. *J. Neurosci.* 16, 2057–2063.

Galtrey, C. M., and Fawcett, J. W (2007). The role of chondroitin sulfate proteoglycans in regeneration and plasticity in the central nervous system. *Brain Res. Rev.* 54, 1–18. doi: 10.1016/j.brainresrev.2006.09.006

Gama, C. I., Tully, S. E., Sotogaku, N., Clark, P. M., Rawat, M., Vaidehi, N., et al. (2006). Sulfation patterns of glycosaminoglycans encode molecular recognition and activity. *Nat. Chem. Biol.* 2, 467–473. doi: 10.1038/nchembio810

Garey, L. J., Ong, W. Y., Patel, T. S., Kanani, M., Davis, A., Mortimer, A. M., et al. (1998). Reduced dendritic spine density on cerebral cortical pyramidal neurons in schizophrenia. *J. Neurol. Neurosurg. Psychiatr.* 65, 446–453. doi: 10.1136/jnnp.65.4.446

Gautam, M., Noakes, P. G., Moscoso, L., Rupp, F., Scheller, R. H., Merlie, J. P., et al. (1996). Defective neuromuscular synaptogenesis in agrin-deficient mutant mice. *Cell* 85, 525–535. doi: 10.1016/s0092-8674(00)81253-2

Gee, S. H., Blacher, R. W., Douville, P. J., Provost, P. R., Yurchenco, P. D., and Carbonetto, S. (1993). Laminin-binding protein 120 from brain is closely related to the dystrophin-associated glycoprotein, dystroglycan and binds with high affinity to the major heparin binding domain of laminin. *J. Biol. Chem.* 268, 14972–14980.

Gehlsen, K. R., Dillner, L., Engvall, E., and Ruoslahti, E. (1988). The human laminin receptor is a member of the integrin family of cell adhesion receptors. *Science* 241, 1228–1229. doi: 10.1126/science.2970671

Glantz, L. A., and Lewis, D. A (2000). Decreased dendritic spine density on prefrontal cortical pyramidal neurons in schizophrenia. *Arch. Gen. Psychiatry* 57, 65–73. doi: 10.1001/archpsyc.57.1.65

Glass, D. J., Bowen, D. C., Stitt, T. N., Radziejewski, C., Bruno, J., Ryan, T. E., et al. (1996). Agrin acts via a MuSK receptor complex. *Cell* 85, 513–523. doi: 10.1016/s0092-8674(00)81252-0

Gogolla, N., Caroni, P., Lüthi, A., and Herry, C. (2009). Perineuronal nets protect fear memories from erasure. *Science* 325, 1258–1261. doi: 10.1126/science.1174146

Gordon, J. A., and Stryker, M. P. (1996). Experience-dependent plasticity of binocular responses in the primary visual cortex of the mouse. *J. Neurosci.* 16, 3274–3286.

Gray, E. G. (1959a). Axo-somatic and axo-dendritic synapses of the cerebral cortex: an electron microscope study. *J. Anat.* 93, 420–433.

Gray, E. G. (1959b). Electron microscopy of synaptic contacts on dendrite spines of the cerebral cortex. *Nature* 183, 1592–1593. doi: 10.1038/1831592a0

Groc, L., Choquet, D., Stephenson, F. A., Verrier, D., Manzoni, O. J., and Chavis, P. (2007). NMDA receptor surface trafficking and synaptic subunit composition are developmentally regulated by the extracellular matrix protein Reelin. *J. Neurosci.* 27, 10165–10175. doi: 10.1523/jneurosci.1772-07.2007

Grutzendler, J., Kasthuri, N., and Gan, W.-B. (2002). Long-term dendritic spine stability in the adult cortex. *Nature* 420, 812–816. doi: 10.1038/nature01276

Gschwend, T. P., Krueger, S. R., Kozlov, S. V., Wolfer, D. P., and Sonderegger, P. (1997). Neurotrypsin, a novel multidomain serine protease expressed in the nervous system. *Mol. Cell. Neurosci.* 9, 207–219. doi: 10.1006/mcne.1997.0616

Gumbiner, B. M. (1996). Cell adhesion: the molecular basis of tissue architecture and morphogenesis. *Cell* 84, 345–357. doi: 10.1016/s0092-8674(00)81279-9

Gundelfinger, E. D., Frischknecht, R., Choquet, D., and Heine, M. (2010). Converting juvenile into adult plasticity: a role for the brain's extracellular matrix. *Eur. J. Neurosci.* 31, 2156–2165. doi: 10.1111/j.1460-9568.2010.07253.x

Gurevicius, K., Gureviciene, I., Valjakka, A., Schachner, M., and Tanila, H. (2004). Enhanced cortical and hippocampal neuronal excitability in mice deficient in the extracellular matrix glycoprotein tenascin-R. *Mol. Cell. Neurosci.* 25, 515–523. doi: 10.1016/j.mcn.2003.12.001

Hack, I., Hellwig, S., Junghans, D., Brunne, B., Bock, H. H., Zhao, S., et al. (2007). Divergent roles of ApoER2 and Vldlr in the migration of cortical neurons. *Development* 134, 3883–3891. doi: 10.1242/dev.005447

Harris, K. M., and Kater, S. B. (1994). Dendritic spines: cellular specializations imparting both stability and flexibility to synaptic function. *Annu. Rev. Neurosci.* 17, 341–371. doi: 10.1146/annurev.neuro.17.1.341

Harris, K. M., and Stevens, J. K. (1988). Dendritic spines of rat cerebellar Purkinje cells: serial electron microscopy with reference to their biophysical characteristics. *J. Neurosci.* 8, 4455–4469.

Harris, K. M., and Stevens, J. K. (1989). Dendritic spines of CA 1 pyramidal cells in the rat hippocampus: serial electron microscopy with reference to their biophysical characteristics. *J. Neurosci.* 9, 2982–2997.

Harris, K. M., and Weinberg, R. J. (2012). Ultrastructure of synapses in the mammalian brain. *Cold Spring Harb. Perspect. Biol.* 4:a005587. doi: 10.1101/cshperspect.a005587

Harvey, C. D., Yasuda, R., Zhong, H., and Svoboda, K. (2008). The spread of Ras activity triggered by activation of a single dendritic spine. *Science* 321, 136–140. doi: 10.1126/science.1159675

Henry, M. D., and Campbell, K. P. (1996). Dystroglycan: an extracellular matrix receptor linked to the cytoskeleton. *Curr. Opin. Cell Biol.* 8, 625–631. doi: 10.1016/s0955-0674(96)80103-7

Hering, H., and Sheng, M. (2001). Dendritic spines: structure, dynamics and regulation. *Nat. Rev. Neurosci.* 2, 880–888. doi: 10.1038/35104061

Higley, M. J., and Sabatini, B. L. (2012). Calcium signaling in dendritic spines. *Cold Spring Harb. Perspect. Biol.* 4:a005686. doi: 10.1101/cshperspect.a005686

Hoffman, K. B., Pinkstaff, J. K., Gall, C. M., and Lynch, G. (1998). Seizure induced synthesis of fibronectin is rapid and age dependent: implications for long-term potentiation and sprouting. *Brain Res.* 812, 209–215. doi: 10.1016/s0006-8993(98)00727-6

Holtmaat, A. J. G. D., Trachtenberg, J. T., Wilbrecht, L., Shepherd, G. M., Zhang, X., Knott, G. W., et al. (2005). Transient and persistent dendritic spines in the neocortex in vivo. *Neuron* 45, 279–291. doi: 10.1016/j.neuron.2005.01.003

Horejs, C.-M., Serio, A., Purvis, A., Gormley, A. J., Bertazzo, S., Poliniewicz, A., et al. (2014). Biologically-active laminin-111 fragment that modulates the epithelial-to-mesenchymal transition in embryonic stem cells. *Proc. Natl. Acad. Sci. U S A* 111, 5908–5913. doi: 10.1073/pnas.1403139111

Horn, K. E., Glasgow, S. D., Gobert, D., Bull, S.-J., Luk, T., Girgis, J., et al. (2013). DCC expression by neurons regulates synaptic plasticity in the adult brain. *Cell Rep.* 3, 173–185. doi: 10.1016/j.celrep.2012.12.005

Horwitz, A., Duggan, K., Buck, C., Beckerle, M. C., and Burridge, K. (1986). Interaction of plasma membrane fibronectin receptor with talin—a transmembrane linkage. *Nature* 320, 531–533. doi: 10.1038/320531a0

Horwitz, A., Duggan, K., Greggs, R., Decker, C., and Buck, C. (1985). The cell substrate attachment (CSAT) antigen has properties of a receptor for laminin and fibronectin. *J. Cell Biol.* 101, 2134–2144. doi: 10.1083/jcb.101.6.2134

Huang, Y. Y., Bach, M. E., Lipp, H. P., Zhuo, M., Wolfer, D. P., Hawkins, R. D., et al. (1996). Mice lacking the gene encoding tissue-type plasminogen activator show a selective interference with late-phase long-term potentiation in both Schaffer collateral and mossy fiber pathways. *Proc. Natl. Acad. Sci. U S A* 93, 8699–8704. doi: 10.1073/pnas.93.16.8699

Huang, Z., Shimazu, K., Woo, N. H., Zang, K., Müller, U., Lu, B., et al. (2006). Distinct roles of the beta 1-class integrins at the developing and the mature hippocampal excitatory synapse. *J. Neurosci.* 26, 11208–11219. doi: 10.1523/jneurosci.3526-06.2006

Hunt, C. A., Schenker, L. J., and Kennedy, M. B. (1996). PSD-95 is associated with the postsynaptic density and not with the presynaptic membrane at forebrain synapses. *J. Neurosci.* 16, 1380–1388.

Hunter, D. D., Porter, B. E., Bulock, J. W., Adams, S. P., Merlie, J. P., and Sanes, J. R. (1989a). Primary sequence of a motor neuron-selective adhesive site in the synaptic basal lamina protein S-laminin. *Cell* 59, 905–913. doi: 10.1016/0092-8674(89)90613-2

Hunter, D. D., Shah, V., Merlie, J. P., and Sanes, J. R. (1989b). A laminin-like adhesive protein concentrated in the synaptic cleft of the neuromuscular junction. *Nature* 338, 229–234. doi: 10.1038/338229a0

Huntley, G. W., Gil, O., and Bozdagi, O. (2002). The cadherin family of cell adhesion molecules: multiple roles in synaptic plasticity. *Neuroscientist* 8, 221–233. doi: 10.1177/1073858402008003008

Iafrati, J., Orejarena, M. J., Lassalle, O., Bouamrane, L., Gonzalez-Campo, C., and Chavis, P. (2014). Reelin, an extracellular matrix protein linked to early onset psychiatric diseases, drives postnatal development of the prefrontal cortex via GluN2B-NMDARs and the mTOR pathway. *Mol. Psychiatry* 19, 417–426. doi: 10.1038/mp.2013.66

Ignatius, M. J., and Reichardt, L. F. (1988). Identification of a neuronal laminin receptor: an Mr 200K/120K integrin heterodimer that binds laminin in a divalent cation-dependent manner. *Neuron* 1, 713–725. doi: 10.1016/0896-6273(88)90170-5

Impagnatiello, F., Guidotti, A. R., Pesold, C., Dwivedi, Y., Caruncho, H., Pisu, M. G., et al. (1998). A decrease of reelin expression as a putative vulnerability factor in schizophrenia. *Proc. Natl. Acad. Sci. U S A* 95, 15718–15723. doi: 10.1073/pnas.95.26.15718

Irintchev, A., Rollenhagen, A., Troncoso, E., Kiss, J. Z., and Schachner, M. (2005). Structural and functional aberrations in the cerebral cortex of tenascin-C deficient mice. *Cereb. Cortex* 15, 950–962. doi: 10.1093/cercor/bhh195

Ishii, N., Wadsworth, W. G., Stern, B. D., Culotti, J. G., and Hedgecock, E. M. (1992). UNC-6, a laminin-related protein, guides cell and pioneer axon migrations in *C. elegans*. *Neuron* 9, 873–881. doi: 10.1016/0896-6273(92)90240-e

Jaworski, J., Biedermann, I. W., Lapinska, J., Szklarczyk, A., Figiel, I., Konopka, D., et al. (1999). Neuronal excitation-driven and AP-1-dependent activation of tissue inhibitor of metalloproteinases-1 gene expression in rodent hippocampus. *J. Biol. Chem.* 274, 28106–28112. doi: 10.1074/jbc.274.40.28106

Jones, F. S., and Jones, P. L. (2000). The tenascin family of ECM glycoproteins: structure, function and regulation during embryonic development and tissue remodeling. *Dev. Dyn.* 218, 235–259. doi: 10.1002/(sici)1097-0177(200006)218:2<235::aid-dvdy2>3.3.co;2-7

Katzman, R. (1989). Alzheimer's disease is a degenerative disorder. *Neurobiol. Aging* 10, 581–582; discussion 588–590. doi: 10.1016/0197-4580(89)90137-1

Keino-Masu, K., Masu, M., Hinck, L., Leonardo, E. D., Chan, S. S., Culotti, J. G., et al. (1996). Deleted in Colorectal Cancer (DCC) encodes a netrin receptor. *Cell* 87, 175–185. doi: 10.1016/s0092-8674(00)81336-7

Kelly, E. A., Tremblay, M.-È., Gahmberg, C. G., Tian, L., and Majewska, A. K. (2014). Subcellular localization of intercellular adhesion molecule-5 (telencephalin) in the visual cortex is not developmentally regulated in the absence of matrix metalloproteinase-9. *J. Comp. Neurol.* 522, 676–688. doi: 10.1002/cne.23440

Kennedy, M. B. (1994). The biochemistry of synaptic regulation in the central nervous system. *Annu. Rev. Biochem.* 63, 571–600. doi: 10.1146/annurev.biochem.63.1.571

Kennedy, M. B. (1997). The postsynaptic density at glutamatergic synapses. *Trends Neurosci.* 20, 264–268. doi: 10.1016/s0166-2236(96)01033-8

Kerrisk, M. E., Greer, C. A., and Koleske, A. J. (2013). Integrin $\alpha 3$ is required for late postnatal stability of dendrite arbors, dendritic spines and synapses and mouse behavior. *J. Neurosci.* 33, 6742–6752. doi: 10.1523/JNEUROSCI.0528-13.2013

Kikkawa, Y., Sasaki, T., Nguyen, M. T., Nomizu, M., Mitaka, T., and Miner, J. H. (2007). The LG1–3 tandem of laminin alpha5 harbors the binding sites of Lutheran/basal cell adhesion molecule and alpha3beta1/alpha6beta1 integrins. *J. Biol. Chem.* 282, 14853–14860. doi: 10.1074/jbc.m611706200

Koleske, A. J. (2013). Molecular mechanisms of dendrite stability. *Nat. Rev. Neurosci.* 14, 536–550. doi: 10.1038/nrn3486

Korobova, F., and Svitkina, T. (2010). Molecular architecture of synaptic actin cytoskeleton in hippocampal neurons reveals a mechanism of dendritic spine morphogenesis. *Mol. Biol. Cell* 21, 165–176. doi: 10.1091/mbc.e09-07-0596

Kruse, J., Keilhauer, G., Faissner, A., Timpl, R., and Schachner, M. (1985). The J1 glycoprotein–a novel nervous system cell adhesion molecule of the L2/HNK-1 family. *Nature* 316, 146–148. doi: 10.1038/316146a0

Ksiazek, I., Burkhardt, C., Lin, S., Seddik, R., Maj, M., Bezakova, G., et al. (2007). Synapse loss in cortex of agrin-deficient mice after genetic rescue of perinatal death. *J. Neurosci.* 27, 7183–7195. doi: 10.1523/jneurosci.1609-07.2007

Kwok, J. C. F., Dick, G., Wang, D., and Fawcett, J. W. (2011). Extracellular matrix and perineuronal nets in CNS repair. *Dev. Neurobiol.* 71, 1073–1089. doi: 10.1002/dneu.20974

Lai, C. S. W., Franke, T. F., and Gan, W.-B. (2012). Opposite effects of fear conditioning and extinction on dendritic spine remodelling. *Nature* 483, 87–91. doi: 10.1038/nature10792

Lai, K.-O., and Ip, N. Y. (2013). Structural plasticity of dendritic spines: the underlying mechanisms and its dysregulation in brain disorders. *Biochim. Biophys. Acta* 1832, 2257–2263. doi: 10.1016/j.bbadis.2013.08.012

Lai Wing Sun, K., Correia, J. P., and Kennedy, T. E. (2011). Netrins: versatile extracellular cues with diverse functions. *Development* 138, 2153–2169. doi: 10.1242/dev.044529

Lander, A. D., Fujii, D. K., and Reichardt, L. F. (1985). Purification of a factor that promotes neurite outgrowth: isolation of laminin and associated molecules. *J. Cell Biol.* 101, 898–913. doi: 10.1083/jcb.101.3.898

Leonardo, E. D., Hinck, L., Masu, M., Keino-Masu, K., Ackerman, S. L., and Tessier-Lavigne, M. (1997). Vertebrate homologues of *C. elegans* UNC-5 are candidate netrin receptors. *Nature* 386, 833–838. doi: 10.1038/386833a0

Lévi, S., Grady, R. M., Henry, M. D., Campbell, K. P., Sanes, J. R., and Craig, A. M. (2002). Dystroglycan is selectively associated with inhibitory GABAergic synapses but is dispensable for their differentiation. *J. Neurosci.* 22, 4274–4285.

Li, Z., Hilgenberg, L. G., O'Dowd, D. K., and Smith, M. A. (1999). Formation of functional synaptic connections between cultured cortical neurons from agrin-deficient mice. *J. Neurobiol.* 39, 547–557. doi: 10.1002/(sici)1097-4695(19990615)39:4<547::aid-neu8>3.0.co;2-c

Liesi, P., Dahl, D., and Vaheri, A. (1984). Neurons cultured from developing rat brain attach and spread preferentially to laminin. *J. Neurosci. Res.* 11, 241–251. doi: 10.1002/jnr.490110304

Lin, B., Arai, A. C., Lynch, G., and Gall, C. M. (2003). Integrins regulate NMDA receptor-mediated synaptic currents. *J. Neurophysiol.* 89, 2874–2878. doi: 10.1152/jn.00783.2002

Lin, Y.-C., and Koleske, A. J. (2010). Mechanisms of synapse and dendrite maintenance and their disruption in psychiatric and neurodegenerative disorders. *Annu. Rev. Neurosci.* 33, 349–378. doi: 10.1146/annurev-neuro-060909-153204

Liston, C., Cichon, J. M., Jeanneteau, F., Jia, Z., Chao, M. V., and Gan, W.-B. (2013). Circadian glucocorticoid oscillations promote learning-dependent synapse formation and maintenance. *Nat. Neurosci.* 16, 698–705. doi: 10.1038/nn.3387

Liu, W. S., Pesold, C., Rodriguez, M. A., Carboni, G., Auta, J., Lacor, P., et al. (2001). Down-regulation of dendritic spine and glutamic acid decarboxylase 67 expressions in the reelin haploinsufficient heterozygous reeler mouse. *Proc. Natl. Acad. Sci. U S A* 98, 3477–3482. doi: 10.1073/pnas.051614698

Lochner, J. E., Honigman, L. S., Grant, W. F., Gessford, S. K., Hansen, A. B., Silverman, M. A., et al. (2006). Activity-dependent release of tissue plasminogen activator from the dendritic spines of hippocampal neurons revealed by live-cell imaging. *J. Neurobiol.* 66, 564–577. doi: 10.1002/neu.20250

Lonskaya, I., Partridge, J., Lalchandani, R. R., Chung, A., Lee, T., Vicini, S., et al. (2013). Soluble ICAM-5, a product of activity dependent proteolysis, increases mEPSC frequency and dendritic expression of GluA1. *PLoS One* 8:e69136. doi: 10.1371/journal.pone.0069136

Madani, R., Hulo, S., Toni, N., Madani, H., Steimer, T., Muller, D., et al. (1999). Enhanced hippocampal long-term potentiation and learning by increased neuronal expression of tissue-type plasminogen activator in transgenic mice. *EMBO J.* 18, 3007–3012. doi: 10.1093/emboj/18.11.3007

Majewska, A. K., Brown, E., Ross, J., and Yuste, R. (2000). Mechanisms of calcium decay kinetics in hippocampal spines: role of spine calcium pumps and calcium diffusion through the spine neck in biochemical compartmentalization. *J. Neurosci.* 20, 1722–1734.

Majewska, A. K., and Sur, M. (2003). Motility of dendritic spines in visual cortex in vivo: changes during the critical period and effects of visual deprivation. *Proc. Natl. Acad. Sci. U S A* 100, 16024–16029. doi: 10.1073/pnas.2636949100

Manthorpe, M., Engvall, E., Ruoslahti, E., Longo, F. M., Davis, G. E., and Varon, S. (1983). Laminin promotes neuritic regeneration from cultured peripheral and central neurons. *J. Cell Biol.* 97, 1882–1890. doi: 10.1083/jcb.97.6.1882

Martin, P. T., Ettinger, A. J., and Sanes, J. R. (1995). A synaptic localization domain in the synaptic cleft protein laminin beta 2 (s-laminin). *Science* 269, 413–416. doi: 10.1126/science.7618109

Mataga, N., Mizuguchi, Y., and Hensch, T. K. (2004). Experience-dependent pruning of dendritic spines in visual cortex by tissue plasminogen activator. *Neuron* 44, 1031–1041. doi: 10.1016/j.neuron.2004.11.028

Mataga, N., Nagai, N., and Hensch, T. K. (2002). Permissive proteolytic activity for visual cortical plasticity. *Proc. Natl. Acad. Sci. U S A* 99, 7717–7721. doi: 10.1073/pnas.102088899

Matsumoto-Miyai, K., Sokolowska, E., Zurlinden, A., Gee, C. E., Lüscher, D., Hettwer, S., et al. (2009). Coincident pre- and postsynaptic activation induces dendritic filopodia via neurotrypsin-dependent agrin cleavage. *Cell* 136, 1161–1171. doi: 10.1016/j.cell.2009.02.034

Matsuzaki, M., Ellis-Davies, G. C., Nemoto, T., Miyashita, Y., Iino, M., and Kasai, H. (2001). Dendritic spine geometry is critical for AMPA receptor expression in hippocampal CA1 pyramidal neurons. *Nat. Neurosci.* 4, 1086–1092. doi: 10.1038/nn736

Matsuzaki, M., Honkura, N., Ellis-Davies, G. C. R., and Kasai, H. (2004). Structural basis of long-term potentiation in single dendritic spines. *Nature* 429, 761–766. doi: 10.1038/nature02617

McCroskery, S., Bailey, A., Lin, L., and Daniels, M. P. (2009). Transmembrane agrin regulates dendritic filopodia and synapse formation in mature hippocampal neuron cultures. *Neuroscience* 163, 168–179. doi: 10.1016/j.neuroscience.2009.06.012

McCroskery, S., Chaudhry, A., Lin, L., and Daniels, M. P. (2006). Transmembrane agrin regulates filopodia in rat hippocampal neurons in culture. *Mol. Cell. Neurosci.* 33, 15–28. doi: 10.1016/j.mcn.2006.06.004

Meighan, S. E., Meighan, P. C., Choudhury, P., Davis, C. J., Olson, M. L., Zornes, P. A., et al. (2006). Effects of extracellular matrix-degrading proteases matrix metalloproteinases 3 and 9 on spatial learning and synaptic plasticity. *J. Neurochem.* 96, 1227–1241. doi: 10.1111/j.1471-4159.2005.03565.x

Michaluk, P., Wawrzyniak, M., Alot, P., Szczot, M., Wyrembek, P., Mercik, K., et al. (2011). Influence of matrix metalloproteinase MMP-9 on dendritic spine morphology. *J. Cell Sci.* 124, 3369–3380. doi: 10.1242/jcs.090852

Missler, M., Südhof, T. C., and Biederer, T. (2012). Synaptic cell adhesion. *Cold Spring Harb. Perspect. Biol.* 4:a005694. doi: 10.1101/cshperspect.a005694

Mitsui, S., Osako, Y., Yokoi, F., Dang, M. T., Yuri, K., Li, Y., et al. (2009). A mental retardation gene, motopsin/neurotrypsin/prss12, modulates hippocampal function and social interaction. *Eur J. Neurosci.* 30, 2368–2378. doi: 10.1111/j.1460-9568.2009.07029.x

Molinari, F., Rio, M., Meskenaite, V., Encha-Razavi, F., Augé, J., Bacq, D., et al. (2002). Truncating neurotrypsin mutation in autosomal recessive non-syndromic mental retardation. *Science* 298, 1779–1781. doi: 10.1126/science.1076521

Morimoto, K., Fahnestock, M., and Racine, R. J. (2004). Kindling and status epilepticus models of epilepsy: rewiring the brain. *Prog. Neurobiol.* 73, 1–60. doi: 10.1016/j.pneurobio.2004.03.009

Moser, M., Legate, K. R., Zent, R., and Fässler, R. (2009). The tail of integrins, talin and kindlins. *Science* 324, 895–899. doi: 10.1126/science.1163865

Mühleisen, T. W., Mattheisen, M., Strohmaier, J., Degenhardt, F., Priebe, L., Schultz, C. C., et al. (2012). Association between schizophrenia and common variation in neurocan (NCAN), a genetic risk factor for bipolar disorder. *Schizophr. Res.* 138, 69–73. doi: 10.1016/j.schres.2012.03.007

Murakoshi, H., Wang, H., and Yasuda, R. (2011). Local, persistent activation of Rho GTPases during plasticity of single dendritic spines. *Nature* 472, 100–104. doi: 10.1038/nature09823

Murakoshi, H., and Yasuda, R. (2012). Postsynaptic signaling during plasticity of dendritic spines. *Trends Neurosci.* 35, 135–143. doi: 10.1016/j.tins.2011.12.002

Nägerl, U. V., Eberhorn, N., Cambridge, S. B., and Bonhoeffer, T. (2004). Bidirectional activity-dependent morphological plasticity in hippocampal neurons. *Neuron* 44, 759–767. doi: 10.1016/j.neuron.2004.11.016

Nagy, V., Bozdagi, O., Matynia, A., Balcerzyk, M., Okulski, P., Dzwonek, J., et al. (2006). Matrix metalloproteinase-9 is required for hippocampal late-phase long-term potentiation and memory. *J. Neurosci.* 26, 1923–1934. doi: 10.1523/jneurosci.4359-05.2006

Nakagami, Y., Abe, K., Nishiyama, N., and Matsuki, N. (2000). Laminin degradation by plasmin regulates long-term potentiation. *J. Neurosci.* 20, 2003–2010.

Nakic, M., Manahan-Vaughan, D., Reymann, K. G., and Schachner, M. (1998). Long-term potentiation in vivo increases rat hippocampal tenascin-C expression. *J. Neurobiol.* 37, 393–404. doi: 10.1002/(sici)1097-4695(19981115)37:3<393::aid-neu5>3.3.co;2-0

Nedivi, E., Hevroni, D., Naot, D., Israeli, D., and Citri, Y. (1993). Numerous candidate plasticity-related genes revealed by differential cDNA cloning. *Nature* 363, 718–722. doi: 10.1038/363718a0

Nicholson, C., and Syková, E. (1998). Extracellular space structure revealed by diffusion analysis. *Trends Neurosci.* 21, 207–215. doi: 10.1016/s0166-2236(98)01261-2

Nicole, O., Docagne, F., Ali, C., Margaill, I., Carmeliet, P., MacKenzie, E. T., et al. (2001). The proteolytic activity of tissue-plasminogen activator enhances NMDA receptor-mediated signaling. *Nat. Med.* 7, 59–64. doi: 10.1038/83358

Nikonenko, A., Schmidt, S., Skibo, G., Brückner, G., and Schachner, M. (2003). Tenascin-R-deficient mice show structural alterations of symmetric perisomatic synapses in the CA1 region of the hippocampus. *J. Comp. Neurol.* 456, 338–349. doi: 10.1002/cne.10537

Nishimune, H., Sanes, J. R., and Carlson, S. S. (2004). A synaptic laminin-calcium channel interaction organizes active zones in motor nerve terminals. *Nature* 432, 580–587. doi: 10.1038/nature03112

Nishimune, H., Valdez, G., Jarad, G., Moulson, C. L., Müller, U., Miner, J. H., et al. (2008). Laminins promote postsynaptic maturation by an autocrine mechanism at the neuromuscular junction. *J. Cell Biol.* 182, 1201–1215. doi: 10.1083/jcb.200805095

Niu, S., Yabut, O., and D'Arcangelo, G. (2008). The Reelin signaling pathway promotes dendritic spine development in hippocampal neurons. *J. Neurosci.* 28, 10339–10348. doi: 10.1523/JNEUROSCI.1917-08.2008

Noguchi, J., Matsuzaki, M., Ellis-Davies, G. C. R., and Kasai, H. (2005). Spine-neck geometry determines NMDA receptor-dependent Ca2+ signaling in dendrites. *Neuron* 46, 609–622. doi: 10.1016/j.neuron.2005.03.015

O'Connor, L. T., Lauterborn, J. C., Gall, C. M., and Smith, M. A. (1994). Localization and alternative splicing of agrin mRNA in adult rat brain: transcripts encoding lsoforms that aggregate acetylcholine receptors are not restricted to cholinergic regions. *J. Neurosci.* 14, 1141–1152.

Oh, W. C., Hill, T. C., and Zito, K. (2013). Synapse-specific and size-dependent mechanisms of spine structural plasticity accompanying synaptic weakening. *Proc. Natl. Acad. Sci. U S A* 110, E305–E312. doi: 10.1073/pnas.1214705110

Oray, S., Majewska, A. K., and Sur, M. (2004). Dendritic spine dynamics are regulated by monocular deprivation and extracellular matrix degradation. *Neuron* 44, 1021–1030. doi: 10.1016/j.neuron.2004.12.001

Orlando, C., Ster, J., Gerber, U., Fawcett, J. W., and Raineteau, O. (2012). Perisynaptic chondroitin sulfate proteoglycans restrict structural plasticity in an integrin-dependent manner. *J. Neurosci.* 32, 18009–18017, 18017a. doi: 10.1523/JNEUROSCI.2406-12.2012

Otey, C. A., and Burridge, K. (1990). Patterning of the membrane cytoskeleton by the extracellular matrix. *Semin. Cell Biol.* 1, 391–399.

Pan, F., Aldridge, G. M., Greenough, W. T., and Gan, W.-B. (2010). Dendritic spine instability and insensitivity to modulation by sensory experience in a mouse model of fragile X syndrome. *Proc. Natl. Acad. Sci. U S A* 107, 17768–17773. doi: 10.1073/pnas.1012496107

Pang, P. T., Teng, H. K., Zaitsev, E., Woo, N. T., Sakata, K., Zhen, S., et al. (2004). Cleavage of proBDNF by tPA/plasmin is essential for long-term hippocampal plasticity. *Science* 306, 487–491. doi: 10.1126/science.1100135

Pappas, G. D., Kriho, V., and Pesold, C. (2001). Reelin in the extracellular matrix and dendritic spines of the cortex and hippocampus: a comparison between wild type and heterozygous reeler mice by immunoelectron microscopy. *J. Neurocytol.* 30, 413–425. doi: 10.1023/A:1015017710332

Patton, B. L., Cunningham, J. M., Thyboll, J., Kortesmaa, J., Westerblad, H., Edström, L., et al. (2001). Properly formed but improperly localized synaptic specializations in the absence of laminin alpha4. *Nat. Neurosci.* 4, 597–604. doi: 10.1038/88414

Patton, B. L., Miner, J. H., Chiu, A. Y., and Sanes, J. R. (1997). Distribution and function of laminins in the neuromuscular system of developing, adult and mutant mice. *J. Cell Biol.* 139, 1507–1521. doi: 10.1083/jcb.139.6.1507

Pawlak, R., Rao, B. S. S., Melchor, J. P., Chattarji, S., McEwen, B., and Strickland, S. (2005). Tissue plasminogen activator and plasminogen mediate stress-induced decline of neuronal and cognitive functions in the mouse hippocampus. *Proc. Natl. Acad. Sci. U S A* 102, 18201–18206. doi: 10.1073/pnas.0509232102

Pizzorusso, T., Medini, P., Berardi, N., Chierzi, S., Fawcett, J. W., and Maffei, L. (2002). Reactivation of ocular dominance plasticity in the adult visual cortex. *Science* 298, 1248–1251. doi: 10.1126/science.1072699

Pizzorusso, T., Medini, P., Landi, S., Baldini, S., Berardi, N., and Maffei, L. (2006). Structural and functional recovery from early monocular deprivation in adult rats. *Proc. Natl. Acad. Sci. U S A* 103, 8517–8522. doi: 10.1073/pnas.0602657103

Pribiag, H., Peng, H., Shah, W. A., Stellwagen, D., and Carbonetto, S. (2014). Dystroglycan mediates homeostatic synaptic plasticity at GABAergic synapses. *Proc. Natl. Acad. Sci. U S A* 111, 6810–6815. doi: 10.1073/pnas.1321774111

Pujadas, L., Gruart, A., Bosch, C., Delgado, L., Teixeira, C. M., Rossi, D., et al. (2010). Reelin regulates postnatal neurogenesis and enhances spine hypertrophy and long-term potentiation. *J. Neurosci.* 30, 4636–4649. doi: 10.1523/JNEUROSCI.5284-09.2010

Pujadas, L., Rossi, D., Andrés, R., Teixeira, C. M., Serra-Vidal, B., Parcerisas, A., et al. (2014). Reelin delays amyloid-beta fibril formation and rescues cognitive deficits in a model of Alzheimer's disease. *Nat. Commun.* 5:3443. doi: 10.1038/ncomms4443

Qian, Z., Gilbert, M. E., Colicos, M. A., Kandel, E. R., and Kuhl, D. (1993). Tissue-plasminogen activator is induced as an immediate-early gene during seizure, kindling and long-term potentiation. *Nature* 361, 453–457. doi: 10.1038/361453a0

Qiu, S., Korwek, K. M., Pratt-Davis, A. R., Peters, M., Bergman, M. Y., and Weeber, E. J. (2006a). Cognitive disruption and altered hippocampus synaptic function in Reelin haploinsufficient mice. *Neurobiol. Learn. Mem.* 85, 228–242. doi: 10.1016/j.nlm.2005.11.001

Qiu, S., and Weeber, E. J. (2007). Reelin signaling facilitates maturation of CA1 glutamatergic synapses. *J. Neurophysiol.* 97, 2312–2321. doi: 10.1152/jn.00869.2006

Qiu, S., Zhao, L. F., Korwek, K. M., and Weeber, E. J. (2006b). Differential reelin-induced enhancement of NMDA and AMPA receptor activity in the adult hippocampus. *J. Neurosci.* 26, 12943–12955. doi: 10.1523/jneurosci.2561-06.2006

Reif, R., Sales, S., Hettwer, S., Dreier, B., Gisler, C., Wölfel, J., et al. (2007). Specific cleavage of agrin by neurotrypsin, a synaptic protease linked to mental retardation. *FASEB J.* 21, 3468–3478. doi: 10.1096/fj.07-8800com

Rivera, S., Tremblay, E., Timsit, S., Canals, O., Ben-Ari, Y., and Khrestchatisky, M. (1997). Tissue inhibitor of metalloproteinases-1 (TIMP-1) is differentially induced in neurons and astrocytes after seizures: evidence for developmental, immediate early gene and lesion response. *J. Neurosci.* 17, 4223–4235.

Rodriguez, M. A., Pesold, C., Liu, W. S., Kriho, V., Guidotti, A., Pappas, G. D., et al. (2000). Colocalization of integrin receptors and reelin in dendritic spine postsynaptic densities of adult nonhuman primate cortex. *Proc. Natl. Acad. Sci. U S A* 97, 3550–3555. doi: 10.1073/pnas.97.7.3550

Rogers, J. T., Rusiana, I., Trotter, J., Zhao, L., Donaldson, E., Pak, D. T. S., et al. (2011). Reelin supplementation enhances cognitive ability, synaptic plasticity and dendritic spine density. *Learn. Mem.* 18, 558–564. doi: 10.1101/lm.2153511

Rogers, J. T., Zhao, L., Trotter, J. H., Rusiana, I., Peters, M. M., Li, Q., et al. (2013). Reelin supplementation recovers sensorimotor gating, synaptic plasticity and associative learning deficits in the heterozygous reeler mouse. *J. Psychopharmacol.* 27, 386–395. doi: 10.1177/0269881112463468

Ruoslahti, E. (1996a). Brain extracellular matrix. *Glycobiology* 6, 489–492. doi: 10.1093/glycob/6.5.489

Ruoslahti, E. (1996b). RGD and other recognition sequences for integrins. *Annu. Rev. Cell Dev. Biol.* 12, 697–715. doi: 10.1146/annurev.cellbio.12.1.697

Ruoslahti, E., and Pierschbacher, M. D. (1987). New perspectives in cell adhesion: RGD and integrins. *Science* 238, 491–497. doi: 10.1126/science.2821619

Sabatini, B. L., Oertner, T. G., and Svoboda, K. (2002). The life cycle of Ca(2+) ions in dendritic spines. *Neuron* 33, 439–452. doi: 10.1016/s0896-6273(02)00573-1

Saghatelyan, A. K., Dityatev, A., Schmidt, S., Schuster, T., Bartsch, U., and Schachner, M. (2001). Reduced perisomatic inhibition, increased excitatory transmission and impaired long-term potentiation in mice deficient for the extracellular matrix glycoprotein tenascin-R. *Mol. Cell. Neurosci.* 17, 226–240. doi: 10.1006/mcne.2000.0922

Saghatelyan, A. K., Gorissen, S., Albert, M., Hertlein, B., Schachner, M., and Dityatev, A. (2000). The extracellular matrix molecule tenascin-R and its HNK-1 carbohydrate modulate perisomatic inhibition and long-term potentiation in the CA1 region of the hippocampus. *Eur. J. Neurosci.* 12, 3331–3342. doi: 10.1046/j.1460-9568.2000.00216.x

Saghatelyan, A. K., Snapyan, M., Gorissen, S., Meigel, I., Mosbacher, J., Kaupmann, K., et al. (2003). Recognition molecule associated carbohydrate inhibits postsynaptic GABA(B) receptors: a mechanism for homeostatic regulation of GABA release in perisomatic synapses. *Mol. Cell. Neurosci.* 24, 271–282. doi: 10.1016/s1044-7431(03)00163-5

Samuel, M. A., Valdez, G., Tapia, J. C., Lichtman, J. W., and Sanes, J. R. (2012). Agrin and synaptic laminin are required to maintain adult neuromuscular junctions. *PLoS One* 7:e46663. doi: 10.1371/journal.pone.0046663

Sanes, J. R. (1982). Laminin, fibronectin and collagen in synaptic and extrasynaptic portions of muscle fiber basement membrane. *J. Cell Biol.* 93, 442–451. doi: 10.1083/jcb.93.2.442

Sanes, J. R., and Lichtman, J. W. (2001). Induction, assembly, maturation and maintenance of a postsynaptic apparatus. *Nat. Rev. Neurosci.* 2, 791–805. doi: 10.1038/35097557

Sappino, A. P., Madani, R., Huarte, J., Belin, D., Kiss, J. Z., Wohlwend, A., et al. (1993). Extracellular proteolysis in the adult murine brain. *J. Clin. Invest.* 92, 679–685. doi: 10.1172/jci116637

Sato, S., Omori, Y., Katoh, K., Kondo, M., Kanagawa, M., Miyata, K., et al. (2008). Pikachurin, a dystroglycan ligand, is essential for photoreceptor ribbon synapse formation. *Nat. Neurosci.* 11, 923–931. doi: 10.1038/nn.2160

Satz, J. S., Ostendorf, A. P., Hou, S., Turner, A., Kusano, H., Lee, J. C., et al. (2010). Distinct functions of glial and neuronal dystroglycan in the developing and adult mouse brain. *J. Neurosci.* 30, 14560–14572. doi: 10.1523/jneurosci.3247-10.2010

Scheetz, A. J., and Constantine-Paton, M. (1994). Modulation of NMDA receptor function: implications for vertebrate neural development. *FASEB J.* 8, 745–752.

Scheff, S. W., and Price, D. A. (2003). Synaptic pathology in Alzheimer's disease: a review of ultrastructural studies. *Neurobiol. Aging* 24, 1029–1046. doi: 10.1016/j.neurobiolaging.2003.08.002

Schneiders, F. I., Maertens, B., Böse, K., Li, Y., Brunken, W. J., Paulsson, M., et al. (2007). Binding of netrin-4 to laminin short arms regulates basement membrane assembly. *J. Biol. Chem.* 282, 23750–23758. doi: 10.1074/jbc.m703137200

Schwartz, M. A. (2010). Integrins and extracellular matrix in mechanotransduction. *Cold Spring Harb. Perspect. Biol.* 2:a005066. doi: 10.1101/cshperspect.a005066

Schwartz, M. A., and Horwitz, A. R. (2006). Integrating adhesion, protrusion, and contraction during cell migration. *Cell* 125, 1223–1225. doi: 10.1016/j.cell.2006.06.015

Seeds, N. W., Basham, M. E., and Ferguson, J. E. (2003). Absence of tissue plasminogen activator gene or activity impairs mouse cerebellar motor learning. *J. Neurosci.* 23, 7368–7375.

Sekine, K., Kawauchi, T., Kubo, K.-I., Honda, T., Herz, J., Hattori, M., et al. (2012). Reelin controls neuronal positioning by promoting cell-matrix adhesion via inside-out activation of integrin $\alpha5\beta1$. *Neuron* 76, 353–369. doi: 10.1016/j.neuron.2012.07.020

Serafini, T., Colamarino, S. A., Leonardo, E. D., Wang, H., Beddington, R., Skarnes, W. C., et al. (1996). Netrin-1 is required for commissural axon guidance in the developing vertebrate nervous system. *Cell* 87, 1001–1014. doi: 10.1016/s0092-8674(00)81795-x

Serafini, T., Kennedy, T. E., Galko, M. J., Mirzayan, C., Jessell, T. M., and Tessier-Lavigne, M. (1994). The netrins define a family of axon outgrowth-promoting proteins homologous to *C. elegans* UNC-6. *Cell* 78, 409–424. doi: 10.1016/0092-8674(94)90420-0

Serpinskaya, A. S., Feng, G., Sanes, J. R., and Craig, A. M. (1999). Synapse formation by hippocampal neurons from agrin-deficient mice. *Dev. Biol.* 205, 65–78. doi: 10.1006/dbio.1998.9112

Sfakianos, M. K., Eisman, A., Gourley, S. L., Bradley, W. D., Scheetz, A. J., Settleman, J., et al. (2007). Inhibition of Rho via Arg and p190RhoGAP in the postnatal mouse hippocampus regulates dendritic spine maturation, synapse and dendrite stability and behavior. *J. Neurosci.* 27, 10982–10992. doi: 10.1523/jneurosci.0793-07.2007

Sheng, M., and Kim, E. (2011). The postsynaptic organization of synapses. *Cold Spring Harb. Perspect. Biol.* 3:a005678. doi: 10.1101/cshperspect.a005678

Shi, Y., and Ethell, I. M. (2006) Integrins control dendritic spine plasticity in hippocampal neurons through NMDA receptor and Ca2+/calmodulin-dependent protein kinase II-mediated actin reorganization. *J. Neurosci.* 26, 1813–1822. doi: 10.1523/jneurosci.4091-05.2006

Sidhu, H., Dansie, L. E., Hickmott, P. W., Ethell, D. W., and Ethell, I. M. (2014). Genetic removal of matrix metalloproteinase 9 rescues the symptoms of fragile x syndrome in a mouse model. *J. Neurosci.* 34, 9867–9879. doi: 10.1523/jneurosci.1162-14.2014

Sloniowski, S., and Ethell, I. M. (2012). Looking forward to EphB signaling in synapses. *Semin. Cell Dev. Biol.* 23, 75–82. doi: 10.1016/j.semcdb.2011.10.020

Smalheiser, N. R., and Schwartz, N. B. (1987). Cranin: a laminin-binding protein of cell membranes. *Proc. Natl. Acad. Sci. U S A* 84, 6457–6461. doi: 10.1073/pnas.84.18.6457

Smith, C. J., Watson, J. D., VanHoven, M. K., Colón-Ramos, D. A., and Miller, D. M. (2012). Netrin (UNC-6) mediates dendritic self-avoidance. *Nat. Neurosci.* 15, 731–737. doi: 10.1038/nn.3065

Soleman, S., Filippov, M. A., Dityatev, A., and Fawcett, J. W. (2013). Targeting the neural extracellular matrix in neurological disorders. *Neuroscience* 253, 194–213. doi: 10.1016/j.neuroscience.2013.08.050

Stanco, A., Szekeres, C., Patel, N., Rao, S., Campbell, K., Kreidberg, J. A., et al. (2009). Netrin-1-alpha3beta1 integrin interactions regulate the migration of interneurons through the cortical marginal zone. *Proc. Natl. Acad. Sci. U S A* 106, 7595–7600. doi: 10.1073/pnas.0811343106

Staubli, U., Vanderklish, P., and Lynch, G. (1990). An inhibitor of integrin receptors blocks long-term potentiation. *Behav. Neural Biol.* 53, 1–5. doi: 10.1016/0163-1047(90)90712-f

Stawarski, M., Stefaniuk, M., and Wlodarczyk, J. (2014). Matrix metalloproteinase-9 involvement in the structural plasticity of dendritic spines. *Front. Neuroanat.* 8:68. doi: 10.3389/fnana.2014.00068

Stephan, A., Mateos, J. M., Kozlov, S. V., Cinelli, P., Kistler, A. D., Hettwer, S., et al. (2008). Neurotrypsin cleaves agrin locally at the synapse. *FASEB J.* 22, 1861–1873. doi: 10.1096/fj.07-100008

Strekalova, T., Sun, M., Sibbe, M., Evers, M., Dityatev, A., Gass, P., et al. (2002). Fibronectin domains of extracellular matrix molecule tenascin-C modulate hippocampal learning and synaptic plasticity. *Mol. Cell. Neurosci.* 21, 173–187. doi: 10.1006/mcne.2002.1172

Strickland, S. (2001). Tissue plasminogen activator in nervous system function and dysfunction. *Thromb. Haemost.* 86, 138–143.

Sung, U., O'Rear, J. J., and Yurchenco, P. D. (1993). Cell and heparin binding in the distal long arm of laminin: identification of active and cryptic sites with recombinant and hybrid glycoprotein. *J. Cell Biol.* 123, 1255–1268. doi: 10.1083/jcb.123.5.1255

Szepesi, Z., Hosy, E., Ruszczycki, B., Bijata, M., Pyskaty, M., Bikbaev, A., et al. (2014). Synaptically released matrix metalloproteinase activity in control of structural plasticity and the cell surface distribution of GluA1-AMPA receptors. *PLoS One* 9:e98274. doi: 10.1371/journal.pone.0098274

Szklarczyk, A., Lapinska, J., Rylski, M., McKay, R. D. G., and Kaczmarek, L. (2002). Matrix metalloproteinase-9 undergoes expression and activation during dendritic remodeling in adult hippocampus. *J. Neurosci.* 22, 920–930.

Takasaki, K., and Sabatini, B. L. (2014). Super-resolution 2-photon microscopy reveals that the morphology of each dendritic spine correlates with diffusive but not synaptic properties. *Front. Neuroanat.* 8:29. doi: 10.3389/fnana.2014.00029

Tamkun, J. W., DeSimone, D. W., Fonda, D., Patel, R. S., Buck, C., Horwitz, A. F., et al. (1986). Structure of integrin, a glycoprotein involved in the transmembrane linkage between fibronectin and actin. *Cell* 46, 271–282. doi: 10.1016/0092-8674(86)90744-0

Tan, C. L., Kwok, J. C. F., Patani, R., Ffrench-Constant, C., Chandran, S., and Fawcett, J. W. (2011). Integrin activation promotes axon growth on inhibitory chondroitin sulfate proteoglycans by enhancing integrin signaling. *J. Neurosci.* 31, 6289–6295. doi: 10.1523/jneurosci.0008-11.2011

Tawil, N., Wilson, P., and Carbonetto, S. (1993). Integrins in point contacts mediate cell spreading: factors that regulate integrin accumulation in point contacts vs. focal contacts. *J. Cell Biol.* 120, 261–271. doi: 10.1083/jcb.120.1.261

Terry, R. D., Masliah, E., Salmon, D. P., Butters, N., DeTeresa, R., Hill, R., et al. (1991). Physical basis of cognitive alterations in Alzheimer's disease: synapse loss is the major correlate of cognitive impairment. *Ann. Neurol.* 30, 572–580. doi: 10.1002/ana.410300410

Tian, L., Stefanidakis, M., Ning, L., Van Lint, P., Nyman-Huttunen, H., Libert, C., et al. (2007). Activation of NMDA receptors promotes dendritic spine development through MMP-mediated ICAM-5 cleavage. *J. Cell Biol.* 178, 687–700. doi: 10.1083/jcb.200612097

Tissir, F., and Goffinet, A. M. (2003). Reelin and brain development. *Nat. Rev. Neurosci.* 4, 496–505. doi: 10.1038/nrn1113

Tønnesen, J., Katona, G., Rózsa, B., and Nägerl, U. V. (2014). Spine neck plasticity regulates compartmentalization of synapses. *Nat. Neurosci.* 17, 678–685. doi: 10.1038/nn.3682

Trachtenberg, J. T., Chen, B. E., Knott, G. W., Feng, G., Sanes, J. R., Welker, E., et al. (2002). Long-term in vivo imaging of experience-dependent synaptic plasticity in adult cortex. *Nature* 420, 788–794. doi: 10.1038/nature01273

Trotter, J. H., Klein, M., Jinwal, U. K., Abisambra, J. F., Dickey, C. A., Tharkur, J., et al. (2011). ApoER2 function in the establishment and maintenance of retinal synaptic connectivity. *J. Neurosci.* 31, 14413–14423. doi: 10.1523/jneurosci.3135-11.2011

Tueting, P., Costa, E., Dwivedi, Y., Guidotti, A., Impagnatiello, F., Manev, R., et al. (1999). The phenotypic characteristics of heterozygous reeler mouse. *Neuroreport* 10, 1329–1334. doi: 10.1097/00001756-199904260-00032

Ventruti, A., Kazdoba, T. M., Niu, S., and D'Arcangelo, G. (2011). Reelin deficiency causes specific defects in the molecular composition of the synapses in the adult brain. *Neuroscience* 189, 32–42. doi: 10.1016/j.neuroscience.2011.05.050

Visse, R., and Nagase, H. (2003). Matrix metalloproteinases and tissue inhibitors of metalloproteinases: structure, function and biochemistry. *Circ. Res.* 92, 827–839. doi: 10.1161/01.res.0000070112.80711.3d

Walikonis, R. S., Jensen, O. N., Mann, M., Provance, D. W., Mercer, J. A., and Kennedy, M. B. (2000). Identification of proteins in the postsynaptic density fraction by mass spectrometry. *J. Neurosci.* 20, 4069–4080.

Wang, X.-B., Bozdagi, O., Nikitczuk, J. S., Zhai, Z. W., Zhou, Q., and Huntley, G. W. (2008). Extracellular proteolysis by matrix metalloproteinase-9 drives dendritic spine enlargement and long-term potentiation coordinately. *Proc. Natl. Acad. Sci. U S A* 105, 19520–19525. doi: 10.1073/pnas.0807248105

Wang, N., Butler, J. P., and Ingber, D. E. (1993). Mechanotransduction across the cell surface and through the cytoskeleton. *Science* 260, 1124–1127. doi: 10.1126/science.7684161

Warren, M. S., Bradley, W. D., Gourley, S. L., Lin, Y.-C., Simpson, M. A., Reichardt, L. F., et al. (2012). Integrin $\beta 1$ signals through Arg to regulate postnatal dendritic arborization, synapse density and behavior. *J. Neurosci.* 32, 2824–2834. doi: 10.1523/JNEUROSCI.3942-11.2012

Washbourne, P., Dityatev, A., Scheiffele, P., Biederer, T., Weiner, J. A., Christopherson, K. S., et al. (2004). Cell adhesion molecules in synapse formation. *J. Neurosci.* 24, 9244–9249. doi: 10.1523/jneurosci.3339-04.2004

Wegner, F., Härtig, W., Bringmann, A., Grosche, J., Wohlfarth, K., Zuschratter, W., et al. (2003). Diffuse perineuronal nets and modified pyramidal cells immunoreactive for glutamate and the GABA(A) receptor alpha1 subunit form a unique entity in rat cerebral cortex. *Exp. Neurol.* 184, 705–714. doi: 10.1016/s0014-4886(03)00313-3

Wiesel, T. N., and Hubel, D. H. (1963). Single cell responses in striate cortex of kittens deprived of vision in one eye. *J. Neurophysiol.* 26, 1003–1017.

Wilczynski, G. M., Konopacki, F. A., Wilczek, E., Lasiecka, Z., Gorlewicz, A., Michaluk, P., et al. (2008). Important role of matrix metalloproteinase 9 in epileptogenesis. *J. Cell Biol.* 180, 1021–1035. doi: 10.1083/jcb.200708213

Wlodarczyk, J., Mukhina, I., Kaczmarek, L., and Dityatev, A. (2011). Extracellular matrix molecules, their receptors, and secreted proteases in synaptic plasticity. *Dev. Neurobiol.* 71, 1040–1053. doi: 10.1002/dneu.20958

Wright, K. M., Lyon, K. A., Leung, H., Leahy, D. J., Ma, L., and Ginty, D. D. (2012). Dystroglycan organizes axon guidance cue localization and axonal pathfinding. *Neuron* 76, 931–944. doi: 10.1016/j.neuron.2012.10.009

Wu, S. H., Arévalo, J. C., Sarti, F., Tessarollo, L., Gan, W.-B., and Chao, M. V. (2009). Ankyrin repeat-rich membrane spanning/kidins220 protein regulates dendritic branching and spine stability in vivo. *Dev. Neurobiol.* 69, 547–557. doi: 10.1002/dneu.20723

Wu, Y., Chen, L., Zheng, P.-S., and Yang, B. B. (2002). beta 1-Integrin-mediated glioma cell adhesion and free radical-induced apoptosis are regulated by binding to a C-terminal domain of PG-M/versican. *J. Biol. Chem.* 277, 12294–12301. doi: 10.1074/jbc.m110748200

Wu, Y. P., Siao, C. J., Lu, W., Sung, T. C., Frohman, M. A., Milev, P., et al. (2000). The tissue plasminogen activator (tPA)/plasmin extracellular proteolytic system regulates seizure-induced hippocampal mossy fiber outgrowth through a proteoglycan substrate. *J. Cell Biol.* 148, 1295–1304. doi: 10.1083/jcb.148.6.1295

Yamada, H., Watanabe, K., Shimonaka, M., and Yamaguchi, Y. (1994). Molecular cloning of brevican, a novel brain proteoglycan of the aggrecan/versican family. *J. Biol. Chem.* 269, 10119–10126.

Yebra, M., Montgomery, A. M. P., Diaferia, G. R., Kaido, T., Silletti, S., Perez, B., et al. (2003). Recognition of the neural chemoattractant Netrin-1 by integrins alpha6beta4 and alpha3beta1 regulates epithelial cell adhesion and migration. *Dev. Cell* 5, 695–707. doi: 10.1016/s1534-5807(03)00330-7

Yousif, L. F., Di Russo, J., and Sorokin, L. (2013). Laminin isoforms in endothelial and perivascular basement membranes. *Cell Adh. Migr.* 7, 101–110. doi: 10.4161/cam.22680

Yuste, R., Majewska, A. K., and Holthoff, K. (2000). From form to function: calcium compartmentalization in dendritic spines. *Nat. Neurosci.* 3, 653–659. doi: 10.1038/76609

Zhai, S., Ark, E. D., Parra-Bueno, P., and Yasuda, R. (2013). Long-distance integration of nuclear ERK signaling triggered by activation of a few dendritic spines. *Science* 342, 1107–1111. doi: 10.1126/science.1245622

Zhou, X. H., Brakebusch, C., Matthies, H., Oohashi, T., Hirsch, E., Moser, M., et al. (2001). Neurocan is dispensable for brain development. *Mol. Cell. Biol.* 21, 5970–5978. doi: 10.1128/mcb.21.17.5970-5978.2001

Zhou, Q., Homma, K. J., and Poo, M.-M. (2004). Shrinkage of dendritic spines associated with long-term depression of hippocampal synapses. *Neuron* 44, 749–757. doi: 10.1016/j.neuron.2004.11.011

Ziv, N. E., and Smith, S. J. (1996). Evidence for a role of dendritic filopodia in synaptogenesis and spine formation. *Neuron* 17, 91–102. doi: 10.1016/s0896-6273(00)80283-4

Zuo, Y., Lin, A., Chang, P., and Gan, W. B. (2005a). Development of long-term dendritic spine stability in diverse regions of cerebral cortex. *Neuron* 46, 181–189. doi: 10.1016/j.neuron.2005.04.001

Zuo, Y., Yang, G., Kwon, E., and Gan, W.-B. (2005b). Long-term sensory deprivation prevents dendritic spine loss in primary somatosensory cortex. *Nature* 436, 261–265. doi: 10.1038/nature03715

13

Barriers in the brain: resolving dendritic spine morphology and compartmentalization

Max Adrian[1], Remy Kusters[2], Corette J. Wierenga[1], Cornelis Storm[2,3], Casper C. Hoogenraad[1] and Lukas C. Kapitein[1]*

[1] Cell Biology, Department of Biology, Faculty of Science, Utrecht University, Utrecht, Netherlands
[2] Department of Applied Physics, Eindhoven University of Technology, Eindhoven, Netherlands
[3] Institute for Complex Molecular Systems, Eindhoven University of Technology, Eindhoven, Netherlands

***Correspondence:**
Lukas C. Kapitein, Cell Biology, Department of Biology, Faculty of Science, Utrecht University, Padualaan 8, Utrecht, 3584 CH, Netherlands
e-mail: l.kapitein@uu.nl

Dendritic spines are micron-sized protrusions that harbor the majority of excitatory synapses in the central nervous system. The head of the spine is connected to the dendritic shaft by a 50–400 nm thin membrane tube, called the spine neck, which has been hypothesized to confine biochemical and electric signals within the spine compartment. Such compartmentalization could minimize interspinal crosstalk and thereby support spine-specific synapse plasticity. However, to what extent compartmentalization is governed by spine morphology, and in particular the diameter of the spine neck, has remained unresolved. Here, we review recent advances in tool development – both experimental and theoretical – that facilitate studying the role of the spine neck in compartmentalization. Special emphasis is given to recent advances in microscopy methods and quantitative modeling applications as we discuss compartmentalization of biochemical signals, membrane receptors and electrical signals in spines. Multidisciplinary approaches should help to answer how dendritic spine architecture affects the cellular and molecular processes required for synapse maintenance and modulation.

Keywords: dendritic spine, super-resolution microscopy, compartment, diffusion, modeling

INTRODUCTION: DENDRITIC SPINES

The dendritic compartment of a neuron receives input from thousands of upstream neurons via synapses. The majority of excitatory inputs in the central nervous system are located at dendritic spines. Spines are micron-sized protrusions along the dendritic shaft and have first been described about a century ago by Ramón y Cajal (1888). They are composed of a spine head and a thin spine neck that connects them to the dendritic shaft. Typical dimensions are ~<1 μm for the head diameter, and a ~100 nm wide and ~1 μm long spine neck, but notable differences in spine morphology exist (Bourne and Harris, 2008). Based on electron microscopy (EM), three shape categories have been defined: thin, filopodia-like protrusions ("thin spines"), short spines without a well-defined spine neck ("stubby spines") and spines with a large bulbous head ("mushroom spines") (Bourne and Harris, 2008). Importantly, spine shape is not static, but can change, even throughout adulthood, reflecting the plastic nature of synaptic connections. For example, neuronal activity *in vitro* and experience *in vivo* can alter spine morphology (Holtmaat and Svoboda, 2009). Changes in spine size are thought to be generally correlated with changes in the strength of the excitatory synapse (Schikorski and Stevens, 1999; Arellano et al., 2007). Such functional and structural changes of spines and synapses are believed to be at the core of learning and memory in the brain (Yuste and Bonhoeffer, 2001; Holtmaat and Svoboda, 2009; Kasai et al., 2010).

The actin cytoskeleton plays a key role in shaping dendritic spines and is critically important for numerous processes that contribute to the plasticity of synaptic function (Matus, 2000; Hering and Sheng, 2001; Luo, 2002; Ethell and Pasquale, 2005; Hotulainen and Hoogenraad, 2010). The rapid polymerization and depolymerization of actin filaments produces protrusive forces that can quickly change neuronal morphology (Kessels et al., 2011). For example, during spine enlargement, rapid actin polymerization provides the mechanical force required for pushing out the spine membrane (Bosch and Hayashi, 2012). In addition, the actin cytoskeleton provides tracks for myosin-based transport of various cellular materials in and out of spines, including AMPA-type glutamate receptors (Kneussel and Wagner, 2013).

The mechanisms through which spine shape affects its function are not yet fully understood. At its minimum, morphological changes associated with synaptic modulation could just be a secondary effect of altered actin dynamics required to more directly modulate synapse functioning or actin-based transport. Nevertheless, modeling studies have often emphasized the interesting effects that shape can have on the diffusion of proteins, calcium ions and other signaling molecules (Holcman and Schuss, 2011). A small neck should slow diffusion and result in functional compartmentalization by preventing signaling molecules to escape from the spine. In addition, more recent modeling studies report that shape should also affect lateral diffusion of proteins embedded in the plasma membrane (Kusters et al., 2013). Several studies have indeed reported evidence for compartmentalization, but the extent to which this was governed by shape alone could often not be directly assessed because the limited resolution of live-cell light microscopy did not allow to directly correlate diffusion dynamics and spine shape. Recent breakthroughs in fluorescence microscopy allow imaging at resolutions below the diffraction limit, allowing to directly explore how spine shape affects diffusion of cytoplasmic or membrane-embedded molecules (Takasaki and Sabatini, 2014; Tønnesen et al., 2014). In this review, we first discuss existing and emerging technologies to image spine morphology. We then present existing evidence for the compartmentalization in spines. Finally, we discuss how different aspects of spine shape contribute to compartmentalization, with an emphasis on recent modeling studies exploring the influence of shape on lateral diffusion in the membrane.

IMAGING SPINE MORPHOLOGY

Ramón y Cajal (1899-1904) discovered dendritic spines using light microscopy of neurons stained using Golgi impregnation and he suggested these small protrusions to be sites of neuronal signal transmission. His hypothesis was confirmed with the development of EM during the interwar, which allowed imaging at much higher resolution (Gray, 1959). Subsequent refinements of this technology, especially the careful analysis of series of thin tissue sections in serial-sectioning EM, allowed a full morphological description of dendritic spines and have provided many beautiful insights into spine architecture (Bourne and Harris, 2008). Serial-sectioning EM directly visualizes all tissue surrounding spines as well as the structure of the postsynaptic specialization and has been used to identify precise morphological changes upon specific stimuli (Bourne and Harris, 2008). However, the use of EM also has several limitations. First of all, sample preparation procedures and imaging conditions prevent imaging of living tissue. In addition, different preparation procedures can easily introduce artifacts (Bourne and Harris, 2012) and also the labeling of specific proteins has so far remained challenging and very inefficient. Therefore, to study dynamics of spines or specific proteins associated with spines, live-cell fluorescence microscopy is the method of choice.

CONVENTIONAL LIVE CELL IMAGING

Both laser-scanning and spinning disk confocal microscopy are standard techniques to study spine dynamics in dissociated neurons. For imaging in tissue, however, these techniques impose several limitations. Visible light penetrates poorly into tissue and is quickly distorted, resulting in a rapid loss of resolution with increased focus depth because the focus size is no longer diffraction-limited. In addition, many focal planes need to be imaged sequentially to reconstruct complete neurons in three dimensions. Because exposure to excitation light is not restricted to the plane in focus, this results in increased phototoxicity and photobleaching, limiting sample life time and signal intensity.

Two-photon microscopy overcomes both of these limitations through the use of a pulsed infrared light source that excites fluorophores by the combined energy of two photons arriving on the sample nearly simultaneously (Denk et al., 1990; Svoboda et al., 1996). Infrared light is much less distorted and penetrates deeper into the sample compared to visible light. As two-photon excitation efficiency scales quadratically with excitation intensity, it is largely limited to the focus plane and prevents photobleaching of out-of-focus planes. Two-photon microscopy rapidly became the method of choice for deep tissue imaging and has even enabled intravital brain imaging in mice (Svoboda and Yasuda, 2006). However, despite its unique advantages, the resolution of two-photon microscopy is still inherently limited by diffraction to 400–500 nm. Therefore, several studies have combined two-photon live imaging with *post hoc* serial sectioning EM to examine the microstructure of spine, for example to directly demonstrate synapse formation associated with the emergence of a new spine during live imaging (Trachtenberg et al., 2002; Holtmaat et al., 2006; Bourne and Harris, 2012). As this requires fixing the sample, this approach might not detect all morphological changes that occur upon specific stimuli and is prone to morphological artifacts. To better study these processes, live-cell imaging beyond the diffraction limit is required.

LIVE-CELL IMAGING BEYOND THE DIFFRACTION BARRIER

The diffraction of light limits the ability of microscopes to resolve the location of two objects that are located closer to each other than approximately half the wavelength of the light used for imaging. For conventional fluorescence microscopy using visible light this limit lays around 200–300 nanometers. Over the last years, different technologies have allowed fluorescence microscopy at a resolution below the diffraction limit (Hell, 2007). Dendritic spines have frequently been used for proof-of-principle applications of these techniques, because of their small size and physiological relevance. Indeed, careful analysis of spine morphologies using superresolution microscopy has demonstrated that conventional light microscopy methods overestimate the amount of stubby spines in acute and organotypical slice cultures (Tønnesen et al., 2014). Here, we highlight several techniques that have recently contributed to novel insights into spine morphodynamics and synapse architecture.

Stimulated Emission Depletion (STED) microscopy was developed as an extension of confocal microscopy. The conventional excitation beam is complemented with a depletion beam that forms a donut shaped spot surrounding the focus of the excitation beam (Klar et al., 2000; Hell, 2007). The wavelength of the depletion beam is chosen within the tail of the emission spectrum of the imaged fluorophore. It brings fluorophores excited by the excitation laser back to their ground-state by inducing stimulated emission at exactly the wavelength of the depletion beam. As a result, fluorescence emission at all other wavelengths of the emission spectrum is restricted to the center of the donut. Importantly, the size of this zone is not limited by diffraction. Therefore, scanning the lasers with very small steps over the sample improves the resolution of the final image up to 50 nm (Klar et al., 2000; Hell, 2007).

The first STED images of spines in organotypical slices expressing yellow fluorescent protein (YFP) in a sparse subset of neurons were published in 2008 (Nägerl et al., 2008).

Neck diameters of spines located at 0–10 μm depth were originally measured to be on average ~40% reduced compared to confocal imaging (Nägerl et al., 2008), whereas more recent measurements have found neck diameters as low as 51 nm in organotypic cultures and 59 nm in acute slices (Tønnesen et al., 2014). Recently, STED microscopy has also been established *in vivo* in mouse brain (Berning et al., 2012).

The STED principle can also be applied to two-photon microscopy (Moneron and Hell, 2009). However, the depletion wavelength needs to be within the (visible) emission spectrum and is therefore prone to distortions. Nevertheless, it has been successfully applied to dendritic spines in organotypical slices, resulting in 60–150 nm lateral resolution at 50–100 μm depths, but without improving the axial resolution (Ding et al., 2009; Bethge et al., 2013; Takasaki et al., 2013). In addition, two-color detection has been established using spectral unmixing of either pairs of organic dyes (Tønnesen et al., 2011) or the fluorescent proteins YFP and GFP (Bethge et al., 2013). None of the techniques described here improve the axial resolution. However, development of three-dimensional depletion patterns and compensation of optical distortions through adaptive optics promise improvements in the near future (Gould et al., 2012; Loew and Hell, 2013).

Inducing stimulated emission requires very high light intensities, which can induce artifacts and phototoxicity in the imaged sample. To circumvent this, a comparable technique reduces the size of the confocal volume using a specifically engineered fluorescent protein that can transition to a non-fluorescent dark state (RESOLFT: reversible saturable/switchable optical transitions; Grotjohann et al., 2011). This approach requires orders of magnitude of less light intensity and has been demonstrated on living brain slices (Testa et al., 2012). Novel probes are currently being developed that should allow two-color RESOLFT of dendritic spines (Lavoie-Cardinal et al., 2014; Shcherbakova et al., 2014).

Another set of powerful techniques to achieve resolutions beyond the diffraction barrier uses switchable fluorophores or special imaging conditions to ensure that only a small, random subset of fluorophores in the sample is emitting at any given time (Huang et al., 2009). Because these fluorophores are then distributed sparsely enough to be clearly separated, their positions can be obtained from their point spread function with 1–10 nm accuracy. Repeating this procedure thousands of times for different subsets of fluorophores in the region of interest eventually allows reconstructing a superresolved image from the calculated positions. This basic concept of repetitive detection of small subsets has been applied in many different ways and these techniques are collectively referred to as single-molecule localization microscopy (SMLM), of which the most prominent variants are known as PALM, STORM and dSTORM (Huang, 2010). These techniques are often used on fixed samples, because the temporal resolution is limited by the repetitive detection and the required excitation intensities are high. Nevertheless, several groups have succeeded in live-imaging of dendritic spines using these techniques: spine morphology has been probed using labeled antibodies against membrane-bound proteins (Giannone et al., 2010; Ries et al., 2012), using genetically encoded fluorophores that either directly label or transiently bind to actin (Frost et al., 2010; Izeddin et al., 2011), or using a lipophilic cyanine dye that labels the plasma membrane (Shim et al., 2012). In all cases, live super-resolution microscopy requires some thoughtful compromises between temporal and spatial resolution (Frost et al., 2012).

DENDRITIC SPINES FORM DYNAMIC COMPARTMENTS

In principle, there may be several advantages of having substructures like dendritic spines containing synapses along the dendrite. First of all, spines might facilitate connectivity by bridging the physical gap between slightly distant axons and dendrites. However, not all neurons have spines (e.g., stellate neurons) and they can receive excitatory input directly on their shafts (Anderson et al., 1994). It is therefore likely that spines have additional functions. Ever since their discovery by Ramón y Cajal (1899-1904), it has been suggested that spines may play a role in the compartmentalization of synaptic signals. Such compartmentalization may facilitate spine-specific plasticity and thereby regulate the individual strength of synaptic connections (Yuste and Denk, 1995; Matsuzaki et al., 2004; Holtmaat and Svoboda, 2009; Araya et al., 2014). Compartmentalization of spines has been reported on three levels that we discuss in detail in this section: (1) from a molecular and cell biological perspective, signaling cascades elicited by synaptic stimulation may be confined to single spines, making them biochemical signaling compartments that confine structural plasticity to individual spines; (2) spines may also compartmentalize neurotransmitter receptors, both by opposing their diffusion out of spines and by maintaining spine-selective intracellular storage pools, in order to directly regulate the sensitivity of a synapse to stimulations; and (3) lastly, spines may serve as an electrical compartment, playing a role in the processing of synaptic depolarization from synapses along the dendrite.

COMPARTMENTALIZATION OF BIOCHEMICAL SIGNALING

The compartmentalization of spines is most easily studied by measuring the extent to which fluorescent dyes, specific proteins or ions exchange between a spine and the parent dendrite. We first discuss studies that examined the cytoplasmic coupling between spines and the dendritic shaft as a general measure of spine head isolation. In addition, we review the evidence for specific biochemical compartmentalization of calcium ions and signaling molecules.

Diffusional coupling between spine and dendrite

Using two-photon fluorescence recovery after photobleaching (FRAP) microscopy on hippocampal neurons filled with fluorescent dyes in cultured slices, early studies found that spines can indeed compartmentalize cytoplasm as fluorescence recovery rates in dendritic spines are significantly lower than in the shaft (Svoboda et al., 1996). Repeated activation of a photo-activatable variant of GFP (PA-GFP) in individual spines showed substantial variation in the cytoplasmic coupling of individual spines over time that may be regulated by neuronal activity. In a small population of spines, no exchange of soluble fluorescent proteins between shaft and spine heads could be measured during a period of several minutes (Bloodgood and Sabatini, 2005). Whereas in these earlier studies the exact relation between spine shape and cytoplasmic coupling could not be resolved, recent experiments have used STED microscopy to correlate spine morphology and cytoplasmic diffusion kinetics (see Section Spine Necks as Barriers).

In addition to the exchange of soluble dyes and fluorescent proteins between spines and dendrites, the diffusion of calcium ions has also been studied extensively (Bloodgood and Sabatini, 2007a). Calcium ions play a crucial role in initiating downstream signaling during long-term potentiation (LTP) and depression (LTD) and influx of calcium is both necessary and sufficient for structural synaptic plasticity (Pettit et al., 1994; Lledo et al., 1995; Otmakhov et al., 2004). Pioneering two-photon microscopy of calcium dynamics in slices of hippocampal neurons revealed that synaptic stimulation results in accumulation of calcium ions in single spines (Yuste and Denk, 1995). The extent to which the diffusion kinetics of calcium ions are regulated by spine morphology and neck width in particular is debated in the literature. Importantly, when calcium is bound to buffering proteins like calmodulin, the diffusion of the resulting complex is more sensitive to spatial constraints than single ions because of its larger size (Sabatini et al., 2002; Tønnesen et al., 2014). In addition to diffusion into the dendritic shaft, calcium can also be removed from spines by absorption into the smooth endoplasmic reticulum located in spines or by Na/Ca exchangers located in the plasma membrane (Sabatini et al., 2002). These processes help to confine transient calcium ions to the spine head. Nevertheless, morphology does play a role, as long and thin necks prevent the diffusion of calcium, whereas shorter and thicker necks allow for better diffusional coupling with the dendrite (Majewska et al., 2000; Holthoff et al., 2002; Sabatini et al., 2002; Korkotian et al., 2004; Noguchi et al., 2005).

Other factors influencing the local calcium concentrations in spines are the surface to volume ratio of spines and the localization of calcium-permeable ion channels (Sabatini et al., 2002). If these ion channels were distributed equally throughout the plasma membrane, one would expect a higher effective concentration of these channels in spines compared to dendrites as the surface-to-volume ratio of the former is higher. This should theoretically lead to a higher influx of calcium in spines than in the surrounding dendrite (Sabatini et al., 2002). Such an effect is strengthened by the existence of classes of voltage gated calcium channels that exclusively localize to spines but not dendrites and cooperate with other calcium channels to shape local depolarization and synaptic plasticity (Bloodgood and Sabatini, 2007b; Bloodgood et al., 2009).

Spatial restriction of signaling domains

Calcium ions in dendritic spines have an important function in activating signaling cascades that underlie and regulate synaptic plasticity (Kennedy et al., 2005). Their retention in an individual stimulated spine may thus be important to induce downstream signaling and structural plasticity in a synapse-specific manner. CaMKII is a calcium-activated kinase involved in structural plasticity by remodeling of the postsynaptic density (Yoshimura et al., 2002), rearrangement of the actin cytoskeleton (Okamoto et al., 2007) and maintenance of spine enlargement (Matsuzaki et al., 2004; Lee et al., 2009). Downstream of CaMKII, Ras and Rho GTPases are important for regulating spine morphology (Ramakers, 2002; Saneyoshi et al., 2010) and synaptic strength (Zhu et al., 2002; Patterson et al., 2010). It is thought that Rho activation causes spine loss and shrinkage by inhibiting actin polymerization, whereas Cdc42 and Rac activation increase the number of spines by promoting actin polymerization. The precise crosstalk and integration is however not completely understood (Kennedy et al., 2005).

To explore the activity of signaling molecules, activity sensors can be used in which the amount of Förster Resonance Energy Transfer (FRET) between two fluorophores is different between active and inactive conformations. FRET is the process in which an excited donor molecule transfers energy to an acceptor fluorophore, whose excitation spectrum overlaps with the emission spectrum of the donor. The efficiency of this energy transfer is very sensitive to the distance between both fluorophores, which should be within the 2–5 nm range. Energy transfer can be detected either by the appearance of red-shifted emission from the acceptor, or by a decrease in the excited state life time of the donor. In a series of papers, Yasuda and co-workers have used activity reporters for different signaling molecules and measured their fluorescence lifetimes by two-photon microscopy (2P-FRET-FLIM) in cultured hippocampal slices. Additionally, using photoactivatable protein tags, the diffusion kinetics of the same proteins could be measured in spines. This combination of techniques allowed recording activity patterns for CaMKII (Lee et al., 2009), Ras (Harvey et al., 2008), RhoA and Cdc42 (Murakoshi et al., 2011) in dendritic spines following local glutamate uncaging. Intriguingly, these signaling molecules show different activity patterns: while CaMKII and Cdc42 activities are confined to the stimulated dendritic spine (Lee et al., 2009; Murakoshi et al., 2011), Ras and RhoA activities spread along the parent dendrite. Ras activity was shown to invade typically 10–20 neighboring spines in a range of 10 μm along the dendrite, whereas RhoA activity only spread 5 μm and rarely invaded neighboring spines (Harvey et al., 2008; Murakoshi et al., 2011). Thus, despite all being triggered by NMDA-dependent calcium influx, these molecules have quite different signaling ranges. The spread of their signaling activity depends on three factors: (1) the extent and persistence of the upstream activation event; (2) the diffusion rate of the signaling molecule; and (3) its inactivation kinetics, see **Figure 1**.

Upon single-spine glutamate uncaging, the activation of CaMKII peaked within 6 s and only lasted for a few minutes (Lee et al., 2009). The diffusional coupling of CaMKII with the dendrite was significantly slower, in the range of several minutes (Lee et al., 2009), and additional modeling studies have shown that the effective CaMKII diffusion constant depends heavily on binding to synaptic scaffolds and the actin cytoskeleton in spine necks (Byrne et al., 2011). Thus, because inactivation of CaMKII has faster kinetics than CaMKII diffusion, activity of the kinase is restricted to stimulated spines. It should be noted that these results based on single spine stimulations contrast earlier

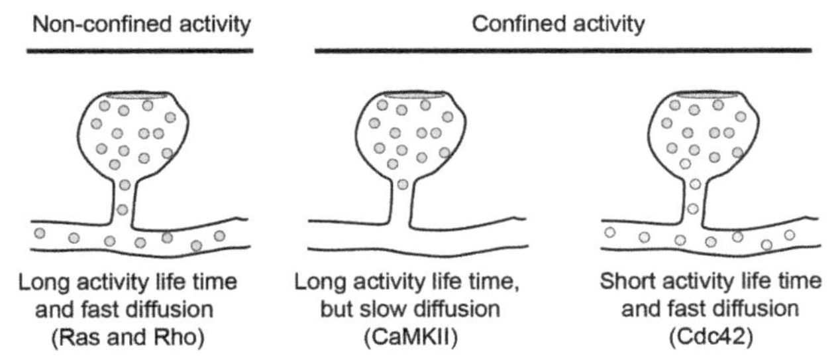

FIGURE 1 | Diffusion models for signaling molecules in spines. The spread of active signaling molecules (green) with long activity life-times depends on their diffusion rate. Limiting the activity life time of signaling molecules is an orthogonal approach to confine signaling activity to individual spines.

biochemical studies that reported persistent phosphorylation of CaMKII upon more global induction of LTP (Fukunaga et al., 1995; Barria et al., 1997; Lisman and Zhabotinsky, 2001).

The activation of Ras measured by FRET-FLIM was dependent on CaMKII activation, peaked later, and recovered to baseline level only after 15 min. Its diffusion rate out of the spine was relatively fast, reaching the dendrite within seconds without leaving any immobile fraction in the spine (Harvey et al., 2008). Together, this explains why Ras activity can spread to neighboring synapses.

Both Cdc42 and Rho showed a rapid activity peak 30 s after stimulation followed by decay over 5 min and a sustained lower activity for more than 30 min. Also the diffusion kinetics of both molecules were comparable and similar to Ras diffusion and showed no immobile fraction left in the spine. Nevertheless, Cdc42 activity remained spatially confined, because it had an intrinsic inactivation time constant of 6 s and therefore depends on continuous activation by CaMKII (Murakoshi et al., 2011). In contrast, Rho inactivated five times slower and could therefore spread into the dendrite. Thus, the specific combinations of activity life-time and diffusion kinetics can explain why CaMKII and Cdc42 activities are restricted to spine heads whereas Ras and Rho activities spread along the dendrite.

From the examples of CaMKII, Ras and Rho it becomes clear that the interplay between diffusion and activity of the signaling proteins is highly coordinated in dendritic spines. This is crucial because these signaling events are thought to coordinate local processes in the stimulated spine. CaMKII-Cdc42-Pak signaling increases spine volume and synaptic strength (Murakoshi et al., 2011), while Rho signaling leads to local AMPA receptor integration in the dendrite (Patterson et al., 2010). In addition, Rho-Rock and Ras-ERK signaling pathways lower the threshold for LTP in neighboring spines (Zhu et al., 2002; Harvey and Svoboda, 2007; Harvey et al., 2008; Lee et al., 2009). In potentiated spines, the structural rearrangement of spine morphology during LTP slows the diffusional coupling between spines and dendrites even further (Tønnesen et al., 2014). Taken together, this highly controlled signaling network allows precise spatiotemporal activation and retention of calcium-induced signaling.

COMPARTMENTALIZATION OF MEMBRANE-BOUND RECEPTORS

Another aspect of compartmentalization in individual spines is the distribution of membrane and membrane-bound proteins. Controlled addition and removal of AMPA-type glutamate receptors from the postsynaptic density is believed to underlie the changes in synaptic strength during learning and memory formation (Malinow and Malenka, 2002; Sheng and Kim, 2002; Bredt and Nicoll, 2003; Collingridge et al., 2004). Whereas reports based on static EM suggested that glutamate receptors are restricted to synapses (Nusser, 2000), live-cell imaging techniques like FRAP and single molecule tracking changed this view radically (Richards et al., 2004; Triller and Choquet, 2005). Lateral diffusion of receptors through the plasma membrane and activity-triggered exocytosis of receptors from internal endosomal compartments have become generally accepted regulation mechanisms for synaptic plasticity, although their respective contributions have remained unresolved (Passafaro et al., 2001; Borgdorff and Choquet, 2002; Adesnik et al., 2005; Ashby et al., 2006; Park et al., 2006; Ehlers et al., 2007; Heine et al., 2008; Newpher and Ehlers, 2008; Yang et al., 2008; Kennedy et al., 2010; Opazo and Choquet, 2011; Czöndör et al., 2012; Czöndör and Thoumine, 2013). Here, we focus on the contribution of lateral diffusion of glutamate receptors and its regulation during structural plasticity of dendritic spines.

The study of bulk AMPA receptor mobility has been greatly facilitated by the generation of a pH sensitive GFP variant, called superecliptic pHluorin (SEP; Miesenböck et al., 1998; Ashby et al., 2004), whose fluorescence is quenched in the acidified endosomal compartments, but not in the extracellular environment after incorporation into the plasma membrane. Studying the FRAP dynamics of a fusion of SEP with the AMPA receptor subunit GluA2 (SEP-GluA2) revealed that receptor turnover in spines is slower compared to non-spinal plasma membrane and that recovery in the spine neck and base is particularly slow (Ashby et al., 2006). Furthermore, fluorescently-tagged plasma membrane probes in spines of different morphologies showed a faster recovery rate in stubby than in mushroom-shaped spines (Richards et al., 2004; Ashby et al., 2006), indicating that mushroom-shaped spines form a membrane compartment in which diffusion is slowed. Combining SEP-GluA1 photobleaching experiments with glutamate uncaging in organotypic slices revealed that synaptic potentiation of AMPA receptors is achieved by restricting their diffusion out of the synaptic membrane (Makino and Malinow, 2009). In addition, a live SMLM study showed reduced diffusion speeds of plasma membrane markers in spine necks (Shim et al., 2012). Together these data indicate that the spine neck is a general diffusion barrier for membrane-bound proteins which, together with the regulated retention of receptors in the synapse, regulates receptor diffusion in the spine compartment.

Another approach to study receptor dynamics in dendritic spines uses single-particle tracking. Membrane-bound receptor movements are followed with extracellular probes, e.g., antibodies or derived fragments, coupled to fluorescent reporters (Triller and Choquet, 2005). The earliest report used latex beads coupled to GluA2 receptors and found that these receptors reversibly stop at synaptic sites. This is modulated by neuronal activity levels that affect calcium transients in the cell. Calcium elevations were shown to generally slow diffusion and locally accumulate AMPA receptors (Borgdorff and Choquet, 2002). However the large size of the beads (~200 nm) precluded a more detailed analysis of receptor motility in spines and synaptic membrane domains. Fluorescently labelled glutamate receptor antibodies were subsequently used to address diffusion kinetics in synaptic and extrasynaptic regions. A pool of synaptic receptors was shown to be immobile while another synaptic pool and extrasynaptic receptors were rapidly moving. Glutamate stimulation enhances the exchange between these pools and increases overall motility of glutamate receptors (Tardin et al., 2003). Long-term tracking of receptor movements was facilitated by using quantum-dots (QD) as fluorescent probes, which have the advantage of relatively small diameters and good photostability allowing bleaching-free imaging over prolonged times (Dahan et al., 2003). AMPA receptors tagged with QDs were reported to selectively reduce their mobility at active synapse while they freely diffused through non-active synapses (Ehlers et al., 2007). The same study observed reduced exchange of single receptor molecules between spines during stimulation. In addition, recent studies have shown that glutamate receptors localize to submicron scale clusters within the synaptic membrane as shown by various techniques ranging from EM to PALM microscopy (Ehlers et al., 2007; MacGillavry et al., 2013; Nair et al., 2013).

How exactly synaptic recruitment and localization of glutamate receptors are regulated is currently under debate. Whereas previously the cytoplasmic tails of GluA receptors have been shown to differentially regulate receptor diffusion and trapping at synapses (Passafaro et al., 2001), a recent study suggests that truncated receptors void of any cytoplasmic tail can rescue the depletion of endogenous GluA1-3 (Granger et al., 2013). Even though the physiological relevance of these experiments has been debated (Sheng et al., 2013), the observed diffusional trapping of truncated receptors in the spine head is interesting as it requires an intrinsic property of the spine to accumulate transmembrane proteins. Based on results from modeling (Renner et al., 2009) it has been suggested that crowding in the spine head may contribute to this phenomenon (Colgan and Yasuda, 2014). In addition, trapping of receptors may be facilitated by the curvature of plasma membrane in spines (Kusters et al., 2013), as discussed in detail below.

COMPARTMENTALIZATION OF ELECTRICAL SIGNALS

In addition to inducing compartmentalization of biochemical signals and receptors, it has been suggested that dendritic spines may also serve as electrical compartments (Segev and Rall, 1998; Yuste, 2013). As small protrusions connected to a large dendrite, spines may be theoretically described as sealed-end cables with an intrinsic asymmetry in conducting electric signals. This means that voltage signals from the dendrite propagate without attenuation into the spines (Holthoff et al., 2010; Carter et al., 2012; Popovic et al., 2014), but synaptic potentials generated inside the spine head are filtered when they travel to the dendrite (Araya et al., 2006, 2014; Harnett et al., 2012). In addition, the high input resistance of spines may further facilitate synaptic potentials inside spines compared to equally strong synapses onto the dendritic shaft. However, how much of these effects contribute to the compartmentalization of synaptic potentials in spines is strongly debated, as most of the relevant parameters, such as spine neck resistance, are simply not known and experimentally inaccessible at present times.

Because voltage and calcium imaging at single spine resolution has long been technically challenging, the majority of available literature either discusses theoretical work or indirectly calculated spine neck resistances based on diffusional coupling of cytoplasm (Shepherd, 1996; Svoboda et al., 1996; Tsay and Yuste, 2004) and often relies on static morphology data from EM (Harris and Stevens, 1988; Koch and Zador, 1993). The resulting values for the spine neck resistance have varied over a wide range and are strongly influenced by the methods and theoretical models used. Most recently, STED microscopy on dendritic spines in organotypic and acute slices suggested that electric compartmentalization is moderate, but not absent, in most spines (Takasaki and Sabatini, 2014; Tønnesen et al., 2014). For the final answer we will probably need to wait until it is possible to directly measure synaptic potentials in spines and nearby dendrites with voltage-sensitive dyes.

Interestingly, induction of plasticity not only results in an increase in spine size (Matsuzaki et al., 2004; Tanaka et al., 2008), but also in changes in spine shape (Grunditz et al., 2008), with consequences for compartmentalization. It was shown that reduction of spine neck length after synaptic potentiation mediates enhanced electric coupling of spine and dendrite, thereby increasing the influence of the potentiated spine on the dendritic and somatic membrane potential (Araya et al., 2014; Tønnesen et al., 2014). Interestingly, it was suggested that the reduction in electrical compartmentalization occurs while chemical compartmentalization is preserved, reflecting two separate functions of spines within the dendrite.

In addition to passive amplification of synaptic potentials, spines are thought to be able to actively contribute to local membrane voltage. Voltage-dependent ion channels are present within spines and activation of these channels results in a change of local membrane potential. Opening of sodium and calcium channels boosts local depolarization (Araya et al., 2007; Bloodgood et al., 2009; Holbro et al., 2010; Carter et al., 2012; Hao and Oertner, 2012), while opening of potassium channels decreases local input resistance and results in smaller synaptic potentials (Ngo-Anh et al., 2005; Giessel and Sabatini, 2010). These active properties of dendritic spines are thought to play an important role in the interactions between multiple synaptic inputs in dendritic computation (Araya et al., 2007; Harnett et al., 2012).

SPINE MORPHOLOGY AS COMPARTMENTALIZATION MECHANISM

We have summarized the evidence for spine-based compartmentalization on three levels: biochemical signaling, membrane-bound receptor dynamics and electrical signaling. All of these levels contribute to proper information processing in the dendritic arbor and are interconnected. However, the exact mechanisms through which spines can regulate different aspects of compartmentalization have remained unclear. Do reduced diffusion rates depend on dedicated barriers imposed by specific protein-based structures, similar to the way in which the axon initial segment forms a barrier for axon entry? Or is the shape of spines sufficient to confine both membrane-based and cytoplasmic diffusion? How exactly do these processes depend on spine neck diameter and spine neck length? In addition, the effect of spine neck constriction on vesicle transport through neck has remained largely unexplored. In this section, we first discuss the role of the spine neck in diffusional coupling with the dendrite and then focus on recent studies showing that spine morphology directly influences lateral diffusion of membrane-bound proteins to and from the synapse. Finally, we discuss the effect of spine shape on vesicular transport into spines.

SPINE NECKS AS BARRIERS

Conventional two-photon microscopy has a limited resolution that prevents accurate description of spine shape. Several pioneering studies have recently used STED microscopy (Ding et al., 2009; Bethge et al., 2013; Takasaki et al., 2013) to overcome this problem and studied the correlation between spine morphology and diffusional coupling to dendrites by analyzing the recovery of fluorescence after photobleaching of soluble fluorophores in the spine (Takasaki and Sabatini, 2014; Tønnesen et al., 2014, see **Figure 2**). Both studies suggest that the recovery time scale τ roughly follows what would be expected if diffusion is governed largely by spine geometry:

$$\tau = \frac{V * L}{D * A}$$

where V denotes the volume of the spine head, D the diffusion coefficient, and L and A the length and cross-sectional area of the neck, respectively. Indeed, both groups find an inverse relation between spine neck diameter d and the recovery time, which appears to follow the predicted inverse quadratic relation ($\tau \propto 1/d^2$). However, whereas the equation suggests a linear increase of the recovery time scale with spine head volume, Takasaki and Sabatini (2014) instead find a weak decrease. Similarly, Tønnesen et al. (2014) report a quadratic dependence on head width w, whereas the model predicts a w^3 dependence (assuming a spherical spine head in which $V \propto w^3$). Interestingly, a fraction of spines strongly deviated from the average trends that were observed (Takasaki and Sabatini, 2014), suggesting that small local constrictions, local protein accumulations and organelle positioning in the neck may create additional diffusion barriers (Arellano et al., 2007; Yuste, 2013). Nonetheless, these important studies demonstrate that the constriction of the spine neck alone has a major impact on crosstalk between spine and dendrite.

Membrane-bound proteins like glutamate receptors are restricted in their passage through the spine neck, as we discussed in the Section Compartmentalization of Membrane-bound Receptors. Such restriction has several causes: in addition to the direct influence of the spine morphology on membrane proteins that we discuss in the next section (Kusters et al., 2013), several cell-biological factors including molecular crowing, corralling and receptor retention in synaptic scaffolds have been studied in recent years. The postsynaptic density is believed to regulate the number of glutamate receptors localized in the synapse and thereby preventing their diffusion out of the spine (Opazo and Choquet, 2011). Additionally, the high density of proteins in the synapse may reduce diffusion rates of all membrane-bound proteins including glutamate receptors due to crowding (Santamaria et al., 2010). Cell adhesion complexes have also been identified as diffusion barriers for membrane proteins (O'Brien et al., 1999; Saglietti et al., 2007). Lastly, the actin cytoskeleton is known to mediate receptor positioning (Gudheti et al., 2013) and its depolymerization was shown to reduce glutamate receptor accumulations in spines (Allison et al., 2000). In the following sections, we discuss the role of spine shape on the passive (diffusive) and active (endosomal) transport of receptors.

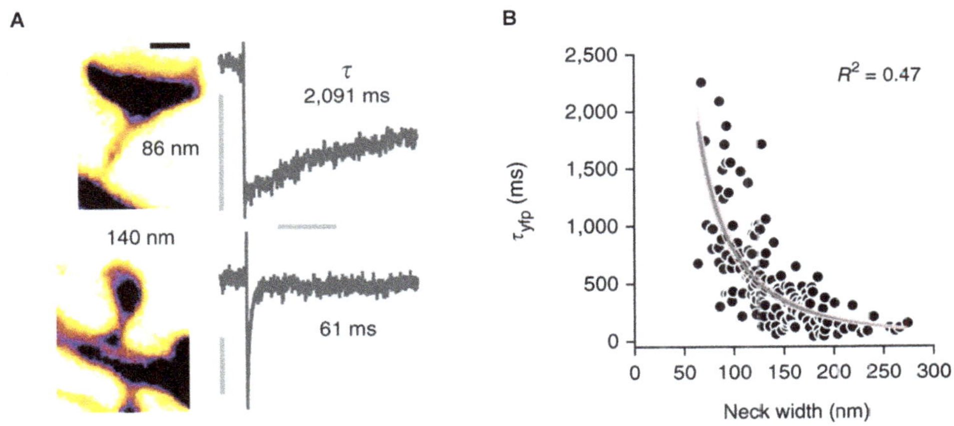

FIGURE 2 | Correlation of spine morphology and diffusional coupling. (A) Left: Two dendritic spines filled with soluble fluorophores were imaged with STED microscopy and neck diameters measured with line scans. Scale bar 500 nm. Right: The rate of diffusional coupling (τ) of these spines was measured by the recovery of photobleaced fluorophores (FRAP). **(B)** τ plotted as function of neck width. Gray line indicates inverse-square fit with 95% confidence interval in pink. Reprinted by permission from Macmillan Publishers Ltd: Nature Neuroscience (Tønnesen et al., 2014).

THE EFFECT OF SPINE SHAPE ON LATERAL DIFFUSION

Several experiments have shown that two-dimensional diffusion of membrane markers and AMPA-type glutamate receptors is sensitive to the morphology of the dendritic spine (Ashby et al., 2006; Shim et al., 2012). Mushroom shaped spines were found to retain AMPA receptors in the vicinity of the synapse for an increased period of time (Ashby et al., 2006; Ehlers et al., 2007; Opazo and Choquet, 2011, see **Figure 3A**). These observations have been rationalized by several modeling studies, which showed that the typical mushroom-like morphology of dendritic spines strongly alters the lateral diffusion of AMPA receptors, demonstrating a pronounced suppression of the receptor exit rate out of spines with decreasing neck radius as well as increasing neck length (Holcman and Schuss, 2011; Kusters et al., 2013; Kusters and Storm, 2014). More specifically, the characteristic timescale for retention, the mean escape time of receptors through the neck of a typical mushroom-shaped spines follows a power-law dependence on neck radius *r*,

$$\tau_{\text{escape}} \sim (r_{\text{neck}})^{-\lambda}$$

as well as neck length *l*,

$$\tau_{\text{escape}} \sim (l_{\text{neck}})^{\eta}$$

where λ and η are positive constants, whose numerical value depends on the actual shape of the spine (Kusters et al., 2013; Kusters and Storm, 2014).

In combination with an exocytic event in the head of the spine, a decreasing neck radius and increasing neck length effectively increase the confinement of receptors at the synapse, as can be seen in **Figure 3B** showing the time-evolution of receptor concentration after the release of 1000 receptors at the top of the spine (Kusters et al., 2013). Mushroom shaped spines with the smallest neck radii are thus significantly more effective at retaining receptors. Moreover, the particular shape of the mushroom-shaped spine in combination with receptor trapping at the synapse further enhances their retention. The timescale for an AMPA receptor reaching the synapse may be up to an order of magnitude faster that the time it takes for a receptor to exit through the neck of the spine. Altogether, this modeling study concluded that mushroom shaped spines with an exocytosis site adjacent to the synapse are privileged over others, because they can rapidly and specifically regulate the synaptic AMPA receptor level (Kusters et al., 2013).

Hydrodynamic interactions of proteins with the plasma membrane and the surrounding liquid significantly reduce their mobility. For flat membranes, Saffman and Delbruck (1975) predicted a logarithmic dependence of the diffusion coefficient with the "size" of the membrane, relative to the size of the protein. Recent experimental studies on membrane tubes show that reducing the radius of a membrane tube, which sets the relevant length scale in the Saffman-Delbruck theory, indeed reduced the mobility of both lipids and proteins with a factor of five compared to planar diffusion (Daniels and Turner, 2007; Domanov et al., 2011). The thin and slender neck, typical for mushroom spines, is in that same range of radii as in these experiments by Domanov et al. (2011) and could therefore reduce the mobility of glutamate receptors, compared to that on the dendritic shaft.

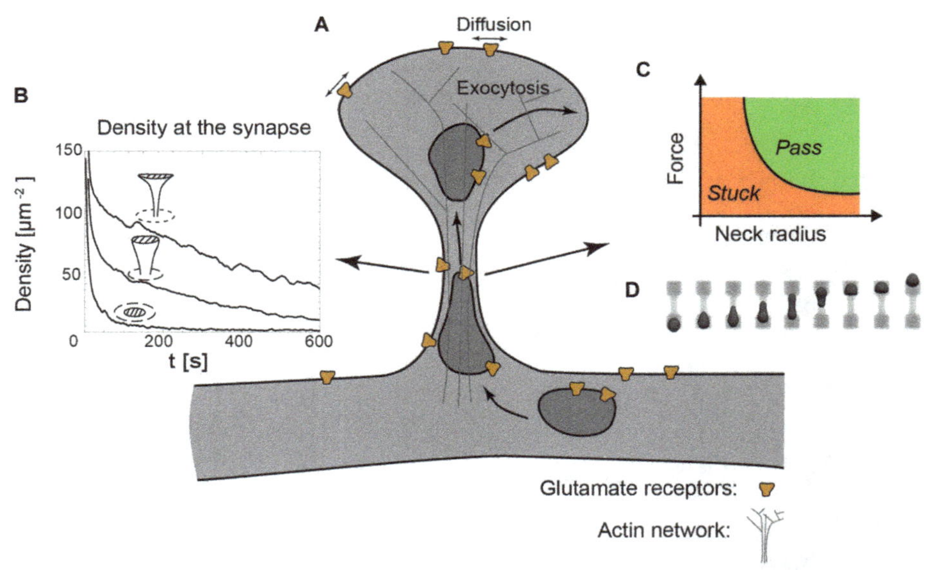

FIGURE 3 | The dendritic spine as a regulatory system. **(A)** Schematic view of a dendritic spine containing recycling endosomes, glutamate receptors and actin cytoskeleton. **(B)** Decreasing the radius of the neck increases the retention of receptors at the synapse, indicated by the time-evolution of the density at the synapse (dashed area) for a planar, stubby and mushroom shaped spine (Kusters et al., 2013). **(C)** Phase diagram indicating that decreasing the neck radius increases the force necessary to transport recycling endosomes through the actin rich constriction. **(D)** Typical sequence of shapes during the translocation of an endosome through the neck, obtained with three-dimensional Lattice-Boltzmann simulations (Kusters et al., 2014b).

The concept of a freely diffusive environment for these receptors, as has been presumed in all the previously described studies, is a very crude approximation of reality. The dendritic membranes on which these receptors reside are, similar to other biological membranes, highly crowded structures (Takamori et al., 2006). Crowding itself is known to significantly decrease the in-plane mobility of proteins (Santamaria et al., 2010). A recent study on the diffusion of steric repulsive particles confined to a cylinder confirmed that, for dense systems, a tubular geometry effectively limits the diffusion of particles along the long axis of the tube (Kusters et al., 2014a). However, how crowding exactly affects the diffusion on highly curved structures remains elusive and will be the focus of future experimental and theoretical studies.

THE EFFECT OF SPINE SHAPE ON VESICULAR TRANSPORT

Besides the effect of shape on lateral mobility, the overall shape of a dendritic spine also impacts the active transport of recycling endosomes. These endosomes, necessary for the delivery and the retrieval of receptors, have been found to operate both close to the synapse, within the head of the spine and in the dendritic shaft (Park et al., 2006; Wang et al., 2008). Endosome-based delivery of receptors into the head of the dendritic spine does come at a cost: to reach the spine head, they have to cross the actin rich neck, which inevitably causes the endosomes to deform. A recent study that explicitly modeled the translocation of vesicles through narrow constrictions has shown that the force produced by a realistic number of molecular motors is capable of transporting an endosome through constrictions with similar dimensions as spine necks (Kusters et al., 2014b). However, this translocation is highly sensitive to the size of the neck and the applied force. This can be shown in a phase diagram indicating whether an endosome passes through the neck or gets stuck in the constriction; see **Figures 3C,D**. Although this study did not explicitly model the actin meshwork in the neck, nor the potential deformation of the spine neck itself, it suggests that decreasing the size of the neck, in contrast to its effect on passive diffusion, could hamper the active transport of receptors (Kusters et al., 2014b). Further development of this model requires a careful experimental analysis of the deformations of both vesicles and the spine neck during spine entry events.

SUMMARY AND OUTLOOK

In this review we have highlighted existing evidence for a role of spine morphology in the compartmentalization of different important processes, such as receptor trafficking and multiple signaling events. Despite the importance for spine functioning, the exact mechanisms that govern compartmentalization are poorly understood. For example, the extent in which protein diffusion is governed by spine shape alone has remained unclear, because most experiments have so far been unable to directly correlate dynamic readouts with exact spine shape. Importantly, two pioneering studies have recently exploited developments in high-resolution light microscopy to more directly map spine morphology in live experiments and examine its effect on diffusion of free molecules (Takasaki and Sabatini, 2014; Tønnesen et al., 2014). Combined with the mathematical modeling approaches that we described (Kusters et al., 2013), this should allow to dissect the interplay between purely shape-based compartmentalization mechanisms and additional cell-biological mechanisms that confine both signaling and receptor localizations. A better understanding of spine compartmentalization and its implication in plasticity will lead to a deepened and refined model on how synaptic strength is regulated on a molecular level.

ACKNOWLEDGMENTS

This work is part of the research programme of the Foundation for Fundamental Research on Matter (FOM), which is part of the Netherlands Organization for Scientific Research (NWO). Corette J. Wierenga was supported by an NWO-VIDI grant.

REFERENCES

Adesnik, H., Nicoll, R. A., and England, P. M. (2005). Photoinactivation of native AMPA receptors reveals their real-time trafficking. *Neuron* 48, 977–985. doi: 10.1016/j.neuron.2005.11.030

Allison, D. W., Chervin, A. S., Gelfand, V. I., and Craig, A. M. (2000). Postsynaptic scaffolds of excitatory and inhibitory synapses in hippocampal neurons: maintenance of core components independent of actin filaments and microtubules. *J. Neurosci.* 20, 4545–4554.

Anderson, J. C., Douglas, R. J., Martin, K. A., and Nelson, J. C. (1994). Map of the synapses formed with the dendrites of spiny stellate neurons of cat visual cortex. *J. Comp. Neurol.* 341, 25–38. doi: 10.1002/cne.903410104

Araya, R., Jiang, J., Eisenthal, K. B., and Yuste, R. (2006). The spine neck filters membrane potentials. *Proc. Natl. Acad. Sci. U S A* 103, 17961–17966. doi: 10.1073/pnas.0608755103

Araya, R., Nikolenko, V., Eisenthal, K. B., and Yuste, R. (2007). Sodium channels amplify spine potentials. *Proc. Natl. Acad. Sci. U S A* 104, 12347–12352. doi: 10.1073/pnas.0705282104

Araya, R., Vogels, T. P., and Yuste, R. (2014). Activity-dependent dendritic spine neck changes are correlated with synaptic strength. *Proc. Natl. Acad. Sci. U S A* 111, E2895–E2904. doi: 10.1073/pnas.1321869111

Arellano, J. I., Benavides-Piccione, R., Defelipe, J., and Yuste, R. (2007). Ultrastructure of dendritic spines: correlation between synaptic and spine morphologies. *Front. Neurosci.* 1:10 doi: 10.3389/neuro.01.1.1.010.2007

Ashby, M. C., De La Rue, S. A., Ralph, G. S., Uney, J., Collingridge, G. L., and Henley, J. M. (2004). Removal of AMPA receptors (AMPARs) from synapses is preceded by transient endocytosis of extrasynaptic AMPARs. *J. Neurosci.* 24, 5172–5176. doi: 10.1523/jneurosci.1042-04.2004

Ashby, M. C., Maier, S. R., Nishimune, A., and Henley, J. M. (2006). Lateral diffusion drives constitutive exchange of AMPA receptors at dendritic spines and is regulated by spine morphology. *J. Neurosci.* 26, 7046–7055. doi: 10.1523/jneurosci.1235-06.2006

Barria, A., Muller, D., Derkach, V., Griffith, L. C., and Soderling, T. R. (1997). Regulatory phosphorylation of AMPA-type glutamate receptors by CaM-KII during long-term potentiation. *Science* 276, 2042–2045. doi: 10.1126/science.276.5321.2042

Berning, S., Willig, K. I., Steffens, H., Dibaj, P., and Hell, S. W. (2012). Nanoscopy in a living mouse brain. *Science* 335:551. doi: 10.1126/science.1215369

Bethge, P., Chéreau, R., Avignone, E., Marsicano, G., and Nägerl, U. V. (2013). Two-photon excitation STED microscopy in two colors in acute brain slices. *Biophys. J.* 104, 778–785. doi: 10.1016/j.bpj.2012.12.054

Bloodgood, B. L., Giessel, A. J., and Sabatini, B. L. (2009). Biphasic synaptic Ca influx arising from compartmentalized electrical signals in dendritic spines. *PLoS Biol.* 7:e1000190. doi: 10.1371/journal.pbio.1000190

Bloodgood, B. L., and Sabatini, B. L. (2005). Neuronal activity regulates diffusion across the neck of dendritic spines. *Science* 310, 866–869. doi: 10.1126/science.1114816

Bloodgood, B. L., and Sabatini, B. L. (2007a). $Ca^{(2+)}$ signaling in dendritic spines. *Curr. Opin. Neurobiol.* 17, 345–351. doi: 10.1016/j.conb.2007.04.003

Bloodgood, B. L., and Sabatini, B. L. (2007b). Nonlinear regulation of unitary synaptic signals by CaV(2.3) voltage-sensitive calcium channels located in dendritic spines. *Neuron* 53, 249–260. doi: 10.1016/j.neuron.2006.12.017

Borgdorff, A. J., and Choquet, D. (2002). Regulation of AMPA receptor lateral movements. *Nature* 417, 649–653. doi: 10.1038/nature00780

Bosch, M., and Hayashi, Y. (2012). Structural plasticity of dendritic spines. *Curr. Opin. Neurobiol.* 22, 383–388. doi: 10.1016/j.conb.2011.09.002

Bourne, J. N., and Harris, K. M. (2008). Balancing structure and function at hippocampal dendritic spines. *Annu. Rev. Neurosci.* 31, 47–67. doi: 10.1146/annurev.neuro.31.060407.125646

Bourne, J. N., and Harris, K. M. (2012). Nanoscale analysis of structural synaptic plasticity. *Curr. Opin. Neurobiol.* 22, 372–382. doi: 10.1016/j.conb.2011.10.019

Bredt, D. S., and Nicoll, R. A. (2003). AMPA receptor trafficking at excitatory synapses. *Neuron* 40, 361–379. doi: 10.1016/s0896-6273(03)00640-8

Byrne, M. J., Waxham, M. N., and Kubota, Y. (2011). The impacts of geometry and binding on CaMKII diffusion and retention in dendritic spines. *J. Comput. Neurosci.* 31, 1–12. doi: 10.1007/s10827-010-0293-9

Carter, B. C., Giessel, A. J., Sabatini, B. L., and Bean, B. P. (2012). Transient sodium current at subthreshold voltages: activation by EPSP waveforms. *Neuron* 75, 1081–1093. doi: 10.1016/j.neuron.2012.08.033

Colgan, L. A., and Yasuda, R. (2014). Plasticity of dendritic spines: subcompartmentalization of signaling. *Annu. Rev. Physiol.* 76, 365–385. doi: 10.1146/annurev-physiol-021113-170400

Collingridge, G. L., Isaac, J. T., and Wang, Y. T. (2004). Receptor trafficking and synaptic plasticity. *Nat. Rev. Neurosci.* 5, 952–962. doi: 10.1038/nrn1556

Czöndör, K., Mondin, M., Garcia, M., Heine, M., Frischknecht, R., Choquet, D., et al. (2012). Unified quantitative model of AMPA receptor trafficking at synapses. *Proc. Natl. Acad. Sci. U S A* 109, 3522–3527. doi: 10.1073/pnas.1109818109

Czöndör, K., and Thoumine, O. (2013). Biophysical mechanisms regulating AMPA receptor accumulation at synapses. *Brain Res. Bull.* 93, 57–68. doi: 10.1016/j.brainresbull.2012.11.001

Dahan, M., Lévi, S., Luccardini, C., Rostaing, P., Riveau, B., and Triller, A. (2003). Diffusion dynamics of glycine receptors revealed by single-quantum dot tracking. *Science* 302, 442–445. doi: 10.1126/science.1088525

Daniels, D. R., and Turner, M. S. (2007). Diffusion on membrane tubes: a highly discriminatory test of the Saffman-Delbruck theory. *Langmuir* 23, 6667–6670. doi: 10.1021/la0635000

Denk, W., Strickler, J. H., and Webb, W. W. (1990). Two-photon laser scanning fluorescence microscopy. *Science* 248, 73–76. doi: 10.1126/science.2321027

Ding, J. B., Takasaki, K. T., and Sabatini, B. L. (2009). Supraresolution imaging in brain slices using stimulated-emission depletion two-photon laser scanning microscopy. *Neuron* 63, 429–437. doi: 10.1016/j.neuron.2009.07.011

Domanov, Y. A., Aimon, S., Toombes, G. E., Renner, M., Quemeneur, F., Triller, A., et al. (2011). Mobility in geometrically confined membranes. *Proc. Natl. Acad. Sci. U S A* 108, 12605–12610. doi: 10.1073/pnas.1102646108

Ehlers, M. D., Heine, M., Groc, L., Lee, M. C., and Choquet, D. (2007). Diffusional trapping of GluR1 AMPA receptors by input-specific synaptic activity. *Neuron* 54, 447–460. doi: 10.1016/j.neuron.2007.04.010

Ethell, I. M., and Pasquale, E. B. (2005). Molecular mechanisms of dendritic spine development and remodeling. *Prog. Neurobiol.* 75, 161–205. doi: 10.1016/j.pneurobio.2005.02.003

Frost, N. A., Lu, H. E., and Blanpied, T. A. (2012). Optimization of cell morphology measurement via single-molecule tracking PALM. *PLoS One* 7:e36751. doi: 10.1371/journal.pone.0036751

Frost, N. A., Shroff, H., Kong, H., Betzig, E., and Blanpied, T. A. (2010). Single-molecule discrimination of discrete perisynaptic and distributed sites of actin filament assembly within dendritic spines. *Neuron* 67, 86–99. doi: 10.1016/j.neuron.2010.05.026

Fukunaga, K., Muller, D., and Miyamoto, E. (1995). Increased phosphorylation of Ca^{2+}/calmodulin-dependent protein kinase II and its endogenous substrates in the induction of long-term potentiation. *J. Biol. Chem.* 270, 6119–6124. doi: 10.1074/jbc.270.11.6119

Giannone, G., Hosy, E., Levet, F., Constals, A., Schulze, K., Sobolevsky, A. I., et al. (2010). Dynamic superresolution imaging of endogenous proteins on living cells at ultra-high density. *Biophys. J.* 99, 1303–1310. doi: 10.1016/j.bpj.2010.06.005

Giessel, A. J., and Sabatini, B. L. (2010). M1 muscarinic receptors boost synaptic potentials and calcium influx in dendritic spines by inhibiting postsynaptic SK channels. *Neuron* 68, 936–947. doi: 10.1016/j.neuron.2010.09.004

Gould, T. J., Burke, D., Bewersdorf, J., and Booth, M. J. (2012). Adaptive optics enables 3D STED microscopy in aberrating specimens. *Opt. Express* 20, 20998–21009. doi: 10.1364/oe.20.020998

Granger, A. J., Shi, Y., Lu, W., Cerpas, M., and Nicoll, R. A. (2013). LTP requires a reserve pool of glutamate receptors independent of subunit type. *Nature* 493, 495–500. doi: 10.1038/nature11775

Gray, E. G. (1959). Axo-somatic and axo-dendritic synapses of the cerebral cortex: an electron microscope study. *J. Anat.* 93, 420–433.

Grotjohann, T., Testa, I., Leutenegger, M., Bock, H., Urban, N. T., Lavoie-Cardinal, F., et al. (2011). Diffraction-unlimited all-optical imaging and writing with a photochromic GFP. *Nature* 478, 204–208. doi: 10.1038/nature10497

Grunditz, A., Holbro, N., Tian, L., Zuo, Y., and Oertner, T. G. (2008). Spine neck plasticity controls postsynaptic calcium signals through electrical compartmentalization. *J. Neurosci.* 28, 13457–13466. doi: 10.1523/jneurosci.2702-08.2008

Gudheti, M. V., Curthoys, N. M., Gould, T. J., Kim, D., Gunewardene, M. S., Gabor, K. A., et al. (2013). Actin mediates the nanoscale membrane organization of the clustered membrane protein influenza hemagglutinin. *Biophys. J.* 104, 2182–2192. doi: 10.1016/j.bpj.2013.03.054

Hao, J., and Oertner, T. G. (2012). Depolarization gates spine calcium transients and spike-timing-dependent potentiation. *Curr. Opin. Neurobiol.* 22, 509–515. doi: 10.1016/j.conb.2011.10.004

Harnett, M. T., Makara, J. K., Spruston, N., Kath, W. L., and Magee, J. C. (2012). Synaptic amplification by dendritic spines enhances input cooperativity. *Nature* 491, 599–602. doi: 10.1038/nature11554

Harris, K. M., and Stevens, J. K. (1988). Dendritic spines of rat cerebellar Purkinje cells: serial electron microscopy with reference to their biophysical characteristics. *J. Neurosci.* 8, 4455–4469.

Harvey, C. D., and Svoboda, K. (2007). Locally dynamic synaptic learning rules in pyramidal neuron dendrites. *Nature* 450, 1195–1200. doi: 10.1038/nature06416

Harvey, C. D., Yasuda, R., Zhong, H., and Svoboda, K. (2008). The spread of Ras activity triggered by activation of a single dendritic spine. *Science* 321, 136–140. doi: 10.1126/science.1159675

Heine, M., Groc, L., Frischknecht, R., Béïque, J. C., Lounis, B., Rumbaugh, G., et al. (2008). Surface mobility of postsynaptic AMPARs tunes synaptic transmission. *Science* 320, 201–205. doi: 10.1126/science.1152089

Hell, S. W. (2007). Far-field optical nanoscopy. *Science* 316, 1153–1158. doi: 10.1126/science.1137395

Hering, H., and Sheng, M. (2001). Dendritic spines: structure, dynamics and regulation. *Nat. Rev. Neurosci.* 2, 880–888. doi: 10.1038/35104061

Holbro, N., Grunditz, A., Wiegert, J. S., and Oertner, T. G. (2010). AMPA receptors gate spine $Ca^{(2+)}$ transients and spike-timing-dependent potentiation. *Proc. Natl. Acad. Sci. U S A* 107, 15975–15980. doi: 10.1073/pnas.1004562107

Holcman, D., and Schuss, Z. (2011). Diffusion laws in dendritic spines. *J. Math. Neurosci.* 1:10. doi: 10.1186/2190-8567-1-10

Holthoff, K., Tsay, D., and Yuste, R. (2002). Calcium dynamics of spines depend on their dendritic location. *Neuron* 33, 425–437. doi: 10.1016/s0896-6273(02)00576-7

Holthoff, K., Zecevic, D., and Konnerth, A. (2010). Rapid time course of action potentials in spines and remote dendrites of mouse visual cortex neurons. *J. Physiol.* 588, 1085–1096. doi: 10.1113/jphysiol.2009.184960

Holtmaat, A., and Svoboda, K. (2009). Experience-dependent structural synaptic plasticity in the mammalian brain. *Nat. Rev. Neurosci.* 10, 647–658. doi: 10.1038/nrn2699

Holtmaat, A., Wilbrecht, L., Knott, G. W., Welker, E., and Svoboda, K. (2006). Experience-dependent and cell-type-specific spine growth in the neocortex. *Nature* 441, 979–983. doi: 10.1038/nature04783

Hotulainen, P., and Hoogenraad, C. C. (2010). Actin in dendritic spines: connecting dynamics to function. *J. Cell Biol.* 189, 619–629. doi: 10.1083/jcb.201003008

Huang, B. (2010). Super-resolution optical microscopy: multiple choices. *Curr. Opin. Chem. Biol.* 14, 10–14. doi: 10.1016/j.cbpa.2009.10.013

Huang, B., Bates, M., and Zhuang, X. (2009). Super-resolution fluorescence microscopy. *Annu. Rev. Biochem.* 78, 993–1016. doi: 10.1146/annurev.biochem.77.061906.092014

Izeddin, I., Specht, C. G., Lelek, M., Darzacq, X., Triller, A., Zimmer, C., et al. (2011). Super-resolution dynamic imaging of dendritic spines using a low-affinity photoconvertible actin probe. *PLoS One* 6:e15611. doi: 10.1371/journal.pone.0015611

Kasai, H., Fukuda, M., Watanabe, S., Hayashi-Takagi, A., and Noguchi, J. (2010). Structural dynamics of dendritic spines in memory and cognition. *Trends Neurosci.* 33, 121–129. doi: 10.1016/j.tins.2010.01.001

Kennedy, M. B., Beale, H. C., Carlisle, H. J., and Washburn, L. R. (2005). Integration of biochemical signalling in spines. *Nat. Rev. Neurosci.* 6, 423–434. doi: 10.1038/nrn1685

Kennedy, M. J., Davison, I. G., Robinson, C. G., and Ehlers, M. D. (2010). Syntaxin-4 defines a domain for activity-dependent exocytosis in dendritic spines. *Cell* 141, 524–535. doi: 10.1016/j.cell.2010.02.042

Kessels, M. M., Schwintzer, L., Schlobinski, D., and Qualmann, B. (2011). Controlling actin cytoskeletal organization and dynamics during neuronal morphogenesis. *Eur. J. Cell Biol.* 90, 926–933. doi: 10.1016/j.ejcb.2010.08.011

Klar, T. A., Jakobs, S., Dyba, M., Egner, A., and Hell, S. W. (2000). Fluorescence microscopy with diffraction resolution barrier broken by stimulated emission. *Proc. Natl. Acad. Sci. U S A* 97, 8206–8210. doi: 10.1073/pnas.97.15.8206

Kneussel, M., and Wagner, W. (2013). Myosin motors at neuronal synapses: drivers of membrane transport and actin dynamics. *Nat. Rev. Neurosci.* 14, 233–247. doi: 10.1038/nrn3445

Koch, C., and Zador, A. (1993). The function of dendritic spines: devices subserving biochemical rather than electrical compartmentalization. *J. Neurosci.* 13, 413–422.

Korkotian, E., Holcman, D., and Segal, M. (2004). Dynamic regulation of spine-dendrite coupling in cultured hippocampal neurons. *Eur. J. Neurosci.* 20, 2649–2663. doi: 10.1111/j.1460-9568.2004.03691.x

Kusters, R., Kapitein, L. C., Hoogenraad, C. C., and Storm, C. (2013). Shape-induced asymmetric diffusion in dendritic spines allows efficient synaptic AMPA receptor trapping. *Biophys. J.* 105, 2743–2750. doi: 10.1016/j.bpj.2013.11.016

Kusters, R., Paquay, S., and Storm, C. (2014a). Confinement without boundaries: anisotropic diffusion on the surface of a cylinder. *ArXiv e-prints.* Available online at: http://adsabs.harvard.edu/abs/2014arXiv1407.3564K. Accessed on July 1, 2014.

Kusters, R., and Storm, C. (2014). Impact of morphology on diffusive dynamics on curved surfaces. *Phys. Rev. E Stat. Nonlin. Soft Matter Phys.* 89:032723. doi: 10.1103/physreve.89.032723

Kusters, R., van der Heijden, T., Kaoui, B., Harting, J., and Storm, C. (2014b). Forced transport of deformable containers through narrow constrictions. *Phys. Rev. E Stat. Nonlin. Soft Matter Phys.* 90:033006. doi: 10.1103/physreve.90.033006

Lavoie-Cardinal, F., Jensen, N. A., Westphal, V., Stiel, A. C., Chmyrov, A., Bierwagen, J., et al. (2014). Two-color RESOLFT nanoscopy with green and red fluorescent photochromic proteins. *Chemphyschem* 15, 655–663. doi: 10.1002/cphc.201301016

Lee, S. J., Escobedo-Lozoya, Y., Szatmari, E. M., and Yasuda, R. (2009). Activation of CaMKII in single dendritic spines during long-term potentiation. *Nature* 458, 299–304. doi: 10.1038/nature07842

Lisman, J. E., and Zhabotinsky, A. M. (2001). A model of synaptic memory: a CaMKII/PP1 switch that potentiates transmission by organizing an AMPA receptor anchoring assembly. *Neuron* 31, 191–201. doi: 10.1016/s0896-6273(01)00364-6

Lledo, P. M., Hjelmstad, G. O., Mukherji, S., Soderling, T. R., Malenka, R. C., and Nicoll, R. A. (1995). Calcium/calmodulin-dependent kinase II and long-term potentiation enhance synaptic transmission by the same mechanism. *Proc. Natl. Acad. Sci. U S A* 92, 11175–11179. doi: 10.1073/pnas.92.24.11175

Loew, L. M., and Hell, S. W. (2013). Superresolving dendritic spines. *Biophys. J.* 104, 741–743. doi: 10.1016/j.bpj.2013.01.011

Luo, L. (2002). Actin cytoskeleton regulation in neuronal morphogenesis and structural plasticity. *Annu. Rev. Cell Dev. Biol.* 18, 601–635. doi: 10.1146/annurev.cellbio.18.031802.150501

MacGillavry, H. D., Song, Y., Raghavachari, S., and Blanpied, T. A. (2013). Nanoscale scaffolding domains within the postsynaptic density concentrate synaptic AMPA receptors. *Neuron* 78, 615–622. doi: 10.1016/j.neuron.2013.03.009

Majewska, A., Brown, E., Ross, J., and Yuste, R. (2000). Mechanisms of calcium decay kinetics in hippocampal spines: role of spine calcium pumps and calcium diffusion through the spine neck in biochemical compartmentalization. *J. Neurosci.* 20, 1722–1734.

Makino, H., and Malinow, R. (2009). AMPA receptor incorporation into synapses during LTP: the role of lateral movement and exocytosis. *Neuron* 64, 381–390. doi: 10.1016/j.neuron.2009.08.035

Malinow, R., and Malenka, R. C. (2002) AMPA receptor trafficking and synaptic plasticity. *Annu. Rev. Neurosci.* 25, 103–126. doi: 10.1146/annurev.neuro.25.112701.142758

Matsuzaki, M., Honkura, N., Ellis-Davies, G. C., and Kasai, H. (2004). Structural basis of long-term potentiation in single dendritic spines. *Nature* 429, 761–766. doi: 10.1038/nature02617

Matus, A. (2000). Actin-based plasticity in dendritic spines. *Science* 290, 754–758. doi: 10.1126/science.290.5492.754

Miesenböck, G., De Angelis, D. A., and Rothman, J. E. (1998). Visualizing secretion and synaptic transmission with pH-sensitive green fluorescent proteins. *Nature* 394, 192–195. doi: 10.1038/28190

Moneron, G., and Hell, S. W. (2009). Two-photon excitation STED microscopy. *Opt. Express* 17, 14567–14573. doi: 10.1364/oe.17.014567

Murakoshi, H., Wang, H., and Yasuda, R. (2011). Local, persistent activation of Rho GTPases during plasticity of single dendritic spines. *Nature* 472, 100–104. doi: 10.1038/nature09823

Nägerl, U. V., Willig, K. I., Hein, B., Hell, S. W., and Bonhoeffer, T. (2008). Live-cell imaging of dendritic spines by STED microscopy. *Proc. Natl. Acad. Sci. U S A* 105, 18982–18987. doi: 10.1073/pnas.0810028105

Nair, D., Hosy, E., Petersen, J. D., Constals, A., Giannone, G., Choquet, D., et al. (2013). Super-resolution imaging reveals that AMPA receptors inside synapses are dynamically organized in nanodomains regulated by PSD95. *J. Neurosci.* 33, 13204–13224. doi: 10.1523/jneurosci.2381-12.2013

Newpher, T. M., and Ehlers, M. D. (2008). Glutamate receptor dynamics in dendritic microdomains. *Neuron* 58, 472–497. doi: 10.1016/j.neuron.2008.04.030

Ngo-Anh, T. J., Bloodgood, B. L., Lin, M., Sabatini, B. L., Maylie, J., and Adelman, J. P. (2005). SK channels and NMDA receptors form a Ca^{2+}-mediated feedback loop in dendritic spines. *Nat. Neurosci.* 8, 642–649. doi: 10.1038/nn1449

Noguchi, J., Matsuzaki, M., Ellis-Davies, G. C., and Kasai, H. (2005). Spine-neck geometry determines NMDA receptor-dependent Ca^{2+} signaling in dendrites. *Neuron* 46, 609–622. doi: 10.1016/j.neuron.2005.03.015

Nusser, Z. (2000). AMPA and NMDA receptors: similarities and differences in their synaptic distribution. *Curr. Opin. Neurobiol.* 10, 337–341. doi: 10.1016/s0959-4388(00)00086-6

O'Brien, R. J., Xu, D., Petralia, R. S, Steward, O., Huganir, R. L., and Worley, P. (1999). Synaptic clustering of AMPA receptors by the extracellular immediate-early gene product Narp. *Neuron* 23, 309–323. doi: 10.1016/s0896-6273(00)80782-5

Okamoto, K., Narayanan, R., Lee, S. H., Murata, K., and Hayashi, Y. (2007). The role of CaMKII as an F-actin-bundling protein crucial for maintenance of dendritic spine structure. *Proc. Natl. Acad. Sci. U S A* 104, 6418–6423. doi: 10.1073/pnas.0701656104

Opazo, P., and Choquet, D. (2011). A three-step model for the synaptic recruitment of AMPA receptors. *Mol. Cell. Neurosci.* 46, 1–8. doi: 10.1016/j.mcn.2010.08.014

Otmakhov, N., Tao-Cheng, J. H., Carpenter, S., Asrican, B., Dosemeci, A., Reese, T. S., et al. (2004). Persistent accumulation of calcium/calmodulin-dependent protein kinase II in dendritic spines after induction of NMDA receptor-dependent chemical long-term potentiation. *J. Neurosci.* 24, 9324–9331. doi: 10.1523/jneurosci.2350-04.2004

Park, M., Salgado, J. M., Ostroff, L., Helton, T. D., Robinson, C. G., Harris, K. M., et al. (2006). Plasticity-induced growth of dendritic spines by exocytic trafficking from recycling endosomes *Neuron* 52, 817–830. doi: 10.1016/j.neuron.2006.09.040

Passafaro, M., Piëch, V., and Sheng, M. (2001). Subunit-specific temporal and spatial patterns of AMPA receptor exocytosis in hippocampal neurons. *Nat. Neurosci.* 4, 917–926. doi: 10.1038/nn0901-917

Patterson, M. A., Szatmari, E. M., and Yasuda, R. (2010). AMPA receptors are exocytosed in stimulated spines and adjacent dendrites in a Ras-ERK-dependent manner during long-term potentiation. *Proc. Natl. Acad. Sci. U S A* 107, 15951–15956. doi: 10.1073/pnas.0913875107

Pettit, D. L., Perlman, S., and Malinow, R. (1994). Potentiated transmission and prevention of further LTP by increased CaMKII activity in postsynaptic hippocampal slice neurons. *Science* 266, 1881–1885. doi: 10.1126/science.7997883

Popovic, M. A., Gao, X., Carnevale, N. T., and Zecevic, D. (2014). Cortical dendritic spine heads are not electrically isolated by the spine neck from membrane potential signals in parent dendrites. *Cereb. Cortex* 24, 385–395. doi: 10.1093/cercor/bhs320

Ramakers, G. J. A. (2002). Rho proteins, mental retardation and the cellular basis of cognition. *Trends Neurosci.* 25, 191–199. doi: 10.1016/s0166-2236(00)02118-4

Ramón y Cajal, S. (1888). Estructura de los centros nerviosos de las aves. *Rev. Trim. Histol. Norm. Patol.* 1, 1–10.

Ramón y Cajal, S. (1899-1904). *Textura del Sistema Nervioso del Hombre y de los Vertebrados.* 2 vols. Madrid: Imprenta y Librería de Nicolás Moya.

Renner, M., Choquet, D., and Triller, A. (2009). Control of the postsynaptic membrane viscosity. *J. Neurosci.* 29, 2926–2937. doi: 10.1523/jneurosci.4445-08.2009

Richards, D. A., De Paola, V., Caroni, P., Gähwiler, B. H., and McKinney, R. A. (2004). AMPA-receptor activation regulates the diffusion of a membrane marker in parallel with dendritic spine motility in the mouse hippocampus. *J. Physiol.* 558, 503–512. doi: 10.1113/jphysiol.2004.062091

Ries, J., Kaplan, C., Platonova, E., Eghlidi, H., and Ewers, H. (2012). A simple, versatile method for GFP-based super-resolution microscopy via nanobodies. *Nat. Methods* 9, 582–584. doi: 10.1038/nmeth.1991

Sabatini, B. L., Oertner, T. G., and Svoboda, K. (2002). The life cycle of $Ca^{(2+)}$ ions in dendritic spines. *Neuron* 33, 439–452. doi: 10.1016/s0896-6273(02)00573-1

Saffman, P. G., and Delbruck, M. (1975). Brownian motion in biological membranes. *Proc. Natl. Acad. Sci. U S A* 72, 3111–3113. doi: 10.1073/pnas.72.8.3111

Saglietti, L., Dequidt, C., Kamieniarz, K., Rousset, M. C., Valnegri, P., Thoumine, O., et al. (2007). Extracellular interactions between GluR2 and N-cadherin in spine regulation. *Neuron* 54, 461–477. doi: 10.1016/j.neuron.2007.04.012

Saneyoshi, T., Fortin, D. A., and Soderling, T. R. (2010). Regulation of spine and synapse formation by activity-dependent intracellular signaling pathways. *Curr. Opin. Neurobiol.* 20, 108–115. doi: 10.1016/j.conb.2009.09.013

Santamaria, F., Gonzalez, J., Augustine, G. J., and Raghavachari, S. (2010). Quantifying the effects of elastic collisions and non-covalent binding on glutamate receptor trafficking in the post-synaptic density. *PLoS Comput. Biol.* 6:e1000780. doi: 10.1371/journal.pcbi.1000780

Schikorski, T., and Stevens, C. F. (1999). Quantitative fine-structural analysis of olfactory cortical synapses. *Proc. Natl. Acad. Sci. U S A* 96, 4107–4112. doi: 10.1073/pnas.96.7.4107

Segev, I., and Rall, W. (1998). Excitable dendrites and spines: earlier theoretical insights elucidate recent direct observations. *Trends Neurosci.* 21, 453–460. doi: 10.1016/s0166-2236(98)01327-7

Shcherbakova, D. M., Sengupta, P., Lippincott-Schwartz, J., and Verkhusha, V. V. (2014). Photocontrollable fluorescent proteins for superresolution imaging. *Annu. Rev. Biophys.* 43, 303–329. doi: 10.1146/annurev-biophys-051013-022836

Sheng, M., and Kim, M. J. (2002). Postsynaptic signaling and plasticity mechanisms. *Science* 298, 776–780. doi: 10.1126/science.1075333

Sheng, M., Malinow, R., and Huganir, R. (2013). Neuroscience: strength in numbers. *Nature* 493, 482–483. doi: 10.1038/493482a

Shepherd, G. M. (1996). The dendritic spine: a multifunctional integrative unit. *J. Neurophysiol.* 75, 2197–2210.

Shim, S. H., Xia, C., Zhong, G., Babcock, H. P., Vaughan, J. C., Huang, B., et al. (2012). Super-resolution fluorescence imaging of organelles in live cells with photoswitchable membrane probes. *Proc. Natl. Acad. Sci. U S A* 109, 13978–13983. doi: 10.1073/pnas.1201882109

Svoboda, K., Tank, D. W., and Denk, W. (1996). Direct measurement of coupling between dendritic spines and shafts. *Science* 272, 716–719. doi: 10.1126/science.272.5262.716

Svoboda, K., and Yasuda, R. (2006). Principles of two-photon excitation microscopy and its applications to neuroscience. *Neuron* 50, 823–839. doi: 10.1016/j.neuron.2006.05.019

Takamori, S., Holt, M., Stenius, K., Lemke, E. A., Gronborg, M., Riedel, D., et al. (2006). Molecular anatomy of a trafficking organelle. *Cell* 127, 831–846. doi: 10.1016/j.cell.2006.10.030

Takasaki, K. T., Ding, J. B., and Sabatini, B. L. (2013). Live-cell superresolution imaging by pulsed STED two-photon excitation microscopy. *Biophys. J.* 104, 770–777. doi: 10.1016/j.bpj.2012.12.053

Takasaki, K., and Sabatini, B. L. (2014). Super-resolution 2-photon microscopy reveals that the morphology of each dendritic spine correlates with diffusive but not synaptic properties. *Front. Neuroanat.* 8:29. doi: 10.3389/fnana.2014.00029

Tanaka, J., Horiike, Y., Matsuzaki, M., Miyazaki, T., Ellis-Davies, G. C., and Kasai, H. (2008). Protein synthesis and neurotrophin-dependent structural plasticity of single dendritic spines. *Science* 319, 1683–1687. doi: 10.1126/science.1152864

Tardin, C., Cognet, L., Bats, C., Lounis, B., and Choquet, D. (2003). Direct imaging of lateral movements of AMPA receptors inside synapses. *EMBO J.* 22, 4656–4665. doi: 10.1093/emboj/cdg463

Testa, I., Urban, N. T., Jakobs, S., Eggeling, C., Willig, K. I., and Hell, S. W. (2012). Nanoscopy of living brain slices with low light levels. *Neuron* 75, 992–1000. doi: 10.1016/j.neuron.2012.07.028

Tønnesen, J., Katona, G., Rozsa, B., and Nagerl, U. V. (2014). Spine neck plasticity regulates compartmentalization of synapses. *Nat. Neurosci.* 17, 678–685. doi: 10.1038/nn.3682

Tønnesen, J., Nadrigny, F., Willig, K. I., Wedlich-Soldner, R., and Nagerl, U. V. (2011). Two-color STED microscopy of living synapses using a single laser-beam pair. *Biophys. J.* 101, 2545–2552. doi: 10.1016/j.bpj.2011.10.011

Trachtenberg, J. T., Chen, B. E., Knott, G. W., Feng, G., Sanes, J. R., Welker, E., et al. (2002). Long-term in vivo imaging of experience-dependent synaptic plasticity in adult cortex. *Nature* 420, 788–794. doi: 10.1038/nature01273

Triller, A., and Choquet, D. (2005). Surface trafficking of receptors between synaptic and extrasynaptic membranes: and yet they do move! *Trends Neurosci.* 28, 133–139. doi: 10.1016/j.tins.2005.01.001

Tsay, D., and Yuste, R. (2004). On the electrical function of dendritic spines. *Trends Neurosci.* 27, 77–83. doi: 10.1016/j.tins.2003.11.008

Wang, Z., Edwards, J. G., Riley, N., Provance, D. W. Jr., Karcher, R., Li, X. D., et al. (2008). Myosin Vb mobilizes recycling endosomes and AMPA receptors for postsynaptic plasticity. *Cell* 135, 535–548. doi: 10.1016/j.cell.2008.09.057

Yang, Y., Wang, X. B., Frerking, M., and Zhou, Q. (2008). Delivery of AMPA receptors to perisynaptic sites precedes the full expression of long-term potentiation. *Proc. Natl. Acad. Sci. U S A* 105, 11388–11393. doi: 10.1073/pnas.0802978105

Yoshimura, Y., Shinkawa, T., Taoka, M., Kobayashi, K., Isobe, T., and Yamauchi, T. (2002). Identification of protein substrates of $Ca^{(2+)}$/calmodulin-dependent protein kinase II in the postsynaptic density by protein sequencing and mass spectrometry. *Biochem. Biophys. Res. Commun.* 290, 948–954. doi: 10.1006/bbrc.2001.6320

Yuste, R. (2013). Electrical compartmentalization in dendritic spines. *Annu. Rev. Neurosci.* 36, 429–449. doi: 10.1146/annurev-neuro-062111-150455

Yuste, R., and Bonhoeffer, T. (2001). Morphological changes in dendritic spines associated with long-term synaptic plasticity. *Annu. Rev. Neurosci.* 24, 1071–1089. doi: 10.1146/annurev.neuro.24.1.1071

Yuste, R., and Denk, W. (1995). Dendritic spines as basic functional units of neuronal integration. *Nature* 375, 682–684. doi: 10.1038/375682a0

Zhu, J. J., Qin, Y., Zhao, M., Van Aelst, L., and Malinow, R. (2002). Ras and Rap control AMPA receptor trafficking during synaptic plasticity. *Cell* 110, 443–455. doi: 10.1016/S0092-8674(02)00897-8

14

Spatiotemporal dynamics of dendritic spines in the living brain

Chia-Chien Chen*[1]*, Ju Lu*[2] *and Yi Zuo*[1]**

[1] *Department of Molecular, Cell and Developmental Biology, University of California at Santa Cruz, Santa Cruz, CA, USA*
[2] *Department of Biological Sciences and James H. Clark Center, Stanford University, Stanford, CA, USA*

Correspondence:
Yi Zuo, Department of Molecular, Cell and Developmental Biology, University of California at Santa Cruz, 1156 High Street, Santa Cruz, CA 95064, USA
e-mail: yizuo@ucsc.edu

Dendritic spines are ubiquitous postsynaptic sites of most excitatory synapses in the mammalian brain, and thus may serve as structural indicators of functional synapses. Recent works have suggested that neuronal coding of memories may be associated with rapid alterations in spine formation and elimination. Technological advances have enabled researchers to study spine dynamics *in vivo* during development as well as under various physiological and pathological conditions. We believe that better understanding of the spatiotemporal patterns of spine dynamics will help elucidate the principles of experience-dependent circuit modification and information processing in the living brain.

Keywords: dendritic spine, *in vivo*, two-photon imaging, experience-dependent plasticity, neural circuit, cerebral cortex

INTRODUCTION

Dendritic spines have fascinated generations of neuroscientists since their initial description by Santiago Ramón y Cajal more than a century ago (Ramon y Cajal, 1888). These delicate protrusions emanate from the dendritic shaft and resemble "bristling thorns or short spines" as described vividly by Cajal. They are the postsynaptic sites of the great majority (>90%) of excitatory glutamatergic synapses in the mammalian brain, and contain essential molecular components for postsynaptic signaling and plasticity. Therefore, spines and their structural dynamics may serve as indicators for synaptic connectivity and modifications thereof (Segal, 2005; Tada and Sheng, 2006; Harms and Dunaevsky, 2007).

Most early studies on the dendritic spine examined fixed neural tissue with light or electron microscopy (Lund et al., 1977; Woolley et al., 1990; Harris and Kater, 1994; Hering and Sheng, 2001; Lippman and Dunaevsky, 2005). Although they provided fundamental information about spine morphology and distribution, these fixed tissue examinations only captured static "snapshots" of spines. The introduction of fluorescent labeling techniques and multi-photon microscopy revolutionized the field. In 2002, the pioneering work from two laboratories (Grutzendler et al., 2002; Trachtenberg et al., 2002) demonstrated the possibility to track the same spine in the living brain over a long period (i.e., weeks) of time. In principle, spine dynamics represent synapse dynamics. While stable spines mostly represent synaptic contacts, only a small fraction of transient spines represent short-lived synaptic contacts, and the rest of them represent failed synaptogenesis (Trachtenberg et al., 2002; Knott et al., 2006; Cane et al., 2014). From such time-lapse imaging studies a dynamic picture of spines has emerged: spines form, enlarge, shrink, and retract throughout the animal's lifespan. Furthermore, their morphology and dynamics vary among neuronal types, across developmental stages, and in response to experiences such as sensory stimulation and deprivation, environmental enrichment, and various paradigms of learning (Holtmaat and Svoboda, 2009; Fu and Zuo, 2011).

This review focuses on results from *in vivo* imaging studies. In characterizing spine dynamics, researchers have mainly considered two aspects: overall changes in spine density, and the specific location along the dendrite where spine formation and elimination occur. While spine density provides an approximate estimate of the total number of excitatory synapses onto the postsynaptic neuron, the location of a spine influences the contribution of its synaptically transmitted electrical and chemical signals to the integrated response at the soma (Nevian et al., 2007; Spruston, 2008). Understanding how spine dynamics correlate with anatomical and physiological features of specific neural circuits in different behavioral contexts is crucial to the elucidation of the information processing and storage mechanisms in the brain.

SPINE DYNAMICS DURING DEVELOPMENT

Spine density varies significantly across diverse populations of neurons, likely reflecting the diversity of neuronal morphology and function (Nimchinsky et al., 2002; Ballesteros-Yanez et al., 2006). The balance between spine formation and elimination determines the change in spine density: a surplus of spine formation over elimination along a dendritic segment increases spine density thereon, and vice versa. In the cerebral cortex, while dendritic branches are mostly stable over time (Trachtenberg et al., 2002; Mizrahi and Katz, 2003; Chow et al., 2009; Mostany and Portera-Cailliau, 2011; Schubert et al., 2013), spines are constantly formed and eliminated. The rates of spine formation and elimination change over time, resulting in non-monotonic alteration in spine density (**Figure 1**). For example, spines on the apical dendrites of layer 2/3 pyramidal neurons in rodent barrel cortex

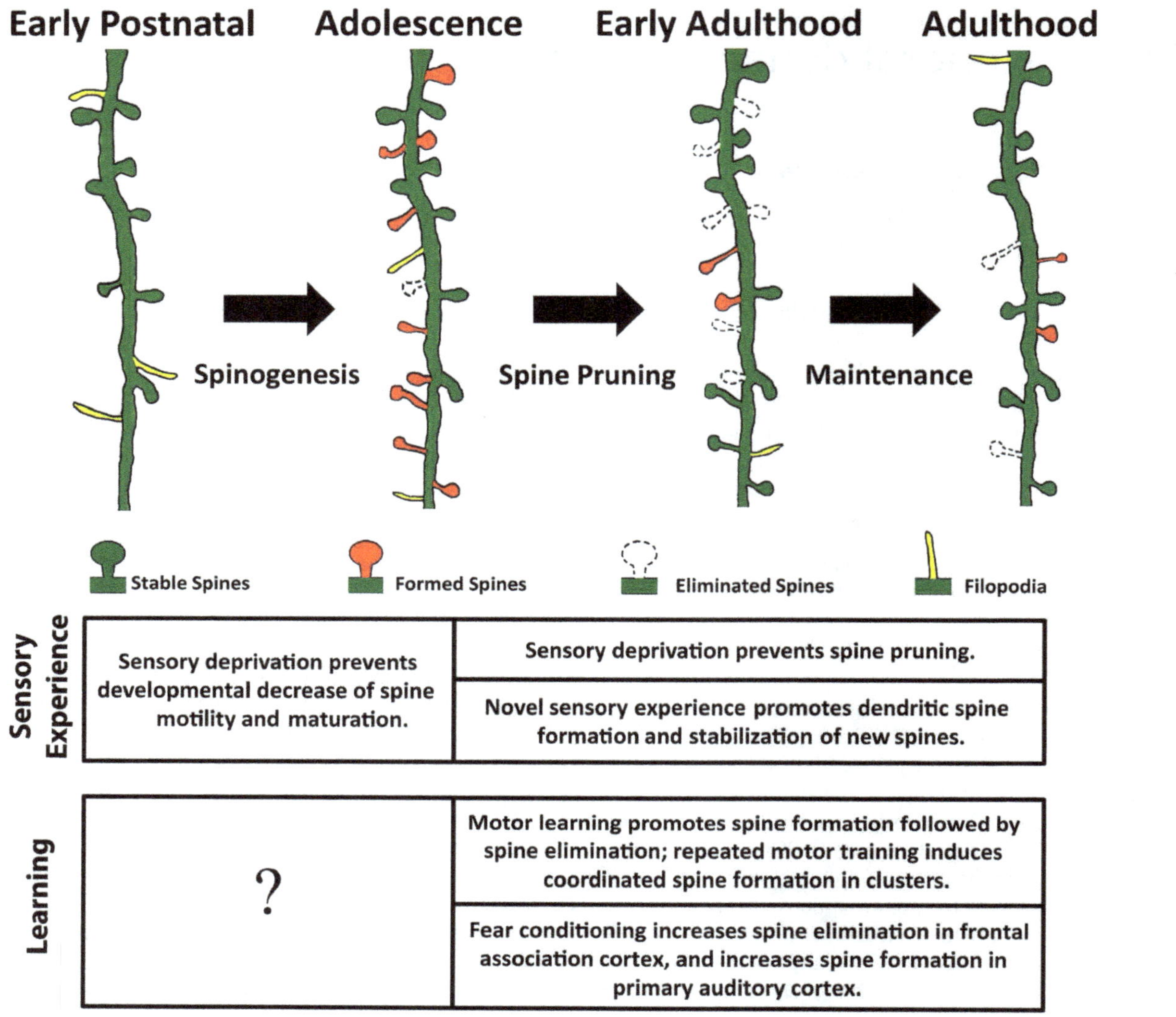

FIGURE 1 | Spine remodeling at different stages of an animal's life. Rapid spinogenesis in early postnatal is followed by a gradual spine pruning in adolescence. In adulthood, spine formation and elimination reach equilibrium, with a small fraction of spines constantly added or removed. Experience affects spine dynamics differently at different developmental stages.

exhibit gradually decreasing motility (elongation and shortening of spines) and turnover rate (defined as the total amount of gains and losses of spines) between postnatal day 7 and 24 (P7-24; Lendvai et al., 2000; Cruz-Martin et al., 2010). Nevertheless, spine density continuously increases over this period of time (Cruz-Martin et al., 2010). After this initial phase of net spine gain, spine elimination starts to outpace formation, leading to an overall reduction of spine density (Holtmaat et al., 2005; Zuo et al., 2005b; Yang et al., 2009). Between P28 and P42, 17% of spines are eliminated along the apical dendrites of layer 5 pyramidal neurons in the mouse barrel cortex, while only 5% of new spines are formed during the same period of time (Zuo et al., 2005a,b). Importantly, not all spines are equally susceptible to elimination: those with large heads are more stable than thin ones. As spine head size correlates with synaptic strength, this phenomenon suggests that stronger synapses are more stable (Holtmaat et al., 2005). Furthermore, newly formed spines are more likely to be eliminated than pre-existing spines (Xu et al., 2009), and the majority of stable spines formed before adolescence remain incorporated in the adult neuronal circuit (Zuo et al., 2005a; Yang et al., 2009; Yu et al., 2013). Finally, in adult animals spine formation and elimination reach equilibrium; spine density remains roughly constant until the onset of aging (Zuo et al., 2005a; Mostany et al., 2013).

SPINE DYNAMICS IN RESPONSE TO SENSORY EXPERIENCE

The cerebral cortex has the amazing ability to reorganize its circuitry in response to experiences. Therefore, how sensory experiences (or lack thereof) impact spine dynamics is of great interest to neuroscientists. Both acute and chronic sensory manipulations have been shown to profoundly impact spine dynamics, but the exact effect depends on the manipulation paradigm and duration, as well as the developmental stage of the animal. During early postnatal period, sensory inputs play instructive roles in the stabilization and maturation of spines. In the mouse visual cortex, depriving visual input from birth prevented the decrease in spine motility and maturation of spine morphology (Majewska and Sur, 2003; Tropea et al., 2010). Genetic deletion of the PirB receptor mimicked the effect of monocular deprivation on spine motility (Djurisic et al., 2013). In mice that had been subjected to visual deprivation previously, light-induced spine maturation could be partially mimicked by pharmacological activation of the GABAergic system, suggesting an important role of inhibitory circuits in the maturation of excitatory synapses (Tropea et al., 2010). Later on, sensory experience drives spine pruning (defined as net loss of spines). Unilateral trimming of all whiskers in 1-month-old mice for 4 or 14 days dramatically reduced spine elimination in the barrel cortex, but left spine formation largely unperturbed (Zuo et al., 2005b; Yu et al., 2013). Pharmacological blockade of NMDA receptors mimicked the effect of whisker trimming, indicating the involvement of the NMDA receptor pathway in such activity-dependent spine elimination (Zuo et al., 2005b).

While complete whisker trimming removes sensory input globally, trimming every other whisker ("chessboard trimming") presumably amplifies any difference in activity levels and patterns of neighboring barrels, thereby introducing a novel sensory experience. Such paradigm has been shown to promote spine turnover and to stabilize newly formed spines selectively in a subclass of cortical neurons (Trachtenberg et al., 2002; Holtmaat et al., 2006). New spines were preferentially added onto layer 5 pyramidal neurons with complex apical tufts, rather than those with simple tufts (Holtmaat et al., 2006). In αCaMKII-T286A defective mice, chessboard trimming failed to increase stabilization of new persistent spines at the border between spared and deprived barrels (Wilbrecht et al., 2010). Recently, an elegant study combining optogenetic stimulation and *in vivo* imaging showed that it is the pattern of neural activity, rather than the magnitude, that determines the stability of dendritic spines (Wyatt et al., 2012).

Similar to chessboard trimming, brief monocular deprivation (MD) increases the disparity between the inputs from two eyes. Thus similar to chessboard trimming, MD has been found to increase spine formation along apical dendritic tufts of layer 5 pyramidal neurons in the binocular zone of the mouse visual cortex. However this effect was not observed in layer 2/3 neurons, or in the monocular zone (Hofer et al., 2009), again indicating a cell type specific synapse remodeling. Interestingly, a second MD failed to increase spine formation further, but selectively enlarged the spines formed during the initial MD, suggesting that new spines formed during the initial MD had functional synapses that were reactivated during the second MD (Hofer et al., 2009).

SPINE DYNAMICS DURING LEARNING

The highly dynamic nature of dendritic spines elicits the prevalent idea that spines may serve as the structural substrate for learning and memory. It has been suggested that newly emerged spines (typically with small heads) underlie memory acquisition, while stable spines (typically with large heads) serve as memory storage sites (Bourne and Harris, 2007). Indeed, *in vivo* imaging studies have shown that in the cerebral cortex, spine dynamics directly correlates with learning. In the mouse motor cortex, spine formation begins immediately as the animal learns a new task. Following this rapid spinogenesis, spine density reverts to the baseline level through elevated spine elimination (Xu et al., 2009; Yu and Zuo, 2011). In song birds, higher baseline spine turnover rate before song learning has been found to correlate with a greater capacity for subsequent song imitation (Roberts et al., 2010). In mice, the amount of spines gained during initial learning closely correlates with the motor performance of learning acquisition (Xu et al., 2009); and survival of new spines correlates with retention of the motor skill (Yang et al., 2009). Furthermore, different motor skills are likely encoded by different subpopulations of synapses in the motor cortex, as learning a novel motor task in pre-trained mice continues to induce robust turnover in the adult motor cortex (Xu et al., 2009). Recently, it has also been found that the glucocorticoid level impacts motor learning-induced spine dynamics. Training mice at glucocorticoid peaks resulted in higher rate of spine formation, whereas glucocorticoid troughs following training was necessary for stabilization of spines formed during training and long-term memory retention (Liston et al., 2013). Addiction, which has been considered as pathological learning (Hyman, 2005), elicits similar temporal changes in spine dynamics as motor learning does. Using a cocaine-conditioned place preference paradigm, a recent imaging study showed that initial cocaine exposure promoted spine formation in the frontal cortex, and that the amount of new persistent spines correlated with the preference for the cocaine-paired context (Munoz-Cuevas et al., 2013). More interestingly, spine dynamics in different cortical regions may vary during the same task. For example, a fear conditioning paradigm that pairs auditory cues with foot shocks has demonstrated opposite effects in auditory and frontal cortex. In the auditory cortex, it was found that increased spine formation was correlated with paired fear conditioning, while unpaired conditioning was associated with increased elimination of spines (Moczulska et al., 2013). In the frontal association cortex, increased spine elimination was found to be associated with learning, while spine formation was associated with fear extinction, and reconditioning eliminated spines formed during extinction (Lai et al., 2012). Taken together, these studies reveal the diversity of temporal rules underlying learning-induced spine dynamics. Whether spines are formed or removed during learning depends on the behavioral paradigm as well as the specific neuronal circuit and cell types participating in the learning process.

It is worth noting that all the examples discussed above refer to non-declarative memory, which does not involve the conscious recollection of specific time, location, and episodic experience (i.e., declarative memory). Exploration of *in vivo* spine dynamics associated with declarative memory proves to be much more challenging. On one hand, hippocampus, the structure crucial for formation of declarative memory, is buried beneath cortex and beyond the reach of standard two-photon microscopy. On the other hand, declarative memory is believed to be diffusely stored in the large neocortical networks, making it difficult for targeted imaging. Therefore, the advancement of deep brain imaging techniques (e.g., microendoscopy, adaptive optics) together with a better understanding of memory allocation in the cortex holds the key to future investigation of spine dynamics underlying declarative memory.

SPINE DYNAMICS IN DISEASES

Alterations in dendritic spine densities have been observed in various neurological and neuropsychiatric diseases. Each disorder presents with its own hallmark abnormalities in spine dynamics, which further corroborates the idea that spines are structural underpinnings for proper cognitive functioning. There is growing consensus that spine abnormality is associated with behavioral deficiency and decline in cognitive functions (for detail see Fiala et al., 2002; Penzes et al., 2011).

In stroke models, it is shown that severe ischemia leads to rapid spine loss, which is reversible after reperfusion if the rescue is performed within a short period of time (20–60 min; Zhang et al., 2005). Following stroke, spine formation and subsequent elimination increase in the peri-infarct region, but not in cortical territories distant from the infarct or in the contralateral hemisphere (Brown et al., 2009; Johnston et al., 2013). This injury-induced plasticity reaches its peak at 1 week post-stroke; from then on the rate of spine formation and elimination steadily decline. This phenomenon suggests the existence of a critical period during which the surviving peri-infarct cortical tissues are most amenable to therapeutic interventions (Brown et al., 2007, 2009). In a mouse model for chronic pain, partial sciatic nerve ligation increases spine formation and elimination. Similar to the stroke model, elevation of spine formation rate precedes that of elimination, leading to an initial increase in spine density followed by its reduction. Such effects could be abolished by tetrodotoxin blockade, indicating that post-lesion spine remodeling is activity-dependent (Kim and Nabekura, 2011).

Altered spine dynamics has also been reported in animal models of degenerative diseases. For example, spine loss is accelerated in the vicinity of β-amyloid plaques in the cerebral cortex (Tsai et al., 2004; Spires et al., 2005). In an animal model of Huntington's disease spine formation rate increases, but newly formed spines do not persist to be incorporated into the local circuitry, which results in a net decrease in spine density (Murmu et al., 2013). While neurodegenerative diseases are usually associated with net spine loss, neurodevelopmental disorders exhibit diverse spine phenotypes. In a mouse model of Fragile X syndrome, spines are more numerous, and a higher percentage of them appear immature upon examination of adult fixed tissues (Comery et al., 1997; Irwin et al., 2000). *In vivo* studies further showed that in such animals spine turnover increased in various cortical areas (Cruz-Martin et al., 2010; Pan et al., 2010; Padmashri et al., 2013), and neither whisker trimming nor motor learning could further alter spine dynamics (Pan et al., 2010; Padmashri et al., 2013). In mice overexpressing MECP2, a Rett Syndrome related gene, it has been found that both spine gains and losses are elevated. However, new spines are more vulnerable to elimination than in wild type mice, resulting in a net loss of spines (Jiang et al., 2013).

GLIAL CONTRIBUTION TO SPINE DYNAMICS

The nervous system comprises two classes of cells: neurons and glia. The most intriguing role of glial cells is their participation at synaptic functioning and dynamics. Recently, a few exciting studies explored the role of glial signaling in spine maturation and plasticity. For example, blockade of astrocytic glutamate uptake has been shown to accelerate experience-dependent spine elimination during adolescent development (Yu et al., 2013). Another type of glial cells, microglia, have also been found to be in close contact with dendritic spines. The motility of microglial processes and spine contact are actively regulated by sensory experience and are involved in spine elimination (Tremblay et al., 2010). In addition, the depletion of microglia resulted in significant reduction of motor learning induced spine formation, and selective removal of brain-derived neurotrophic factor (BDNF) in microglia recapitulated the effects of microglial depletion (Parkhurst et al., 2013).

SPATIAL MANIFESTATION OF SPINE DYNAMICS

Structural imaging of spines has suggested that the emergence and disappearance of spines are neither uniform nor random along dendrites, but rather occur at spatially selective "hot spots." In the mouse motor cortex, new spines that form during repeated training with the same motor task tend to cluster. Furthermore, addition of the second new spine in the cluster is often associated with the enlargement of the first new spine. In contrast, spines formed during tandem execution of different motor tasks or during motor enrichment do not cluster (Fu et al., 2012). Taken together, these observations suggest that repeated re-activation of the first new spine is required for the clustered emergence of the second new spine. Similar spatial selectivity of spine dynamics has been observed in the fear conditioning paradigm: a spine eliminated during fear conditioning is usually replaced by a spine in its vicinity (within 2 μm) during fear extinction (Lai et al., 2012). Interestingly, spine dynamics are also influenced by dynamics of inhibitory synapses. Monocular deprivation significantly increases coordinated dynamics of spines and the inhibitory synapses nearby in layer 2/3 pyramidal neurons (Chen et al., 2012). These findings support the clustered plasticity model, which postulates that clustered synapses are more likely to participate in encoding the same information than synapses dispersed throughout the dendritic arbor (Govindarajan et al., 2006).

Combining *in vivo* whole-cell patch recording and single spine calcium imaging, a recent work has shown that spines tuned for different peak frequencies are interspersed along dendrites of pyramidal neurons in the mouse auditory cortex (Chen et al., 2011). This finding raises an interesting question: do clustered new spines correspond to inputs with similar or different characteristics (e.g., activity patterns, tuning properties)? In order to address this question, it will be necessary to sample spines over a broad area of the dendritic arbor, identify "hotspots" of spine remodeling, and combine structural imaging of spines with real-time functional imaging. Such experiments will not only help elucidate the cellular mechanisms of activity-dependent spine remodeling, but also provide clues to information representation and storage in neurons.

FUTURE DIRECTIONS

In this article, we have reviewed recent investigations on the dynamics of dendritic spines in the living brain. Although these studies have significantly advanced our understanding of how spine dynamics alter temporally and spatially, many questions remain on various fronts. For example, are there molecular markers that distinguish stable spines from newly formed spines and spines to be eliminated? Is the total number of spines maintained through a homeostatic mechanism, so that the dendrite may sustain the metabolic demand of synaptic transmission? Does clustering of new spines reflect changes in the strength of existing connections with the same axon (while maintaining the same network topology), or does it indicate the establishment of additional connections with previously unconnected axons nearby? It is worth noting that all works discussed above have focused on the postsynaptic side, which is only half of the story. The other major determinant of spine distribution and dynamics lies at the presynaptic side: the identity and geometry of presynaptic axons and the availability of axonal boutons. Knowing such presynaptic information is crucial in resolving many of the questions arising from observations of spine dynamics. However, identification of the presynaptic partner of an imaged dendritic spine remains a technical challenge, as the presynaptic axon may originate from a plethora of sources, and is usually intermingled with many other axonal processes. In addition, much remains to be learned about the sequence of structural remodeling that occurs at the contact site between the axonal bouton and the spine, and how such sequence associates with formation and elimination of synapses. Simultaneous imaging of axonal boutons and their partnering spines in the context of behavioral manipulation will provide abundant information to address this question. Retrospective ultrastructural examinations such as electron microscopy (Knott et al., 2009) and Array Tomography (Micheva and Smith, 2007; Micheva et al., 2010) may also complement *in vivo* imaging to validate the presence of synapses, and to reveal molecular fingerprints of imaged structures.

The temporal sequence and spatially selective rearrangements of neuronal connections, and how these changes collectively contribute to alterations of behavior as the result of experiences, is one of the fundamental questions in neuroscience. Advancement in imaging techniques, together with development in electrophysiology, molecular genetics and optogenetics, will help reveal the blueprint of neuronal circuitry at the microscopic level, as well as the mechanisms of information encoding, integration and storage in the brain.

AUTHOR CONTRIBUTIONS

Chia-Chien Chen made the figure. Chia-Chien Chen, Ju Lu, and Yi Zuo wrote the manuscript.

ACKNOWLEDGMENT

This work is supported by a grant (R01MH094449) from the National Institute of Mental Health to Yi Zuo.

REFERENCES

Ballesteros-Yanez, I., Benavides-Piccione, R., Elston, G. N., Yuste, R., and Defelipe, J. (2006). Density and morphology of dendritic spines in mouse neocortex. *Neuroscience* 138, 403–409. doi: 10.1016/j.neuroscience.2005.11.038

Bourne, J., and Harris, K. M. (2007). Do thin spines learn to be mushroom spines that remember? *Curr. Opin. Neurobiol.* 17, 381–386. doi: 10.1016/j.conb.2007.04.009

Brown, C. E., Aminoltejari, K., Erb, H., Winship, I. R., and Murphy, T. H. (2009). In vivo voltage-sensitive dye imaging in adult mice reveals that somatosensory maps lost to stroke are replaced over weeks by new structural and functional circuits with prolonged modes of activation within both the peri-infarct zone and distant sites. *J. Neurosci.* 29, 1719–1734. doi: 10.1523/JNEUROSCI.4249-08.2009

Brown, C. E., Li, P., Boyd, J. D., Delaney, K. R., and Murphy, T. H. (2007). Extensive turnover of dendritic spines and vascular remodeling in cortical tissues recovering from stroke. *J. Neurosci.* 27, 4101–4109. doi 10.1523/JNEUROSCI.4295-06.2007

Cane, M., Maco, B., Knott, G., and Holtmaat, A. (2014). The relationship between PSD-95 clustering and spine stability in vivo. *J. Neurosci.* 34, 2075–2086. doi: 10.1523/JNEUROSCI.3353-13.2014

Chen, J. L., Villa, K. L., Cha, J. W., So, P. T., Kubota, Y., and Nedivi, E. (2012). Clustered dynamics of inhibitory synapses and dendritic spines in the adult neocortex. *Neuron* 74, 361–373. doi: 10.1016/j.neuron.2012.02.030

Chen, X., Leischner, U., Rochefort, N. L., Nelken, I., and Konnerth, A. (2011). Functional mapping of single spines in cortical neurons in vivo. *Nature* 475, 501–505. doi: 10.1038/nature10193

Chow, D. K., Groszer, M., Pribadi, M., Machniki, M., Carmichael, S. T., Liu, X., et al. (2009). Laminar and compartmental regulation of dendritic growth in mature cortex. *Nat. Neurosci.* 12, 116–118. doi: 10.1038/nn.2255

Comery, T. A., Harris, J. B., Willems, P. J., Oostra, B. A., Irwin, S. A., Weiler, I. J., et al. (1997). Abnormal dendritic spines in fragile X knockout mice: maturation and pruning deficits. *Proc. Natl. Acad. Sci. U.S.A.* 94, 5401–5404. doi: 10.1073/pnas.94.10.5401

Cruz-Martin, A., Crespo, M., and Portera-Cailliau, C. (2010). Delayed stabilization of dendritic spines in fragile X mice. *J. Neurosci.* 30, 7793–7803. doi: 10.1523/JNEUROSCI.0577-10.2010

Djurisic, M., Vidal, G. S., Mann, M., Aharon, A., Kim, T., Ferrao Santos, A., et al. (2013). PirB regulates a structural substrate for cortical plasticity. *Proc. Natl. Acad. Sci. U.S.A.* 110, 20771–20776. doi: 10.1073/pnas.1321092110

Fiala, J. C., Spacek, J., and Harris, K. M. (2002). Dendritic spine pathology: cause or consequence of neurological disorders? *Brain Res. Brain Res. Rev.* 39, 29–54. doi: 10.1016/S0165-0173(02)00158-3

Fu, M., Yu, X., Lu, J., and Zuo, Y. (2012). Repetitive motor learning induces coordinated formation of clustered dendritic spines in vivo. *Nature* 483, 92–95. doi: 10.1038/nature10844

Fu, M., and Zuo, Y. (2011). Experience-dependent structural plasticity in the cortex. *Trends Neurosci.* 34, 177–187. doi: 10.1016/j.tins.2011.02.001

Govindarajan, A., Kelleher, R. J., and Tonegawa, S. (2006). A clustered plasticity model of long-term memory engrams. *Nat. Rev. Neurosci.* 7, 575–583. doi: 10.1038/nrn1937

Grutzendler, J., Kasthuri, N., and Gan, W. B. (2002). Long-term dendritic spine stability in the adult cortex. *Nature* 420, 812–816. doi: 10.1038/nature01276

Harms, K. J., and Dunaevsky, A. (2007). Dendritic spine plasticity: looking beyond development. *Brain Res.* 1184, 65–71. doi: 10.1016/j.brainres.2006.02.094

Harris, K. M., and Kater, S. B. (1994). Dendritic spines: cellular specializations imparting both stability and flexibility to synaptic function. *Annu. Rev. Neurosci.* 17, 341–371. doi: 10.1146/annurev.ne.17.030194.002013

Hering, H., and Sheng, M. (2001). Dendritic spines: structure, dynamics and regulation. *Nat. Rev. Neurosci.* 2, 880–888. doi: 10.1038/35104061

Hofer, S. B., Mrsic-Flogel, T. D., Bonhoeffer, T., and Hubener, M. (2009). Experience leaves a lasting structural trace in cortical circuits. *Nature* 457, 313–317. doi: 10.1038/nature07487

Holtmaat, A., and Svoboda, K. (2009). Experience-dependent structural synaptic plasticity in the mammalian brain. *Nat. Rev. Neurosci.* 10, 647–658. doi: 10.1038/nrn2699

Holtmaat, A. J., Trachtenberg, J. T., Wilbrecht, L., Shepherd, G. M., Zhang, X., Knott, G. W., et al. (2005). Transient and persistent dendritic spines in the neocortex in vivo. *Neuron* 45, 279–291. doi: 10.1016/j.neuron.2005.01.003

Holtmaat, A., Wilbrecht, L., Knott, G. W., Welker, E., and Svoboda, K. (2006). Experience-dependent and cell-type-specific spine growth in the neocortex. *Nature* 441, 979–983. doi: 10.1038/nature04783

Hyman, S. E. (2005). Addiction: a disease of learning and memory. *Am. J. Psychiatry* 162, 1414–1422. doi: 10.1176/appi.ajp.162.8.1414

Irwin, S. A., Galvez, R., and Greenough, W. T. (2000). Dendritic spine structural anomalies in fragile-X mental retardation syndrome. *Cereb. Cortex* 10, 1038–1044. doi: 10.1093/cercor/10.10.1038

Jiang, M., Ash, R. T., Baker, S. A., Suter, B., Ferguson, A., Park, J., et al. (2013). Dendritic arborization and spine dynamics are abnormal in the mouse model of MECP2 duplication syndrome. *J. Neurosci.* 33, 19518–19533. doi: 10.1523/JNEUROSCI.1745-13.2013

Johnston, D. G., Denizet, M., Mostany, R., and Portera-Cailliau, C. (2013). Chronic in vivo imaging shows no evidence of dendritic plasticity or functional remapping in the contralesional cortex after stroke. *Cereb. Cortex* 23, 751–762. doi: 10.1093/cercor/bhs092

Kim, S. K., and Nabekura, J. (2011). Rapid synaptic remodeling in the adult somatosensory cortex following peripheral nerve injury and its association with neuropathic pain. *J. Neurosci.* 31, 5477–5482. doi: 10.1523/JNEUROSCI.0328-11.2011

Knott, G. W., Holtmaat, A., Trachtenberg, J. T., Svoboda, K., and Welker, E. (2009). A protocol for preparing GFP-labeled neurons previously imaged in vivo and in slice preparations for light and electron microscopic analysis. *Natl. Protoc.* 4, 1145–1156. doi: 10.1038/nprot.2009.114

Knott, G. W., Holtmaat, A., Wilbrecht, L., Welker, E., and Svoboda, K. (2006). Spine growth precedes synapse formation in the adult neocortex in vivo. *Nat. Neurosci.* 9, 1117–1124. doi: 10.1038/nn1747

Lai, C. S., Franke, T. F., and Gan, W. B. (2012). Opposite effects of fear conditioning and extinction on dendritic spine remodelling. *Nature* 483, 87–91. doi: 10.1038/nature10792

Lendvai, B., Stern, E. A., Chen, B., and Svoboda, K. (2000). Experience-dependent plasticity of dendritic spines in the developing rat barrel cortex in vivo. *Nature* 404, 876–881. doi: 10.1038/35009107

Lippman, J., and Dunaevsky, A. (2005). Dendritic spine morphogenesis and plasticity. *J. Neurobiol.* 64, 47–57. doi: 10.1002/neu.20149

Liston, C., Cichon, J. M., Jeanneteau, F., Jia, Z., Chao, M. V., and Gan, W. B. (2013). Circadian glucocorticoid oscillations promote learning-dependent synapse formation and maintenance. *Nat. Neurosci.* 16, 698–705. doi: 10.1038/nn.3387

Lund, J. S., Boothe, R. G., and Lund, R. D. (1977). Development of neurons in the visual cortex (area 17) of the monkey (*Macaca nemestrina*): a Golgi study from fetal day 127 to postnatal maturity. *J. Comp. Neurol.* 176, 149–188. doi: 10.1002/cne.901760203

Majewska, A., and Sur, M. (2003). Motility of dendritic spines in visual cortex in vivo: changes during the critical period and effects of visual deprivation. *Proc. Natl. Acad. Sci. U.S.A.* 100, 16024–16029. doi: 10.1073/pnas.2636949100

Micheva, K. D., Busse, B., Weiler, N. C., O'Rourke, N., and Smith, S. J. (2010). Single-synapse analysis of a diverse synapse population: proteomic imaging methods and markers. *Neuron* 68, 639–653. doi: 10.1016/j.neuron.2010.09.024

Micheva, K. D., and Smith, S. J. (2007). Array tomography: a new tool for imaging the molecular architecture and ultrastructure of neural circuits. *Neuron* 55, 25–36. doi: 10.1016/j.neuron.2007.06.014

Mizrahi, A., and Katz, L. C. (2003). Dendritic stability in the adult olfactory bulb. *Nat. Neurosci.* 6, 1201–1207. doi: 10.1038/nn1133

Moczulska, K. E., Tinter-Thiede, J., Peter, M., Ushakova, L., Wernle, T., Bathellier, B., et al. (2013). Dynamics of dendritic spines in the mouse auditory cortex during memory formation and memory recall. *Proc. Natl. Acad. Sci. U.S.A.* 110, 18315–18320. doi: 10.1073/pnas.1312508110

Mostany, R., Anstey, J. E., Crump, K. L., Maco, B., Knott, G., and Portera-Cailliau, C. (2013). Altered synaptic dynamics during normal brain aging. *J. Neurosci.* 33, 4094–4104. doi: 10.1523/JNEUROSCI.4825-12.2013

Mostany, R., and Portera-Cailliau, C. (2011). Absence of large-scale dendritic plasticity of layer 5 pyramidal neurons in peri-infarct cortex. *J. Neurosci.* 31, 1734–1738. doi: 10.1523/JNEUROSCI.4386-10.2011

Munoz-Cuevas, F. J., Athilingam, J., Piscopo, D., and Wilbrecht, L. (2013). Cocaine-induced structural plasticity in frontal cortex correlates with conditioned place preference. *Nat. Neurosci.* 16, 1367–1369. doi: 10.1038/nn.3498

Murmu, R. P., Li, W., Holtmaat, A., and Li, J. Y. (2013). Dendritic spine instability leads to progressive neocortical spine loss in a mouse model of Huntington's disease. *J. Neurosci.* 33, 12997–13009. doi: 10.1523/JNEUROSCI.5284-12.2013

Nevian, T., Larkum, M. E., Polsky, A., and Schiller, J. (2007). Properties of basal dendrites of layer 5 pyramidal neurons: a direct patch-clamp recording study. *Nat. Neurosci.* 10, 206–214. doi: 10.1038/nn1826

Nimchinsky, E. A., Sabatini, B. L., and Svoboda, K. (2002). Structure and function of dendritic spines. *Annu. Rev. Physiol.* 64, 313–353. doi: 10.1146/annurev.physiol.64.081501.160008

Padmashri, R., Reiner, B. C., Suresh, A., Spartz, E., and Dunaevsky, A. (2013). Altered structural and functional synaptic plasticity with motor skill learning in a mouse model of fragile x syndrome. *J. Neurosci.* 33, 19715–19723. doi: 10.1523/JNEUROSCI.2514-13.2013

Pan, F., Aldridge, G. M., Greenough, W. T., and Gan, W. B. (2010). Dendritic spine instability and insensitivity to modulation by sensory experience in a mouse model of fragile X syndrome. *Proc. Natl. Acad. Sci. U.S.A.* 107, 17768–17773. doi: 10.1073/pnas.1012496107

Parkhurst, C. N., Yang, G., Ninan, I., Savas, J. N., Yates, J. R. III, Lafaille, J. J., et al. (2013). Microglia promote learning-dependent synapse formation through brain-derived neurotrophic factor. *Cell* 155, 1596–1609. doi: 10.1016/j.cell.2013.11.030

Penzes, P., Cahill, M. E., Jones, K. A., Vanleeuwen, J. E., and Woolfrey, K. M. (2011). Dendritic spine pathology in neuropsychiatric disorders. *Nat. Neurosci.* 14, 285–293. doi: 10.1038/nn.2741

Ramon y Cajal, S. (1888). Estructura de los centros nerviosos de las aves Rev. *Trim. Histol. Norm. Pat.* 1, 1–10.

Roberts, T. F., Tschida, K. A., Klein, M. E., and Mooney, R. (2010). Rapid spine stabilization and synaptic enhancement at the onset of behavioural learning. *Nature* 463, 948–952. doi: 10.1038/nature08759

Schubert, V., Lebrecht, D., and Holtmaat, A. (2013). Peripheral deafferentation-driven functional somatosensory map shifts are associated with local, not large-scale dendritic structural plasticity. *J. Neurosci.* 33, 9474–9487. doi: 10.1523/JNEUROSCI.1032-13.2013

Segal, M. (2005). Dendritic spines and long-term plasticity. *Nat. Rev. Neurosci.* 6, 277–284. doi: 10.1038/nrn1649

Spires, T. L., Meyer-Luehmann, M., Stern, E. A., Mclean, P. J., Skoch, J., Nguyen, P. T., et al. (2005). Dendritic spine abnormalities in amyloid precursor protein transgenic mice demonstrated by gene transfer and intravital multiphoton microscopy. *J. Neurosci.* 25, 7278–7287. doi: 10.1523/JNEUROSCI.1879-05.2005

Spruston, N. (2008). Pyramidal neurons: dendritic structure and synaptic integration. *Nat. Rev. Neurosci.* 9, 206–221. doi: 10.1038/nrn2286

Tada, T., and Sheng, M. (2006). Molecular mechanisms of dendritic spine morphogenesis. *Curr. Opin. Neurobiol* 16, 95–101. doi: 10.1016/j.conb.2005.12.001

Trachtenberg, J. T., Chen, B. E., Knott, G. W., Feng, G., Sanes, J. R., Welker, E., et al. (2002). Long-term in vivo imaging of experience-dependent synaptic plasticity in adult cortex. *Nature* 420, 788–794. doi: 10.1038/nature01273

Tremblay, M. E., Lowery, R. L., and Majewska, A. K. (2010). Microglial interactions with synapses are modulated by visual experience. *PLoS Biol.* 8:e1000527. doi: 10.1371/journal.pbio.1000527

Tropea, D., Majewska, A. K., Garcia, R., and Sur, M. (2010). Structural dynamics of synapses in vivo correlate with functional changes during experience-dependent plasticity in visual cortex. *J. Neurosci.* 30, 11086–11095. doi: 10.1523/JNEUROSCI.1661-10.2010

Tsai, J., Grutzendler, J., Duff, K., and Gan, W. B. (2004). Fibrillar amyloid deposition leads to local synaptic abnormalities and breakage of neuronal branches. *Nat. Neurosci.* 7, 1181–1183. doi: 10.1038/nn1335

Wilbrecht, L., Holtmaat, A., Wright, N., Fox, K., and Svoboda, K. (2010). Structural plasticity underlies experience-dependent functional plasticity of cortical circuits. *J. Neurosci.* 30, 4927–4932. doi: 10.1523/JNEUROSCI.6403-09.2010

Woolley, C. S., Gould, E., Frankfurt, M., and Mcewen, B. S. (1990). Naturally occurring fluctuation in dendritic spine density on adult hippocampal pyramidal neurons. *J. Neurosci.* 10, 4035–4039.

Wyatt, R. M., Tring, E., and Trachtenberg, J. T. (2012). Pattern and not magnitude of neural activity determines dendritic spine stability in awake mice. *Nat. Neurosci.* 15, 949–951. doi: 10.1038/nn.3134

Xu, T., Yu, X., Perlik, A. J., Tobin, W. F., Zweig, J. A., Tennant, K., et al. (2009). Rapid formation and selective stabilization of synapses for enduring motor memories. *Nature* 462, 915–919. doi: 10.1038/nature08389

Yang, G., Pan, F., and Gan, W. B. (2009). Stably maintained dendritic spines are associated with lifelong memories. *Nature* 462, 920–924. doi: 10.1038/nature08577

Yu, X., Wang, G., Gilmore, A., Yee, A. X., Li, X., Xu, T., et al. (2013). Accelerated experience-dependent pruning of cortical synapses in ephrin-A2 knockout mice. *Neuron* 80, 64–71. doi: 10.1016/j.neuron.2013.07.014

Yu, X., and Zuo, Y. (2011). Spine plasticity in the motor cortex. *Curr. Opin. Neurobiol.* 21, 169–174. doi: 10.1016/j.conb.2010.07.010

Zhang, S., Boyd, J., Delaney, K., and Murphy, T. H. (2005). Rapid reversible changes in dendritic spine structure in vivo gated by the degree of ischemia. *J. Neurosci.* 25, 5333–5338. doi: 10.1523/JNEUROSCI.1085-05.2005

Zuo, Y., Lin, A., Chang, P., and Gan, W. B. (2005a). Development of long-term dendritic spine stability in diverse regions of cerebral cortex. *Neuron* 46, 181–189. doi: 10.1016/j.neuron.2005.04.001

Zuo, Y., Yang, G., Kwon, E., and Gan, W. B. (2005b). Long-term sensory deprivation prevents dendritic spine loss in primary somatosensory cortex. *Nature* 436, 261–265. doi: 10.1038/nature03715

15

Input transformation by dendritic spines of pyramidal neurons

Roberto Araya *

Department of Neurosciences, Faculty of Medicine, University of Montreal, Montreal, QC, Canada

***Correspondence:**
Roberto Araya, Department of Neurosciences, Faculty of Medicine, University of Montreal, C.P. 6128 Succursale Centre-Ville, Montreal, QC H3C 3J7, Canada
e-mail: roberto.araya@umontreal.ca

In the mammalian brain, most inputs received by a neuron are formed on the dendritic tree. In the neocortex, the dendrites of pyramidal neurons are covered by thousands of tiny protrusions known as dendritic spines, which are the major recipient sites for excitatory synaptic information in the brain. Their peculiar morphology, with a small head connected to the dendritic shaft by a slender neck, has inspired decades of theoretical and more recently experimental work in an attempt to understand how excitatory synaptic inputs are processed, stored and integrated in pyramidal neurons. Advances in electrophysiological, optical and genetic tools are now enabling us to unravel the biophysical and molecular mechanisms controlling spine function in health and disease. Here I highlight relevant findings, challenges and hypotheses on spine function, with an emphasis on the electrical properties of spines and on how these affect the storage and integration of excitatory synaptic inputs in pyramidal neurons. In an attempt to make sense of the published data, I propose that the *raison d'etre* for dendritic spines lies in their ability to undergo activity-dependent structural and molecular changes that can modify synaptic strength, and hence alter the gain of the linearly integrated sub-threshold depolarizations in pyramidal neuron dendrites before the generation of a dendritic spike.

Keywords: spine neck, synaptic transmission, plasticity, synaptic integration, biophysical processes, two-photon uncaging, dendritic computation, input-output transformation

INTRODUCTION

The fundamental operation of a neuron is to integrate synaptic inputs and decide whether and when to fire an action potential. Neocortical neurons, which may be subdivided into glutamatergic pyramidal neurons and GABAergic interneurons, form complex networks that are ultimately responsible for the production of higher cognitive functions (Kandel et al., 2000). The pyramidal neuron is the most abundant neuron in the cerebral cortex, yet how it processes, stores, and integrates its thousands of inputs remains ill-defined. A notable characteristic of pyramidal neurons is that their dendrites are covered by tiny protrusions called dendritic spines (**Figures 1A,B**). Since their discovery by Santiago Ramon y Cajal in 1888 (Cajal, 1888) we have learned a great deal about their morphological, molecular and biophysical properties. Dendritic spines are the main gateway of excitatory synaptic transmission in the brain (Gray, 1959), with almost all (~95%) of excitatory synaptic input to pyramidal neurons being received by spines (Spacek and Harris, 1998; Arellano et al., 2007b; Chen et al., 2012a) (**Figure 1B**). In addition, it has been shown that GABAergic inputs target not only dendritic shafts but also some dendritic spines (Somogyi and Cowey, 1981; Freund et al., 1986; DeFelipe et al., 1989; Chen et al., 2012a), with recent evidence indicating that GABAergic synapses from somatostatin-expressing interneurons can be directed to some spine heads, exerting a local inhibition of Ca^{2+} signals (Chiu et al., 2013).

Although excitatory input to GABAergic interneurons does not show the same exclusivity for spines, these structures are also present on various classes of interneurons (Feldman and Peters, 1978; Freund and Buzsaki, 1996; Kawaguchi et al., 2006) and share some of the functional properties of spines found on pyramidal neurons (Scheuss and Bonhoeffer, 2013). The issue of why the prevalence of dendritic spines varies between interneuron subtypes is intriguing but is not covered in this review; the reader is referred to the following references for further information (Feldman and Peters, 1978; Kawaguchi, 1993; Pitkanen and Amaral, 1993; McBain et al., 1994; Freund and Buzsaki, 1996; Kawaguchi et al., 2006; Keck et al., 2011; Scheuss and Bonhoeffer, 2013).

Importantly, spines are believed to be the preferential site for the induction of synaptic long-term potentiation (LTP) (Lang et al., 2004; Matsuzaki et al., 2004; Harvey et al., 2008; Araya et al., 2014) and can undergo structural remodeling. In addition, several studies have demonstrated that dendritic spines are the fundamental substrates of pathogenesis in neuropsychiatric disorders such as the autism spectrum disorders, schizophrenia, and neurodegenerative disorders such as Alzheimer's disease (Selemon and Goldman-Rakic, 1999; Glantz and Lewis, 2000; Tackenberg et al., 2009; Hutsler and Zhang, 2010; Portera-Cailliau, 2012), which are characterized by impairments in spine structure and/or density (Penzes et al., 2011).

Although the importance of spines is acknowledged, the biophysical and molecular mechanisms controlling their function in health and disease remain poorly understood. Their small size (<1 fL volume) has allowed us only indirect access

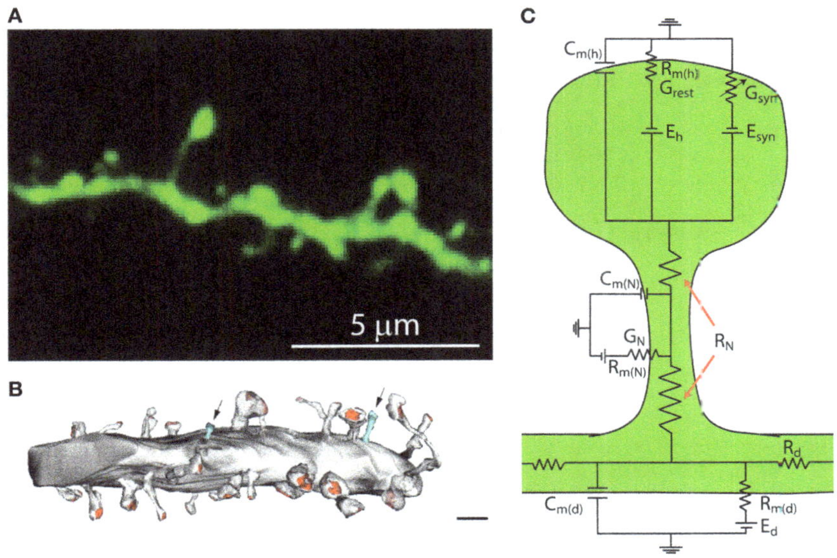

FIGURE 1 | Dendritic spines are tiny protrusions that cover the dendrites of pyramidal neurons and are the sites at which excitatory connections are made. (A) Confocal scanning image of a representative dendrite, covered with dendritic spines, of a layer 5 pyramidal neuron from a thy1-YFP-H transgenic mouse expressing the yellow fluorescent protein. **(B)** Synaptic contacts occur at spines. Reconstruction of electron micrographs taken from serial sections of dendritic segments from neocortical pyramidal neurons. Note the distribution of postsynaptic contacts (PSD, red; excitatory asymmetric contacts). Only a few percent of dendritic protrusions are devoid of synaptic contacts (blue). Note that the shaft lacks excitatory synaptic contacts. Scale bar = 2 μm (Modified with permission from Arellano et al., 2007b). **(C)** Simplified circuit diagram of a passive dendritic spine. $C_{m(h)}$, capacitance of the spine head membrane; $C_{m(N)}$, capacitance of the spine neck membrane; $C_{m(d)}$, dendritic membrane capacitance; $R_{m(h)}$, membrane resistance of the spine head; $R_{m(N)}$, membrane resistance of the spine neck; $R_{m(d)}$, membrane resistance of the dendrite; E_h, reversal potential at the spine head; E_{syn}, synaptic reversal potential; E_d, reversal potential at the dendrite; R_N, neck resistance; R_d dendritic resistance; G_{rest}, spine's conductance at rest; G_{syn}, spine's synaptic conductance; G_N, spine neck's conductance.

for measurement using standard electrophysiological techniques. However, with the advent of two-photon (2P) microscopy (Denk et al., 1990), and the development of 2P glutamate uncaging—with which it is possible to image and photo-activate live dendritic spines deep in tissue with high spatial resolution (Matsuzaki et al., 2001; Araya et al., 2006b; Bloodgood and Sabatini, 2007; Harvey et al., 2008)—some experimental challenges posed by the small size of dendritic spines have been bypassed. In combination with virally delivered or genetically encoded fluorescent Ca^{2+} indicators (Nakai et al., 2001), voltage sensitive dyes (Peterka et al., 2011), fluorescence resonance energy transfer (FRET)-based sensors (Yasuda, 2006; Lee et al., 2009; Murakoshi et al., 2011), and optogenetic activation and inactivation techniques (Fenno et al., 2011), we have begun to gather important information as to how spine function relates to the input/output properties of excitatory neurons. Here I will review what we know about spines, with an emphasis on their electrical properties and how passive (e.g., spine morphology) and active mechanisms (recruitment of voltage-gated spine channels) might affect the storage and integration of excitatory inputs in pyramidal neurons.

STRUCTURAL PROPERTIES OF SPINES IN PYRAMIDAL NEURONS: USE OF NANOSCOPY METHODS

The peculiar morphology of spines (Cajal, 1888), with their small head (~1 μm in diameter and <1 fL volume) separated from the main dendrite by a slender neck (<0.2 μm in diameter) (Sorra and Harris, 2000; Arellano et al., 2007b; Takasaki and Sabatini, 2014; Tonnesen et al., 2014) (**Figure 1**), has inspired decades of theoretical work that has, in the past 25 years, been complemented by much needed experimental work. Together, these efforts have been aimed at understanding how a synaptic current at the spine head, and the voltage signal generated by it, are delivered to the parent dendrite, as well as the effect that spine morphological properties have on the integration of excitatory inputs (Chang, 1952; Rall, 1964; Llinás and Hillman, 1969; Jack et al., 1975; Koch and Poggio, 1983a,b; Segev and Rall, 1988). In addition, the extent to which the morphological, molecular and biophysical properties of spines transform synaptic inputs (Miller et al., 1985; Araya et al., 2006b; Harnett et al., 2012), support synaptic plasticity (Matsuzaki et al., 2004; Harvey et al., 2008; Araya et al., 2014), and affect the integration of excitatory synaptic inputs (Llinás and Hillman, 1969; Araya et al., 2006a) have been intensively investigated.

Ultrastructural studies using electron microscopy (EM) or super-resolution light microscopy (see below) have shown that different spine shapes co-exist in the dendrites of pyramidal neurons (see **Table 1**). Spines can be classified morphologically as "stubby" (lacking a neck), "thin" (thin, long neck with an apparent head), or "mushroom" (big head with thick neck) (Peters and Kaiserman-Abramof, 1970), and activity-dependent changes in their morphology (Lang et al., 2004; Matsuzaki et al., 2004; Harvey et al., 2008; Tanaka et al., 2008; Araya et al., 2014) and/or internal biochemistry (Matsuzaki et al., 2004; Yasuda and Murakoshi, 2011; Sala and Segal, 2014) are thought to

Table 1 | Dimensions of individual spines with electron microscopy and STED imaging.

CA1 pyramidal cell	EM (fixed tissue)	STED (live tissue)
Neck length (μm)	–	0.157–1.8 (0.689)*
Neck width (μm)	0.038–0.46[b]	0.059–0.292 (0.167)*
Head width (μm)	–	0.262–1.104 (0.583)*
Head volume (μm^3)	0.003–0.55[b]	–
Cortical pyramidal cell		
Neck length (μm)	0.1–2.21 (0.66)[a]	–
Neck width (μm)	0.09–0.51 (0.2)[a]	–
Head width (μm)	–	–
Head volume (μm^3)	0.01–0.38 (0.07)[a]	–

**Tonnesen et al. (2014).*
[a]Arellano et al. (2007a).
[b]Sorra et al., (Sorra and Harris, 2000).

affect synaptic efficacy. In this way, spines may serve as substrates for synaptic plasticity and be a means through which the input/output properties of pyramidal neurons are altered (Lang et al., 2004; Matsuzaki et al., 2004; Harvey et al., 2008; Araya et al., 2014). In electron microscopy (EM), electrons are the source of illumination and hence the resolving power is much higher than with light microscopy; this has allowed us to learn a great deal about spine architecture and spine morphological variability at the nanoscale (Gray, 1959; Spacek and Harris, 1998; Sorra and Harris, 2000; Arellano et al., 2007a). However, the use of EM necessitates using fixed tissue, since the sample needs to be permeabilized, fixated, dehydrated, and placed under high vacuum. In addition, fixation and embedding protocols may cause structural artifacts (compare the morphological discrepancies of images from live spines with their respective images gathered using EM in Knott et al., 2006 and Chen et al., 2012a).

Recent developments in super-resolution light microscopy techniques have enabled us to perform sub diffraction-limited imaging of live dendritic spines (for review see Huang et al., 2010; Maglione and Sigrist, 2013). Among the main nanoscopy methods utilized to study brain structures are stimulated emission depletion (STED) microscopy, photoactivatable localization microscopy (PALM) (Betzig et al., 2006; Hess et al., 2006) and stochastic optical reconstruction microscopy (STORM) (Rust et al., 2006). In stimulated emission depletion (STED) microscopy the fluorescence emission at the border of the point-spread function (PSF) of the microscope is depleted by creating an annulus of high intensity light overlaying the outer edge of the PSF, through a process known as stimulated emission depletion. This leaves a fluorescence volume only at the center of the PSF, providing lateral and axial resolutions of 30–50 nm and ~30–600 nm, respectively (Huang et al., 2010; Maglione and Sigrist, 2013). In photoactivated localization microscopy (PALM) (Betzig et al., 2006; Hess et al., 2006) and stochastic optical reconstruction microscopy (STORM) (Rust et al., 2006), detection of images beyond the diffraction-limited resolution is achieved by using photoswitching or other mechanisms to stochastically activate individual fluorophores that are separated by a distance greater than the diffraction-limited resolution of the microscope, allowing their individual localization. Image reconstruction is obtained by superimposing a large number of wide-field images, each containing only a few individually detected fluorophores (Huang et al., 2010; Maglione and Sigrist, 2013). PALM uses fluorophores in the form of photoactivatable fluorescence proteins, while STORM uses immunolabeling with cyanine-tagged dyes (Huang et al., 2010; Maglione and Sigrist, 2013). Although some laboratories have successfully used PALM and STORM to image live brain tissue (Dani and Huang, 2010) and spines (Lu et al., 2014), their low imaging speed hinder the collection of high resolution images in live samples. However with STED, small fields of view can be imaged rapidly, and when combined with 2P-excitation optical sectioning one can image at considerable depths (~80–100 μm) in thick acute brain slices (Bethge et al., 2013; Takasaki et al., 2013). Thus, STED allows imaging of live dendritic spines, providing a super-resolution view of the spine neck (length and diameter) and head (see **Table 1**) (Nagerl et al., 2008; Nagerl and Bonhoeffer, 2010; Maglione and Sigrist, 2013; Takasaki and Sabatini, 2014; Tonnesen et al., 2014) and thus enabling an improved assessment of the spine structure–function relationship. Although the benefits of STED and PALM/STORM are evident, their current disadvantage is the need for high fluorescence labeling density in order to collect many photons per pixel to provide an acceptable signal-to-noise ratio (Maglione and Sigrist, 2013). In STED microscopy, the use of continuous wave lasers requires higher depletion beam power than with pulsed lasers, resulting in more severe photobleaching of the sample (Willig et al., 2007). Some of these constrains have been bypassed by the use of Switching Laser Mode (SLAM) microscopy, in which switching between laser modes in a confocal microscope provides a way for diffraction-limited resolution images of spines and other structures to be enhanced by a factor of two. To obtain images of sub-diffraction resolution and contrast, it is necessary to subtract the images obtained in dark (laser mode having a dark spot at its center) and bright modes (laser mode having a peak of intensity at its center) in order to observe the sub-diffraction dimensions of the dark spot on the azimuthally polarized beam (doughnut-shaped light) (Dehez et al., 2013).

BIOCHEMICAL COMPARTMENTALIZATION IN THE SPINE: A FOCUS ON Ca^{2+}

Due to their small size, dendritic spines are well suited to the compartmentalization of biochemical and electrical signals. Indeed, biochemical signals, such as a buildup of intracellular Ca^{2+} after activation of glutamatergic receptors, have been shown to be compartmentalized in the spine head for several milliseconds (Yuste and Denk, 1995). The assumption that the spine morphology predicts biochemical compartmentalization is justified by a simplified compartmental model where the passive diffusional coupling of a molecule x, τ_x, through the spine neck is given by,

$$\tau_x = \frac{Vl}{DA} \tag{1}$$

where V is the volume of the spine, l is the neck length, D the diffusion coefficient of the molecule x, and A the cross-sectional area of the spine neck (A is defined as πr^2, with r being the radius of the spine neck).

Recently, direct measurements of spine morphology in live tissue with STED imaging in combination with fluorescence recovery times after photobleaching (FRAP) (experimental τ, τ_{exp}) of free diffusible fluorescence proteins (Tonnesen et al., 2014) or Alexa dyes (Takasaki and Sabatini, 2014; Tonnesen et al., 2014) indicated that τ_{exp} is determined by spine structure. As predicted by equation (1), τ_{exp} is negatively correlated with spine neck width, with small variations in neck diameter having significant effects on compartmentalization of fluorescent proteins and Alexa dyes (Takasaki and Sabatini, 2014; Tonnesen et al., 2014). Furthermore, it has been shown that τ_{exp} is positively correlated with spine neck length (strong linear correlation, $r = 0.75$, Takasaki and Sabatini, 2014; weak correlation, $r = 0.42$, Tonnesen et al., 2014) and spine head width (Tonnesen et al., 2014) (although see, Takasaki and Sabatini, 2014). In addition, using confocal microscopy and fluorescence loss in photobleaching (FLIP) it has been shown that τ_{exp} of membrane-bound fluorescent proteins is positively correlated with spine neck length and head size (Hugel et al., 2009). In agreement with these experimental findings, recent theoretical calculations using refined equations for the diffusion across the spine neck of a Brownian particle that is either inside the spine head or bound to its membrane suggest a strong dependency (negative correlation) between the diffusional coupling of a particle and (1) the spine neck length, and (2) the curvature of the connection between the spine head–neck (Holcman and Schuss, 2011). Hence, these experimental and theoretical results indicate that spine morphology predicts the compartmentalization of freely diffusible proteins, dyes and membrane-bound fluorescent proteins. Is this conclusion applicable for the spine–dendrite diffusion of ions and molecules such as Ca^{2+}?

The development of Ca^{2+} imaging techniques such as 2P Ca^{2+} imaging (Denk et al., 1990) and the use of fluorescent Ca^{2+} indicators (Tsien, 1988) has opened up a means to explore neuronal activity with high spatial and temporal detail, providing a better understanding of the signaling pathways and function of subthreshold and suprathreshold spine Ca^{2+} signaling in synaptic transmission, storage and integration. Recently, the development of methods for data acquisition at high frame rates and low-excitation laser power has allowed researchers to perform 2P calcium imaging of dendritic spines *in vivo* (Chen et al., 2012b).

These advances have permitted imaging of the spatiotemporal calcium dynamics in single dendritic spines. For example, it has been reported that the decay time of Ca^{2+} in the spine head, τ_{Ca}, has a positive correlation with the spine neck length (Majewska et al., 2000). In addition, combining electrical stimulation of dendritic spines with 2P monitoring of τ_{Ca} in the spine head and computer simulations has suggested that the amplitude of spine Ca^{2+} transients is positively correlated with the diffusional resistance of the spine neck (Grunditz et al., 2008), implying that the spine neck geometry can control the amplitude of the Ca^{2+} signal in the spine head as well as τ_{Ca}, as predicted by simulations (Gold and Bear, 1994). Furthermore, it has been suggested that the spine head volume is negatively correlated with the amplitude of the glutamate uncaging-generated spine $[Ca^{2+}]_i$, but positively correlated with the $[Ca^{2+}]_i$ in the adjacent dendritic shaft (Noguchi et al., 2005). This suggests that spine neck and head morphologies are likely important determinants of the amplitude and diffusion of Ca^{2+} through the spine neck. In contrast, it has been shown using 2P uncaging of glutamate over single spines in combination with 2P calcium imaging that spine morphology cannot predict the amplitude of Ca^{2+} signals in spines (Sobczyk et al., 2005; Araya et al., 2006b, 2014). Moreover, a recent study using the same technical approach but also complemented by STED imaging showed the absence of a correlation between the peak Ca^{2+} amplitude and neck diameter or length (Takasaki and Sabatini, 2014). The reason for the discrepancy between these studies might be the fact that the spatiotemporal confinement of the Ca^{2+} signal is believed to rely not only on spine morphology but also on the characteristics of the synaptic input (Yuste and Denk, 1995; Sabatini et al., 2002), the variability and distribution of endogenous Ca^{2+} sensors (Baimbridge et al., 1992; Raghuram et al., 2012), the Ca^{2+} diffusion coefficient (Murthy et al., 2000), the presence and mobility of endogenous buffers (Gold and Bear, 1994; Murthy et al., 2000) and their Ca^{2+} binding ratios (Sabatini et al., 2002), as well as on active transport mechanisms, membrane potential and local spine activation of voltage-sensitive calcium channels (VSCCs) (Bloodgood and Sabatini, 2007), and the mechanisms for Ca^{2+} release from intracellular stores located within the spine head (Finch and Augustine, 1998; Takechi et al., 1998). However, the interplay between the various spine Ca^{+2} sensors and buffers (Raghuram et al., 2012), Ca^{2+} extrusion mechanisms (Ca^{2+} exit from the spine and/or sequestration into intracellular stores) (Yuste et al., 2000; Higley and Sabatini, 2012), activation of VSCCs (Bloodgood and Sabatini, 2007) and morphological spine features that explain Ca^{2+} compartmentalization and signaling in spines, as well as the compartmentalization of an array of other biochemical signals (Colgan and Yasuda, 2014; Sala and Segal, 2014), remain somewhat ill-defined.

WHAT ARE THE PATHWAYS BY WHICH Ca^{2+} ACCUMULATES IN THE SPINE HEAD OF PYRAMIDAL NEURONS?

The main pathways by which glutamate release from presynaptic terminals triggers a Ca^{2+} transient in the spine head are the following: First, the binding of glutamate to postsynaptic AMPA and NMDA glutamate receptors, followed by AMPA receptor-mediated membrane depolarization and Mg^{2+} unblock from the NMDA receptor, leads to the influx of both Na^{+} and Ca^{2+} into the spine head. Second, the depolarization provided by currents flowing through glutamate receptors has been suggested to lead to the activation of spine VSCCs (Bloodgood and Sabatini, 2007), which might provide an additional source of Ca^{2+} to the spine head. Third, Ca^{2+} can be released from internal stores via the metabotropic glutamate receptor (mGluR)-triggered production of inositol trisphosphate (IP_3) in the spine head and the subsequent activation of IP_3 receptors (Holbro et al., 2009; Oh et al., 2013) (**Figure 2**).

The activation of spine IP_3 receptors and consequent release of Ca^{2+} from internal stores is required for long-term synaptic depression (LTD) (Holbro et al., 2009; Oh et al., 2013) and LTP (Raymond and Redman, 2006; de Sevilla and Buno, 2010). In addition, spine synapse-dependent Ca^{2+} transients are believed to be responsible for mediating LTP (Chittajallu et al., 1998; Lang

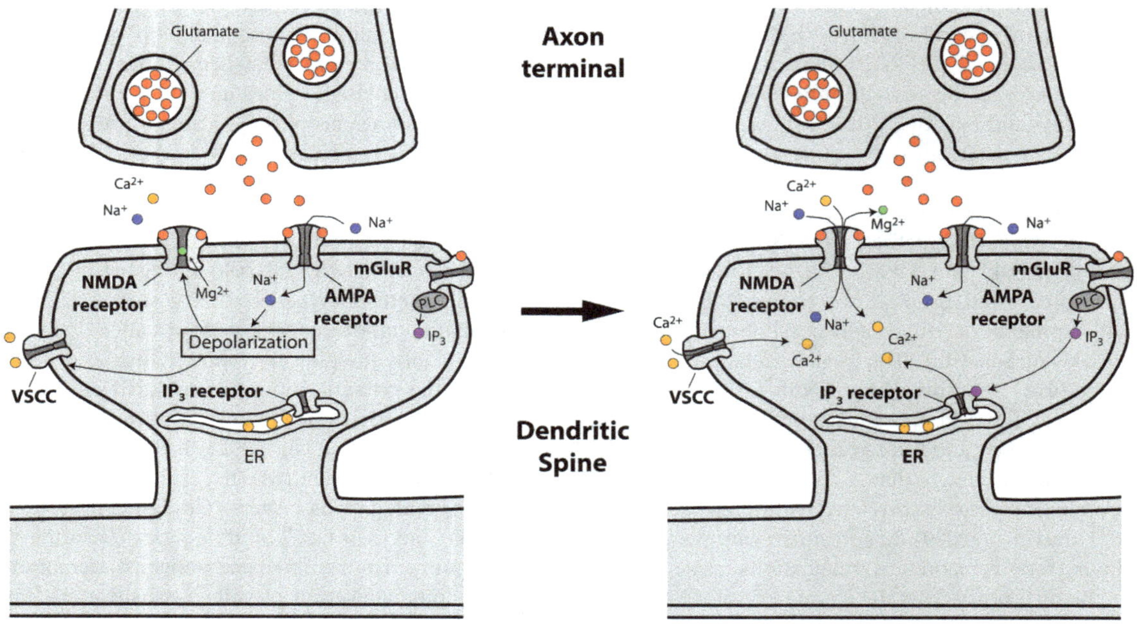

FIGURE 2 | Schematic representing excitatory synaptic transmission and the sources of Ca^{2+} accumulations at the spine head in pyramidal neurons. Left, drawing showing how presynaptically released glutamate activates glutamate (AMPA, NMDA and mGluR) receptors leading to spine head depolarization. **Right**, spine depolarization will generate Ca^{2+} transients at the spine by removing the magnesium block from NMDA receptors, triggering the activation of voltage-sensitive Ca^{2+} channels (VSCCs) and the generation of second messengers like IP_3 (for details see text).

et al., 2004; Matsuzaki et al., 2004; Harvey et al., 2008). The mechanisms through which this occurs include the activation of calcium/calmodulin-dependent protein kinase II (CaMKII) and modification of the AMPA receptor conductance, plasma membrane insertion of AMPA receptors and recruitment of surface AMPA receptors into the synapse (Lisman et al., 2012), modifications to the internalization of spine voltage-gated channels (Kim et al., 2007), and alterations in spine actin dynamics (Fortin et al., 2012; Sala and Segal, 2014). The generation of LTP in individual spines by repetitive 2P uncaging of glutamate has been shown to produce increases in spine head volume that are associated with a Ca^{2+}- and calmodulin-dependent actin reorganization process (Matsuzaki et al., 2004). In addition, studies in which LTD was triggered using low-frequency electrical stimulation or 2P uncaging of glutamate have demonstrated that spine heads may shrink in volume (Zhou et al., 2004; Oh et al., 2013; Wiegert and Oertner, 2013) via a mechanism dependent on mGluRs, IP_3Rs and Ca^{2+} (Oh et al., 2013), or that spines may even retract completely (Nagerl et al., 2004; Wiegert and Oertner, 2013). The activity-dependent structural spine changes observed after LTP and LTD are thought to contribute to the experience-dependent brain changes associated with learning and memory (Lynch, 2004; Holtmaat and Svoboda, 2009; Kasai et al., 2010). Recently, it has been demonstrated that changes in synaptic strength via LTP and LTD are linked with memory formation (Nabavi et al., 2014), suggesting that spines are indeed the functional unit of learning and memory.

In both LTP and LTD, the activation of NMDA receptors and the subsequent increase in spine Ca^{2+} has been suggested to be differentially regulated by the recruitment of separate molecular pathways (Malenka and Bear, 2004). These separate pathways are initiated by the different spatiotemporal Ca^{2+} signals generated by protocols that trigger LTP [high-frequency stimulation (HFS)] or LTD [low-frequency stimulation (LFS)], with LTP being triggered by fast and large spine Ca^{2+} signals within the spine head and LTD triggered by Ca^{2+} signals with differing magnitude and/or duration (i.e., small Ca^{2+} signals) (Malenka and Bear, 2004). Furthermore, NMDA receptor activation and increases in spine Ca^{2+} are required for a process known as spike-timing dependent plasticity (STDP). STDP is a variation of LTP and LTD that has been described in pyramidal cells and involves the pairing of pre- and postsynaptic action potentials (Magee and Johnston, 1997; Markram et al., 1997; Bi and Poo, 1998; Debanne et al., 1998; Zhang et al., 1998). In this process, the relative timing of pre- and postsynaptic action potentials determines the polarity and magnitude of the change in synaptic strength (Zhang et al., 1998). These timing rules are altered in mouse models of Rett and Fragile-X syndromes, two X-linked neurological disorders (Desai et al., 2006; Meredith et al., 2007). Thus, STDP is an important model for understanding learning and memory and is of key importance for understanding developmental and neurodegenerative disorders in which spine structure is impaired (Fiala et al., 2002). Many questions regarding the induction paradigms and molecular cascades responsible for the generation of STDP in the spines of pyramidal neurons remain to be determined.

The fact that spines exist in a variety of head and neck morphologies (Spacek and Harris, 1998; Sorra and Harris, 2000; Arellano et al., 2007b; Takasaki and Sabatini, 2014; Tonnesen et al., 2014) and that the spine neck seems to be important in controlling the amplitude and diffusion of Ca^{2+} out of the spine head (Gold and Bear, 1994; Majewska et al., 2000; Noguchi et al., 2005; Grunditz et al., 2008) is suggestive of a process in which spine morphology not only determines the amplitude and spatiotemporal confinement of Ca^{2+} in the spine head, but also the generation of plasticity. In agreement with this notion, recent modeling studies showed that the relationship between Ca^{2+} influx and spine head morphology is key for determining synaptic stability (O'Donnell et al., 2011). Another important determinant of Ca^{2+} influx in the spine head might be related to the electrical properties of spines (see below) (Grunditz et al., 2008; Bloodgood et al., 2009), in particular how variations in spine neck morphology affect neck resistance (R_N, see below) and synaptic amplification and ion influx in the spine head. Although there is evidence linking spine geometry with the compartmentalization of Ca^{2+} signals in the spine head, how spine geometry affects the molecular machinery and synaptic efficacy during plasticity remains ill-defined. The plethora of functions exerted by Ca^{2+} in the spine is most readily explained by the ability of synaptic inputs and backpropagating action potentials to generate Ca^{2+} signals with different amplitude, kinetics, and spatiotemporal confinement (Sabatini et al., 2002). These features enable the differential activation of signaling pathways (Malenka and Bear, 2004) and lead to structural rearrangements, thereby modifying the close relationship between spine structure and function.

ELECTRICAL COMPARTMENTALIZATION OF THE SPINE

ROLE IN SYNAPTIC TRANSMISSION

Theoretical studies looking at the electrical behavior of spines have suggested that their electrical properties may result in the generation of large excitatory post-synaptic potentials (EPSPs) at the spine head (Jack et al., 1975; Segev and Rall, 1988) that are sufficient to activate spine voltage-gated channels and thus modify synaptic efficacy (Miller et al., 1985; Perkel and Perkel, 1985; Shepherd et al., 1985; Segev and Rall, 1988). These predictions are based on Ohm's law ($V = I * R$, where V is the potential, R the resistance and I the current) and can be understood by considering the spine in the form of an equivalent circuit, consisting of a spine head connected to the dendrite by a slender neck. Each of these membrane compartments can be represented by a resistance–capacitance (RC) circuit (**Figure 1C**). Hence, a useful simplified model to study the generation and propagation of excitatory postsynaptic potentials from the spine head to the dendritic shaft considers the capacitance of the spine head ($C_{m(h)}$), neck ($C_{m(N)}$) and dendrite ($C_{m(d)}$); their membrane resistance ($R_{m(h)}$, $R_{m(N)}$, $R_{m(d)}$) and the synaptic conductance at the spine head (G_{syn}), as well as other conductances at the spine head, neck (G_N), and dendrite (G_d). In addition, the overall spine neck resistance (R_N, see below) and dendritic resistance (R_d) are important factors in controlling the spread of synaptic potentials (**Figure 1C**). Since the spine head and neck have a small surface area their capacitance is negligible. Hence, in this model, the excitatory postsynaptic potential at the spine head ($EPSP_{spHead}$) is represented by

$$EPSP_{spHead} \approx I_{syn} * (R_N + Z) \quad (2)$$

Where I_{syn} is the synaptic current, R_N the spine neck resistance, and Z the dendritic impedance (a property dependent on the resistance and capacitance). Based on dendritic dimensions, Z is expected to be both much smaller than, and not as easily modified as, R_N. In addition, R_N is determined by

$$R_N = 4\rho l/\pi d^2 \quad (3)$$

Where l is the spine neck length, d its diameter and ρ the axial resistivity (Koch, 2004). It is important to note that although it is possible to experimentally measure spine l and d (**Table 1**), the current technologies prevents us measuring the spine neck ρ , hence calculations of R_N using arbitrary values of spine neck ρ (Tonnesen et al., 2014) might not be adequate. Thus, the amplitude of the EPSP at the spine head ($EPSP_{spHead}$) and the degree of passive spine voltage amplification may be drastically modified by changes in R_N, as determined by the neck length l, diameter d and axial resistivity ρ (Koch, 2004). In addition, these predictions indicate that a high R_N will generate large and fast EPSPs at the spine head, which has been suggested to diminish the location-dependent variability of spine potentials (Gulledge et al., 2012) that would otherwise be expected if inputs impinged directly onto the dendritic shaft (Rinzel and Rall, 1974). Furthermore, theoretical studies have proposed that the slender spine neck has an R_N high enough to significantly attenuate the synaptic potential between the spine head and its parent dendrite, therefore affecting synaptic efficacy (Chang, 1952; Llinás and Hillman, 1969; Diamond et al., 1970; Rall, 1974; Jack et al., 1975; Koch and Poggio, 1983a; Koch et al., 1983; Segev and Rall, 1988; Koch, 2004).

Is R_N sufficient to control synaptic weight and thereby modify somatic EPSPs?

Synaptic inputs in individual spines can be mimicked via 2P uncaging of caged glutamate (Matsuzaki et al., 2001; Araya et al., 2006a, 2014; Bloodgood and Sabatini, 2007; Harvey et al., 2008; Harnett et al., 2012). Using this technique, it has been shown in cortical pyramidal neurons that the amplitude of the uncaging evoked spine potentials recorded at the soma are inversely proportional to the length of the spine neck (Araya et al., 2006b; Richardson et al., 2009) (**Figure 3**). In addition, a recent report, using STED-2P imaging and 2P uncaging of glutamate in individual spines of CA1 hippocampal pyramidal neurons, showed an inverse correlation between spine neck length and uncaging potentials recorded at the soma, but with a weaker correlation ($p = 0.09$) than that found in cortical pyramidal neurons (Takasaki and Sabatini, 2014). This apparent discrepancy might depend on dissimilarities between cortical and hippocampal pyramidal spines, or simply because the data from Takasaki and Sabatini (2014) explored spines with a narrower range of neck lengths (~0.2–1.2 μm) than that from Araya et al. (~ 0.2–2 μm) (Araya et al., 2006b). Furthermore, we recently used minimal synaptic stimulation of identified spines and confirmed that EPSP amplitudes are indeed inversely correlated with spine neck lengths, although no significant changes occur in the amplitude of the spine Ca^{2+} response, as measured using 2-photon glutamate uncaging (Araya et al., 2014). This is similar to the reported

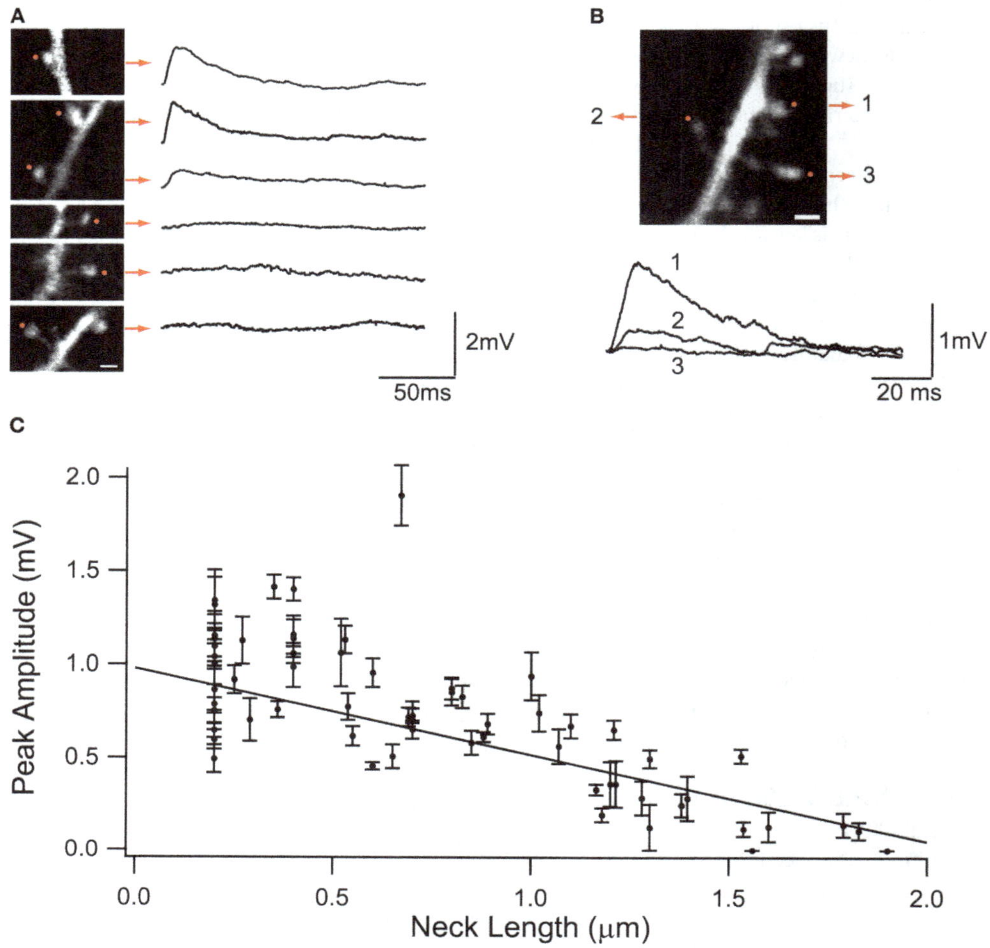

FIGURE 3 | Effect of the spine neck on spine uncaging potentials. (A) Examples of two-photon glutamate uncaging potentials in spines with different neck lengths. Red dots indicate the site of uncaging, and traces correspond to averages of 10 uncaging potentials from each spine. **(B)** Three neighboring spines with different neck lengths. Note the different uncaging potentials generated at the soma of the neuron. **(C)** Plot of the uncaging potential peak amplitude versus neck length. Line is the linear regression of the data with a weighted fit. Standard errors are provided for each point (Figure taken with permission from Araya et al., 2006b).

lack of correlation between spine Ca^{2+} and neck length when using glutamate uncaging at single spines together with 2P STED imaging (Takasaki and Sabatini, 2014).

An intuitive way of capturing the essence of the relation between somatic EPSP and R_N can be obtained by using the voltage divider equation for inputs impinging onto a spine or dendrite (Johnston and Wu, 1995)

$$EPSP_{dend(sp)} = E_{syn} * \frac{R_d}{\frac{1}{Gsyn} + R_N + R_d} \quad (4)$$

$$EPSP_{dend(dend)} = E_{syn} * \frac{R_d}{\frac{1}{Gsyn} + R_d} \quad (5)$$

where $EPSP_{dend(sp)}$ is the amplitude of the voltage generated in the dendrite at the place where the spine is attached, when the synapse occurs at the spine head, and $EPSP_{dend(dend)}$ is the amplitude of the voltage in the dendrite when the synapse is located in the dendrite. R_d represents the input resistance of the dendrite at the place where the spine is attached to the dendrite; G_{syn}, the synaptic conductance; R_N, the spine neck resistance; and E_{syn}, the synaptic reversal potential. Using equations (4) and (5) we can arrive at a simplified formula that depicts the relative effectiveness of a synapse on a spine compared with one directed onto the dendrite

$$\frac{EPSP_{dend(sp)}}{EPSP_{dend(dend)}} = \frac{1}{1+P} \quad (6)$$

in which P is the product of G_{syn} and R_N. For simplicity, I assume a negligible value of R_d. This assumption relies on the fact that the cross sectional area (A) of a dendrite is much larger than that of the spine neck, and hence R_d is much smaller than R_N (see **Figure 4C** for estimated values of R_N and R_d). Second, the assumption is made because the goal of the formulation is to evaluate the effect of the spine neck on synaptic transmission from the spine head to the dendrite through the neck. This fit reveals that provided P is much less than 1, there should be no effect of R_N on dendritic or somatic EPSPs, and a synapse onto a spine could be approximated as a constant current source of amplitude $G_{syn} * E_{syn}$. It is important to note that due to the differential input resistance of the spine head and dendrite, the voltage at the spine head is not the same as the voltage observed in the parent dendrite, with an attenuation factor given by

$$\frac{EPSP_{dend(sp)}}{EPSP_{dend(dend)}} = \frac{R_d}{R_N + R_d} \tag{7}$$

At the other extreme, if $P >> 1$, then the EPSP at the spine head will start to reach E_{syn} and the spine will act as a voltage source, where changes in spine neck length will affect the amount of current entering the spine, and as a consequence the somatic EPSP and the neck length l should be reciprocally related (Koch and Poggio, 1983b) (**Figure 3**). The rate of somatic voltage attenuation with neck length, obtained from the slope of the linear fit to the experimental data from spines from neocortical pyramidal neurons (Araya et al., 2006b, 2014), implies under these assumptions that $P \sim 1$, therefore suggesting that R_N is appreciable.

What is the value of G_{syn} for individual pyramidal neuron spines?

Unfortunately, this value cannot be measured directly at the spine head. However, indirect measurements of AMPA and NMDA receptor unitary synaptic conductances and their content per spine can prove useful when trying to estimate G_{syn} in single dendritic spines. Indeed, non-stationary fluctuation analysis from EPSCs obtained by 2P uncaging of glutamate over individual CA1 pyramidal neuron spines gave an estimated average AMPA receptor unitary current of 0.6 pA and an AMPA receptor number per spine of 46–147 (mean 82) (Matsuzaki et al., 2001). Thus, the conductance of a single AMPA channel (γ) located in a spine can be calculated by dividing the unitary current (0.6 pA) by the driving force at a resting membrane potential of the recorded cells (clamped at −65 mV in Matsuzaki et al., 2001). This gives a value of $\gamma = 9.2$ pS, similar to the calculated AMPA receptor γ value of ~8 pS obtained from non-stationary fluctuation analyses of synaptic responses in CA1 pyramidal neurons (Benke et al., 1998). Although there was some variability in the unitary synaptic conductance reported in both articles, most of the inputs triggered small unitary synaptic conductances [(Benke et al., 1998), mean value for γ of 7.7 ± 0.7 pS; (Matsuzaki et al., 2001), mean AMPA unitary current of 0.6 ± 0.1 (or 9 pS)]. By multiplying the number of AMPA receptors per spine by γ, the total estimated AMPA receptor dependent synaptic conductance per spine is ~0.4–1.4 nS (mean 0.8 nS) for a CA1 pyramidal neuron. Given these estimated AMPA-only G_{syn} values, the addition of NMDA receptors and active conductances could easily produce G_{syn} values of ≥1 nS. At such G_{syn} values and with the simplified assumption of $P \sim 1$, (this) supports the somatic voltage attenuation with spine neck length observed experimentally (Araya et al., 2006b, 2014), and implies R_N values of ~1 GΩ.

Furthermore, as predicted by modeling studies (Miller et al., 1985), voltage-gated ion channels in the spine are recruited independently of those in the dendritic shaft (Araya et al., 2007; Bloodgood et al., 2009), thereby affecting synaptic efficacy (Miller et al., 1985; Araya et al., 2007; Allen et al., 2011). These data suggest that spines have an appreciable R_N that allows them to act as electrical compartments with active conductances, but it is unclear if the experimentally observed correlation between spine neck length and EPSP amplitude recorded at the soma can be explained entirely or only partly by the passive attenuation of synaptic potentials through the spine neck. The explanation as to why this question remains unresolved resides in the experimental limitations of current electrophysiological techniques, which are incapable of directly measuring R_N or absolute spine voltage responses. However, different experimental strategies have been implemented to estimate R_N, providing values ranging from just a few MΩ (Svoboda et al., 1996; Grunditz et al., 2008; Palmer and Stuart, 2009; Tonnesen et al., 2014) up to ~500 MΩ (Palmer and Stuart, 2009; Harnett et al., 2012) or 1 GΩ (Bloodgood and Sabatini, 2005; Grunditz et al., 2008). A recent study by Magee and colleagues used a clever experimental design in which 2P Ca^{2+} imaging, glutamate uncaging, and dual dendritic patch-clamp recording and current injection were combined to estimate the R_N of spines belonging to CA1 pyramidal neurons using the voltage divider equation (**Figure 4**) (Harnett et al., 2012). Their data showed that all spines they analyzed had high R_N (spines with an apparent short neck), with an average value of ~500 MΩ—sufficient to amplify spine potentials to ~25 mV for an average unitary event and to enhance input cooperativity (Harnett et al., 2012). Their experimental design and the variables recorded in order to estimate R_N can be seen in **Figure 4**.

Are R_N values of ~500 MΩ sufficient to influence somatic EPSP amplitude and thereby provide a mechanism for controlling synaptic efficacy?

Experimental evidence therefore indicates that relatively high values of R_N can lead to amplification of synaptic inputs at the spine head. The question then arises as to whether similar R_N values may be sufficient to influence somatic EPSP amplitude. In this regard, numerical simulations of spines using a G_{syn} of 500 pS have shown that an R_N of 500 MΩ can cause a reduction in somatic EPSP amplitude of only ~15% (Palmer and Stuart, 2009). In addition, our own simulations using morphologically realistic multi-compartmental models to explore the passive spine properties and R_N values required to reproduce the experimentally obtained inverse correlation between neck length and somatic EPSP amplitude (Araya et al., 2006b, 2014; Richardson et al., 2009; Vogels et al., 2009) gave us R_N values that are at odds with previous R_N estimates (Harnett et al., 2012). Thus, it is unlikely that R_N values of ~500 MΩ can significantly influence somatic EPSP amplitude and explain the neck length control of somatic EPSP amplitude. Instead, the inverse correlation we observed may result from a combination of passive (e.g., through a reduction in driving force for the synaptic current entering the spine head with increasing R_N, see above) and active spine mechanisms (e.g., active dampening of EPSPs by the engagement of spine voltage-gated potassium channels) and/or

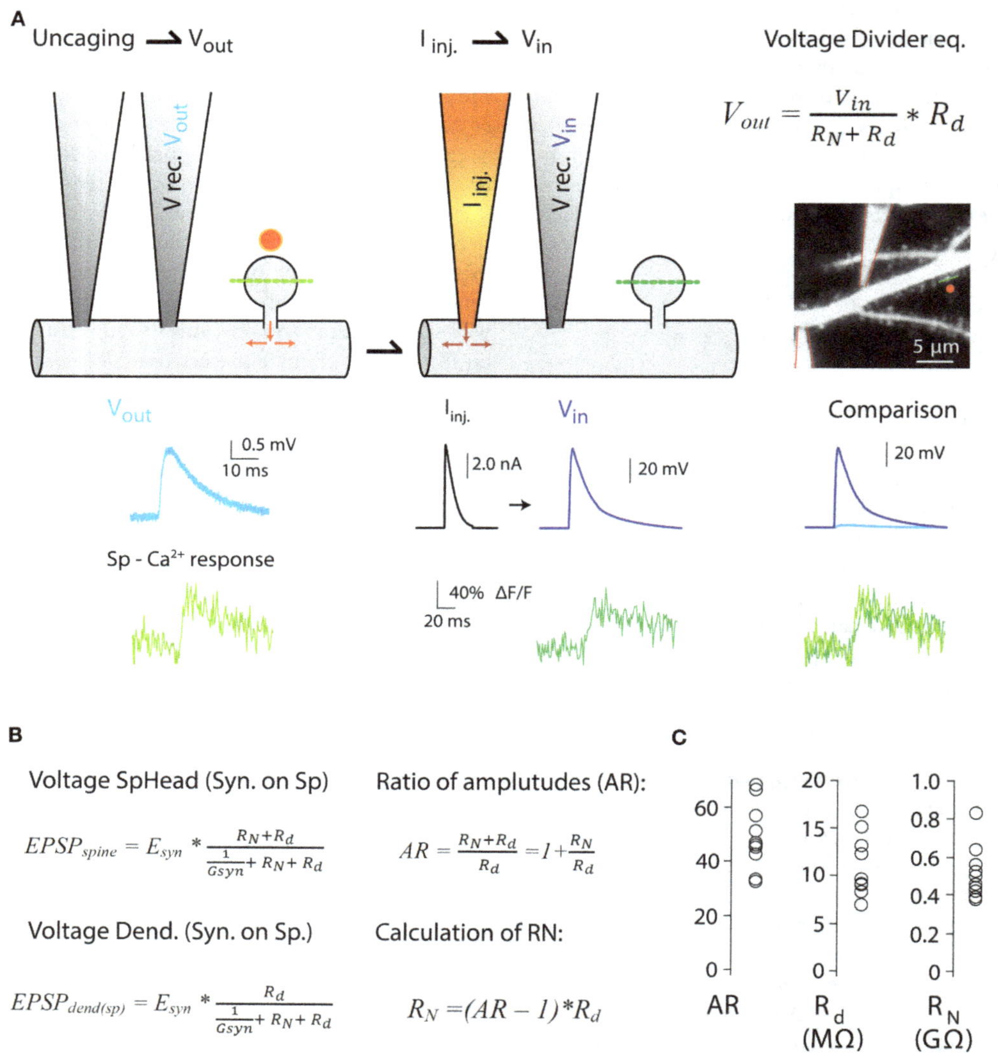

FIGURE 4 | Measurements of the ratio of spine-to-dendrite voltage amplitude, to estimate R_N using the voltage divider equation. Harnett et al. (2012) estimated R_N by combining two-photon Ca^{2+} imaging and glutamate uncaging with dual dendritic patch-clamp current injection and voltage recording from hippocampal CA1 pyramidal neurons in acute slices. **(A)** Uncaging potential [light blue trace in **(A)**] was produced by uncaging onto a single spine and recording in the dendrite (V rec. V_{out}) while measuring spine head Ca^{2+} responses (Sp-Ca^{2+} response, light green trace) mediated exclusively by voltage-sensitive Ca^{2+} channels (VSCC) (see Harnett et al., 2012 for details). Next, current injection ($I_{inj.}$) into the dendrite was performed to depolarize the spine to a level that triggers Ca^{2+} responses in the spine head (dark green traces) similar to the ones produced by glutamate uncaging (V_{in} in voltage divider equation. Also see comparison of V_{in} and V_{out} spine head Ca^{2+} responses). Assuming a lack of voltage attenuation from the dendrite to the spine, the uncaging potential and the voltage generated by I_{inj} provide a good estimate of the spine head potentials (V_{in}). Two-photon image of a dendrite patched with two patch electrodes, and the voltage and calcium traces were taken from Harnett et al. (2012). **(B)** The amount of electrical compartmentalization produced by the spine can be measured as the amplitude ratio (AR) of the voltage at the spine head when an input impinges on the spine ($EPSP_{spine}$), to the voltage at the dendrite when the synapse impinges on the spine ($EPSP_{dend(sp)}$). **(C)** Calculation of R_N was obtained by the equation depicted in **(B)**. Modified with permission from Harnett et al. (2012). See Harnett et al. (2012) for details.

the differential control of AMPA receptor content between spines of different neck lengths.

Recently, by inducing LTP with an STDP protocol in which 2P uncaging of glutamate over individual spines was paired with bAPs (Tanaka et al., 2008), it was demonstrated that activated spines undergo activity-dependent structural changes (Tanaka et al., 2008; Araya et al., 2014), with long- and short-necked spines experiencing a rapid shrinkage in spine neck length that correlated with an increase in the somatically recorded uncaging potential (Araya et al., 2014). These results could provide an explanation as to why pyramidal neuron dendrites are covered with long-necked spines, providing a reservoir of connectivity that can be called into action upon activity, without the need to rewire the neuronal network.

To better understand the electrical properties of spines and the implications for synaptic transmission and plasticity, further experiments devoted to understanding the passive and active mechanisms controlling synaptic efficacy and synaptic amplification at the spine head are required. In addition, it seems likely that to achieve a full understanding of these issues, strategies that allow neural electrode size to be substantially reduced—capable of recording directly from the spine head and parent dendrite—as well as proper optical voltage-sensing probes must be developed to directly measure absolute spine potentials, neck resistivity ρ and R_N.

ROLE OF SPINES IN SYNAPTIC INTEGRATION AND PLASTICITY: CLUSTERED vs DISTRIBUTED CONNECTIVITY

Two fundamental questions in neuroscience are (1) what is the spatiotemporal pattern of the multitude of excitatory inputs impinging on a pyramidal neuron? and (2) how can structural and molecular remodeling at the synaptic level support synaptic plasticity, modify the strength of individual synapses and change the input/output properties of a pyramidal neuron?

Two main models exist for the possible distribution of synaptic inputs: clustered, in which synchronous or asynchronous synaptic inputs arrive at a spatially restricted zone in the dendrites of the postsynaptic neuron; and distributed, in which inputs are spread along the dendritic arbor of the postsynaptic neuron. Related to this are the concepts of random and structured connectivity. Random connectivity naturally implies that connections between two neurons occur by chance, and inputs should therefore be distributed approximately randomly over the dendritic tree (Peters and Feldman, 1976). Structured connectivity, however, allows for clustered inputs (although inputs may also be "structured" to achieve distributed inputs), which implies that there is a choice by the presynaptic neuron as to where to form a synaptic connection. Clearly, the fact that excitatory inputs are directed to spines rather than shaft locations implies that connectivity is not entirely random. The level of randomness within a structured connectivity paradigm could then be defined at the next level—how excitatory inputs, directed to spines, are placed along the dendritic tree of the postsynaptic pyramidal neuron; are they distributed or clustered? What are the functional consequences and computational power conferred by having inputs distributed or clustered in the dendrites? Single-synapse resolution reconstructions of axons and dendrites from connected pairs of layer V thick-tufted pyramidal neurons of the somatosensory cortex have suggested that axons touch all neighboring dendrites in a distributed manner without any bias (Kalisman et al., 2005). Consistent with this, a more recent study from the Konnerth laboratory using high speed *in vivo* 2P imaging of dendrites and electrophysiological recordings from Layer II pyramidal neurons revealed that orientation-tuned neurons received spatially distributed synaptic inputs to generate their characteristic firing pattern (Jia et al., 2010). Moreover, in a follow-up paper, the same group performed *in vivo* imaging of spine activity in the dendrites of Layer II pyramidal neurons and demonstrated that a sound stimulus activated spines that were broadly distributed on basal and apical dendrites (Chen et al., 2011).

However, not all studies have found such spatially distributed connectivity, instead obtaining evidence for clustered connectivity. Recently, experiments performed in neuronal hippocampal slice cultures and in Layer II/III barrel cortex pyramidal neurons *in vivo* showed that activity frequently occurred in neighboring spines (Takahashi et al., 2012), a finding that was also observed during the development of hippocampal pyramidal neurons (Kleindienst et al., 2011, for review see DeBello et al., 2014).

But how would distributed or clustered connectivity affect neuronal output?

The first to propose that the mode of integration of coincident synaptic inputs impinging directly on the dendrite will depend greatly upon their dendritic location was Rall (1964), who stated:

> "*These results show that, although the departure from linearity* [linearity meaning the arithmetic sum of the synaptic events] *can become quite large when perturbations are superimposed upon the same compartment, the departure from linearity can be surprisingly small when brief perturbations occur in separate portions of the dendritic periphery.*"

Theoretical predictions and experimental studies—in which numerous spines are activated almost simultaneously by means of 2P uncaging of glutamate—have shown that the activation of a small number of neighboring spines results in linear integration (Poirazi et al., 2003; Araya et al., 2006a; Losonczy and Magee, 2006; Gomez Gonzalez et al., 2011) (**Figure 5**), but that the addition of clustered excitatory inputs causes a threshold to be reached for the generation of a non-linear, suprathreshold integrative voltage response—or spike—generated in the dendrites (Gasparini and Magee, 2006; Losonczy and Magee, 2006; Harnett et al., 2012) (**Figure 5**). Indeed, it is well known that neocortical pyramidal neuron dendrites are capable of triggering sodium, calcium, and NMDA spikes (Larkum and Nevian, 2008; Major et al., 2008; Larkum et al., 2009; Murayama et al., 2009; Polsky et al., 2009). Thus, the presence of clustered inputs and the generation of non-linear responses can increase the computational power of dendrites (Losonczy et al., 2008), for example by changing the threshold for LTP at local (to the input) spines (Harvey et al., 2008) and selectively enhancing excitability in dendrites (Losonczy et al., 2008), as well as serving as a mechanism to overcome the distance dependence of synaptic efficacy (Williams and Stuart, 2003; Spruston, 2008). However, in a fully distributed network, this level of structural and functional dendritic fitness would not be necessary for neuronal and network computations, and synaptic transmission and storage will mainly be controlled by the biochemical and electrical properties of spines (**Figure 6**).

In conclusion, significant evidence has accumulated in favor of both the distributed and clustered input hypotheses. However, whether these are mutually exclusive has not yet been resolved, and the divergent results may be due to different regimes being recruited under different circumstances. In addition, how dendrites and spines transform different spatiotemporal input sequences into different output patterns, and how these inputs can trigger changes in synapse strength and affect experience-dependent learning, remain ill-defined.

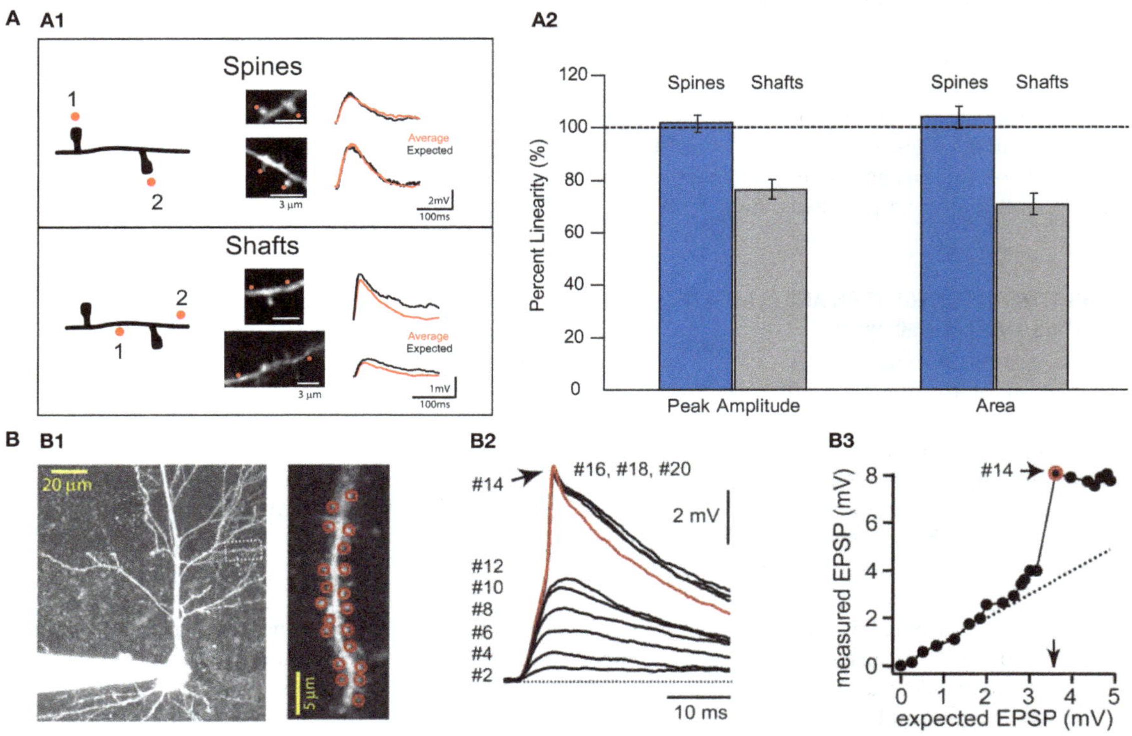

FIGURE 5 | Summation of excitatory uncaging potentials on spines and dendritic shafts. (A1) Left, drawing of a dendrite from a layer V pyramidal cell showing the protocol for testing summation in spines and shafts. Red dots indicate the sites of uncaging in spines or shafts. Middle, two-photon images showing the uncaging locations in spines or shafts (red dots). Right, voltage responses were recorded with a patch electrode in current-clamp configuration. Two-photon uncaging of glutamate was performed first at each spine or shaft location (1 or 2) and then in either both spines together or in both shaft locations (1 + 2). Summation in spines: Red trace corresponds to an average of 10 depolarizations caused by uncaging over the two spines, and black traces correspond to the expected algebraic (linear) sum of the individual events of each spine. Summation in shafts: Data are presented as for spines. Note how the average uncaging response when spines are activated is close to the expected value. However, when inputs impinge on shaft locations, the integration is sublinear (Image modified from Araya et al., 2006a). **(A2)** Summary of results from Araya et al. (2006a). Data are presented as averages ± s.e.m. **(B)** Data taken with permission from Losonczy and Magee (2006). **(B1)** Two-photon image stack from a CA1 pyramidal neuron. Inset, red circles indicate the site of uncaging in spines—up to 20 spines in this example. **(B2)** Two-photon uncaging potentials evoked at a 0.1 ms interval, ranging from 2 to 20 activated spines. **(B3)** Input/output plot for the experiment. Note how inputs onto spines integrate linearly before additional inputs generate a dendritic spike.

A HYPOTHESIS FOR THE *RAISON D'ETRE* OF DENDRITIC SPINES

In 1969, Llinás and Hillman (1969) suggested that if synaptic inputs are directed simultaneously to dendritic spines with high R_N, the synapses would be converted into a near constant current system that protects the length constant of the dendrite by preventing variations in input resistance, producing a more linear summation of synaptic potentials in spines that belong to the same dendritic compartment. In addition, they predicted that if synaptic inputs are instead directed toward the dendritic shaft, the inputs would summate in a more non-linear fashion (Llinás and Hillman, 1969). Indeed, as pointed out before, experiments using nearly simultaneous 2P uncaging of glutamate to activate 2–3 (Araya et al., 2006b), 7–10 (Gasparini and Magee, 2006) or up to ~20 spines (Losonczy and Magee, 2006) located in the same dendritic compartment (covering <20 µm of the dendrite) demonstrated that excitatory inputs onto spines integrate linearly before additional inputs generate a dendritic spike (Losonczy and Magee, 2006) (**Figure 5B**), whereas inputs delivered to the same compartment but onto the dendritic shaft integrate sublinearly (Araya et al., 2006a) (**Figure 5A**), most likely due to a local decrease in driving force or shunting interactions between the excitatory inputs, as proposed by Llinás and Hillman (1969) (**Figures 5, 6**). These results and predictions suggest that the departure from linearity in pyramidal neurons (and other neurons) should be small or negligible when excitatory inputs are directed to separate portions of the dendritic shaft (Rall, 1974) (**Figure 6**). Indeed, the degree of linear summation between converging EPSPs on fast spiking (FS) cells correlates with the distance between the nearest neighboring synapses impinging on the dendritic shaft of FS cells (Tamas et al., 2002).

IS THE OBSERVED SUBTHRESHOLD LINEAR SUMMATION OF SYNCHRONOUS EXCITATORY INPUTS PROTECTED BY THE SPINE R_N?

Numerical simulations have indicated that two neighboring, simultaneously active spine synapses could reproduce the linear integration observed experimentally (Araya et al., 2006a) by building spines with R_N of 600 MΩ (Grunditz et al., 2008),

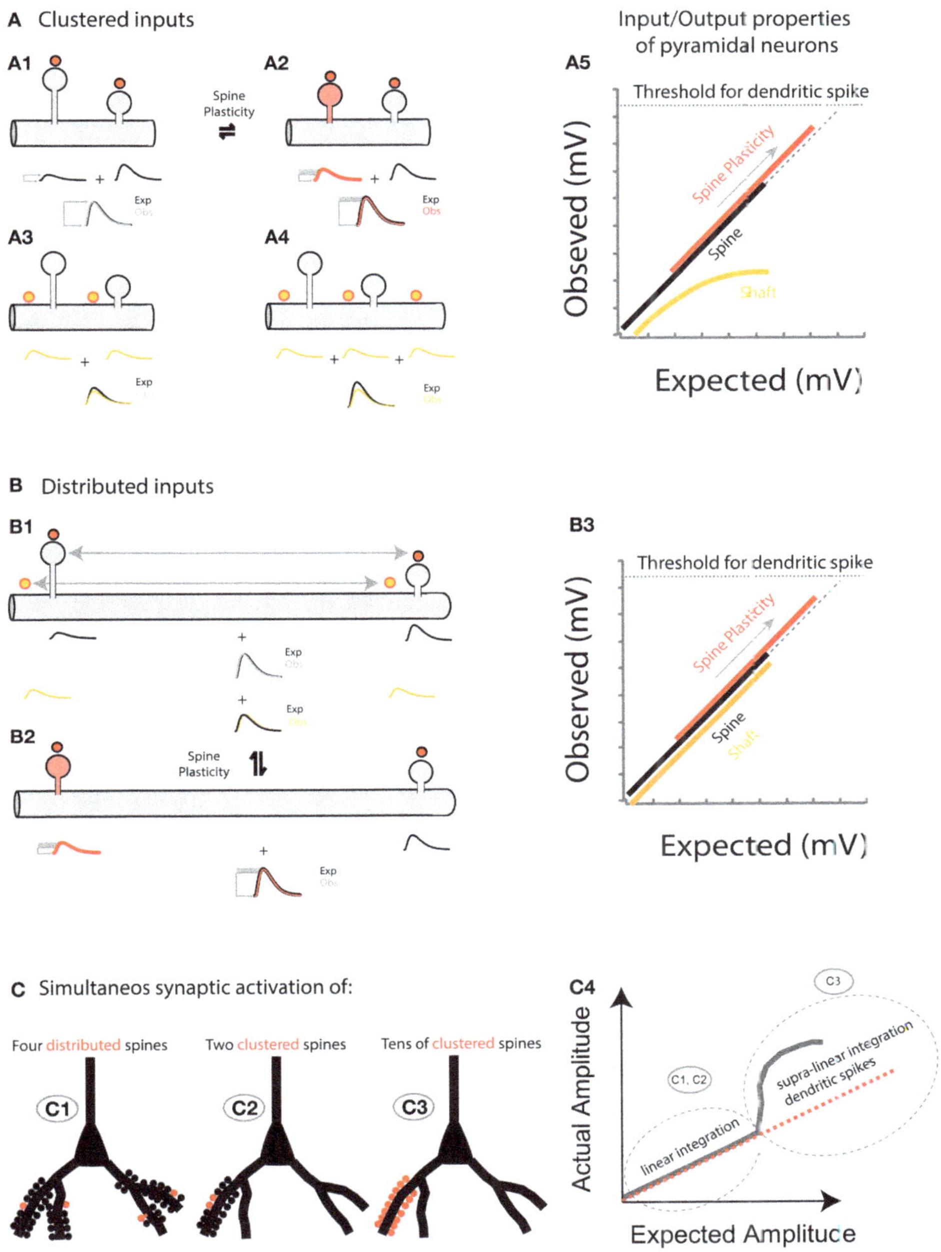

FIGURE 6 | (A) Spatially clustered inputs: Excitatory inputs directed to clustered spines add linearly (**A1**, compare the expected algebraic (linear) sum (Exp., black trace) of the individual events of each spine with the observed response after simultaneous activation of all spines (Obs., gray trace)) before the generation of a dendritic spike (**A5**, dotted line indicates the threshold for triggering a dendritic spike). In contrast, excitatory inputs directed to clustered shaft locations will shunt each other (**A3** for 2 inputs, and **A4** for 3 inputs). Note that more shunting is expected if more clustered inputs are directed to the shaft (compare Exp. (black trace) vs. Obs. (yellow trace) in **A3**,**A4**). **A5**, Plot of the observed vs. expected amplitude (mV) for uncaging events in spines (black) or shafts (yellow) along the dendrite of layer 5 pyramidal neurons. Plasticity (for simplicity I only focus here on neck plasticity as reported in Araya et al., 2014): Spine-STDP will generate a significant change in the neck length (and probably a conductance change) of the stimulated spine (**A2**, red spine) with a concomitant change in synaptic weight (red trace, gray box shows the amplitude change from control). Single spine-STDP will increase the input/output gain (**A5**, red trace and arrow indicating the change in gain from the control (black) trace) of the neuron without affecting the linear integration of subthreshold excitatory inputs. **(B)** Spatially distributed inputs: Distributed excitatory inputs directed to spine (red dots) or shaft locations (yellow dots) will integrate linearly (**B1**, compare Exp. Vs. Obs.) by preventing large variations in the input impedance of the dendrite, thus avoiding shunting interactions that would otherwise be expected if clustered inputs are directed to the dendritic shaft (**A3**,**A4**). **B3** same as **A5** but with distributed inputs onto spine and shaft locations. **(C)** Representation of the summation of excitatory inputs directed to spines of a pyramidal neuron. The simultaneous synaptic activation of a few distributed (**C1**) or clustered (**C2**) spines (red) would trigger a voltage response that matches the arithmetic linear sum of each spine's voltage contribution. If tens of spines are activated simultaneously within the same branch (**C3**), then a supralinear response, or dendritic spike, will be generated.

similar to the R_N values calculated from the spines of CA1 pyramidal neurons (Harnett et al., 2012). In addition, these simulations showed that the same synapses can experience sublinear integration when R_N is lowered to 100 MΩ (Grunditz et al., 2008), resembling the experimentally observed sublinear integration when neighboring shaft locations were activated (Araya et al., 2006a) (**Figure 5A**). In these simulations the high spine R_N-dependent linear summation of excitatory inputs depends on electrical amplification and the recruitment of voltage-gated channels at the spine head (Grunditz et al., 2008). These experimental results (Araya et al., 2006a; Gasparini and Magee, 2006; Losonczy and Magee, 2006), together with modeling predictions (Grunditz et al., 2008), imply that most if not all spines with short- and long necks act as electrical compartments, having R_N values that exceed the critical threshold for promoting the linear integration of excitatory inputs (**Figures 5, 6**). However, the precise passive and active spine mechanisms that promote the linear summation of subthreshold inputs remains unknown. Thus, subthreshold depolarizations in the dendrites that arise from multiple synchronously activated spines—either spatially clustered (Araya et al., 2006a; Gasparini and Magee, 2006; Losonczy and Magee, 2006) or distributed (Gasparini and Magee, 2006; Losonczy and Magee, 2006)—summate linearly before the generation of a dendritic spike (**Figures 5, 6**).

SPINES AS ACTIVITY-DEPENDENT GAIN MODULATORS: A HYPOTHESIS ON THE TRUE *RAISON D'ETRE* FOR SPINES

If one of the important functions of spines is to promote the linear integration of subthreshold dendritic depolarizations that are triggered by synchronous, clustered excitatory inputs, then why are excitatory inputs still directed to spines in circumstances when the distance between synapses is large enough to allow linear summation if the inputs were directed directly to the dendritic shaft? One possible reason, and perhaps the true *raison d'etre* for spines, is that they can undergo transient and persistent activity-dependent structural [spine head enlargement (Lang et al., 2004; Matsuzaki et al., 2004; Harvey et al., 2008), spine head reduction (Zhou et al., 2004; Oh et al., 2013; Wiegert and Oertner, 2013), and neck plasticity (Bloodgood and Sabatini, 2005; Grunditz et al., 2008; Tanaka et al., 2008; Araya et al., 2014; Tonnesen et al., 2014)] and molecular changes (Malenka and Bear, 2004; Yasuda, 2006; Harvey et al., 2008; Lee et al., 2009; Murakoshi et al., 2011; Yasuda and Murakoshi, 2011; Lisman et al., 2012) that can modify synaptic strength (Matsuzaki et al., 2004; Araya et al., 2014), and hence alter the gain of pyramidal neuron input/output properties without the need to rewire the network.

Hence, the hypothesis I put forth is that: (1) Subthreshold depolarizations in the dendrites, arising from multiple synchronously activated spines—either spatially clustered or distributed—summate linearly before the generation of a dendritic spike (**Figures 5, 6**); and (2) that spine plasticity triggers rapid and reversible changes in synaptic weight and hence in the gain of pyramidal neuron input/output properties, providing an effective and rapid control of the threshold (number of spines activated) required to generate a dendritic or somatic spike (**Figure 6**).

This more economical way of modifying a neuron's computational power would rely on the ability to modify the passive (e.g., spine morphology) and active (recruitment of voltage-gated channels) properties of spines, influencing the neuron's electrical and biochemical compartmentalization capabilities and providing a fast and effective control of synaptic transmission, storage and integration.

Another prediction for this hypothesis is that the activity-dependent spine changes, although sufficient to change synaptic efficacy, might not be drastic enough to disrupt the linearly integrated sub-threshold dendritic depolarization. This would prevent the sublinear integration of synchronous and clustered inputs that would be observed if inputs impinged on spines with a low R_N or directly onto the dendritic shaft. I based this prediction on the experimental observations showing that linearity of subthreshold depolarization is protected even when the uncaging of glutamate was directed to clustered spines of different morphologies (Araya et al., 2006a; Gasparini and Magee, 2006; Losonczy and Magee, 2006).

To test this hypothesis, a spatially multiplexed imaging/uncaging tool such as a spatial light modulator (SLM) (Nikolenko et al., 2008) could be employed. This would allow the simultaneous uncaging of glutamate (with single spine resolution) at several spines (up to 30 in a 2P regime) and facilitate study of the role of spines in spatial summation, as well as how plasticity paradigms might affect the input/output gain and/or integration algorithm of sub-threshold depolarizations.

SPINES AND DISEASE

In his seminal article "Dendritic spine 'dysgenesis' and mental retardation," Dr. Purpura described the perfect correlation between the degree of mental retardation and the extent of spine morphological aberrations, with dendrites from cortical neurons of retarded children being covered with abnormally long and thin dendritic spines (Purpura, 1974). Since then, many studies have indicated that an important phenotype in many brain disorders is the abnormal shape and density of dendritic spines (see below). As pointed out before, the correlation between form and function of dendritic spines is well accepted; thus the notion that alterations in spine morphology affect synaptic transmission, integration and information storage is not challenged.

Fragile X syndrome (FXS) is the most frequent form of inherited mental retardation (Jacquemont et al., 2007; Hagerman et al., 2010) and the most common known single-gene cause of autism (Wang et al., 2012). FXS is caused by inactivation of the Fragile X Mental retardation 1 (FMR1) gene, which encodes the Fragile X Mental Retardation Protein (FMRP) (Bassell and Warren, 2008; De Rubeis and Bagni, 2010) an RNA-binding protein that has a major role in inhibiting the translation of bound mRNAs, especially at neuronal synapses (Darnell et al., 2011; Wang et al., 2012). At a gross scale the post-mortem brains of FXS patients are almost intact (Reiss et al., 1995; Hallahan et al., 2011). However, at the micro-anatomical level it has been found that FXS is characterized by major alterations to dendritic spines, with abnormally long-necked spines with prominent heads mixed with normal looking spines (Rudelli et al., 1985; Irwin et al., 2001). The assumption was that since these spine aberrations resemble immature spines, the phenotype could be indicative of developmental dendritic deficits. A similar spine phenotype—with long, thin and tortuous spines—was evident in a mouse model of FXS, the Fmr1 KO mice (Irwin et al., 2002; Galvez and Greenough, 2005). In addition, there is evidence in the Fmr1 KO mice that not only is spine morphology impaired, but that spine density is increased (Comery et al., 1997; Galvez and Greenough, 2005; McKinney et al., 2005). Furthermore, it has been demonstrated in these mice that stronger neuronal activity is required to trigger STDP in Fmr1 KO mice (Meredith et al., 2007). The reader is referred to the following reviews on spine density, maturity and plasticity in FXS for further information (Portera-Cailliau, 2012; He and Portera-Cailliau, 2013). Moreover, in Rett syndrome, a disease caused by mutations in the X-linked methyl CpG binding protein 2 (MECP2) and associated with intellectual disabilities (Amir et al., 1999), patients exhibit a drastic reduction in cortical pyramidal neuron spine density (for review see Xu et al., 2014).

A reduction in the number of spines and dendritic impairments has also been observed in aging, psychiatric disorders such as schizophrenia and major depressive disorder, and in neurodegenerative disorders such as Alzheimer's disease (Peters et al., 1998; Fiala et al., 2002; Penzes et al., 2011; Koleske, 2013). The list of diseases in which spine morphology and density have proven important is vast, including not only neurodegenerative or psychiatric disorders, but also diseases like epilepsy in which spine loss is evident (Scheibel et al., 1974; Isokawa, 1997). This is perhaps not surprising since spines are the main gateway of excitatory and some inhibitory information in the brain, and alterations in spine structure and function will likely have huge effects on input transformation in the brain.

In conclusion, the study of spines has proven to be essential for the understanding of synaptic processing, plasticity and integration in pyramidal neurons. In addition, these tiny protrusions are believed to be the pathogenic substrate in neuropsychiatric disorders in which spine structure, density and/or function are impaired. Thus, understanding spine function will not only shed light on how pyramidal neurons and the circuits in which they reside work, but will also provide a new framework for understanding the contribution of spines to various diseases. This may in turn aid the development of novel therapeutic approaches for neurodegenerative disorders such as Alzheimer's disease and Fragile X-syndrome, illnesses in which spine structure and function are impaired.

ACKNOWLEDGMENT

I would like to thank Dr. Alan Woodruff for comments and discussion.

REFERENCES

Allen, D., Bond, C. T., Lujan, R., Ballesteros-Merino, C., Lin, M. T., Wang, K., et al. (2011). The SK2-long isoform directs synaptic localization and function of SK2-containing channels. *Nat. Neurosci.* 14, 744–749. doi: 10.1038/nn.2832

Amir, R. E., Van den Veyver, I. B., Wan, M., Tran, C. Q., Francke, U., and Zoghbi, H. Y. (1999). Rett syndrome is caused by mutations in X-linked MECP2, encoding methyl-CpG-binding protein 2. *Nat. Genet.* 23, 185–188. doi: 10.1038/13810

Araya, R., Eisenthal, K. B., and Yuste, R. (2006a). Dendritic spines linearize the summation of excitatory potentials. *Proc. Natl. Acad. Sci. U.S.A.* 103, 18799–18804. doi: 10.1073/pnas.0609225103

Araya, R., Jiang, J., Eisenthal, K. B., and Yuste, R. (2006b). The spine neck filters membrane potentials. *Proc. Natl. Acad. Sci. U.S.A.* 103, 17961–17966. doi: 10.1073/pnas.0608755103

Araya, R., Nikolenko, V., Eisenthal, K. B., and Yuste, R. (2007). Sodium channels amplify spine potentials. *Proc. Natl. Acad. Sci. U.S.A.* 104, 12347–12352. doi: 10.1073/pnas.0705282104

Araya, R., Vogels, T. P., and Yuste, R. (2014). Activity-dependent dendritic spine neck changes are correlated with synaptic strength. *Proc. Natl. Acad. Sci. U.S.A.* 111, E2895–E2904. doi: 10.1073/pnas.1321869111

Arellano, J. I., Benavides-Piccione, R., Defelipe, J., and Yuste, R. (2007a). Ultrastructure of dendritic spines: correlation between synaptic and spine morphologies. *Front. Neurosci.* 1, 131–143. doi: 10.3389/neuro.01.1.1.010.2007

Arellano, J. I., Espinosa, A., Fairen, A., Yuste, R., and DeFelipe, J. (2007b). Non-synaptic dendritic spines in neocortex. *Neuroscience* 145, 464–469. doi: 10.1016/j.neuroscience.2006.12.015

Baimbridge, K. G., Celio, M. R., and Rogers, J. H. (1992). Calcium-binding proteins in the nervous system. *Trends Neurosci.* 15, 303–308. doi: 10.1016/0166-2236(92)90081-I

Bassell, G. J., and Warren, S. T. (2008). Fragile X syndrome: loss of local mRNA regulation alters synaptic development and function. *Neuron* 60, 201–214. doi: 10.1016/j.neuron.2008.10.004

Benke, T. A., Luthi, A., Isaac, J. T., and Collingridge, G. L. (1998). Modulation of AMPA receptor unitary conductance by synaptic activity. *Nature* 393, 793–797. doi: 10.1038/31709

Bethge, P., Chereau, R., Avignone, E., Marsicano, G., and Nagerl, U. V. (2013). Two-photon excitation STED microscopy in two colors in acute brain slices. *Biophys. J.* 104, 778–785. doi: 10.1016/j.bpj.2012.12.054

Betzig, E., Patterson, G. H., Sougrat, R., Lindwasser, O. W., Olenych, S., Bonifacino, J. S., et al. (2006). Imaging intracellular fluorescent proteins at nanometer resolution. *Science* 313, 1642–1645. doi: 10.1126/science.1127344

Bi, G. Q., and Poo, M. M. (1998). Synaptic modifications in cultured hippocampal neurons: dependence on spike timing, synaptic strength, and postsynaptic cell type. *J. Neurosci.* 18, 10464–10472.

Bloodgood, B. L., Giessel, A. J., and Sabatini, B. L. (2009). Biphasic synaptic Ca influx arising from compartmentalized electrical signals in dendritic spines. *PLoS Biol.* 7:e1000190. doi: 10.1371/journal.pbio.1000190

Bloodgood, B. L., and Sabatini, B. L. (2005). Neuronal activity regulates diffusion across the neck of dendritic spines. *Science* 310, 866–869. doi: 10.1126/science.1114816

Bloodgood, B. L., and Sabatini, B. L. (2007). Nonlinear regulation of unitary synaptic signals by CaV(2.3) voltage-sensitive calcium channels located in dendritic spines. *Neuron* 53, 249–260. doi: 10.1016/j.neuron.2006.12.017

Cajal, S. R. (1888). Estructura de los centros nerviosos de las aves. *Rev. Trim. Histol. Norm. Patol.* 1, 1–10.

Chang, H. T. (1952). Cortical neurons with particular reference to the apical dendrite. *Cold Spring Harb. Symp. Quant. Biol.* 17, 189–202. doi: 10.1101/SQB.1952.017.01.019

Chen, J. L., Villa, K. L., Cha, J. W., So, P. T., Kubota, Y., and Nedivi, E. (2012a). Clustered dynamics of inhibitory synapses and dendritic spines in the adult neocortex. *Neuron* 74, 361–373. doi: 10.1016/j.neuron.2012.02.030

Chen, X., Leischner, U., Rochefort, N. L., Nelken, I., and Konnerth, A. (2011). Functional mapping of single spines in cortical neurons *in vivo*. *Nature* 475, 501–505. doi: 10.1038/nature10193

Chen, X., Leischner, U., Varga, Z., Jia, H., Deca, D., Rochefort, N. L., and Konnerth, A. (2012b). LOTOS-based two-photon calcium imaging of dendritic spines *in vivo*. *Nat. Protoc.* 7, 1818–1829. doi: 10.1038/nprot.2012.106

Chittajallu, R., Alford, S., and Collingridge, G. L. (1998). Ca2+ and synaptic plasticity. *Cell Calcium* 24, 377–385. doi: 10.1016/S0143-4160(98)90061-6

Chiu, C. Q., Lur, G., Morse, T. M., Carnevale, N. T., Ellis-Davies, G. C., and Higley, M. J. (2013). Compartmentalization of GABAergic inhibition by dendritic spines. *Science* 340, 759–762. doi: 10.1126/science.1234274

Colgan, L. A., and Yasuda, R. (2014). Plasticity of dendritic spines: subcompartmentalization of signaling. *Annu. Rev. Physiol.* 76, 365–385. doi: 10.1146/annurev-physiol-021113-170400

Comery, T. A., Harris, J. B., Willems, P. J., Oostra, B. A., Irwin, S. A., Weiler, I. J., et al. (1997). Abnormal dendritic spines in fragile X knockout mice: maturation and pruning deficits. *Proc. Natl. Acad. Sci. U.S.A.* 94, 5401–5404. doi: 10.1073/pnas.94.10.5401

Dani, A., and Huang, B. (2010). New resolving power for light microscopy: applications to neurobiology. *Curr. Opin. Neurobiol.* 20, 648–652. doi: 10.1016/j.conb.2010.07.006

Darnell, J. C., Van Driesche, S. J., Zhang, C., Hung, K. Y., Mele, A., Fraser, C. E., et al. (2011). FMRP stalls ribosomal translocation on mRNAs linked to synaptic function and autism. *Cell* 146, 247–261. doi: 10.1016/j.cell.2011.06.013

De Rubeis, S., and Bagni, C. (2010). Fragile X mental retardation protein control of neuronal mRNA metabolism: insights into mRNA stability. *Mol. Cell Neurosci.* 43, 43–50. doi: 10.1016/j.mcn.2009.09.013

de Sevilla, D. F., and Buno, W. (2010). The muscarinic long-term enhancement of NMDA and AMPA receptor-mediated transmission at schaffer collateral synapses develop through different intracellular mechanisms. *J. Neurosci.* 30, 11032–11042. doi: 10.1523/JNEUROSCI.1848-10.2010

Debanne, D., Gahwiler, B. H., and Thompson, S. M. (1998). Long-term synaptic plasticity between pairs of individual CA3 pyramidal cells in rat hippocampal slice cultures. *J. Physiol. Lond.* 507, 237–247. doi: 10.1111/j.1469-7793.1998.237bu.x

DeBello, W. M., McBride, T. J., Nichols, G. S., Pannoni, K. E., Sanculi, D., and Totten, D. J. (2014). Input clustering and the microscale structure of local circuits. *Front. Neural Circuits* 8:112. doi: 10.3389/fncir.2014.00112

DeFelipe, J., Hendry, S. H., and Jones, E. G. (1989). Synapses of double bouquet cells in monkey cerebral cortex visualized by calbindin immunoreactivity. *Brain Res.* 503, 49–54. doi: 10.1016/0006-8993(89)91702-2

Dehez, H., Piche, M., and De Koninck, Y. (2013). Resolution and contrast enhancement in laser scanning microscopy using dark beam imaging. *Optics Express* 21, 15912–15925. doi: 10.1364/OE.21.015912

Denk, W., Strickler, J. H., and Webb, W. W. (1990). Two-photon laser scanning fluorescence microscopy. *Science* 248, 73–76. doi: 10.1126/science.2321027

Desai, N. S., Casimiro, T. M., Gruber, S. M., and Vanderklish, P. W. (2006). Early postnatal plasticity in neocortex of Fmr1 knockout mice. *J. Neurophysiol.* 96, 1734–1745. doi: 10.1152/jn.00221.2006

Diamond, J., Gray, E. G., and Yasagril, G. M. (1970). "The function of the dendritic spine: an hypothesis," in *Excitatory Synaptic Mechanisms*, eds P. Andersen and J. K. S. Jansen Jr. (Oslo: Universitetsforlaget), 213–222.

Feldman, M. L., and Peters, A. (1978). The forms of non-pyramidal neurons in the visual cortex of the rat. *J. Comp. Neurol.* 179, 761–793. doi: 10.1002/cne.901790406

Fenno, L., Yizhar, O., and Deisseroth, K. (2011). The development and application of optogenetics. *Annu. Rev. Neurosci.* 34, 389–412. doi: 10.1146/annurev-neuro-061010-113817

Fiala, J. C., Spacek, J., and Harris, K. M. (2002). Dendritic spine pathology: cause or consequence of neurological disorders? *Brain Res. Rev.* 39, 29–54. doi: 10.1016/S0165-0173(02)00158-3

Finch, E. A., and Augustine, G. J. (1998). Local calcium signalling by inositol-1,4,5-trisphosphate in Purkinje cell dendrites. *Nature* 396, 753–756. doi: 10.1038/25541

Fortin, D. A., Srivastava, T., and Soderling, T. R. (2012). Structural modulation of dendritic spines during synaptic plasticity. *Neuroscientist* 18, 326–341. doi: 10.1177/1073858411407206

Freund, T. F., and Buzsaki, G. (1996). Interneurons of the hippocampus. *Hippocampus* 6, 347–470.

Freund, T. F., Magloczky, Z., Soltesz, I., and Somogyi, P. (1986). Synaptic connections, axonal and dendritic patterns of neurons immunoreactive for cholecystokinin in the visual cortex of the cat. *Neuroscience* 19, 1133–1159. doi: 10.1016/0306-4522(86)90129-6

Galvez, R., and Greenough, W. T. (2005). Sequence of abnormal dendritic spine development in primary somatosensory cortex of a mouse model of the fragile X mental retardation syndrome. *Am. J. Med. Genet. A* 135, 155–160. doi: 10.1002/ajmg.a.30709

Gasparini, S., and Magee, J. C. (2006). State-dependent dendritic computation in hippocampal CA1 pyramidal neurons. *J. Neurosci.* 26, 2088–2100. doi: 10.1523/JNEUROSCI.4428-05.2006

Glantz, L. A., and Lewis, D. A. (2000). Decreased dendritic spine density on prefrontal cortical pyramidal neurons in schizophrenia. *Arch. Gen. Psychiatry* 57, 65–73. doi: 10.1001/archpsyc.57.1.65

Gold, J. I., and Bear, M. F. (1994). A model of dendritic spine Ca2+ concentration exploring possible bases for a sliding synaptic modification threshold. *Proc. Natl. Acad. Sci. U.S.A.* 91, 3941–3945. doi: 10.1073/pnas.91.9.3941

Gomez Gonzalez, J. F., Mel, B. W., and Poirazi, P. (2011). Distinguishing linear vs. non-linear integration in CA1 radial oblique dendrites: it's about time. *Front. Comput. Neurosci.* 5:44. doi: 10.3389/fncom.2011.00044

Gray, E. G. (1959). Electron microscopy of synaptic contacts on dendrite spines of the cerebral cortex. *Nature* 183, 1592–1593. doi: 10.1038/1831592a0

Grunditz, A., Holbro, N., Tian, L., Zuo, Y., and Oertner, T. G. (2008). Spine neck plasticity controls postsynaptic calcium signals through electrical compartmentalization. *J. Neurosci.* 28, 13457–13466. doi: 10.1523/JNEUROSCI.2702-08.2008

Gulledge, A. T., Carnevale, N. T., and Stuart, G. J. (2012). Electrical advantages of dendritic spines. *PLoS ONE* 7:e36007. doi: 10.1371/journal.pone.0036007

Hagerman, R., Hoem, G., and Hagerman, P. (2010). Fragile X and autism: intertwined at the molecular level leading to targeted treatments. *Mol. Autism* 1:12. doi: 10.1186/2040-2392-1-12

Hallahan, B. P., Craig, M. C., Toal, F., Daly, E. M., Moore, C. J., Ambikapathy, A., et al. (2011). *In vivo* brain anatomy of adult males with Fragile X syndrome: an MRI study. *Neuroimage* 54, 16–24. doi: 10.1016/j.neuroimage.2010.08.015

Harnett, M. T., Makara, J. K., Spruston, N., Kath, W. L., and Magee, J. C. (2012). Synaptic amplification by dendritic spines enhances input cooperativity. *Nature* 491, 599–602. doi: 10.1038/nature11554

Harvey, C. D., Yasuda, R., Zhong, H. N., and Svoboda, K. (2008). The spread of Ras activity triggered by activation of a single dendritic spine. *Science* 321, 136–140. doi: 10.1126/science.1159675

He, C. X., and Portera-Cailliau, C. (2013). The trouble with spines in fragile X syndrome: density, maturity and plasticity. *Neuroscience* 251, 120–128. doi: 10.1016/j.neuroscience.2012.03.049

Hess, S. T., Girirajan, T. P. K., and Mason, M. D. (2006). Ultra-high resolution imaging by fluorescence photoactivation localization microscopy. *Biophys. J.* 91, 4258–4272. doi: 10.1529/biophysj.106.091116

Higley, M. J., and Sabatini, B. L. (2012). Calcium signaling in dendritic spines. *Cold Spring Harb. Perspect. Biol.* 4:a005686. doi: 10.1101/cshperspect.a005686

Holbro, N., Grunditz, A., and Oertner, T. G. (2009). Differential distribution of endoplasmic reticulum controls metabotropic signaling and plasticity at hippocampal synapses. *Proc. Natl. Acad. Sci. U.S.A.* 106, 15055–15060. doi: 10.1073/pnas.0905110106

Holcman, D., and Schuss, Z. (2011). Diffusion laws in dendritic spines. *J. Math. Neurosci.* 1:10. doi: 10.1186/2190-8567-1-10

Holtmaat, A., and Svoboda, K. (2009). Experience-dependent structural synaptic plasticity in the mammalian brain. *Nat. Rev. Neurosci.* 10, 647–658. doi: 10.1038/nrn2699

Huang, B., Babcock, H., and Zhuang, X. (2010). Breaking the diffraction barrier: super-resolution imaging of cells. *Cell* 143, 1047–1058. doi: 10.1016/j.cell.2010.12.002

Hugel, S., Abegg, M., de Paola, V., Caroni, P., Gahwiler, B. H., and McKinney, R. A. (2009). Dendritic spine morphology determines membrane-associated protein exchange between dendritic shafts and spine heads. *Cereb. Cortex* 19, 697–702. doi: 10.1093/cercor/bhn118

Hutsler, J. J., and Zhang, H. (2010). Increased dendritic spine densities on cortical projection neurons in autism spectrum disorders. *Brain Res.* 1309, 83–94. doi: 10.1016/j.brainres.2009.09.120

Irwin, S. A., Idupulapati, M., Gilbert, M. E., Harris, J. B., Chakravarti, A. B., Rogers, E. J., et al. (2002). Dendritic spine and dendritic field characteristics of layer V pyramidal neurons in the visual cortex of fragile-X knockout mice. *Am. J. Med. Genet.* 111, 140–146. doi: 10.1002/ajmg.10500

Irwin, S. A., Patel, B., Idupulapati, M., Harris, J. B., Crisostomo, R. A., Larsen, B. P., et al. (2001). Abnormal dendritic spine characteristics in the temporal and visual cortices of patients with fragile-X syndrome: a quantitative examination. *Am. J. Med. Genet.* 98, 161–167. doi: 10.1002/1096-8628(20010115)98:2<161::AID-AJMG1025>3.0.CO;2-B

Isokawa, M. (1997). Preservation of dendrites with the presence of reorganized mossy fiber collaterals in hippocampal dentate granule cells in patients with temporal lobe epilepsy. *Brain Res.* 744, 339–343. doi: 10.1016/S0006-8993(96)01067-0

Jack, J. J. B., Noble, D., and Tsien, R. W. (1975). *Electric Current Flow in Excitable Cells.* Oxford, Clarendon Press.

Jacquemont, S., Hagerman, R. J., Hagerman, P. J., and Leehey, M. A. (2007). Fragile-X syndrome and fragile X-associated tremor/ataxia syndrome: two faces of FMR1. *Lancet Neurol.* 6, 45–55. doi: 10.1016/S1474-4422(06)70676-7

Jia, H., Rochefort, N. L., Chen, X., and Konnerth, A. (2010). Dendritic organization of sensory input to cortical neurons *in vivo*. *Nature* 464, 1307–1312. doi: 10.1038/nature08947

Johnston, D., and Wu, S. (1995). *Foundations of Cellular Neurophysiology.* Cambridge, MA: MIT Press.

Kalisman, N., Silberberg, G., and Markram, H. (2005). The neocortical microcircuit as a tabula rasa. *Proc. Natl. Acad. Sci. U.S.A.* 102, 880–885. doi: 10.1073/pnas.0407088102

Kandel, E. R., Schwartz, J. H., and Jessell, T. M. (2000). *Principles of Neural Science, 4th Edn.* New York, NY: McGraw-Hill.

Kasai, H., Fukuda, M., Watanabe, S., Hayashi-Takagi, A., and Noguchi, J. (2010). Structural dynamics of dendritic spines in memory and cognition. *Trends Neurosci.* 33, 121–129. doi: 10.1016/j.tins.2010.01.001

Kawaguchi, Y. (1993). Groupings of nonpyramidal and pyramidal cells with specific physiological and morphological characteristics in rat frontal cortex. *J. Neurophysiol.* 69, 416–431.

Kawaguchi, Y., Karube, F., and Kubota, Y. (2006). Dendritic branch typing and spine expression patterns in cortical nonpyramidal cells. *Cereb. Cortex* 16, 696–711. doi: 10.1093/cercor/bhj015

Keck, T., Scheuss, V., Jacobsen, R. I., Wierenga, C. J., Eysel, U. T., Bonhoeffer, T., et al. (2011). Loss of sensory input causes rapid structural changes of inhibitory neurons in adult mouse visual cortex. *Neuron* 71, 869–882. doi: 10.1016/j.neuron.2011.06.034

Kim, J. Y., Jung, S. C., Clemens, A. M., Petralia, R. S., and Hoffman, D. A. (2007). Regulation of dendritic excitability by activity-dependent trafficking of the A-type K(+) channel subunit Kv4.2 in hippocampal neurons. *Neuron* 54, 933–947. doi: 10.1016/j.neuron.2007.05.026

Kleindienst, T., Winnubst, J., Roth-Alpermann, C., Bonhoeffer, T., and Lohmann, C. (2011). Activity-dependent clustering of functional synaptic inputs on developing hippocampal dendrites. *Neuron* 72, 1012–1024. doi: 10.1016/j.neuron.2011.10.015

Knott, G. W., Holtmaat, A., Wilbrecht, L., Welker, E., and Svoboda, K. (2006). Spine growth precedes synapse formation in the adult neocortex *in vivo*. *Nat. Neurosci.* 9, 1117–1124. doi: 10.1038/nn1747

Koch, C. (2004). *Biophysics of Computation Information Processing in Single Neurons.* New York, NY, Oxford University Press.

Koch, C., and Poggio, T. (1983a). Electrical-properties of dendritic spines. *Trends Neurosci.* 6, 80–83. doi: 10.1016/0166-2236(83)90043-7

Koch, C., and Poggio, T. (1983b). A theoretical-analysis of electrical-properties of spines. *Proc. R. Soc. Lond. B Biol. Sci.* 218, 455–477. doi: 10.1098/rspb.1983.0051

Koch, C., Poggio, T., and Torre, V. (1983). Nonlinear interactions in a dendritic tree: localization, timing, and role in information processing. *Proc. Natl. Acad. Sci. U.S.A.* 80, 2799–2802. doi: 10.1073/pnas.80.9.2799

Koleske, A. J. (2013). Molecular mechanisms of dendrite stability. *Nat. Rev. Neurosci.* 14, 536–550. doi: 10.1038/nrn3486

Lang, C., Barco, A., Zablow, L., Kandel, E. R., Siegelbaum, S. A., and Zakharenko, S. S. (2004). Transient expansion of synaptically connected dendritic spines upon induction of hippocampal long-term potentiation. *Proc. Natl. Acad. Sci. U.S.A.* 101, 16665–16670. doi: 10.1073/pnas.0407581101

Larkum, M. E., and Nevian, T. (2008). Synaptic clustering by dendritic signalling mechanisms. *Curr. Opin. Neurobiol.* 18, 321–331. doi: 10.1016/j.conb.2008.08.013

Larkum, M. E., Nevian, T., Sandler, M., Polsky, A., and Schiller, J. (2009). Synaptic integration in tuft dendrites of layer 5 pyramidal neurons: a new unifying principle. *Science* 325, 756–760. doi: 10.1126/science.1171958

Lee, S. J., Escobedo-Lozoya, Y., Szatmari, E. M., and Yasuda, R. (2009). Activation of CaMKII in single dendritic spines during long-term potentiation. *Nature* 458, 299–304. doi: 10.1038/nature07842

Lisman, J., Yasuda, R., and Raghavachari, S. (2012). Mechanisms of CaMKII action in long-term potentiation. *Nat. Rev. Neurosci.* 13, 169–182. doi: 10.1038/nrn3192

Llinás, R., and Hillman, D. E. (1969). "Physiological and morphological organization of the cerebellar circuits in various vertebrates," in *Neurobiology of Cerebellar Evolution and Development*, ed R. Llinas (Chicago: American Medical Association), 43–73.

Losonczy, A., and Magee, J. C. (2006). Integrative properties of radial oblique dendrites in hippocampal CA1 pyramidal neurons. *Neuron* 50, 291–307. doi: 10.1016/j.neuron.2006.03.016

Losonczy, A., Makara, J. K., and Magee, J. C. (2008). Compartmentalized dendritic plasticity and input feature storage in neurons. *Nature* 452, 436–441. doi: 10.1038/nature06725

Lu, H. E., MacGillavry, H. D., Frost, N. A., and Blanpied, T. A. (2014). Multiple spatial and kinetic subpopulations of CaMKII in spines and dendrites as resolved by single-molecule tracking PALM. *J. Neurosci.* 34, 7600–7610. doi: 10.1523/JNEUROSCI.4364-13.2014

Lynch, M. A. (2004). Long-term potentiation and memory. *Physiol. Rev.* 84, 87–136. doi: 10.1152/physrev.00014.2003

Magee, J. C., and Johnston, D. (1997). A synaptically controlled, associative signal for Hebbian plasticity in hippocampal neurons. *Science* 275, 209–213. doi: 10.1126/science.275.5297.209

Maglione, M., and Sigrist, S. J. (2013). Seeing the forest tree by tree: super-resolution light microscopy meets the neurosciences. *Nat. Neurosci.* 16, 790–797. doi: 10.1038/nn.3403

Majewska, A., Tashiro, A., and Yuste, R. (2000). Regulation of spine calcium dynamics by rapid spine motility. *J. Neurosci.* 20, 8262–8268.

Major, G., Polsky, A., Denk, W., Schiller, J., and Tank, D. W. (2008). Spatiotemporally graded NMDA spike/plateau potentials in basal dendrites of neocortical pyramidal neurons. *J. Neurophysiol.* 99, 2584–2601. doi: 10.1152/jn.00011.2008

Malenka, R. C., and Bear, M. F. (2004). LTP and LTD: an embarrassment of riches. *Neuron* 44, 5–21. doi: 10.1016/j.neuron 2004.09.012

Markram, H., Lubke, J., Frotscher, M., and Sakmann, B. (1997). Regulation of synaptic efficacy by coincidence of postsynaptic APs and EPSPs. *Science* 275, 213–215. doi: 10.1126/science.275.5297.213

Matsuzaki, M., Ellis-Davies, G. C. R., Nemoto, T., Miyashita, Y., Iino, M., and Kasai, H. (2001). Dendritic spine geometry is critical for AMPA receptor expression in hippocampal CA1 pyramidal neurons. *Nat. Neurosci.* 4, 1086–1092. doi: 10.1038/nn736

Matsuzaki, M., Honkura, N., Ellis-Davies, G. C. R., and Kasai, H. (2004). Structural basis of long-term potentiation in single dendritic spines. *Nature* 429, 761–766. doi: 10.1038/nature02617

McBain, C. J., DiChiara, T. J., and Kauer, J. A. (1994). Activation of metabotropic glutamate receptors differentially affects two classes of hippocampal interneurons and potentiates excitatory synaptic transmission. *J. Neurosci.* 14, 4433–4445.

McKinney, B. C., Grossman, A. W., Elisseou, N. M., and Greenough, W. T. (2005). Dendritic spine abnormalities in the occipital cortex of C57BL/6 Fmr1 knockout mice. *Am. J. Med. Genet. B Neuropsychiatr. Genet.* 136B, 98–102. doi: 10.1002/ajmg.b.30183

Meredith, R. M., Holmgren, C. D., Weidum, M., Burnashev, N., and Mansvelder, H. D. (2007). Increased threshold for spike-timing-dependent plasticity is caused by unreliable calcium signaling in mice lacking fragile X gene Fmr1. *Neuron* 54, 627–638. doi: 10.1016/j.neuron.2007.04.028

Miller, J. P., Rall, W., and Rinzel, J. (1985). Synaptic amplification by active membrane in dendritic spines. *Brain Res.* 325, 325–330. doi: 10.1016/0006-8993(85)90333-6

Murakoshi, H., Wang, H., and Yasuda, R. (2011). Local, persistent activation of Rho GTPases during plasticity of single dendritic spines. *Nature* 472, 100–104. doi: 10.1038/nature09823

Murayama, M., Perez-Garci, E., Nevian, T, Bock, T., Senn, W., and Larkum, M. E. (2009). Dendritic encoding of sensory stimuli controlled by deep cortical interneurons. *Nature* 457, 1137–1141. doi: 10.1038/nature07663

Murthy, V. N., Sejnowski, T. J., and Stevens, C. F. (2000). Dynamics of dendritic calcium transients evoked by quantal release at excitatory hippocampal synapses. *Proc. Natl. Acad. Sci. U.S.A.* 97, 901–906. doi: 10.1073/pnas.97.2.901

Nabavi, S., Fox, R., Proulx, C. D., Lin, J. Y., Tsien, R. Y., and Malinow, R. (2014). Engineering a memory with LTD and LTP. *Nature* 511, 348–352. doi: 10.1038/nature13294

Nagerl, U. V., and Bonhoeffer, T. (2010). Imaging living synapses at the nanoscale by STED microscopy. *J. Neurosci.* 30, 9341–9346. doi: 10.1523/JNEUROSCI.0990-10.2010

Nagerl, U. V., Eberhorn, N., Cambridge, S. B., and Bonhoeffer, T. (2004). Bidirectional activity-dependent morphological plasticity in hippocampal neurons. *Neuron* 44, 759–767. doi: 10.1016/j.neuron.2004.11.016

Nagerl, U. V., Willig, K. I., Hein, E., Hell, S. W., and Bonhoeffer, T. (2008). Live-cell imaging of dendritic spines by STED microscopy. *Proc. Natl. Acad. Sci. U.S.A.* 105, 18982–18987. doi: 10.1073/pnas.0810028105

Nakai, J., Ohkura, M., and Imoto, K. (2001). A high signal-to-noise Ca(2+) probe composed of a single green fluorescent protein. *Nat. Biotechnol.* 19, 137–141. doi: 10.1038/84397

Nikolenko, V., Watson, B. O., Araya, R., Woodruff, A., Peterka, D. S., and Yuste, R. (2008). SLM Microscopy: scanless two-photon imaging and photostimulation with spatial light modulators. *Front. Neural Circuits* 2:5. doi: 10.3389/neuro.04.005.2008

Noguchi, J., Matsuzaki, M., Ellis-Davies, G. C. R., and Kasai, H. (2005). Spine-neck geometry determines NMDA receptor-dependent Ca2+ signaling in dendrites. *Neuron* 46, 609–622. doi: 10.1016/j.neuron.2005.03.015

O'Donnell, C., Nolan, M. F., and van Rossum, M. C. (2011). Dendritic spine dynamics regulate the long-term stability of synaptic plasticity. *J. Neurosci.* 31, 16142–16156. doi: 10.1523/JNEUROSCI.2520-11.2011

Oh, W. C., Hill, T. C., and Zito, K. (2013). Synapse-specific and size-dependent mechanisms of spine structural plasticity accompanying synaptic weakening. *Proc. Natl. Acad. Sci. U.S.A.* 110, E305–E312. doi: 10.1073/pnas.1214705110

Palmer, L. M., and Stuart, G. J. (2009). Membrane potential changes in dendritic spines during action potentials and synaptic input. *J. Neurosci.* 29, 6897–6903. doi: 10.1523/JNEUROSCI.5847-08.2009

Penzes, P., Cahill, M. E., Jones, K. A., VanLeeuwen, J. E., and Woolfrey, K. M. (2011). Dendritic spine pathology in neuropsychiatric disorders. *Nat. Neurosci.* 14, 285–293. doi: 10.1038/nn.2741

Perkel, D. H., and Perkel, D. J. (1985). Dendritic spines: role of active membrane in modulating synaptic efficacy. *Brain Res.* 325, 331–335. doi: 10.1016/0006-8993(85)90334-8

Peterka, D. S., Takahashi, H., and Yuste, R. (2011). Imaging voltage in neurons. *Neuron* 69, 9–21. doi: 10.1016/j.neuron.2010.12.010

Peters, A., and Feldman, M. L. (1976). The projection of the lateral geniculate nucleus to area 17 of the rat cerebral cortex. I. General description. *J. Neurocytol.* 5, 63–84. doi: 10.1007/BF01176183

Peters, A., and Kaiserman-Abramof, I. R. (1970). The small pyramidal neuron of the rat cerebral cortex. The perikaryon, dendrites and spines. *Am. J. Anat.* 127, 321–355. doi: 10.1002/aja.1001270402

Peters, A., Sethares, C., and Moss, M. B. (1998). The effects of aging on layer 1 in area 46 of prefrontal cortex in the rhesus monkey. *Cereb. Cortex* 8, 671–684. doi: 10.1093/cercor/8.8.671

Pitkanen, A., and Amaral, D. G. (1993). Distribution of parvalbumin-immunoreactive cells and fibers in the monkey temporal lobe: the hippocampal formation. *J. Comp. Neurol.* 331, 37–74. doi: 10.1002/cne.903310104

Poirazi, P., Brannon, T., and Mel, B. W. (2003). Pyramidal neuron as two-layer neural network. *Neuron* 37, 989–999. doi: 10.1016/S0896-6273(03)00149-1

Polsky, A., Mel, B., and Schiller, J. (2009). Encoding and decoding bursts by NMDA spikes in basal dendrites of layer 5 pyramidal neurons. *J. Neurosci.* 29, 11891–11903. doi: 10.1523/JNEUROSCI.5250-08.2009

Portera-Cailliau, C. (2012). Which comes first in fragile X syndrome, dendritic spine dysgenesis or defects in circuit plasticity? *Neuroscientist* 18, 28–44. doi: 10.1177/1073858410395322

Purpura, D. P. (1974). Dendritic spine "dysgenesis" and mental retardation. *Science* 186, 1126–1128. doi: 10.1126/science.186.4169.1126

Raghuram, V., Sharma, Y., and Kreutz, M. R. (2012). Ca(2+) sensor proteins in dendritic spines: a race for Ca(2+). *Front. Mol. Neurosci.* 5:61. doi: 10.3389/fnmol.2012.00061

Rall, W. (1964). "Theoretical significance of dendritic trees for neuronal input-output relations," in *Neural Theory and Modeling*, ed R. F. Reiss (Palo Alto, CA: Stanford University Press), 73.

Rall, W. (1974). *Dendritic Spines, Synaptic Potency and Neuronal Plasticity.* Los Angeles, CA: University of California, Brain Information Service Research Report #3.

Raymond, C. R., and Redman, S. J. (2006). Spatial segregation of neuronal calcium signals encodes different forms of LTP in rat hippocampus. *J. Physiol.* 570, 97–111. doi: 10.1113/jphysiol.2005.098947

Reiss, A. L., Abrams, M. T., Greenlaw, R., Freund, L., and Denckla, M. B. (1995). Neurodevelopmental effects of the FMR-1 full mutation in humans. *Nat. Med.* 1, 159–167. doi: 10.1038/nm0295-159

Richardson, R. J., Blundon, J. A., Bayazitov, I. T., and Zakharenko, S. S. (2009). Connectivity patterns revealed by mapping of active inputs on dendrites of thalamorecipient neurons in the auditory cortex. *J. Neurosci.* 29, 6406–6417. doi: 10.1523/JNEUROSCI.0258-09.2009

Rinzel, J., and Rall, W. (1974). Transient response in a dendritic neuron model for current injected at one branch. *Biophys. J.* 14, 759–790. doi: 10.1016/S0006-3495(74)85948-5

Rudelli, R. D., Brown, W. T., Wisniewski, K., Jenkins, E. C., Laure-Kamionowska, M., Connell, F., et al. (1985). Adult fragile X syndrome. Clinico-neuropathologic findings. *Acta Neuropathol.* 67, 289–295. doi: 10.1007/BF00687814

Rust, M. J., Bates, M., and Zhuang, X. W. (2006). Sub-diffraction-limit imaging by stochastic optical reconstruction microscopy (STORM). *Nat. Methods* 3, 793–795. doi: 10.1038/nmeth929

Sabatini, B. L., Oertner, T. G., and Svoboda, K. (2002). The life cycle of Ca(2+) ions in dendritic spines. *Neuron* 33, 439–452. doi: 10.1016/S0896-6273(02)00573-1

Sala, C., and Segal, M. (2014). Dendritic spines: the locus of structural and functional plasticity. *Physiol. Rev.* 94, 141–188. doi: 10.1152/physrev.00012.2013

Scheibel, M. E., Crandall, P. H., and Scheibel, A. B. (1974). The hippocampal-dentate complex in temporal lobe epilepsy. A Golgi study. *Epilepsia* 15, 55–80. doi: 10.1111/j.1528-1157.1974.tb03997.x

Scheuss, V., and Bonhoeffer, T. (2013). Function of dendritic spines on hippocampal inhibitory neurons. *Cereb. Cortex* 24, 3142–3153. doi: 10.1093/cercor/bht171

Segev, I., and Rall, W. (1988). Computational study of an excitable dendritic spine. *J. Neurophysiol.* 60, 499–523.

Selemon, L. D., and Goldman-Rakic, P. S. (1999). The reduced neuropil hypothesis: a circuit based model of schizophrenia. *Biol. Psychiatry* 45, 17–25. doi: 10.1016/S0006-3223(98)00281-9

Shepherd, G. M., Brayton, R. K., Miller, J. P., Segev, I., Rinzel, J., and Rall, W. (1985). Signal enhancement in distal cortical dendrites by means of interactions between active dendritic spines. *Proc. Natl. Acad. Sci. U.S.A.* 82, 2192–2195. doi: 10.1073/pnas.82.7.2192

Sobczyk, A., Scheuss, V., and Svoboda, K. (2005). NMDA receptor subunit-dependent [Ca2+] signaling in individual hippocampal dendritic spines. *J. Neurosci.* 25, 6037–6046. doi: 10.1523/JNEUROSCI.1221-05.2005

Somogyi, P., and Cowey, A. (1981). Combined Golgi and electron microscopic study on the synapses formed by double bouquet cells in the visual cortex of the cat and monkey. *J. Comp. Neurol.* 195, 547–566. doi: 10.1002/cne.901950402

Sorra, K. E., and Harris, K. M. (2000). Overview on the structure, composition, function, development, and plasticity of hippocampal dendritic spines. *Hippocampus* 10, 501–511. doi: 10.1002/1098-1063(2000)10:5<501::AID-HIPO1>3.3.CO;2-K

Spacek, J., and Harris, K. M. (1998). Three-dimensional organization of cell adhesion junctions at synapses and dendritic spines in area CA1 of the rat hippocampus. *J. Comp. Neurol.* 393, 58–68.

Spruston, N. (2008). Pyramidal neurons: dendritic structure and synaptic integration. *Nat. Rev. Neurosci.* 9, 206–221. doi: 10.1038/nrn2286

Svoboda, K., Tank, D. W., and Denk, W. (1996). Direct measurement of coupling between dendritic spines and shafts. *Science* 272, 716–719. doi: 10.1126/science.272.5262.716

Tackenberg, C., Ghori, A., and Brandt, R. (2009). Thin, stubby or mushroom: spine pathology in Alzheimer's disease. *Curr. Alzheimer Res.* 6, 261–268. doi: 10.2174/156720509788486554

Takahashi, N., Kitamura, K., Matsuo, N., Mayford, M., Kano, M., Matsuki, N., et al. (2012). Locally synchronized synaptic inputs. *Science,* 335, 353–356. doi: 10.1126/science.1210362

Takasaki, K., and Sabatini, B. L. (2014). Super-resolution 2-photon microscopy reveals that the morphology of each dendritic spine correlates with diffusive but not synaptic properties. *Front. Neuroanat.* 8:29. doi: 10.3389/fnana.2014.00029

Takasaki, K. T., Ding, J. B., and Sabatini, B. L. (2013). Live-cell superresolution imaging by pulsed STED two-photon excitation microscopy. *Biophys. J.* 104, 770–777. doi: 10.1016/j.bpj.2012.12.053

Takechi, H., Eilers, J., and Konnerth, A. (1998). A new class of synaptic response involving calcium release in dendritic spines. *Nature* 396, 757–760. doi: 10.1038/25547

Tamas, G., Szabadics, J., and Somogyi, P. (2002). Cell type- and subcellular position-dependent summation of unitary postsynaptic potentials in neocortical neurons. *J. Neurosci.* 22, 740–747.

Tanaka, J. I., Horiike, Y., Matsuzaki, M., Miyazaki, T., Ellis-Davies, G. C. R., and Kasai, H. (2008). Protein synthesis and neurotrophin-dependent structural plasticity of single dendritic spines. *Science* 319, 1683–1687. doi: 10.1126/science.1152864

Tonnesen, J., Katona, G., Rozsa, B., and Nagerl, U. V. (2014). Spine neck plasticity regulates compartmentalization of synapses. *Nat. Neurosci.* 17, 678–685. doi: 10.1038/nn.3682

Tsien, R. Y. (1988). Fluorescence measurement and photochemical manipulation of cytosolic free calcium. *Trends Neurosci.* 11, 419–424. doi: 10.1016/0166-2236(88)90192-0

Vogels, T., Araya, R., and Yuste, R. (2009). Modeling the electrical function of dendritic spines. *Front. Syst. Neurosci. Conference Abstract: Computational and Systems Neuroscience 2009*. doi: 10.3389/conf.neuro.06.2009.03.119

Wang, T., Bray, S. M., and Warren, S. T. (2012). New perspectives on the biology of fragile X syndrome. *Curr. Opin. Genet. Dev.* 22, 256–263. doi: 10.1016/j.gde.2012.02.002

Wiegert, J. S., and Oertner, T. G. (2013). Long-term depression triggers the selective elimination of weakly integrated synapses. *Proc. Natl. Acad. Sci. U.S.A.* 110, E4510–E4519. doi: 10.1073/pnas.1315926110

Williams, S. R., and Stuart, G. J. (2003). Role of dendritic synapse location in the control of action potential output. *Trends Neurosci.* 26, 147–154. doi: 10.1016/S0166-2236(03)00035-3

Willig, K. I., Harke, B., Medda, R., and Hell, S. W. (2007). STED microscopy with continuous wave beams. *Nat. Methods* 4, 915–918. doi: 10.1038/nmeth1108

Xu, X., Miller, E. C., and Pozzo-Miller, L. (2014). Dendritic spine dysgenesis in Rett syndrome. *Front. Neuroanat.* 8:97. doi: 10.3389/fnana.2014.00097

Yasuda, R. (2006). Imaging spatiotemporal dynamics of neuronal signaling using fluorescence resonance energy transfer and fluorescence lifetime imaging microscopy. *Curr. Opin. Neurobiol.* 16, 551–561. doi: 10.1016/j.conb.2006.08.012

Yasuda, R., and Murakoshi, H. (2011). The mechanisms underlying the spatial spreading of signaling activity. *Curr. Opin. Neurobiol.* 21, 313–321. doi: 10.1016/j.conb.2011.02.008

Yuste, R., and Denk, W. (1995). Dendritic spines as basic functional units of neuronal integration. *Nature* 375, 682–684. doi: 10.1038/375682a0

Yuste, R., Majewska, A., and Holthoff, K. (2000). From form to function: calcium compartmentalization in dendritic spines. *Nat. Neurosci.* 3, 653–659. doi: 10.1038/76609

Zhang, L. I., Tao, H. W., Holt, C. E., Harris, W. A., and Poo, M. M. (1998). A critical window for cooperation and competition among developing retinotectal synapses. *Nature* 395, 37–44. doi: 10.1038/25665

Zhou, Q., Homma, K. J., and Poo, M. M. (2004). Shrinkage of dendritic spines associated with long-term depression of hippocampal synapses. *Neuron* 44, 749–757. doi: 10.1016/j.neuron.2004.11.011

16

Measuring F-actin properties in dendritic spines

Mikko Koskinen and Pirta Hotulainen *

Neuroscience Center, University of Helsinki, Helsinki, Finland

****Correspondence:***
Pirta Hotulainen, Neuroscience Center, University of Helsinki, Viikinkaari 4, 00790 Helsinki, Finland
e-mail: pirta.hotulainen@helsinki.fi

During the last decade, numerous studies have demonstrated that the actin cytoskeleton plays a pivotal role in the control of dendritic spine shape. Synaptic stimulation rapidly changes the actin dynamics and many actin regulators have been shown to play roles in neuron functionality. Accordingly, defects in the regulation of the actin cytoskeleton in neurons have been implicated in memory disorders. Due to the small size of spines, it is difficult to detect changes in the actin structures in dendritic spines by conventional light microscopy imaging. Instead, to know how tightly actin filaments are bundled together, and how fast the filaments turnover, we need to use advanced microscopy techniques, such as fluorescence recovery after photobleaching (FRAP), photoactivatable green fluorescent protein (PAGFP) fluorescence decay and fluorescence anisotropy. Fluorescence anisotropy, which measures the Förster resonance energy transfer (FRET) between two GFP fluorophores, has been proposed as a method to measure the level of actin polymerization. Here, we propose a novel idea that fluorescence anisotropy could be more suitable to study the level of actin filament bundling instead of actin polymerization. We validate the method in U2OS cell line where the actin structures can be clearly distinguished and apply to analyze how actin filament organization in dendritic spines changes during neuronal maturation. In addition to fluorescence anisotropy validation, we take a critical look at the properties and limitations of FRAP and PAGFP fluorescence decay methods and offer our proposals for the analysis methods for these approaches. These three methods complement each other, each providing additional information about actin dynamics and organization in dendritic spines.

Keywords: actin, FRAP, PAGFP, FRET, dendritic spine

INTRODUCTION

Dendritic spines are small bulbous protrusions from the dendritic shafts of neurons. These distinct cellular compartments house the majority of the postsynaptic terminals of excitatory synapses. Synaptic function has a strong coupling to the morphology and dynamics of dendritic spines (Alvarez and Sabatini, 2007; Bhatt et al., 2009). The plasticity of the synaptic terminals found in dendritic spines enables them to shape the function of the neuronal network. This has led to the hypothesis that dendritic spines are the sites of memory formation and maintenance in the brain (Kasai et al., 2010; Chen et al., 2014). Abnormalities in the shape and size or the development and distribution of dendritic spines have been linked to several neurological diseases such as Autism spectrum disorders (ASD), Schizophrenia, Alzheimers disease (AD) (Penzes et al., 2011), Down syndrome and mental retardation (Kaufmann and Moser, 2000).

The main cytoskeletal component of dendritic spines is actin (Hotulainen and Hoogenraad, 2010). Dendritic spines are enriched with actin, containing approximately 6 times more actin than dendritic shafts (Honkura et al., 2008). Actin monomers (globular actin, G-actin) polymerize to form actin filaments (filamentous actin, F-actin). Most of the actin in dendritic spines is F-actin with only about 12% of the total actin being monomeric (Star et al., 2002; Honkura et al., 2008). Single actin filaments undergo constant exchange of monomers from the ends of the filaments. The filaments are polar containing a barbed (plus)-end and a pointed (minus)-end. Polymerization and depolymerization rates for the ends are different leading to a constant flow of actin monomers through the filaments from barbed to pointed ends. This process is called treadmilling (Pollard and Cooper, 2009). Actin filaments can control cell shape by exerting a mechanical force on the cell membrane through polymerization (Pollard and Cooper, 2009; Blanchoin et al., 2014).

F-actin structures range from branched filament network to thick actin bundles of several cross-linked filaments (Blanchoin et al., 2014). These structures have highly variable lifetimes. Filaments forming the actin mesh at the leading edge of a migrating cell can change very rapidly whereas thick actin bundles called stress fibers can remain stable for a long time. The three-dimensional structure and dynamics of actin filament network are regulated by actin binding proteins (ABPs) (Dos Remedios et al., 2003; Pollard and Cooper, 2009). ABPs can affect the treadmilling rate of the filaments as well as their stability and organization. ABPs have a multitude of different functions; they can initiate polymerization, induce branching of filaments, cap filaments and block polymerization, sever filaments to shorter pieces, depolymerize filaments, bundle or cross-link filaments, produce contractile force or protect filaments from depolymerization (Dos Remedios et al., 2003).

A number of studies have investigated the roles of different ABPs in regulating the dynamics and organization of dendritic spine actin (Hotulainen and Hoogenraad, 2010). Numerous ABPs have been shown to influence neurophysiological function (Lamprecht, 2014). For example, myosin IIb, which binds actin and can induce contractility into a network, has been indicated in long-term potentiation (LTP) stabilization and memory consolidation (Rex et al., 2010). The loss of Arp2/3, the protein complex known for nucleating actin filaments and the induction of branched actin filament network, has been shown to lead to cognitive, psychomotor and social disturbances in aging mice (Kim et al., 2013). Cofilin-1, which severs and depolymerizes actin filaments, has been suggested to be involved in late-LTP (L-LTP) induction and associative learning (Rust et al., 2010) as well as in memory extinction (Wang et al., 2013). In line with these results, defects in the regulation of the actin cytoskeleton in neurons have been implicated in memory disorders (Penzes et al., 2011; Caroni et al., 2012).

In order to be able to study the dendritic spine F-actin organization and dynamics we need to have suitable microscopy techniques. Different actin structures can be relatively easily visualized by conventional fluorescent microscopy techniques in fibroblasts. However, the average size of dendritic spines themselves is close to the physical resolution limit of conventional light microscopy and therefore more advanced light microscopy techniques or electron microscopy methods are necessary to image and measure actin organization and dynamics in these compartments. With electron microscopy, actin spinoskeleton has been shown to consist of a combination of short and branched filaments and longer bundles of actin filaments (Korobova and Svitkina, 2010). However, visualizing actin filaments by electron microscopy approaches is feasible only in a few laboratories. In addition, electron microscopy is possible only with fixed samples and is thus not applicable to measure actin dynamics. Therefore, several light-microscopy methods have been applied to measure the properties of actin filaments in dendritic spines. These techniques involve fluorescence recovery after photobleaching (FRAP), photo activated green fluorescent protein (PAGFP) fluorescence decay, photo-activation localization microscopy (PALM), Förster resonance energy transfer (FRET) and stimulated emission depletion (STED) fluorescence microscopy.

FRAP and PAGFP decay experiments have shown that spine F-actin can be divided into two pools based on their turnover rate: the fast turnover rate dynamic pool with a time constant <1 min and a slower turnover rate stable pool with a time constant of $\sim$17 min (Star et al., 2002; Honkura et al., 2008). Honkura and colleagues also detected an enlargement pool that formed into dendritic spines following LTP induction. LTP stabilization was found to be dependent on the retention of the enlargement pool of actin inside the dendritic spine head (Honkura et al., 2008). Single molecule tracking (PALM) has revealed that actin filaments in dendritic spines are relatively short ($\sim$200 nm) and that they exhibit very heterogeneous treadmilling rates (Frost et al., 2010).

The organization of actin filament structures also plays an important role in the regulation of actin filament turnover rate as well as in determining the overall function of the spinoskeleton. Conventional two-color FRET experiments have revealed that LTP formation causes a shift of F-actin/G-actin equilibrium toward F-actin (Okamoto et al., 2004). Recently, a fluorescence anisotropy-based FRET method (only one fluorophore i.e., homoFRET) was proposed as an alternative way to probe actin polymerization state (Vishwasrao et al., 2012). It is important to note that fluorescent molecules are typically expressed in very low levels in neurons. The probability for FRET to occur drops to less than 1% when the fluorophore pair is further than 10 nm apart. If every tenth actin monomer in a single filament is coupled to GFP, there would be GFP in every fifth monomer in an actin double helix. This distance is already $\sim$20 nm, meaning that GFP molecules are too far away from each other to carry out FRET. For this reason, we wanted to test whether the fluorescence anisotropy reflects the inter-filament rather than intra-filament FRET. In other words, if fluorescence anisotropy can be used to measure the level of F-actin bundling instead of the level of F-actin polymerization.

In addition to fluorescence anisotropy validation, we take a critical look at the properties and limitations of FRAP and PAGFP fluorescence decay methods and offer our proposals for the optimal application of these approaches. These three methods complement each other, each providing additional information about actin dynamics and organization. Optimally these methods could be used together or in combination with super-resolution approaches to improve our understanding on the organization and dynamics of the dendritic spine actin filaments.

MATERIALS AND METHODS

NEURONAL CELL CULTURES, TRANSFECTION AND FIXED SAMPLE PREPARATION

Rat hippocampal neuron cultures were prepared as described previously (Bertling et al., 2012). Briefly, the hippocampi of embryonal day 17 Wistar rat fetuses were dissected and the meninges were removed. The cells were dissociated with 0.05% papain along with mechanical trituration. The plating density of the cells was 1,00,000 cells/coverslip (diameter 13 mm). The coverslips were coated with Poly-L-Lysine (0.1 mg/ml) (Sigma). Cells were plated in neurobasal medium (Gibco) supplemented with B-27 (Invitrogen), L-glutamine (Invitrogen) and penicillin-streptomycin (Lonza). Transfections were performed as described previously (Hotulainen et al., 2009) at days *in vitro* (DIV) 10–13 or DIV20 using Lipofectamine 2000 (Invitrogen). Plasmids pEGFP-N1 (GFP) and mCherry-C1 (mCherry) were purchased from Clontech Laboratories, Inc. Human GFP-β-actin (GFP-actin) (Choidas et al., 1998), PAGFP-actin and GFP-GFP (Dopie et al., 2012) were gifts from Maria Vartiainen (University of Helsinki, Finland). mCherry-palladin was a gift from Gergana Gateva and Pekka Lappalainen (University of Helsinki, Finland). mCherry-MHCIIb and mCherry-MHCIIb-R709C were kind gifts from Alan Rick Horwitz (University of Virginia, USA). siRNA oligonucleotides against MHCIIb (target sequence CCGGGATGAAGTGATCAAGCA) were purchased from Ambion. U2OS cells were cultured, plated and transfected as described earlier in Hotulainen and Lappalainen (2006). Cells were fixed with 4% PFA. F-actin was stained using phalloidin conjugated to Alexa 594 (dilution 1:400, Molecular Probes).

CONFOCAL IMAGING

Confocal imaging was performed with Leica TCS SP5 or Leica SP5 MP SMD FLIM upright confocal microscopes. For fixed sample imaging a 63 × 1.3 NA objective lens was used. Live-cell recordings were performed using a 63 × 0.9 NA water-dipping objective. For all live-cell experiments the microscopes were equipped with temperature controlled chamber and CO_2 supply. Live-cell experiments were performed at 37°C and 5% CO_2. The image files were processed with LAS AF (Leica microsystems, Germany), Photoshop CS6 (Adobe) and ImageJ softwares.

FRAP

FRAP experiments were performed as described previously (Koskinen et al., 2012). Briefly, neurons were transfected with GFP-actin at DIV13. Only mature mushroom type spines were used for the experiments. The frame including the ROI (measured whole spine) was imaged three times before bleaching. Photobleaching was achieved with five scans (total bleach time 3.117 s) of the region of interest with ~2.2 mW laser power at the sample (488 nm). Imaging of the area was resumed immediately after photo-bleaching and continued every 2–20 s for ~100–300 s. All the post-bleach values were divided by the values from the non-bleached area of the cells and normalized to the first pre-bleach value. The first post-bleach measurement was set to 0 s. The analysis of the FRAP recovery data was performed as described in the text using LAS AF (Leica Microsystems, Germany), Excel (Microsoft) and Origin8.6 (OriginLab) software.

PAGFP FLUORESCENCE DECAY

PAGFP fluorescence decay experiments were performed as described previously (Koskinen et al., 2012). Briefly, neurons were co-transfected with PAGFP-actin and mCherry at DIV10. Only mushroom spines of similar size were used for the experiments. Photo-activation was induced with one scan (0.78 s) of moderate intensity (~0.4 mW at the sample) 405 nm laser over the ROI (a single spine). Imaging of the area was resumed immediately following photo-activation and continued every 5–60 s for ~1000 s. For the analysis purposes the last pre-activation frame intensity was first subtracted from all post-activation values to exclude background and possible channel cross-talk. All post activation values were normalized to the first measured value. The activation frame was set as 0 s. For illustration figures the contour images were acquired from mCherry images by using Matlab 2010a (Mathworks, US). The data were processed with a 3 × 3 medial filter to reduce the noise. After this, the images were intensity-thresholded at a value of 25 to remove the background. The morphological "open" operation was performed on the resulting binary image to further smooth the edges. Finally the edges were calculated from these binary images using Canny edge detector (Canny, 1986). The analysis of the data was performed with LAS AF (Leica Microsystems, Germany), Excel (Microsoft) and Origin8.6 (OriginLab) Software as described in the text and figure and table legends.

FLUORESCENCE ANISOTROPY

Förster resonance energy transfer between two GFP-molecules, i.e., homoFRET, was quantified by measuring the fluorescence anisotropy. The experiments were carried out with a Leica SP5 MP SMD FLIM microscope (Leica Microsystems, Germany) using a 63 × 0.9 NA dipping objective. An argon laser (488 nm) was used to excite the fluorophores. A polarization prism (Leica Microsystems, Germany) was used to divide the emission signal into two channels, one parallel and the other perpendicular to the excitation laser. Both signals were measured using MPD PDM/C single-photon avalanche diodes (PicoQuant GmbH, Germany) and a photon counting mode to accurately measure the intensity variations within the sample.

The data were processed with Las AF software (Leica Microsystems, Germany) and Excel (Microsoft) using the equation presented by Bader et al. (2011):

$$r_{ani} = \frac{I_{\parallel} - I_{\perp}}{I_{\parallel} + 2I_{\perp}}$$

Equation 1: Anisotropy at a given pixel, or any given region of interest, is calculated as a ratio of detected emission on channels measuring light parallel and perpendicular to the excitation laser.

Average anisotropies were calculated from either whole cell images of U2OS cells transfected with GFP, GFP-GFP, GFP-Actin, or GFP-actin + palladin-mCherry or from selected regions of interest (ROIs) from the images of spines acquired from neurons transfected with free GFP, GFP-actin (at DIV14 and DIV21) or GFP-actin together with myosin heavy chain IIb WT-mCherry (MHC WT), MHC IIb siRNA or a non-contractile mutant MHC IIb R709C-mCherry (MHC IIb R709C). Anisotropy images shown in **Figures 6C,E** were calculated from the raw data as in equation 1, and subsequently processed with a 3 × 3 median filter to reduce noise. The resulting images were thresholded so that any values smaller than 0.1× the brightest pixel were set to zero. This processing was carried out with Matlab software (MathWorks, USA).

STATISTICAL TESTS

Statistical analyses were performed with SPSS software package (IBM). A paired sample *t*-test, Mann–Whitney test and ANOVA were used as applicable. All values in the text and figures represent mean ± standard deviation (SD) unless otherwise indicated.

MEASURING ACTIN TURNOVER RATE IN DENDRITIC SPINES

The active turnover of actin structures is a fundamental property of the filaments. Many of the ABPs function by manipulating the actin turnover rate to regulate different cellular processes such as cell division, cell motility (Pollard and Cooper, 2009), spinogenesis (Hotulainen et al., 2009) and spine morphology (Hodges et al., 2011). Therefore, measuring the actin turnover rate provides an important insight into the roles of different ABPs in dendritic spines. In the following paragraphs, we describe how actin turnover rate can be measured with FRAP and PAGFP fluorescence decay. We discuss what parameters should be taken into account when these methods are applied, possible obstacles to the application of these methods and finally the analysis of the data.

FLUORESCENCE RECOVERY AFTER PHOTOBLEACHING (FRAP)

FRAP is the most commonly used bulk kinetics approach method to study the dynamics of actin structures. In FRAP, a fluorescent protein is bleached from a small volume inside the cell with high-power laser. The recovery of the fluorescence is followed by time-lapse imaging. The fluorescence recovery is then used to elucidate the dynamics of the protein of interest (Star et al., 2002; Hotulainen et al., 2009; Koskinen et al., 2012; Kim et al., 2013; Stamatakou et al., 2013). When using FRAP to measure actin turnover, the recovery of the fluorescence represents addition of new non-bleached monomers onto the filaments and the depolymerization and diffusion of the bleached monomers. In other words, FRAP estimates the turnover rate by measuring the rate of actin filament assembly (Koskinen et al., 2012).

When using FRAP to determine the actin turnover rate in dendritic spines certain assumptions are usually made which are valid when the whole spine is bleached: first, the actin filaments do not diffuse through the spine neck, and second, actin monomer diffusion in and out of the spine is fast with a time constant of under 1 s (range 5–670 ms) (Star et al., 2002; Honkura et al., 2008). Therefore, the G-actin diffusion is not a rate limiting step. As an exception to these assumptions, filament diffusion out of the spine has been observed in special cases such as in failure to stabilize LTP (Honkura et al., 2008). When the whole spine area is bleached and measured, the actin network flow (Honkura et al., 2008; Frost et al., 2010) inside the spine does not affect the results.

Parameters to consider when using FRAP

Key points to consider when using FRAP are a strict timescale of bleaching and recovery follow-up as well as the power of the laser used for bleaching. In general it is good to keep all settings the same throughout the experimental setup. All live-cell fluorescence imaging leads to phototoxic effects (Magidson and Khodjakov, 2013). In photobleaching, some phototoxic effects are by definition unavoidable. It is better to use a short powerful laser pulse, than to increase the bleaching time. The turnover time constant for G-actin inside the dendritic spine is <1 s. To minimize the effect on the whole cell fluorescence level, bleach times should be kept as short as possible. How long bleaching is necessary for proper bleaching depends on the imaging setup and the sample. Bleaching laser power should not be increased to levels where noticeable, acute, effects on the cell are apparent, such as no recovery of fluorescence or cell death. The shortest possible bleach time minimizes the amount of G-actin diffusing in and out of the spine during bleaching thus minimizing the effect on the initial recovery in the form of bleached monomers diffusing back into the spine. The experiments described in the following paragraphs have been carried out with 2.2 mW laser power at the sample.

A critical look at the properties and limitations of FRAP

In FRAP we are measuring a change in fluorescence intensity as it recovers from the photo-bleaching. This means that any intrinsic fluctuation of the fluorescence intensity in the system is compromising the accuracy of the measurements. Dendritic spines, especially in neuron cultures, are highly dynamic (Korkotian and Segal, 2001; Bertling et al., 2012). Thus, actin filaments in the dendritic spines are continuously re-organized. This is detected as constant increase and decrease of the GFP-actin fluorescence found in nearly all spines (**Figures 1A,B**). On average, the GFP-actin fluorescence intensity of a single spine of a cultured rat DIV14 hippocampal neuron fluctuates at an amplitude of 8 ± 1.7% of the mean value (**Figure 1B**).

Bleaching of the GFP-molecules requires a considerable dose of radiation concentrated to a single spine. The effects of this

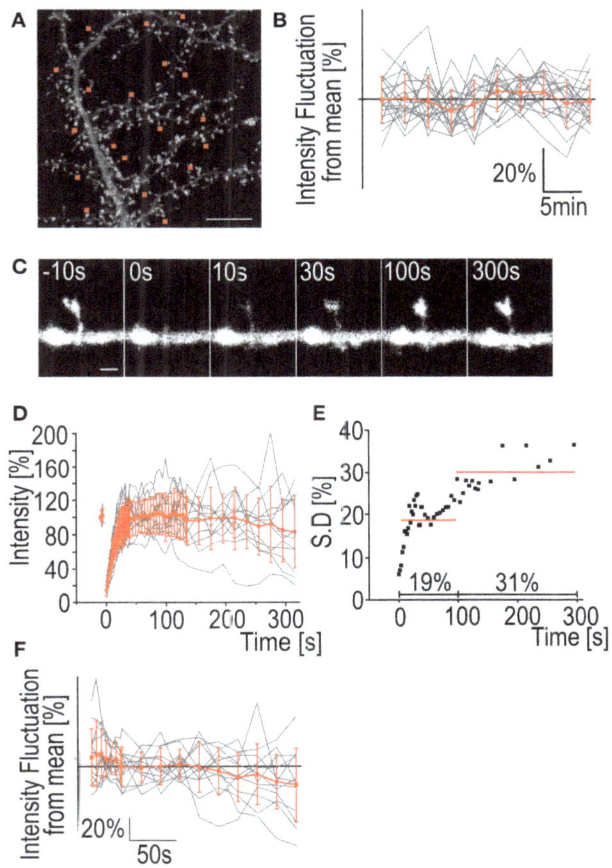

FIGURE 1 | Fluctuation of F-actin fluorescence and FRAP standard deviation. (A) A maximum projection of a DIV14 rat hippocampal neuron transfected with GFP-actin. Image is the first in a 3D time-lapse series of 10 images with 3 min intervals. The red squares mark the spines whose fluorescence intensity was followed during the series. Scale bar, 10 μm. **(B)** The fluorescence intensity of spines from the hippocampal neuron represented in **(A)**. Gray traces represent the individual spines and the red trace is mean ± SD. Mean spine intensity over all timepoints was set to 100%. $n = 19$ spines. **(C)** A time-lapse series of a DIV14 rat hippocampal neuron transfected with GFP-actin. The GFP fluorescence was bleached and the recovery followed. Numbers on top of the images are time after bleaching. Time $t = 0$ s is the first measurement post bleaching. Scale bar, 1 μm. **(D)** GFP-actin FRAP recovery curves from DIV14 rat hippocampal neuron spines. The gray traces represent individual spines and the red is mean ± SD, $n = 12$ spines. **(E)** The standard deviation of the mean FRAP recovery curve from **(D)**. The red lines represent the average of 19% during the first 100 s of recovery and 31% during the recovery between 100 and 315 s. **(F)** The fluorescence intensity fluctuation from the FRAP data in **(D)** after 100 s recovery. Mean spine intensity over all timepoints was set to 100%. Gray traces are individual spines and the red trace is mean ± SD.

radiation on the spine morphology and actin dynamics are difficult to quantify but it seems evident that bleaching increases fluorescence intensity fluctuation (and spine dynamics). If we look at the standard deviation of the actin fluorescence after bleaching we can see that the average SD of the measurements is 19% during the first 100 s of the recovery. The fluctuation becomes even greater when the recovery reaches a plateau with the average SD 100–315 s after bleaching being 31% (**Figures 1C–E**). The fluorescence values for single spines 100 s after bleaching fluctuate at an amplitude of 17 ± 8.1% from the mean (**Figure 1F**). Comparison to fluctuation of non-bleached neurons reveals that the GFP-actin intensity exhibits larger fluctuation in bleached spines (**Figures 1B** vs. **F**). Fluorescence fluctuation makes accurate determination of intensity value difficult, both before bleaching as well as after full recovery. SD especially increases after the 100 s mark. We therefore decided to image recovery for only up to 100 s after bleaching. Consequently, FRAP is not suitable to measure the properties of the stable actin pool in dendritic spines. It can be used to estimate the stable pool size but it is better to use PAGFP fluorescence decay to confirm results, especially if the change in the stable pool size between different treatments is small (see next section).

Another phenomenon we have observed is the enlargement of spines following bleaching (**Figure 2**). In 9/12 cases the spine head was enlarged 315 s after bleaching as measured by full-width-at-half-maximum of the GFP-actin fluorescence (**Figures 2A,B**). The average enlargement was 27% of pre-bleach value, almost twice the average fluctuation of spine head width previously reported (Bertling et al., 2012). In 3/12 cases the spines shrunk by an average of 7.8%. Mean spine width was increased from 0.95 ± 0.25 μm to 1.1 ± 0.34 μm ($p < 0.05$ Paired samples t-test) (**Figure 2C**). In the neighboring control spines 17/35 were found enlarged. The average enlargement was 16%. The average spine shrinkage found in 18/35 cases was 17%. Counting all the spines showed that neighboring spines stayed on average the same size as before bleaching, with an average size change of −0.70 ± 3.6%, as opposed to bleached spines which were enlarged by 19 ± 29% ($p < 0.05$ Mann–Whitney test) (**Figure 2D**). The cause of this spine enlargement is not known but it seems that it is most obvious when a high laser power is used (our unpublished observations). So although high laser power enables the use of short bleaching time, it might have stronger undesirable effects on the cell than long bleaching with a low laser power. Spine enlargement after bleaching makes it difficult to estimate the ratio of the dynamic and stable actin pools; the amount of total actin in spines increases resulting in the fluorescence intensity overshooting the initial pre-bleach value.

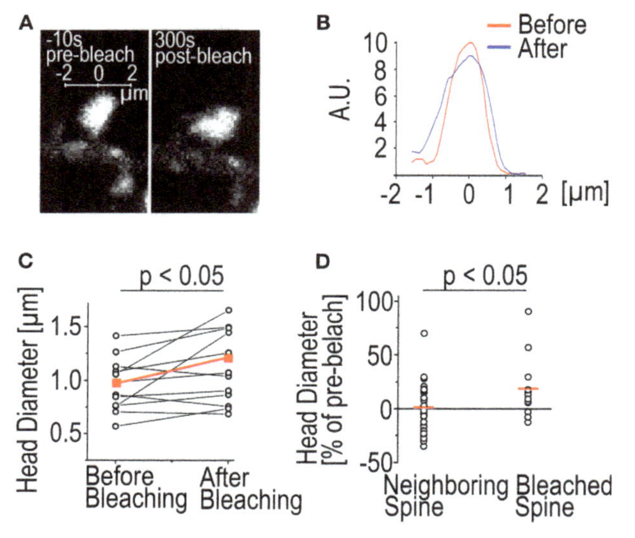

FIGURE 2 | Spine enlargement following photo-bleaching. **(A)** A DIV14 rat hippocampal neuron spine imaged 10 s before and 300 s after photo-bleaching. **(B)** The fluorescence profiles of the spine in **(A)** through the middle of the spines along the axis shown in **(A)**. The red trace represents the profile before bleaching and the blue after bleaching. Profile was averaged over 0.5 μm along the axis. **(C)** Spine head diameter before and after bleaching. Black traces are individual spines, red trace is the mean. The mean spine size as full width at half maximum through the center of the spine changes from 0.95 ± 0.25 to 1.12 ± 0.34 μm, $p < 0.05$ Paired samples t-test, $n = 12$ spines. **(D)** Spine enlargement affects only the bleached spines and not the neighboring ones. Black circles represent individual spines, mean indicated by a red line. Size change: Neighboring −0.70 ± 3.6%; bleached 19 ± 29%, $p < 0.05$ Mann–Whitney test, $n = 35$ neighboring spines, 12 bleached.

Due to different laser power and different bleaching times used in different microscopy setups, it is difficult to directly compare FRAP values from different laboratories. In addition, values from different model systems (cultured neurons/ slice cultures) cannot be directly compared.

Analysis of FRAP data

FRAP data is usually analyzed by measuring the fluorescence at the ROI (spine) at time intervals, dividing this with a reference fluorescence value from elsewhere in the cell to correct for general fluctuation (usually bleaching caused by imaging + detector error) of the fluorescence, and normalizing to fluorescence values at the ROI before bleaching (Star et al., 2002; Koskinen et al., 2012). Several different strategies have been employed to interpret the resulting fluorescence recovery data. Most common strategies have been (a) fitting the individual measurement data to a single exponent equation (Star et al., 2002) and (b) determining the recovery half-time from averaged data and using that to calculate the first order rate constant

$$\left(k_{obs} = \frac{\ln(2)}{t_{1/2}}\right)$$

Equation 2. Calculation of the first order rate constant of the fluorescence recovery.

Hotulainen et al. (2009); Kim et al. (2013); Stamatakou et al. (2013); Koskinen et al. (2014). To evaluate the fitting method we used the FRAP data presented in **Figure 1**. We fitted each individual spine data to a single component equation (**Table 1**, **Figure 3A**).

Two features stand out from these results: (1) the wide range of recovery time constants (t_1) and, (2) the negative stable component values (y_0). The heterogeneity of the time constants undermines the sensitivity of the method. Our experiments resulted in a mean time constant of 17 ± 10 s with a 95% confidence interval of 11–23 s. This means that small differences in time constant are not reliably detected unless n is considerably large. If all conditions would follow the same distribution of time constants, these twelve measurements would be enough to acquire a statistical power for 50% change (8.5 s difference) in turnover rate. To detect a 2 s difference in mean time constants with 90% statistical power, n would need to exceed ~200 measurements. Thus, FRAP is only suitable for analyzing large changes in actin dynamics.

The negative values for the stable component are the result of the fluorescence intensity overshooting the initial pre-bleach values, due to intrinsic and/or bleaching-induced fluctuations in intensity and/or spine enlargement.

The signal quality of the measurements was determined by looking at the residuals from the fits (**Figure 3B**). Residual is the difference between the each data point and fit at that point. The smaller the range of residuals is, the better is the signal quality and fit to the used equation. The residuals of individual FRAP experiments spread roughly between −40 and 40%. The mean of all absolute residual values was 5.5 ± 5.0%.

Averaging the data from all spines before fitting leads to a better fit to single component equation (**Table 2, Figure 3C**) but still results in a negative stable component value.

The difficulties in determining the stable component size and distinguishing the recovery of the stable and dynamic components through automated curve fitting can be overcome by employing a simpler analysis of the mean curve. Using the mean recovery curve, the size of the stable component can be manually approximated by determining the slope of the curve segment after ~5 times the time constant of the dynamic pool. At this point > 99% of the dynamic pool fluorescence has been recovered (**Figure 1D**). Interpolating a straight line with this slope to the timepoint corresponding to the first post-bleach measurement gives an approximation of the stable pool size (Honkura et al., 2008) (**Figure 3C**, lower panel). The recovery half-time of

Table 1 | Results of fitting curves from individual FRAP experiments to the equation $y(t) = y_0 - A_1 e^{-\frac{t}{t_1}}$ where y_0 is the stable component, A_1 is the dynamic component and t_1 is the time constant, inverse of the rate constant.

Spine	y_0 Value	y_0 SE	A_1 Value	A_1 SE	t_1 Value	t_1 SE	Statistics Reduced Chi-Sqr	Statistics Adj. R-Square
d1s1	−0.12	0.023	1.1	0.071	9.1	1.2	0.0085	0.89
d1s2	0.30	0.013	0.58	0.036	10	1.2	0.0024	0.91
d1s3	−0.32	0.034	1.2	0.054	20	2.2	0.0075	0.94
d2s1	−0.10	0.035	1.1	0.12	7.5	1.6	0.023	0.76
d2s2	−0.034	0.021	0.88	0.035	19	1.7	0.0030	0.95
d2s3	−0.73	0.060	1.6	0.052	43	3.9	0.0033	0.98
d2s4	0.059	0.013	0.81	0.027	16	1.1	0.0016	0.97
d3s1	0.091	0.020	0.68	0.047	13	1.8	0.0046	0.88
d3d2	−0.23	0.026	1.1	0.076	9.8	1.4	0.010	0.88
d3s3	0.10	0.0088	0.75	0.022	12	0.72	9.3E-04	0.98
d4s1	−0.14	0.044	1.1	0.053	26	3.3	0.0074	0.93
d4s2	0.18	0.015	0.80	0.029	16	1.3	0.0019	0.96
Average	−0.078	0.026	0.97	0.052	17	1.8	0.0061	0.92

Table 2 | Result of fitting average FRAP curve to the equation $y(t) = y_0 - A_1 e^{-\frac{t}{t_1}}$ where y_0 is the stable component, A_1 is the dynamic component and t_1 is the time constant, inverse of the rate constant.

	y_0 Value	y_0 *SE*	A_1 Value	A_1 *SE*	t_1 Value	t_1 *SE*	Statistics Reduced Chi-Sqr	Statistics Adj. R-Square
Average	−0.034	0.0053	0.92	0.011	15	0.38	2.82E-04	0.9956

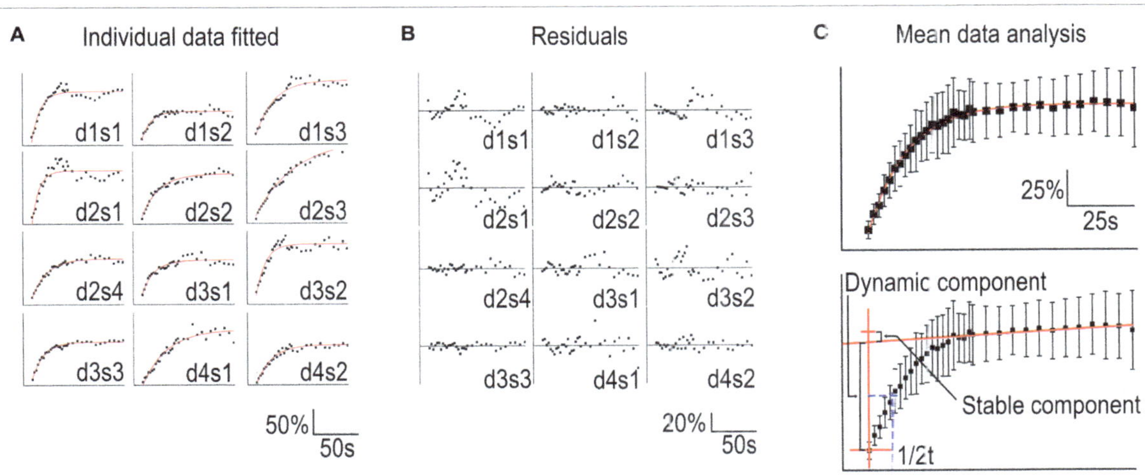

FIGURE 3 | Analysis of FRAP curves. (A) Individual FRAP data measured from GFP-actin transfected, DIV14, rat hippocampal neuron spines fitted to the equation in **Table 1**. Data were labeled as spines (s) 1–4 belonging to a specific dendrite (d) 1–4. **(B)** The residuals corresponding to the fits in **(A)**. **(C)** Upper panel: Mean ± SD curve from data in **(A)** fitted to a single component equation as in **(A)**. Lower panel: The same mean ± SD curve as in the upper panel with the time = 0 and the linear approximation of the stable component marked by red lines and the dynamic component recovery half time in blue.

the dynamic component can then be determined between the first measurement and the stable pool fraction and used to calculate the first order rate constant of the recovery (**Figure 3C**). This manual analysis of the measured values results in a stable component of 8.5% and a recovery half-time of 9.5 s which corresponds to a time constant of 14 s.

It is important to note that the stable component refers here to the actual coefficient of the immobile or slower F-actin pool. The stable pool can also be defined as a fraction of total F-actin (Star et al., 2002; Honkura et al., 2008).

$$\left(\frac{F_{stable}}{F_{stable} + F_{dynamic}}\right).$$

The main obstacle in the analyses of FRAP data was the enlargement of spines after bleaching. Obviously, spine enlargement should be minimized by optimizing bleach settings. Alternatively, the reference color (such as mCherry-actin) could be used to make it possible to correct for intrinsic fluctuation or increased actin fluorescent intensity during imaging. Using two colors is technically more challenging but can give more accurate results. Averaging whenever possible can also improve the results.

PHOTO-ACTIVATABLE GFP FLUORESCENCE DECAY

Photo-activatable GFP is essentially a GFP-molecule with a point mutation resulting in a very low GFP fluorescence intensity prior to activation. Brief illumination by a 405 nm laser increases fluorescence 100 fold (Patterson and Lippincott-Schwartz, 2002). Approximation of the F-actin turnover rate using PAGFP is similar to FRAP except that the decay of the activated PAGFP fluorescence from the spine is followed (Honkura et al., 2008). At an ideal steady state, where actin polymerization and depolymerization rates are the same, FRAP and PAGFP fluorescence decay mirror one another resulting in identical time constants. However, the two methods do give different results in the presence of fluctuations in polymerization and depolymerization. For example, an increase in polymerization within the spine would be more evident in FRAP rather than in PAGFP fluorescence decay, and increase in depolymerization and filament disassembly would be more visible in PAGFP fluorescent decay. In dendritic spines, polymerization and depolymerization rates fluctuate constantly, which can also be seen in the intrinsic fluctuation of the GFP-actin fluorescence (**Figures 1A,B**).

Parameters to consider when using PAGFP fluorescence decay

When performing PAGFP-decay experiments the key points to control are: (a) the time scale, (b) the imaging settings, and (c) spine size. The stable pool size is often calculated as a fraction of the total fluorescence at the first imaged frame after PAGFP activation (Honkura et al., 2008; Koskinen et al., 2014). Therefore, the time interval from activation to the first frame has to be kept constant in order to compare different measurements. Imaging settings need to be optimized to keep the activated fluorescence in the linear range of the detector and avoid detector saturation. If planning to pool results from single spines to study the size of the stable pool, spine size must be taken into account as the size of the stable pool is correlated to spine size (Honkura et al., 2008).

Differences to FRAP

The most notable difference in using PAGFP decay instead of FRAP to measure the actin turnover rate is the smaller variation in fluorescence change rate. The activation of the PAGFP only requires a very short, millisecond-range, pulse of the 405 nm laser. The fast activation results in a "freeze frame" image of the F-actin at one moment and the observed decay is only affected by the filament depolymerization and disassembly rates (**Figures 4A,B**). This can be seen as the low average standard deviation of the decay curves (2.2%) (**Figure 4C**). It is also possible to follow fluorescence decay much longer than fluorescence recovery. The decaying fluorescence signal does not need to compete with intrinsic signal fluctuation so a stable recording can be maintained even at very low levels of fluorescence.

Analysis of the PAGFP fluorescence decay data

Due to the stable decay characteristics of the PAGFP-actin fluorescence individual measurements can be well fitted to an equation. The longer recordings also make it possible to determine the turnover rate for the slowly recovering actin pool. Additionally, no change in spine size was observed following PAGFP activation with 405 nm laser (mean spine size was 0.98 ± 0.083 μm before and 0.88 ± 0.086 μm after activation, $p > 0.05$, paired t-test).

Before fitting the individual spine data to an equation the number of differently regulated components can be evaluated. A mean decay curve from several measured spines of similar sizes (spine head width 0.98 ± 0.083 μm) was fitted to single-, bi-, or triexponential decay equations (**Figure 5A**). The accuracy of the fits can be estimated from the mean residuals (**Figure 5B**). First the distribution of the residuals was examined. All residual are normally distributed (Shapiro-Wilk test

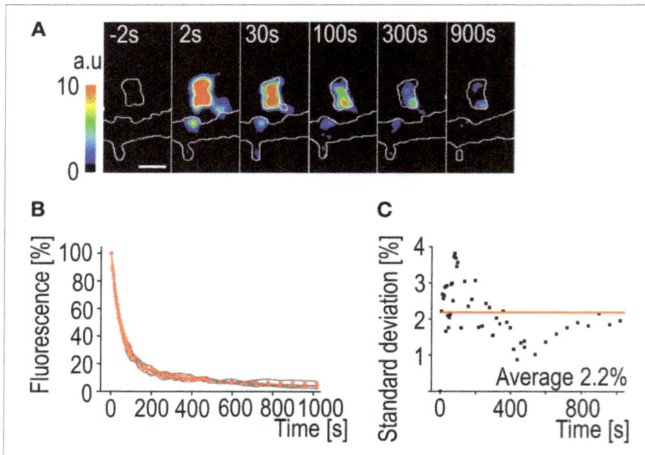

FIGURE 4 | PAGFP fluorescence decay standard deviation. (A) A time-lapse series of a DIV14 rat hippocampal neuron transfected with PAGFP-actin and mCherry. The numbers represent time after photo-activation. The image is pseudocolored according to the scale on the left. The outlines of the cell were derived from mCherry fluorescence. Scale bar, 1 μm. **(B)** The PAGFP-actin fluorescence decay data from DIV14 hippocampal neuron spines. The gray traces represent individual spines and the red mean ± SD, $n = 5$ spines. **(C)** The standard deviation of the mean PAGFP fluorescence decay curve from **(B)**. The red line represents the average of 2.2%.

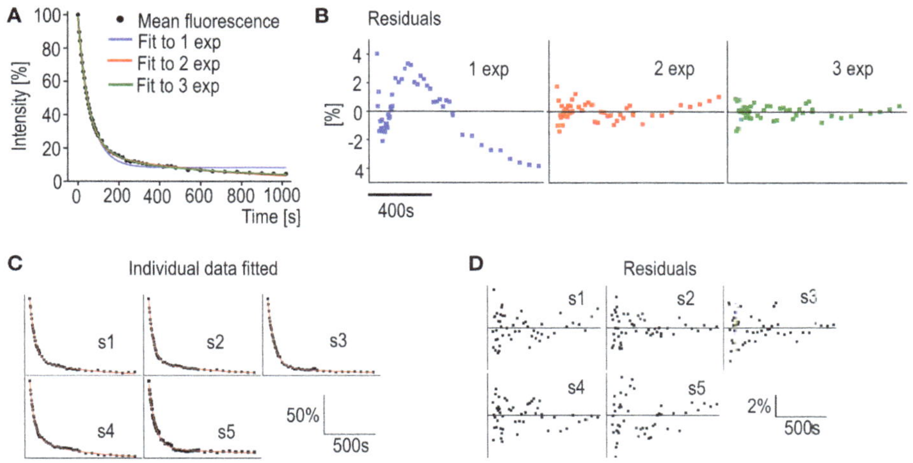

FIGURE 5 | Analysis of PAGFP decay curves. (A) Averaged PAGFP-actin fluorescence data from DIV14 rat hippocampal neuron spines fitted to equations with a different number of components. Blue trace = 1 component equation, red trace = 2 component equation and green trace = 3 component equation. $n = 5$ spines. **(B)** The regular residual means from the fit curves from **(A)**. **(C)** Individual PAGFP fluorescence decay data measured from DIV14 rat hippocampal neuron spines fitted to the 2-component equation as in **(A)**. Curves were named as spines (s) 1–5. **(D)** Residuals corresponding to the fits in **(C)**.

significance values >0.05) and therefore fulfill the first criterion. In **Figure 5B** it is seen that when the mean curve is fitted to a one-component exponential decay equation the residuals are not randomly distributed along the timescale. This indicates a poor fit. When a biexponential decay equation is used, the residuals are more randomly distributed along the timescale except for a few final values, which might indicate a third even slower turnover rate component. Using a triexponential decay equation does lead to randomly distributed residuals with smaller values but the standard errors of the time constant values increase (**Table 3**).

Moreover, the two faster component time-constants in three component fit are fairly close to each other (40 vs. 91 s) and as such do not present new biological insight and can be seen as overfitting. These observations, taken together with the prior knowledge from Honkura et al. (2008) of the two differently regulated components of spine F-actin, led us to conclude that, with measurements of this timescale, the decay of the PAGFP-actin fluorescence from spines is best described by an equation of two differently regulated components.

Fitting the data from individual measurements resulted in a mean stable component size of 18 ± 5.8% as well as mean time constants of 51 ± 8.4 s and 840 ± 390 s for the dynamic and stable components, respectively (**Figure 5C**, **Table 4**). The residuals of the fits confirm the low noise level of the measurements (**Figure 5D**); the residuals spread between −4 and 4%, with a mean absolute value of 1.1 ± 0.84%. This range is five-fold smaller than in FRAP measurements. The narrower range of time constants allows for a lower number of n to be used. To detect a 6 s difference in dynamic pool time constants (6 s is percentually the same order change from PAGFP-obtained time constant as 2 s is in FRAP-obtained time constants) with a 90% statistical power only requires an n of 17 measurements.

Table 3 | PAGFP-actin averaged data fitted to one $\left(y(t) = y_0 + Ae^{-\frac{t}{t_1}}\right)$, two $\left(y(t) = A_1e^{-\frac{t}{t_1}} + A_2e^{-\frac{t}{t_2}}\right)$ and three $\left(y(t) = A_1e^{-\frac{t}{t_1}} + A_2e^{-\frac{t}{t_2}} + A_3e^{-\frac{t}{t_3}}\right)$ -component equations.

Parameter		1 exp	2 exp	3 exp
y_0*	Value	8.4	–	–
y_0	*SE*	0.42	–	–
A_1	Value	89	82	57
A_1	*SE*	1.2	0.62	17
t_1	Value	62	50	40
t_1	*SE*	1.6	0.74	5.0
A_2	Value		18	30
A_2	*SE*		0.61	16
t_2	Value		630	91
t_2	*SE*		32	28
A_3	Value			14
A_3	*SE*			1.5
t_3	Value			830
t_3	*SE*			110
Statistics	Reduced Chi-Sqr	4.0262	0.3950	0.2552
Statistics	Adj. R-Square	0.9937	0.9994	0.9996

A_x represents the component coefficient and t_x the time constant, inverse of the rate constant.

** y_0 is a constant depicting an immobile pool used only in fitting to 1 exp due to the curve not reaching zero.*

MEASURING THE ACTIN FILAMENT ORGANIZATION IN DENDRITIC SPINES

Due to the small size of the dendritic spines, actin filament organization has been very difficult to determine. With the recently developed fluorescence anisotropy assay (Vishwasrao et al., 2012), we can measure how densely GFP molecules are packed in cells. GFP-actin fluorescence normally retains the polarization of the

Table 4 | PAGFP data curve fitted to the two-component equation $\left(y(t) = A_1 e^{-\frac{t}{t_1}} + A_2 e^{-\frac{t}{t_2}}\right)$ where A_1 and A_2 are the coefficients of the components and t_1 and t_2 the time constants.

Spine	A_1 Value	A_1 SE	t_1 Value	t_1 SE	A_2 Value	A_2 SE	t_2 Value	t_2 SE	Statistics Reduced Chi-Sqr	Statistics Adj. R-Square
S1	82.3	1.41	50.0	1.60	20.0	1.43	522	50.9	1.656	0.9976
S2	83.4	1.00	43.4	1.08	17.6	0.912	671	59.6	1.265	0.9979
S3	89.0	1.14	61.3	1.56	10.3	1.06	1150	278	1.780	0.9975
S4	73.6	1.33	41.1	1.46	27.3	1.35	422	26.4	1.479	0.9976
S5	84.0	1.53	60.4	2.24	13.4	1.37	1440	425	3.656	0.9942
Average	82.5	1.28	51.2	1.59	17.7	1.22	841	168	1.967	0.9969
SD	4.97	0.190	8.38	0.374	5.82	0.202	390	157	0.8622	0.001374

excitation light. This polarization information is lost when GFP-actin undergoes FRET with other nearby localized GFP-actin molecules (distance < 10 nm). The ratio of detected parallel and perpendicular emission light (anisotropy) can be used to derive information about F-actin structures (**Figures 6A,B**).

$$E = \frac{1}{1 + \left(\frac{r}{R_0}\right)^6}$$

Equation 3: FRET efficiency r = distance between the fluorophores R_0 = Förster distance.

Equation 3 represents the FRET efficiency as a function of the distance between the fluorophores. The Förster radius R_0, the distance at which the energy transfer efficiency between the fluorophore pair is 50%, for GFP-GFP interaction is 4.58 nm (Vishwasrao et al., 2012). The probability for FRET to occur drops to less than 1% when the fluorophore pair is further than 10 nm apart. It is also indicated in the Vishwasrao et al. (2012) that in compartments of dense actin the inter-filamentary FRET can be equal or dominant form of energy transfer.

We wanted to evaluate the method and to investigate whether the signal observed is the result of intra- or inter-filament interactions of GFP-actin molecules. It is important to note that GFP-actin expression levels 24 h after transfection are typically low [6% of total actin has been estimated to be GFP-labeled (Westphal et al., 1997)], which is important to minimize over-expression artifacts and improve overall neuronal health. We estimated that under these conditions maximally every 10th actin monomer carries GFP. Thus, the probability for intra-filament FRET is low although not impossible (Vishwasrao et al., 2012). We conclude that the mathematical reasoning strongly supports the hypothesis that with fluorescence anisotropy we mainly detect inter-filament FRET.

To experimentally test whether the fluorescence anisotropy measures intra- or inter-filament FRET, we first calibrated the fluorescence anisotropy boarder values from U2 osteosarcoma cells (U2OS) expressing either free GFP or GFP dimers [two GFP molecules fused together via a molecular linker allowing for efficient energy transfer between fluorophores (Dopie et al., 2012)]. The free GFP resulted in average values of 0.27 (dimensionless ratio) whereas the GFP dimers resulted in a value of 0.16 (**Figures 6C,D**). Thus, with GFP-actin we should obtain values within this range, where values close to 0.27 indicate actin monomers or actin filaments where two GFP molecules do not get close enough for FRET to occur. We next tested the fluorescence anisotropy values in U2OS cells expressing GFP-actin. Low anisotropy values were only detected along stress fibers (**Figure 6C**). Stress fibers are tightly cross-linked thick bundles of myosin II and actin filaments. To further enhance actin cross-linking and to test if enhanced cross-linking can decrease the fluorescence anisotropy, we over-expressed palladin, an actin bundling protein, the over-expression of which leads to the formation of unusually robust actin-stress fibers in cells (Rachlin and Otey, 2006; Dixon et al., 2008). The whole cell fluorescence anisotropy was decreased in cells expressing palladin together with GFP-actin (0.27 vs. 0.22, respectively) (**Figures 6C,D**). Stress fibers could be clearly distinguished from the fluorescence anisotropy images of cells expressing GFP-actin with palladin (**Figure 6C**). We further tested the idea of measuring actin bundling with fluorescence anisotropy by comparing the fluorescence anisotropy values in lamellipodia and along stress fibers (**Figure 6C**). Lamellipodia are composed of actin filament networks. These networks are densely packed but filaments are not aligned as bundles (Svitkina and Borisy, 1999). We first obtained images of GFP-actin anisotropy from live U2OS cells that were subsequently fixed and the F-actin was visualized with phalloidin staining (**Figure 6C**, lower panel). The phalloidin staining shows clearly both lamellipodium (red arrow) as well as stress fibers (pink arrow). Anisotropy decreases along stress fibers but not in the lamellipodium (**Figure 6C**, lower panel). The anisotropy results indicate that the anisotropy decreases significantly only when actin filaments are tightly bundled together, as in stress fibers. Taken together, these results indicate that in cells expressing low levels of GFP-actin the anisotropy values represent the level of actin filament bundling. The fact that the average fluorescence anisotropy value in the area of lamellipodium with a lot of F-actin was similar to values detected with free GFP indicates that the intra-filament FRET is actually under the detection level. Thus, we conclude that fluorescence anisotropy is a potentially highly useful tool for actin bundling measurements.

We next applied this method to analyze how actin filament organization changes during neuronal maturation. We first measured the mean anisotropy from the dendritic spines of neurons

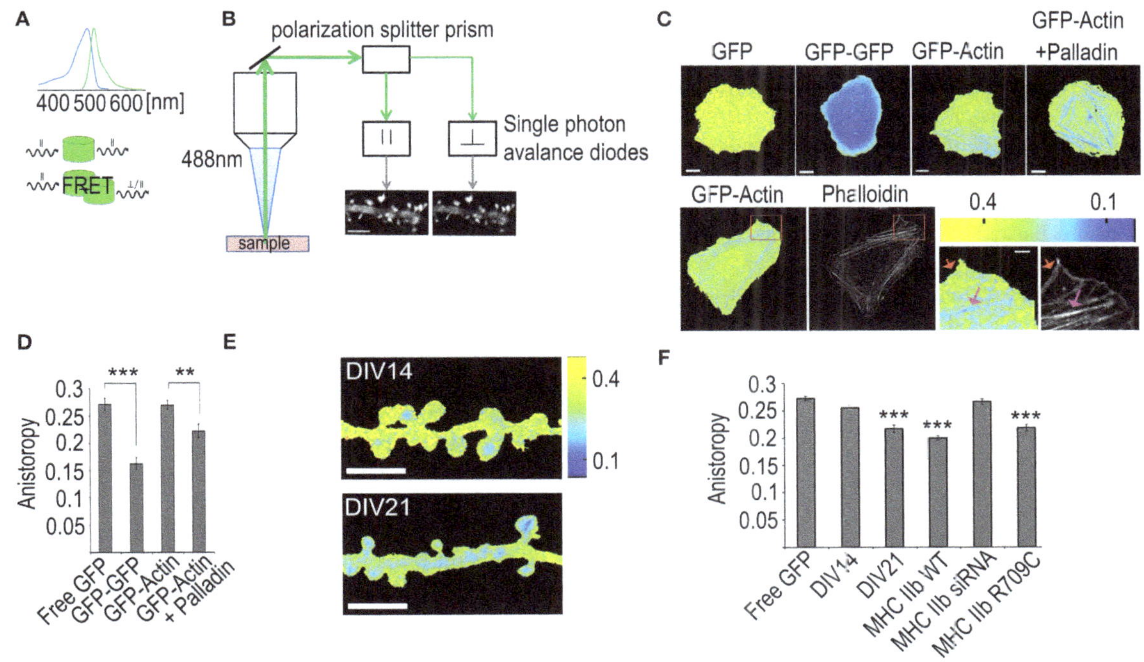

FIGURE 6 | Using fluorescence anisotropy measurements to study actin bundling. (A) Upper panel: the absorption and emission spectra of GFP. Lower panel: a schematic of the differences between direct emission and FRET-mediated emission where the polarization information is lost. **(B)** The signal path of the emission. The emission signal is first directed to a polarization splitter prism that separates the signal having polarization parallel to the excitation laser from the perpendicular one. The signal is then directed to two single photon avalanche diode detectors that form accurate intensity images of the sample. Scale bar, 5 μm. **(C)** Upper panel: Fluorescence anisotropy images of U2OS cells transfected with GFP, GFP-GFP, GFP-actin or GFP-actin + palladin-mCherry, Scale bars 10 μm. Lower panel: first frame: a fluorescence anisotropy image of a U2OS cell transfected with GFP-actin, second frame: the same cell with F-actin stained with phalloidin-Alexa 594. The two last frames: enlargements of the area indicated by the red rectangle in the fluorescence anisotropy and the phalloidin images, red arrows indicate the non-bundled F-actin in the cell cortex and the pink arrows indicate the bundled stress fibers. Scale bars: whole cell images 10 μm, enlarged sections 2 μm. All the fluorescence anisotropy images are pseudocolored according to the scale in the upper right corner of the lower panel. **(D)** Mean GFP anisotropy values of whole U2OS cells transfected with free GFP ($n = 18$ cells), GFP-GFP ($n = 15$ cells), GFP-actin ($n = 23$ cells) or GFP-actin with palladin-mCherry ($n = 13$ cells). ANOVA shows that there are statistically significant differences between groups in fluorescence anisotropy $F_{(3, 65)} = 24.335$, $p < 0.0001$. Free GFP ($M = 0.27$) had statistically significant ($p < 0.0001$) higher values than GFP-GFP ($M = 0.16$), likewise GFP-actin ($M = 0.27$) had higher values than GFP-GFP. Free GFP had statistically significant ($p < 0.01$) higher values than GFP-actin + palladin ($M = 0.22$), likewise GFP-actin + Palladin had higher values than GFP-GFP and, GFP-actin had higher values than GFP-actin + Palladin. All graphs mean ± s.e.m. **(E)** Anisotropy images of DIV14 and DIV21 rat hippocampal neurons color-coded according to the scale on the right. Scale bar, 5 μm. **(F)** Comparison of the mean anisotropy values from dendritic spines of DIV14 hippocampal neurons or DIV21 hippocampal neurons (DIV21). DIV21 neurons were transfected with GFP-actin $n = 66$ spines. DIV14 neurons were transfected with various constructs (1) free GFP (marked as free GFP) $n = 49$ spines, (2) GFP-actin (marked as DIV14) $n = 77$ spines, (3) GFP-actin and mCherry-MHC IIb $n = 61$ spines, (4) GFP-actin and MHC IIb siRNA $n = 69$ spines, (5) GFP-actin and mCherry-MHC IIb R709C $n = 41$ spines, (6) ANOVA showed that there are statistically significant differences in anisotropy between groups $F_{(8, 574)} = 20.641$, $p < 0.0001$. DIV14 ($M = 0.25$) had higher values ($p < 0.0001$) than DIV21 ($M = 0.21$), MHC-WT ($M = 0.20$), MHC IIb R709C ($M = 0.21$). All graphs mean ± s.e.m. $^{**}p < 0.01$, $^{***}p < 0.001$.

transfected with GFP-actin at DIV14 and DIV21 and found the mean anisotropy from DIV21 neuron spines to be significantly lower than that from DIV14 neuron spines (0.22 vs. 0.26, respectively) (**Figures 6E,F**), indicating an increase in actin bundling. This is consistent with our previous study, where we described—using FRAP and PAGFP fluorescence decay—that the size of the F-actin stable pool increases during neuronal maturation and hypothesized that the stable F-actin pool is increased by enhanced cross-linking of the actin filaments (Koskinen et al., 2014). Furthermore, no significant difference was found between DIV14 anisotropy values and free GFP (0.26 and 0.27 respectively) (**Figure 6F**), indicating very low levels of bundled actin in immature spines. This also indicates that F-actin polymerization itself is not sufficient to decrease the anisotropy values. Based on our previous FRAP and PAGFP fluorescence decay results, we proposed that myosin IIb cross-links the actin filaments in dendritic spines independent of its motor activity. Thus, to further test the fluorescence anisotropy method, we tested how myosin IIb over-expression, depletion and expression of the non-contractile myosin IIb mutant construct (R709C) affect fluorescence anisotropy values. The expression of MHC IIb or MHC IIb R709C both resulted in significantly lower levels of anisotropy (0.20 and 0.22, respectively) compared to control, suggesting their function in actin cross-linking. Furthermore, no significant difference was found between control neurons and MHC siRNA-transfected ones (0.26 and 0.27 respectively) (**Figure 6F**), indicating no or very few cross-linked actin filaments in myosin IIb depleted DIV14 neurons. This data fits well with our previous FRAP and PAGFP fluorescence decay data showing that myosin IIb overexpression (both wild-type and non-contractile mutant constract) significantly increased the size of the stable actin pool while the depletion of myosin IIb using siRNA completely abolished the stable actin pool (Koskinen et al., 2014).

With fluorescence anisotropy we can measure how closely GFP molecules are packed in cells in different cell areas. Our mathematical reasoning as well as experimental evidence suggest that this method measures mainly the GFP-actin:GFP-actin FRET between closely packed actin filaments, and thus can be used as a method to measure values for actin filament bundling. The closer the actin filaments are to each other, the smaller is the fluorescence anisotropy value.

DISCUSSION

FRAP has been extensively used and refined in studies of actin dynamics especially in fibroblasts. So far only a few studies utilized this method for studying actin dynamics in neurons and especially dendritic spines, but it is clear that there is an increasing interest. It is, therefore, worthwhile to consider what parameters need to be taken into account to get the best results. The main drawbacks of using FRAP in dendritic spines are the large variation between measurements, fast dendritic spine dynamics and changes in GFP-actin intensity as well as spine enlargement following photo-bleaching (**Figures 1B,D**). Currently, the reasons underlying spine enlargement are not clear but it is plausible that photo-bleaching increases the rate of actin polymerization. High laser power illumination can cause severing of actin filaments and rapid creation of new barbed ends (Jacobson et al., 2008; Reymann et al., 2011). This could explain the rapid increase in spine size, the overshoot of the fluorescence from pre-bleach levels and the high fluctuation of the post-bleaching fluorescence. If this is the case and the newly formed barbed ends lead to increased net polymerization of the filaments then the rate constants obtained using FRAP overestimate the turnover rate of the dynamic actin pool. It seems that this effect is not uniformly manifested across all conditions or imaging systems. Manipulating ABP levels or activity seems to affect the magnitude of the observed effect. For example, the knockdown of a capping protein could lead to a prolonged increase in bulk polymerization compared to control due to the inability to control the polymerization by capping the newly formed filament barbed ends. This emphasizes the need to control and test the laser power used for photo-bleaching. There have been attempts to improve the method, such as dual color FRAP (Dunn et al., 2002). Use of two colors could be useful also in spines. The reference color would allow normalization against intrinsic fluctuations of the dendritic spine of interest.

In control conditions and especially in young neurons, the stable actin pool often comprises only a few percent of the total F-actin, depending on spine size (Star et al., 2002; Honkura et al., 2008). Due to GFP-actin fluorescence fluctuation, particularly when the recovery has reached the plateau level (**Figure 1B**), the size and the turnover rate of the stable actin pool are difficult to determine from single FRAP measurements. Averaging frees the analysis from many of the problems posed by high fluctuation of the values (**Figures 3B–F**). On the other hand, averaging makes statistical testing impossible. It could be useful to look into methods to estimate how "different" two average curves are. One such method is the Kullback-Leiber divergence (Kullback and Leibler, 1951). However, using this method to compare two curves does not directly lead to a *p*-value but the significance is estimated by other means. More elaborate means of analysis are also found where fitting is performed to a stochastic model of actin treadmilling (Halavatyi et al., 2010). These models work well in *in silico* simulations but fitting measured data to six different parameters without fixed values is not feasible.

Using PAGFP-actin fluorescence decay has the advantage of a more stable signal compared to FRAP experiments in dendritic spines (**Figure 3**). The brief, moderate intensity, pulse needed for the photo-activation minimizes the adverse effects of laser illumination. The stable recordings are easy to fit to an equation. This allows to treat spines as individual units and compare several parameters, such as spine head size, in addition to the actin turnover data. Compared to FRAP, the PAGFP fluorescence decay is a bit more difficult technique to use. It requires the co-transfection of another fluorophore to visualize the cell and more optimization is needed to determine the expression level of the PAGFP-actin and to standardize imaging settings.

One of the main questions regarding the actin turnover is the distinction between filament treadmilling and actin structure assembly/disassembly. This question has been addressed in studies of actin dynamics in lamellipodia, a structure consisting of highly dynamic actin filament network (McGrath et al., 1998; Lai et al., 2008; Miyoshi and Watanabe, 2013; Smith et al., 2013). According to models based on single molecule tracking results it is unlikely that filament treadmilling alone is responsible for the fast turnover of actin structures in lamellipodia (Miyoshi and Watanabe, 2013). A new type of actin structure, a slow diffusing oligomere, resulting from a cleavage of an actin filament, which polymerizes to filaments along the lamellipodia and itself depolymerizes according to a distinct rate has been proposed as an explanation for the discrepancy between single molecule tracking and bulk kinetics experiments (Smith et al., 2013). It is plausible that rebinding of actin monomers/oligomers also happens to some extend in dendritic spines. This should be taken into considerations if absolute values of the structure turnover rate are needed. It is also possible that the rebinding of monomers and oligomers are at least partly responsible for the stable component observed in FRAP and PAGFP decay experiments.

Okamoto et al. (2004) first took advantage of FRET between actin monomers labeled with cyan fluorescent protein (CFP) and yellow fluorescent protein (YFP) in living neurons. The method used to measure energy transfer was fluorescence intensity based. Increase in energy transfer was interpreted as a shift in the G-actin/F-actin ratio. This was based on the assumption that energy transfer was only possible if CFP- and YFP-actin were found one after another in filamentous actin. For this to happen, at a noticeable frequency, the amount of labeled actin inside the cell must be very high (Vishwasrao et al., 2012). Also, FRET between two GFP fluorophores has been proposed as a method to measure the level of actin polymerization (Vishwasrao et al., 2012). Here, we propose a novel idea that these FRET assays would be more suitable to study the level of actin filament bundling instead of actin polymerization. Although the method is theoretically feasible and our experiments support this idea, it is important to note that in cells the intra- and inter-filament FRET cannot be completely separated as they form a continuum along the labeling density. Nevertheless, the probability of intra-filament FRET is completely determined by a sufficient labeling density of the individual filaments. Inter-filament FRET, on the other hand, depends on the bundlling of filaments. Increase of bundling will always result in an increase in local F-actin concentration and therefore units of GFP-actin inside a given volume, without an increase in labeling density of individual filaments. Furthermore, it is difficult to produce direct evidence for actin bundling vs. polymerization in cells because we can neither block polymerization without affecting actin bundles (no filaments—no bundles) nor can we block bundling without affecting the G-/F-actin ratio (if actin filaments are not bundled they are more vulnerable for cofilin induced depolymerization). Therefore, the methodological development would benefit from *in vitro* evaluation, such as actin *in vitro* polymerization and bundling assays. Regardless of whether fluorescence anisotropy measures polymerization or bundling, our results show that actin monomers are more closely packed in dendritic spines of 3 week old neurons, compared to 2-week old neurons. Based on our earlier results (Koskinen et al., 2014) and other literature, it is plausible that this tighter packing of actin reflects a higher level of actin filament bundling.

Although GFP-actin has widely been used for live-cell imaging in various model systems (Fischer et al., 1998; Schneider et al., 2002; Honkura et al., 2008), in all methods utilizing GFP-actin it is important to remember that especially highly over-expressed GFP-actin may influence actin dynamics (Aizawa et al., 1997; Feng et al., 2005; Deibler et al., 2011). Moreover, GFP-actin might be excluded from formin-assembled actin filaments, as GFP-actin expressed in fission yeast does not incorporate into the contractile ring assembled primarily by formin homology protein Cdc12p (Chen et al., 2012). Formins play critical roles in assembling various actin structures, including tightly bundled stress fibers in fibroblasts (Hotulainen and Lappalainen, 2006; Tojkander et al., 2011). Thus, it is possible that the fluorescence anisotropy will overlook some formin assembled actin bundles. Similarly, FRAP and photoactivation assays may ignore formin-based actin dynamics.

CONCLUSIONS

FRAP is a fast and easy technique to use but - especially in dendritic spines—there are aspects that need to be considered in its application and analysis. The bleaching laser pulse may have its own effect of increasing spine size and dynamics. As such, FRAP is most suitable for studying differences in dynamic pool turnover rate. In addition, FRAP can detect clear differences in the sizes of the F-actin stable pool. The use of a dual color approach could help to tackle the difficulties but is technically more challenging. Single FRAP measurements are difficult to fit to equations and several measurements need to be taken in order to obtain reliable results. The comparison of two average curves from FRAP measurements seems to be the best way to show the differences between test groups or conditions but demonstrating the statistical significance requires advanced statistics.

PAGFP fluorescence decay offers the possibility for longer, more stable measurements. PAGFP fluorescence decay is especially useful for measuring the size and turnover rate of the stable actin pool. Small differences in dynamic pool turn-over rate may be lost due to longer time interval in imaging often utilized compared to FRAP. The big advantage of this method is that the measurements can be analyzed individually and there is much less variance in decay measurements than in FRAP measurements. The possibility of individual spine measurements without averaging enables comparison of single spines to one another.

Fluorescence anisotropy is an easy and fast method. Fluorescence anisotropy is particularly useful in providing information about structures that can not be examined in detail using conventional methods, such as dendritic spines.

If only one method is used to measure actin turnover rate, PAGFP fluorescence decay seems to be more reliable than FRAP. However, it is important to remember that FRAP is measuring the F-actin assembly whereas PAGFP decay is measuring the F-actin disassembly. Thus, these methods complement each other and should optimally be used together. In combination with FRAP and PAGFP decay, fluorescence anisotropy provides an additional method to improve our understanding on the organization and dynamics of dendritic spine actin filaments.

AUTHOR CONTRIBUTIONS

Mikko Koskinen and Pirta Hotulainen designed the experiments and wrote the manuscript. Mikko Koskinen performed the experiments.

ACKNOWLEDGMENTS

The authors would like to acknowledge Outi Nikkilä and Seija Lågas for primary neuron cultures. Marko Crivaro is acknowledged for the help in setting up the fluorescence anisotropy method. We thank Risto Hotulainen for the help with statistical tests. Maria Vartiainen is acknowledged for providing the PAGFP-actin and the GFP-GFP tandem constructs and Pekka Lappalainen together with Gergana Gateva for the Palladin-mCherry construct. We thank Rick Horwitz for the MHC IIb wild-type and mutant constructs. Imaging was performed at the Light microscopy unit (Institute of biotechnology, Helsinki University). Enni Bertling, Amr Abou Elezz and Marko Crivaro are acknowledged for critical reading of the manuscript. Mikko Koskinen is supported by the University of Helsinki. Pirta Hotulainen is supported by Academy of Finland, Neuroscience Center and the University of Helsinki.

REFERENCES

Aizawa, H., Sameshima, M., and Yahara, I. (1997). A green fluorescent protein-actin fusion protein dominantly inhibits cytokinesis, cell spreading, and locomotion in Dictyostelium. *Cell Struct. Funct.* 22, 335–345.

Alvarez, V. A., and Sabatini, B. L. (2007). Anatomical and physiological plasticity of dendritic spines. *Annu. Rev. Neurosci.* 30, 79–97. doi: 10.1146/annurev.neuro.30.051606.094222

Bader, A. N., Hoetzl, S., Hofman, E. G., Voortman, J., Van Bergen En Henegouwen, P. M., Van Meer, G., et al. (2011). Homo-FRET imaging as a tool to quantify protein and lipid clustering. *Chemphyschem* 12, 475–483. doi: 10.1002/cphc.201000801

Bertling, E., Ludwig, A., Koskinen, M., and Hotulainen, P. (2012). Methods for three-dimensional analysis of dendritic spine dynamics. *Meth. Enzymol.* 506, 391–406. doi: 10.1016/B978-0-12-391856-7.00043-3

Bhatt, D. H., Zhang, S., and Gan, W. B. (2009). Dendritic spine dynamics. *Annu. Rev. Physiol.* 71, 261–282. doi: 10.1146/annurev.physiol.010908.163140

Blanchoin, L., Boujemaa-Paterski, R., Sykes, C., and Plastino, J. (2014). Actin dynamics, architecture, and mechanics in cell motility. *Physiol. Rev.* 94, 235–263. doi: 10.1152/physrev.00018.2013

Canny, J. (1986). A computational approach to edge detection. *IEEE Trans. Pattern Anal. Mach. Intell.* 8, 679–698.

Caroni, P., Donato, F., and Muller, D. (2012). Structural plasticity upon learning: regulation and functions. *Nat. Rev. Neurosci.* 13, 478–490. doi: 10.1038/nrn3258

Chen, C.-C., Lu, J., and Zuo, Y. (2014). Spatiotemporal dynamics of dendritic spines in the living brain. *Front. Neuroanat.* 8:28. doi: 10.3389/fnana.2014.00028

Chen, N., Nag, S., and Pollard, T. D. (2012). Formins filter modified actin subunits during processive elongation. *J. Struc. Biol.* 177, 32–39. doi: 10.1016/j.jsb.2011.10.005

Choidas, A., Jungbluth, A., Sechi, A., Murphy, J., Ullrich, A., and Marriott, G. (1998). The suitability and application of a GFP-actin fusion protein for long-term imaging of the organization and dynamics of the cytoskeleton in mammalian cells. *Eur. J. Cell Biol.* 77, 81–90. doi: 10.1016/S0171-9335(98)80075-7

Deibler, M., Spatz, J. P., and Kemkemer, R. (2011). Actin fusion proteins alter the dynamics of mechanically induced cytoskeleton rearrangement. *PLoS ONE* 6:e22941. doi: 10.1371/journal.pone.0022941

Dixon, R. D., Arneman, D. K., Rachlin, A. S., Sundaresan, N. R., Costello, M. J., Campbell, S. L., et al. (2008). Palladin is an actin cross-linking protein that uses immunoglobulin-like domains to bind filamentous actin. *J. Biol. Chem.* 283, 6222–6231. doi: 10.1074/jbc.M707694200

Dopie, J., Skarp, K. P., Rajakyla, E. K., Tanhuanpaa, K., and Vartiainen, M. K. (2012). Active maintenance of nuclear actin by importin 9 supports transcription. *Proc. Natl. Acad. Sci. U.S.A.* 109, E544–E552. doi: 10.1073/pnas.1118880109

Dos Remedios, C. G., Chhabra, D., Kekic, M., Dedova, I. V., Tsubakihara, M., Berry, D. A., et al. (2003). Actin binding proteins: regulation of cytoskeletal microfilaments. *Physiol. Rev.* 83, 433–473. doi: 10.1152/physrev.00026.2002

Dunn, G. A., Dobbie, I. M., Monypenny, J., Holt, M. R., and Zicha, D. (2002). Fluorescence localization after photobleaching (FLAP): a new method for studying protein dynamics in living cells. *J. Microsc.* 205, 109–112. doi: 10.1046/j.0022-2720.2001.001007.x

Feng, Z., Ning Chen, W., Vee Sin Lee, P., Liao, K., and Chan, V. (2005). The influence of GFP-actin expression on the adhesion dynamics of HepG2 cells on a model extracellular matrix. *Biomaterials* 26, 5348–5358. doi: 10.1016/j.biomaterials.2005.01.069

Fischer, M., Kaech, S., Knutti, D., and Matus, A. (1998). Rapid actin-based plasticity in dendritic spines. *Neuron* 20, 847–854.

Frost, N. A., Shroff, H., Kong, H., Betzig, E., and Blanpied, T. A. (2010). Single-molecule discrimination of discrete perisynaptic and distributed sites of actin filament assembly within dendritic spines. *Neuron* 67, 86–99. doi: 10.1016/j.neuron.2010.05.026

Halavatyi, A. A., Nazarov, P. V., Al Tanoury, Z., Apanasovich, V. V., Yatskou, M., and Friederich, E. (2010). A mathematical model of actin filament turnover for fitting FRAP data. *Eur. Biophys. J.* 39, 669–677. doi: 10.1007/s00249-009-0558-2

Hodges, J. L., Newell-Litwa, K., Asmussen, H., Vicente-Manzanares, M., and Horwitz, A. R. (2011). Myosin IIb activity and phosphorylation status determines dendritic spine and post-synaptic density morphology. *PLoS ONE* 6:e24149. doi: 10.1371/journal.pone.0024149

Honkura, N., Matsuzaki, M., Noguchi, J., Ellis-Davies, G. C., and Kasai, H. (2008). The subspine organization of actin fibers regulates the structure and plasticity of dendritic spines. *Neuron* 57, 719–729. doi: 10.1016/j.neuron.2008.01.013

Hotulainen, P., and Hoogenraad, C. C. (2010). Actin in dendritic spines: connecting dynamics to function. *J. Cell Biol.* 189, 619–629. doi: 10.1083/jcb.201003008

Hotulainen, P., and Lappalainen, P. (2006). Stress fibers are generated by two distinct actin assembly mechanisms in motile cells. *J. Cell Biol.* 173, 383–394. doi: 10.1083/jcb.200511093

Hotulainen, P., Llano, O., Smirnov, S., Tanhuanpaa, K., Faix, J., Rivera, C., et al. (2009). Defining mechanisms of actin polymerization and depolymerization during dendritic spine morphogenesis. *J. Cell Biol.* 185, 323–339. doi: 10.1083/jcb.200809046

Jacobson, K., Rajfur, Z., Vitriol, E., and Hahn, K. (2008). Chromophore-assisted laser inactivation in cell biology. *Trends Cell Biol.* 18, 443–450. doi: 10.1016/j.tcb.2008.07.001

Kasai, H., Fukuda, M., Watanabe, S., Hayashi-Takagi, A., and Noguchi, J. (2010). Structural dynamics of dendritic spines in memory and cognition. *Trends Neurosci.* 33, 121–129. doi: 10.1016/j.tins.2010.01.001

Kaufmann, W. E., and Moser, H. W. (2000). Dendritic anomalies in disorders associated with mental retardation. *Cereb. Cortex* 10, 981–991. doi: 10.1093/cercor/10.10.981

Kim, I. H., Racz, B., Wang, H., Burianek, L., Weinberg, R., Yasuda, R., et al. (2013). Disruption of Arp2/3 results in asymmetric structural plasticity of dendritic spines and progressive synaptic and behavioral abnormalities. *J. Neurosci.* 33, 6081–6092. doi: 10.1523/JNEUROSCI.0035-13.2013

Korkotian, E., and Segal, M. (2001). Regulation of dendritic spine motility in cultured hippocampal neurons. *J. Neurosci.* 21, 6115–6124.

Korobova, F., and Svitkina, T. (2010). Molecular architecture of synaptic actin cytoskeleton in hippocampal neurons reveals a mechanism of dendritic spine morphogenesis. *Mol. Biol. Cell* 21, 165–176. doi: 10.1091/mbc.E09-07-0596

Koskinen, M., Bertling, E., and Hotulainen, P. (2012). Methods to measure actin treadmilling rate in dendritic spines. *Meth. Enzymol.* 505, 47–58. doi: 10.1016/B978-0-12-388448-0.00011-5

Koskinen, M., Bertling, E., Hotulainen, R., Tanhuanpää, K., and Hotulainen, P. (2014). Myosin IIb controls actin dynamics underlying the dendritic spine maturation. *Mol. Cell. Neurosci.* 61, 56–64. doi: 10.1016/j.mcn.2014.05.008

Kullback, S., and Leibler, R. A. (1951). On information and sufficiency. *Ann. Math. Stat.* 22, 79–86. doi: 10.1214/aoms/1177729694

Lai, F. P. L., Szczodrak, M., Block, J., Faix, J., Breitsprecher, D., Mannherz, H. G., et al. (2008). Arp2/3 complex interactions and actin network turnover in lamellipodia. *EMBO J.* 27, 982–992. doi: 10.1038/emboj.2008.34

Lamprecht, R. (2014). The actin cytoskeleton in memory formation. *Prog. Neurobiol.* 117C, 1–19. doi: 10.1016/j.pneurobio.2014.02.001

Magidson, V., and Khodjakov, A. (2013). Circumventing photodamage in live-cell microscopy. *Methods Cell Biol.* 114, 545–560. doi: 10.1016/B978-0-12-407761-4.00023-3

McGrath, J. L., Tardy, Y., Dewey, C. F. Jr., Meister, J. J., and Hartwig, J. H. (1998). Simultaneous measurements of actin filament turnover, filament fraction, and monomer diffusion in endothelial cells. *Biophys. J.* 75, 2070–2078. doi: 10.1016/S0006-3495(98)77649-0

Miyoshi, T., and Watanabe, N. (2013). Can filament treadmilling alone account for the F-actin turnover in lamellipodia? *Cytoskeleton* 70, 179–190. doi: 10.1002/cm.21098

Okamoto, K., Nagai, T., Miyawaki, A., and Hayashi, Y. (2004). Rapid and persistent modulation of actin dynamics regulates postsynaptic reorganization underlying bidirectional plasticity. *Nat. Neurosci.* 7, 1104–1112. doi: 10.1038/nn1311

Patterson, G. H., and Lippincott-Schwartz, J. (2002). A photoactivatable GFP for selective photolabeling of proteins and cells. *Science* 297, 1873–1877. doi: 10.1126/science.1074952

Penzes, P., Cahill, M. E., Jones, K. A., Vanleeuwen, J. E., and Woolfrey, K. M. (2011). Dendritic spine pathology in neuropsychiatric disorders. *Nat. Neurosci.* 14, 285–293. doi: 10.1038/nn.2741

Pollard, T. D., and Cooper, J. A. (2009). Actin, a central player in cell shape and movement. *Science* 326, 1208–1212. doi: 10.1126/science.1175862

Rachlin, A. S., and Otey, C. A. (2006). Identification of palladin isoforms and characterization of an isoform-specific interaction between Lasp-1 and palladin. *J. Cell Sci.* 119, 995–1004. doi: 10.1242/jcs.02825

Rex, C. S., Gavin, C. F., Rubio, M. D., Kramar, E. A., Chen, L. Y., Jia, Y., et al. (2010). Myosin IIb regulates actin dynamics during synaptic plasticity and memory formation. *Neuron* 67, 603–617. doi: 10.1016/j.neuron.2010.07.016

Reymann, A. C., Suarez, C., Guerin, C., Martiel, J. L., Staiger, C. J., Blanchoin, L., et al. (2011). Turnover of branched actin filament networks by stochastic fragmentation with ADF/cofilin. *Mol. Biol. Cell* 22, 2541–2550. doi: 10.1091/mbc.E11-01-0052

Rust, M. B., Gurniak, C. B., Renner, M., Vara, H., Morando, L., Gorlich, A., et al. (2010). Learning, AMPA receptor mobility and synaptic plasticity depend on n-cofilin-mediated actin dynamics. *EMBO J.* 29, 1889–1902. doi: 10.1038/emboj.2010.72

Schneider, M. E., Belyantseva, I. A., Azevedo, R. B., and Kachar, B. (2002). Rapid renewal of auditory hair bundles. *Nature* 418, 837–838. doi: 10.1038/418837a

Smith, M. B., Kiuchi, T., Watanabe, N., and Vavylonis, D. (2013). Distributed actin turnover in the lamellipodium and FRAP kinetics. *Biophys. J.* 104, 247–257. doi: 10.1016/j.bpj.2012.11.3819

Stamatakou, E., Marzo, A., Gibb, A., and Salinas, P. C. (2013). Activity-dependent spine morphogenesis: a role for the actin-capping protein Eps8. *J. Neurosci.* 33, 2661–2670. doi: 10.1523/JNEUROSCI.0998-12.2013

Star, E. N., Kwiatkowski, D. J., and Murthy, V. N. (2002). Rapid turnover of actin in dendritic spines and its regulation by activity. *Nat. Neurosci.* 5, 239–246. doi: 10.1038/nn811

Svitkina, T. M., and Borisy, G. G. (1999). Arp2/3 complex and actin depolymerizing factor/cofilin in dendritic organization and treadmilling of actin filament array in lamellipodia. *J. Cell Biol.* 145, 1009–1026.

Tojkander, S., Gatewa, G., Schevzov, G., Hotulainen, P., Naumanen, P., Martin, C., et al. (2011). A molecular pathway for myosin II recruitment to stress fibers. *Curr. Biol.* 7, 539–550. doi: 10.1016/j.cub.2011.03.007

Vishwasrao, H. D., Trifilieff, P., and Kandel, E. R. (2012). *In vivo* imaging of the actin polymerization state with two-photon fluorescence anisotropy. *Biophys. J.* 102, 1204–1214. doi: 10.1016/j.bpj.2012.01.031

Wang, Y., Dong, Q., Xu, X. F., Feng, X., Xin, J., Wang, D. D., et al. (2013). Phosphorylation of cofilin regulates extinction of conditioned aversive memory via AMPAR trafficking. *J. Neurosci.* 33, 6423–6433. doi: 10.1523/JNEUROSCI.5107-12.2013

Westphal, M., Jungbluth, A., Heidecker, M., Mühlbauer, B., Heizer, C., Schwartz, J.-M., et al. (1997). Microfilament dynamics during cell movement and chemotaxis monitored using a GFP-actin fusion protein. *Curr. Biol.* 7, 176–183. doi: 10.1016/S0960-9822(97)70088-5

17

The dendritic spine story: an intriguing process of discovery

Javier DeFelipe[1,2]*

[1] Instituto Cajal (CSIC), Madrid, Spain
[2] Laboratorio Cajal de Circuitos Corticales (Centro de Tecnología Biomédica: UPM), and CIBERNED, Madrid, Spain

Correspondence:
Javier DeFelipe, Laboratorio Cajal de Circuitos Corticales (Centro de Tecnología Biomédica: UPM), and CIBERNED, Campus Montegancedo S/N, Pozuelo de Alarcón, 28223 Madrid, Spain
e-mail: defelipe@cajal.csic.es

Dendritic spines are key components of a variety of microcircuits and they represent the majority of postsynaptic targets of glutamatergic axon terminals in the brain. The present article will focus on the discovery of dendritic spines, which was possible thanks to the application of the Golgi technique to the study of the nervous system, and will also explore the early interpretation of these elements. This discovery represents an interesting chapter in the history of neuroscience as it shows us that progress in the study of the structure of the nervous system is based not only on the emergence of new techniques but also on our ability to exploit the methods already available and correctly interpret their microscopic images.

Keywords: pyramidal cells, granule cells, Purkinje cells, Cajal, Golgi, reticular theory, neuron doctrine, history of neuroscience

INTRODUCTION

In 1873, a revolution began in the world of neuroscience with the discovery by Camillo Golgi of a new technique to stain the nervous system which allowed neurons and glia to be visualized with all their processes and in great detail. Since these cells were labeled in black, Golgi referred to this technique as the "*reazione near*" (black reaction). Golgi was very enthusiastic about this discovery as reflected in a letter that he sent to his friend Niccolò Manfredi, where he outlined the new method (Mazzarello, 1999):

> I spend long hours at the microscope. I am delighted that I have found a new reaction to demonstrate even to the blind the structure of the interstitial stroma of the cerebral cortex. I let the silver nitrate react with pieces of brain hardened in potassium dichromate. I have obtained magnificent results and hope to do even better in the future.

The method, named the Golgi method after its discoverer, was published in the *Gazzeta Medica Italiani* on the 2nd of August, 1873 (Golgi, 1873): *Sulla struttura della sostanza grigia del cervello* (On the structure of the gray substance of the cerebrum). Thanks to a very simple staining protocol, requiring a "prolonged immersion of the tissue, previously hardened with potassium or ammonium dichromate, in a 0.50 or 1.0% solution of silver nitrate", it was possible for the first time to observe neurons and glia in a histological preparation (**Figure 1**) with all their parts (cell body, dendrites and axon, in the case of neurons; cell body and processes in the case of glia DeFelipe, 2002). Golgi used this method to examine many regions of the nervous system, providing new insights into the neuroanatomy of these structures and he illustrated the findings with beautiful drawings, as shown in **Figures 1, 2. Figure 1** shows the organization of the olfactory bulb (nerve cells and pathways), whereas **Figure 2** shows different types of neurons in the cerebellar cortex, in great morphological detail, albeit with some important exceptions, like the dendritic arborizations of Purkinje cells which appear free of dendritic spines (see below for further discussion on this).

The introduction of this method was a very important advance since, before this development, the visualization of neurons with the available histological techniques had been incomplete; it was only feasible to observe the cell body and the proximal portions of the dendrites and axon. Thus, it was not possible to follow the trajectory of the thin axons or to visualize the terminal axonal arbors as occurred with the Golgi method (**Figures 1, 2**). Indeed, at that time, the prevailing hypothesis about the organization of the nervous system was in fact the reticular theory, which proposed that the nerve cells of the nervous system formed a continuum, rather than existing as individual elements (later called the neuron doctrine). It was Joseph von Gerlach who really developed the reticular theory and thus, he is considered the father of this theory (von Gerlach, 1872). Interestingly, when Golgi examined the silver impregnated preparations, he concluded that the reticular theory supported by Gerlach was wrong, since Golgi thought that dendrites ended freely and that only the axons and their collaterals anastomose. Therefore, he suggested that the nervous system consisted of a "*rete nervosa diffusa*" (diffuse nervous network), an idea that he supported even

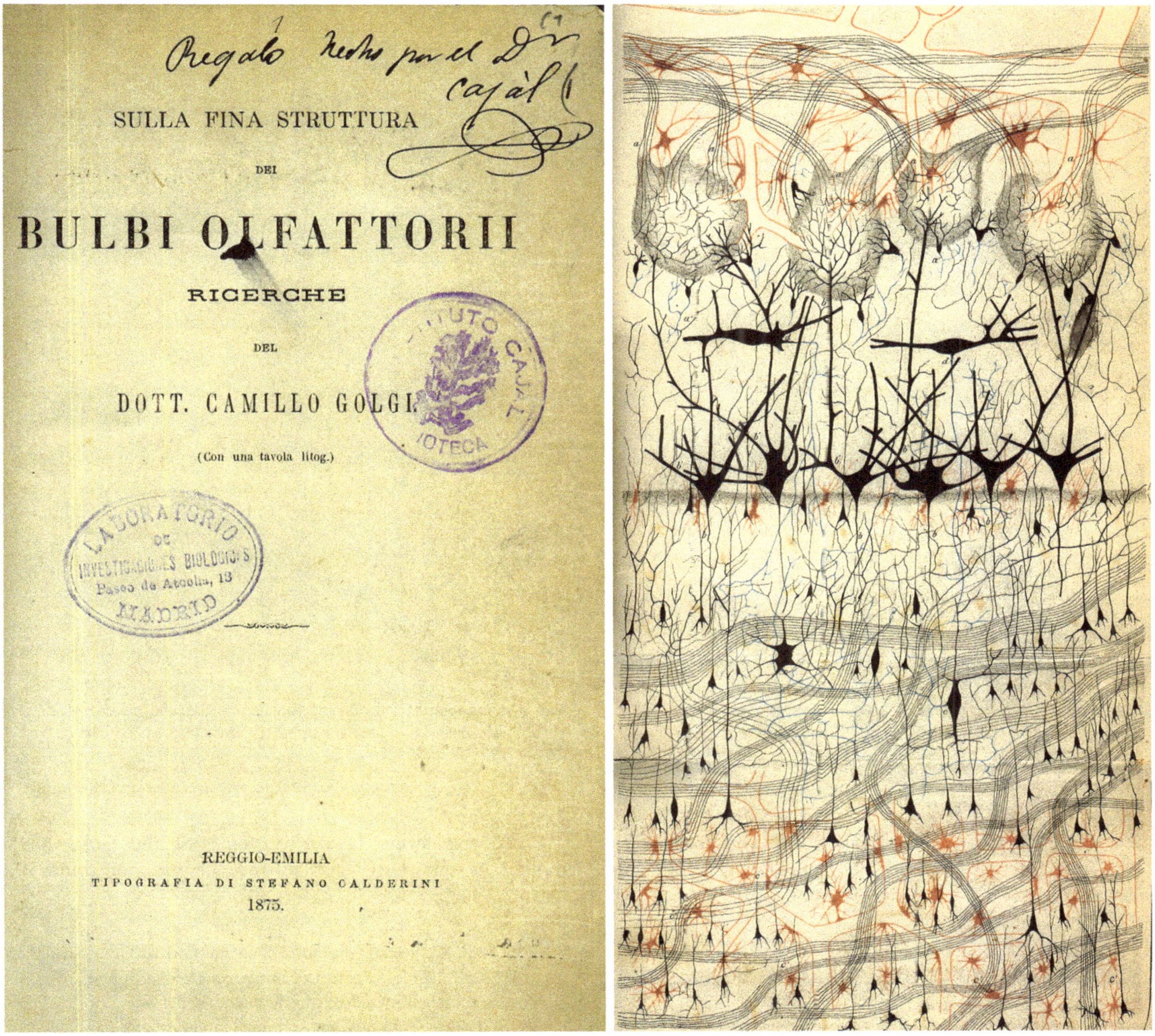

FIGURE 1 | The first illustration by Golgi of a Golgi impregnated preparation of the nervous system. *"Semi-schematic drawing of a fragment of a vertical section of the olfactory bulb of a dog"* (Golgi, 1875). Taken from DeFelipe (2010).

as late as 1906 during his Nobel Price lecture. In contrast, Santiago Ramón y Cajal, using the same methods and microscopes as Golgi, strongly supported the neuron doctrine as he found that all processes of nerve cells end "freely" (i.e., nerve cells are individual elements) and that connections between them are by contact. Since Cajal contributed more than any other researcher of his time to support this theory, he is considered the father of the neuron doctrine (DeFelipe, 2002). As we will see below, dendritic spines of Purkinje cells and pyramidal cells were considered as good examples of transmission by contact.

The present article will focus on the discovery of dendritic spines, which was possible thanks to the application of the Golgi technique to the study of the nervous system, and will also explore the early interpretation of these elements. This discovery represents an interesting page in the history of neuroscience as it shows us that progress in the study of the structure of the nervous system is based not only on the introduction of new techniques but also on the ability to exploit the methods already available and the correct interpretation of their microscopic images. This review is largely based on several of my previously-published articles and books about the structure of the nervous system in the times of Cajal, and it has been divided into three sections: (1) First critical discoveries using the Golgi method: the neuron theory and visualization of dendritic spines;

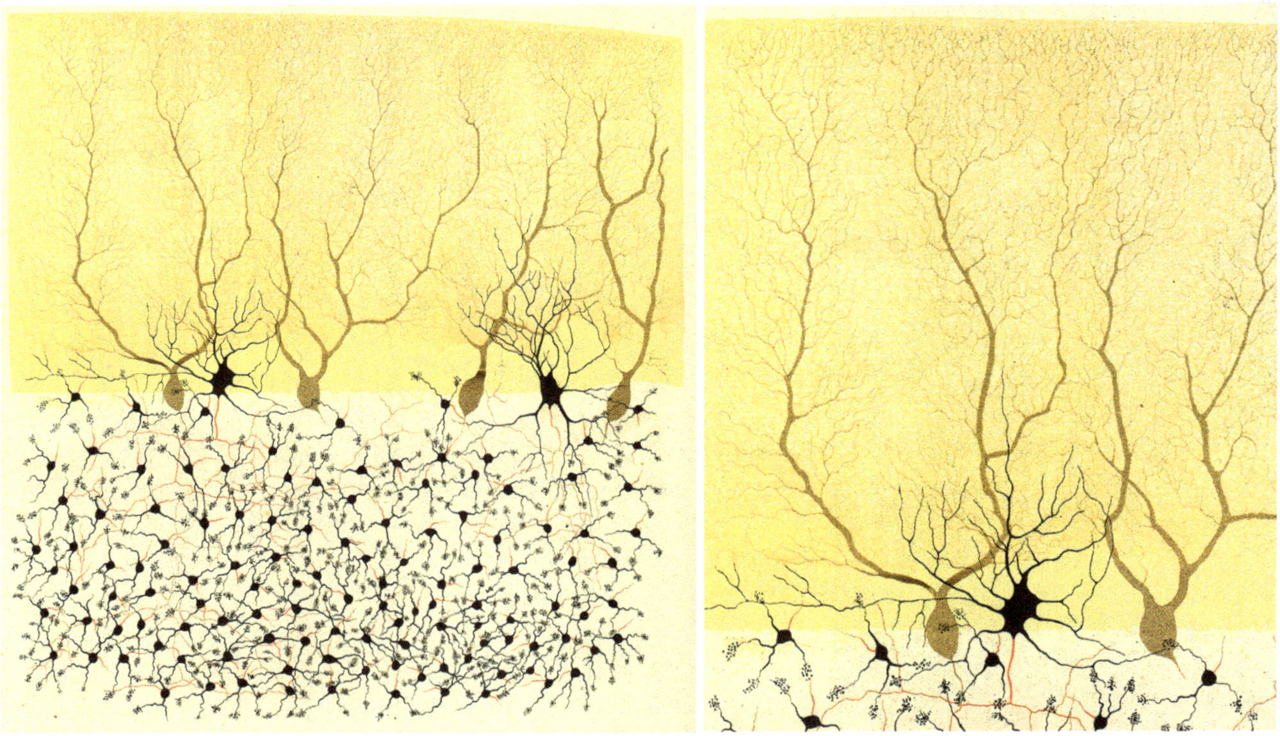

FIGURE 2 | Illustration by Golgi of a Golgi impregnated preparation of the cerebellum. *"Fragment of a vertical section of a cerebellar convolution of the rabbit".* *Left*, panoramic view. *Right*, a high magnification of the drawing to illustrate that the dendrites of the Purkinje cells are smooth, without dendritic spines. Taken from Golgi (1882–1883).

(2) Dendritic spines: true anatomical dispositions vs. artifacts; and (3) Other interpretations of the dendritic spines and final considerations.

FIRST CRITICAL DISCOVERIES USING THE GOLGI METHOD: THE NEURON THEORY AND VISUALIZATION OF DENDRITIC SPINES

Interestingly, for a long time after the discovery of the Golgi method in 1873, the method went virtually unnoticed. This was really unfortunate since this new powerful tool was practically not exploited by the scientific community and many discoveries had to wait for years to see the light of day. This situation was highlighted well by Cajal himself in *Recuerdos de mi vida* (Cajal, 1917):

> I have already expressed above the surprise I felt when I saw with my own eyes the wonderful revelatory power of the chrome-silver reaction [Golgi method] and the indifference of the scientific community regarding this discovery. How could this disinterest be explained? Today, as I better understand the psychology of scholars, I find it very natural. In France, as in Germany, and more in the latter than in the former, a severe school discipline reigns. Out of respect for their master, it is common that disciples do not use research methods that have not been passed on by him. As for the great investigators, they would consider themselves dishonored if they worked with the methods of others.

Cajal was aware of the existence of the Golgi method, though he had not tested it since he did not think it was useful:

> But, as I mentioned, the admirable method of Golgi was then (1887–1888) unknown to the immense majority of neurologists or was underestimated by the few who had precise information about it. Ranvier's book, my technical bible of those days, devoted only a few descriptive lines of to it, written in an indifferent style. It was evident that the French savant had not tried it. Naturally, the readers of Ranvier, like myself, thought this method to be unworthy to be used.

Cajal's interest in using this silver chromate method was thanks to Luis Simarro (1851–1921), a psychiatrist and neurologist who was also an enthusiast of histology. Interestingly, Simarro learned this method from Louis Antoine Ranvier (1835–1922), and introduced some modifications (Fernandez and Breathnach, 2001). It was in 1887 during a visit to Madrid that Cajal—who was living in Valencia at the time—was invited into Simarro's own house, where he first saw a Golgi impregnated preparation (Cajal, 1917):

> I owe to Luis Simarro the unforgettable favor of having been shown the first good preparations made by the method of silver chromate that I ever saw, and of his having called my attention

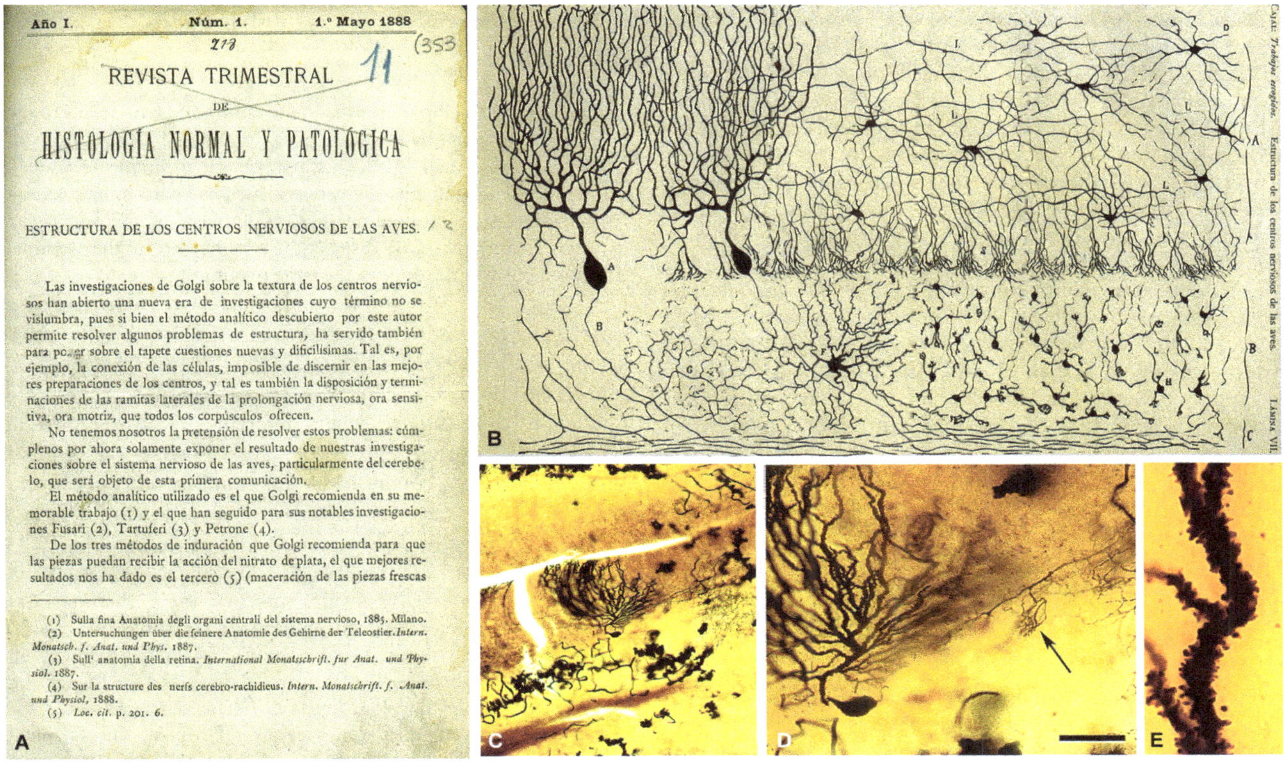

FIGURE 3 | First illustration by Cajal (1888) of a Golgi impregnated preparation of the nervous system. **(A)** First page of the article and **(B)** illustration whose legend states: "*Vertical section of a cerebellar convolution of a hen. Impregnation by the Golgi method. A represents the molecular zone, B designates the granular layer and C the white matter*". **(C)** photomicrograph from one of Cajal's preparations of the cerebellum of an adult bird stained with the Golgi method. **(D)** higher magnification of **(C)** to illustrate a Purkinje cell and a basket formation (arrow). **(E)** dendrite of the Purkinje cell which is covered with dendritic spines. The histological images were obtained by Pablo García-López, Virginia García-Marín, and Miguel Freire (Legado Cajal, Instituto Cajal). Scale bar: 200 μm in **(C)**; 60 μm in **(D)**; 8,4 μm in **(E)**. Taken from DeFelipe (2014).

> to the exceptional importance of the book of the Italian savant devoted to the examination of the fine structure of the gray matter.

Cajal was captivated by this marvelous staining method and he immediately started to use it to analyze practically the entire nervous system in several species. One year after his meeting with Simarro, Cajal published his first important article based on results obtained with this method in the avian cerebellum (**Figure 3**). In this study entitled *Estructura de los centros nerviosos de las aves* (Cajal, 1888), Cajal made two great contributions:

-First, he confirmed Golgi's conclusion that dendrites end freely but, in contrast to Golgi, Cajal added the decisive conclusion that this also applies to axons and their branches:

> We have carried out detailed studies to investigate the course and connections of the nerve fibers in the cerebral and cerebellar convolutions of the human, monkey, dog, etc. We have not been able to see an anastomosis between the ramifications of two different nervous prolongations, nor between the filaments emanating from the same expansion of Deiters [axons]. While the fibers are interlaced in a very complicated manner, engendering an intricate and dense plexus, they never form a net [...] it could be said that each [nerve cell] is an absolutely autonomous physiological canton [unit]

In the years that followed, he provided many examples from throughout the nervous system to support his observation that dendrites and axons end freely. The reticular and the neuron theories are obviously radically divergent regarding the interpretation of how nerve currents flow through a continuous rather than a discontinuous network of neuronal processes. Thus, the new ideas about the connections between neurons led to novel theories on the relationship between neuronal circuits and brain function. Cajal wrote in volume I of *Histologie du système nerveux de l'homme et des vertébrés* (Cajal, 1909–1911):

> The cell bodies, [dendrites and axons] terminate freely but nevertheless, the flow of currents is not impeded in such an infinitely interrupted, fragmented nervous system. How can such currents flow? There can be only one answer, by contact, in much the same way that electric current crosses a splice between two wires.

These early studies with the Golgi method regarding the connections of neurons were so decisive that they represented the main core of the review published by Wilhelm von Waldeyer-Hartz in the journal *Deutsche Medizinische Wochenschrift* in 1891. In this article, the term "neuron" was introduced to denominate the nerve cells and the so-called neuron doctrine became popular. By the end of the XIXth century, this theory was the most accepted theory to explain the organization of the nervous system, in which the neuron was considered as the anatomical, physiological, genetic and metabolic unit of the nervous system. The many, fundamental contributions of Cajal to the neuron doctrine were summarized by himself in several articles and books, and especially in *¿Neuronismo o Reticularismo?* published in 1933 (Cajal, 1933). Cajal distinguished two main types of contacts between nerve cells: connections with the cell body and connections with the dendrites. In 1897, these contacts, also called "articulations" by Cajal, were baptized by Charles Sherrington (1857–1952) with the name of "synapses" (Foster and Sherrington, 1897). In his classic book *The Integrative Action of the Nervous System*, Sherrington masterfully described the hypothetical one-way contact between axon terminals and somata or dendrites, and the possible exceptions of the neuron theory (Sherrington, 1947):

> As to the existence or non-existence of a surface of separation or membrane between neurone and neurone, that is a structural question on which histology might be competent to give valuable information. In certain cases, especially in Invertebrata, observation (Apathy, Bethe, etc.) indicates that many nerve-cells are actually continuous one with another. It is noteworthy that in several of these cases the irreversibility of direction of conduction which is characteristic of spinal reflex-arcs is not demonstrable [...]. But in the neurone-chains on the gray-centred system of vertebrates, histology on the whole furnishes evidence that a surface of separation does exist between neurone and neurone. [...] It seems therefore likely that the nexus between neurone and neurone in the reflex-arc, at least in the spinal arc of the vertebrate, involves a surface of separation between neurone and neurone; and this as a transverse membrane across the conductor must be an important element in intercellular conduction. [...] In view, therefore, of the probable importance physiologically of this mode of nexus between neurone and neurone it is convenient to have a term for it. The term introduced has been *synapse* (Foster and Sherrington, 1897).

-Cajal's second contribution was his description of the existence of dendritic spines (which he also named):

> ...the surface [of the dendrites of Purkinje cells] appears to be covered with thorns or short spines...(At the beginning, we thought that these eminences were the result of a tumultuous precipitation of the silver but the constancy of its existence and its presence, even in preparations in which the reaction appears to be very delicate in the remaining elements, incline us to believe this to be a normal condition).

However, in this article he did not discuss the possible function of dendritic spines. Two years later, Cajal described the existence of these structures in the pyramidal cells of the cerebral cortex and interpreted them as possible targets of axons (Cajal, 1890):

> Layer of the small pyramids —We will only add two details to the description given by Golgi: first, the peripheral arborizations of the ascending shaft bristles with short spines ending in a small swelling. The gulfs that are between such collateral spines receive the impression of innumerable small fibers of the superficial layer. Exactly the same disposition is possessed by the terminal peripheral arborizations of the large pyramids.

It was not until 1892 that he more specifically referred to the dendritic spines as key elements for transmission by contact in both the cerebellar and cerebral cortices (Cajal, 1892). In this article, when referring to the connections between the axonal plexus of layer I with the ascending dendritic tufts of pyramidal cells ending in this layer, he wrote:

> It is impossible not to consider this singular arrangement, which, by the way, is found with the same characteristics in all vertebrates, as an important example of neural transmission by contact, comparable to that occurring in the cerebellum between the tiny parallel fibers and the [dendritic] arborizations of the Purkinje cells. This contact would be transverse or oblique, on account of which the terminal [dendritic] branches of the pyramidal cells possess short collateral spines, in the gaps between which the thinnest small axonal fibers bereft of myelin seem to be tightly caught.

Furthermore, in 1893, he also discovered and named the typical thorny excrescences of hippocampal pyramidal cells of CA3 (Cajal, 1893). He proposed that these large and often branched structures served as points of contact with the mossy fibers from the dentate gyrus (**Figure 4**), an observation that is well established at present (Andersen et al., 2007). In addition, Cajal observed in the immature nervous system the presence of short dendritic protrusions that were different to dendritic spines and that he described as "irregular projections very seldom ending as bulbs" and that were most likely transitory (Cajal, 1933). Later, these transitory protrusions were called "filopodia". After these studies, numerous researchers confirmed the existence of spines (e.g., Retzius, 1891; Schaffer, 1892; Edinger, 1893; Demoor, 1896; Stefanowska, 1897, 1901; Hatai, 1903). Among the later researchers, it is interesting to highlight the studies of Micheline Stefanowska—one of the very few female neuroscientists of that time. Her work was based on the 1890s hypothesis of amoeboid movement of neurons to explain possible changes in brain circuits as plastic responses of the normal brain or after experimental manipulation. For example, it was proposed that inactivity during sleep could be explained by a retraction of dendritic processes (theory of the histophysiology of sleep). This retraction would considerably reduce the number of contacts and thus "the association of the individual cellular activities" (DeFelipe, 2006). Stefanowska focused on the "piriform appendages", the name used by

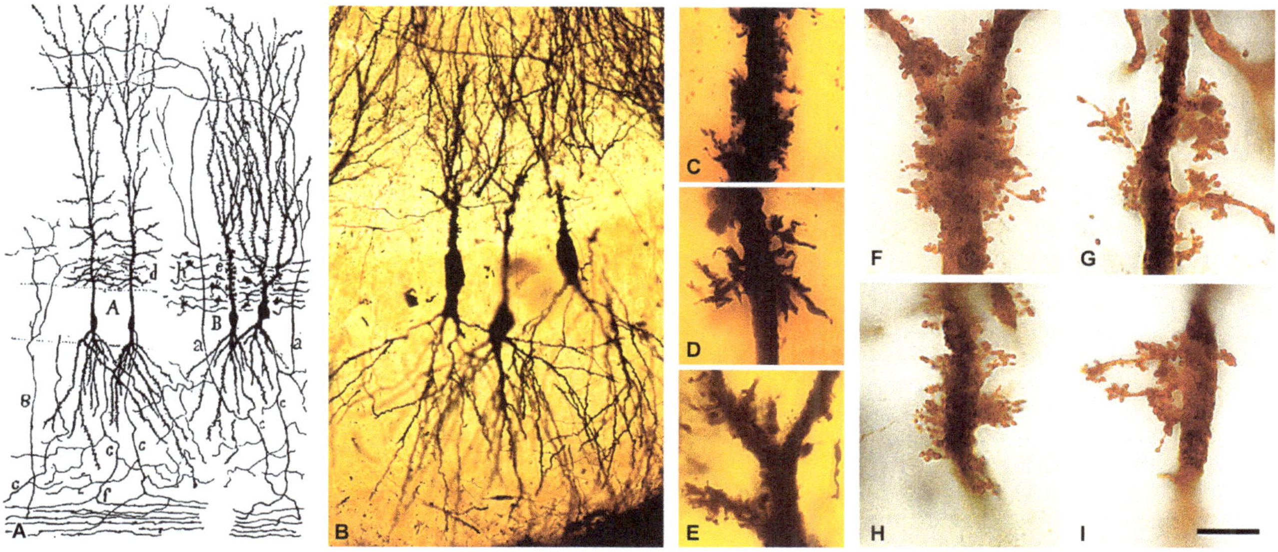

FIGURE 4 | Complex dendritic spines (thorny excrescences) of CA3 pyramidal neurons. **(A)** Cajal's drawing showing pyramidal cells with thorny excrescences in the CA3 (Cajal, 1893). **(B–I)** photomicrographs of Cajal's original histological preparations housed at the Cajal Institute. **(B)** CA3 pyramidal cells of the rabbit stained by the Golgi method. **(C–I)** Examples of thorny excrescences on CA3 pyramidal neurons. **(C–E)** Dendrites from a newborn child's CA3 pyramidal neurons stained by the Golgi method; **(F–I)** Dendrites of rabbit CA3 pyramidal neurons stained by Kenyon's variant of the Golgi method. Scale bar: **(B)** 55 μm; **(C–I)**, 11 μm. Taken from Blazquez-Llorca et al. (2011).

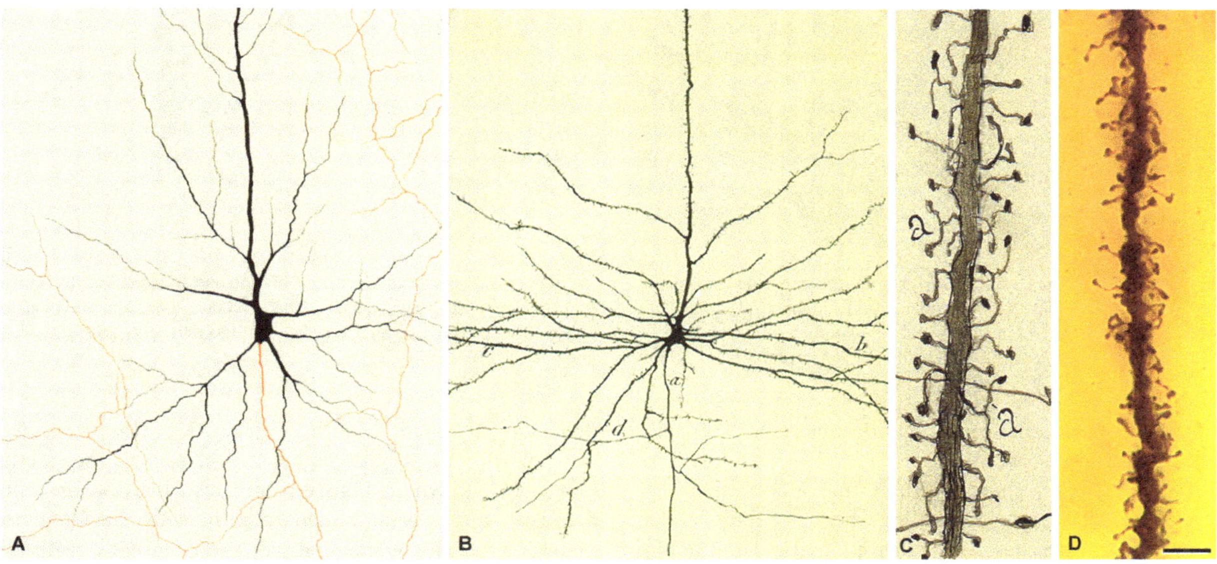

FIGURE 5 | Pyramidal cells of the human cerebral cortex. **(A)** Drawing made by Golgi to illustrate a pyramidal cell of the human motor cortex stained with the Golgi method. The axon appears in red. Taken from Golgi (1882–1883). **(B)** Drawing made by Cajal to illustrate a pyramidal cell of the human motor cortex. *a*, initial part of the axon; *b*, dendrites; *d*, axonal collaterals. Taken from Cajal (1899). **(C)** Drawing by Cajal to illustrate the dendritic spines of pyramidal cells (cerebral cortex of a 2-month-old child). Taken from Cajal (1933). Note that Golgi does not draw dendritic spines. However, in the drawing of Cajal shown in **(B)** it can be seen that the surface of the dendrites are covered with dendrites spines. **(D)** photomicrograph of a preparation of Cajal of the human motor cortex (15-day-old child) stained using the Golgi method. The image illustrates an apical dendrite of a layer V pyramidal cell covered with spines. Scale bar (in **D**): **8** μm. The histological image was obtained by Pablo García-López, Virginia García-Marín and Miguel Freire (Legado Cajal, Instituto Cajal). Taken from DeFelipe (2014).

her to refer to the dendritic spines. She proposed that these piriform appendages could temporarily change both their shape and number in the brain during normal activity and that similar changes may occur in the brain of experimental

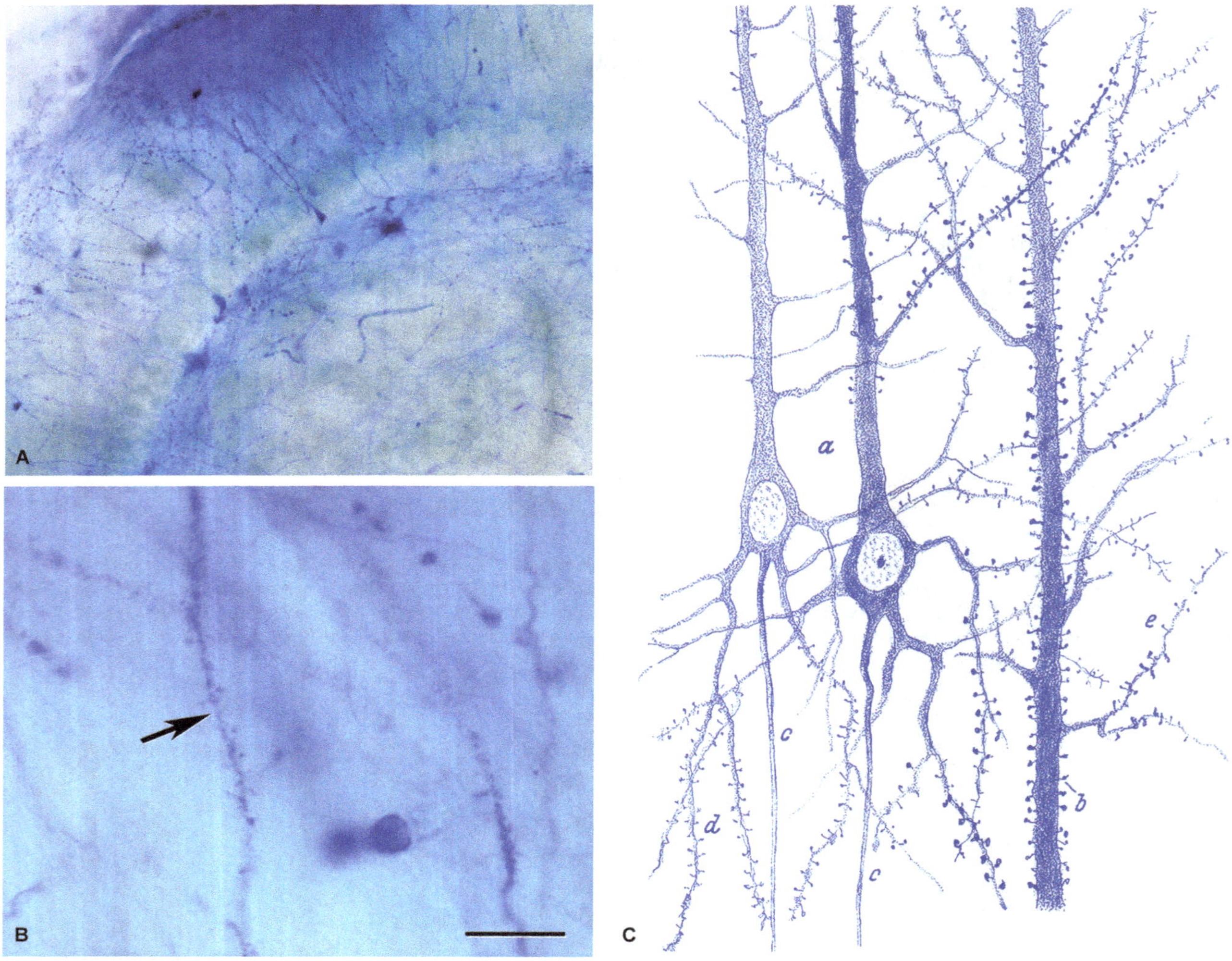

FIGURE 6 | Dendritic spines stained with the methylene blue method. **(A,B)** Low and high magnification photomicrographs, respectively, of a preparation by Cajal of the hippocampus stained with the methylene blue method (preparation housed at the Cajal Institute). These photomicrographs are from unpublished material from DeFelipe and Jones (1988). Scale bar (in **B**): **(A)** 120 μm; **(B)** 10 μm. **(C)** Drawing used by Cajal to show the existence of dendritic spines on pyramidal cells with the methylene blue method. Taken from Cajal (1899–1904).

animals under certain experimental conditions such as electrical stimulation of the cerebral cortex or after the administration of sedatives (morphine, chloral hydrate and chloroform), etc. In general, the conclusions regarding the activity-dependent changes in dendritic spines have received particular attention again in recent times as many of these ideas have been confirmed with modern techniques (e.g., DeFelipe, 2006; Yuste, 2010).

DENDRITIC SPINES: TRUE ANATOMICAL DISPOSITIONS VS. ARTIFACTS

However, for some time, other prestigious authors such as Kölliker (1896), and even Golgi himself, considered that dendritic spines were artifacts, like needle-shaped crystallizations of silver chromate on the surface of neurons, and therefore these structures were not included in their early drawings and consequently dendrites appeared smooth (**Figure 5A**). This skepticism was not only due to the different interpretation of the microscopic images, as shown in **Figure 5**, but also because, at that time, dendritic spines were visualized only with the Golgi method or with a variant of this method, the Golgi-Cox method (Cox, 1891: tissue samples are immersed in a mixture of potassium dichromate and mercuric chloride). Furthermore, in 1895 Meyer published an article reporting that by using a variant of the methylene blue technique he could not verify the existence of these structures (Meyer, 1895, 1896, 1897). The methylene blue technique was introduced by Ehrlich (1881) as a bacteriological stain (Ehrlich, 1881) but it was in 1886 that Ehrlich found that peripheral nerve fibers could be stained by injecting the stain into the blood vessels of living animals (Ehrlich, 1886). This approach became popular as it rendered images comparable to those obtained with Golgi impregnation. The

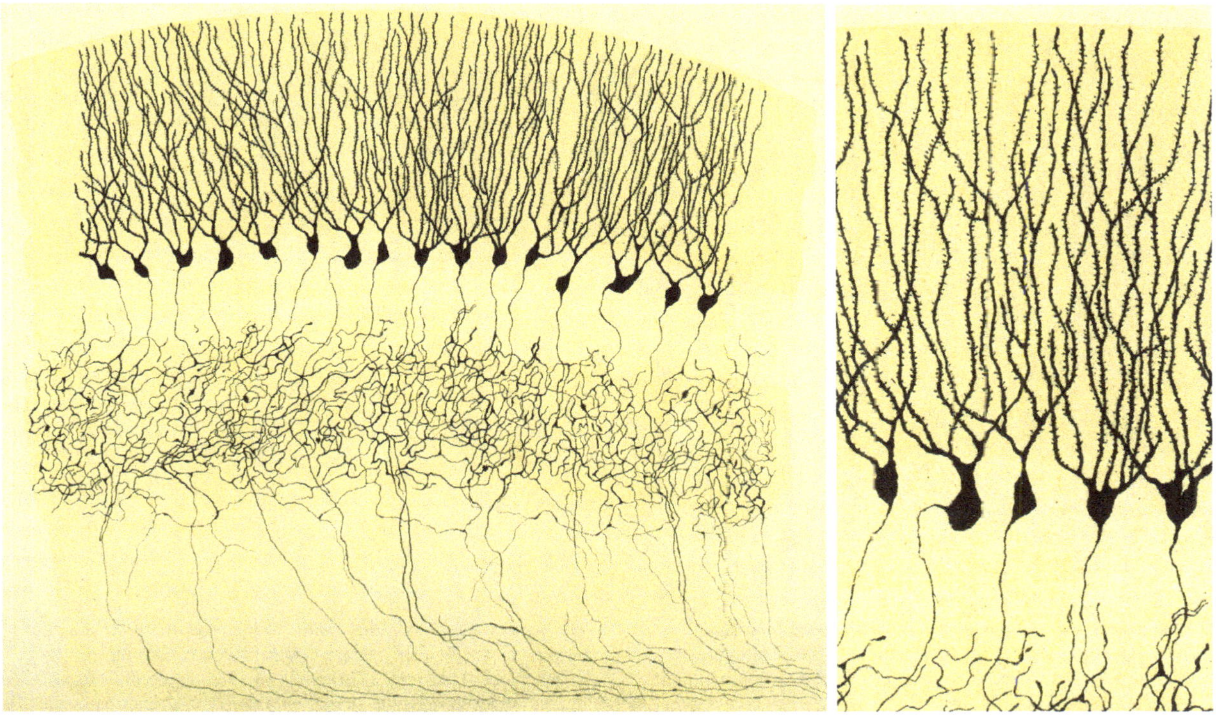

FIGURE 7 | Illustration by Golgi of a Golgi impregnated preparation of the dentate gyrus. "*Fascia dentata del grande piede di Hippocampo*". **Left**, panoramic view. Golgi used this drawing to illustrate that the axons of granule cells formed a very complex nervous network ("*rete nervosa*"). **Right**, High magnification of the drawing to illustrate that Golgi recognized the presence of dendritic spines. Taken from Golgi (1901).

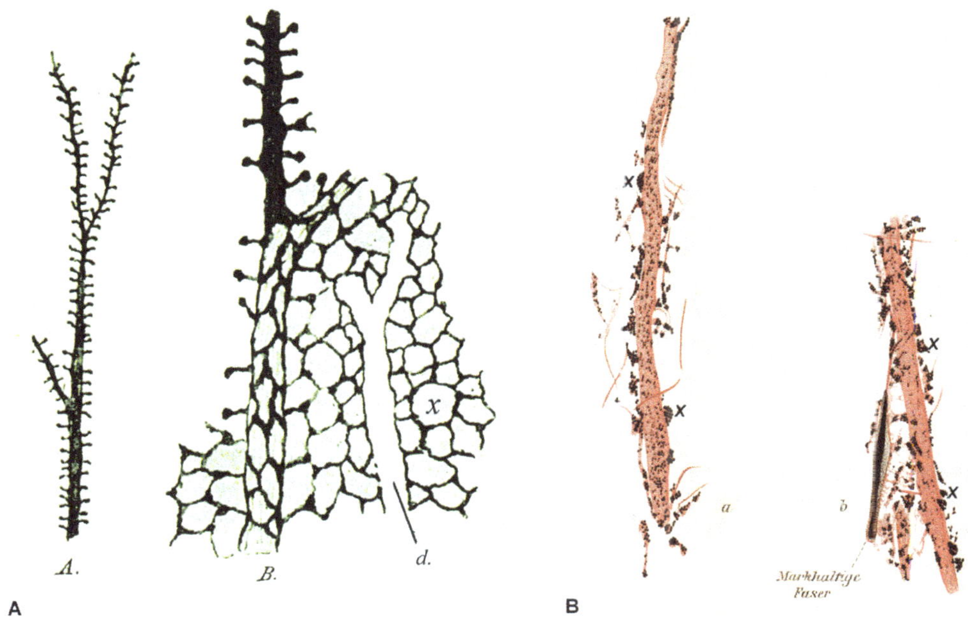

FIGURE 8 | Different interpretation of dendritic spines. (A) Drawings made by Bethe (1903) to illustrate dendritic spines stained with the ammonium molybdate method. *A*, an apical dendrite of a pyramidal cell covered with dendritic spines. *B*, schematic representation to illustrate his hypothesis that dendritic spines were the starting points of an interstitial network of the gray matter. *d*, unstained apical dendrite. **(B)** Drawings made by Held (1897b) to show dendrites innervated by end-feet or axon terminals (some of them are marked with an x). See text for further details.

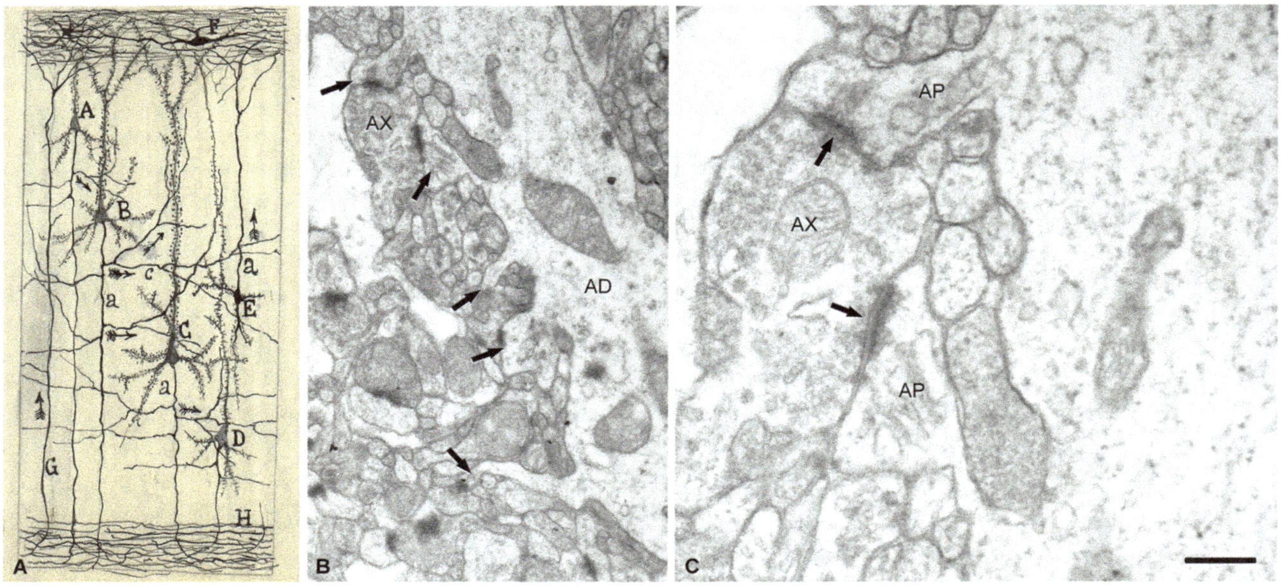

FIGURE 9 | Drawing and images showing dendritic spines as postsynaptic structures. (A) Schematic drawing by Cajal to show synaptic connections and the possible flow of information through neural circuits in the cerebral cortex. The legend states: *A, small pyramid; B, and C, medium and giant pyramids, respectively; a, axon; [c], nervous collaterals that appear to cross and touch the dendrites and the trunks [apical dendrites] of the pyramids; H, white matter;* [*E,* Martinotti cell with ascending axon]; *F, special cells of the first layer of cerebral cortex; G, fiber coming from the white matter. The arrows mark the supposed direction of the nervous current"*. Taken from *¿Neuronismo o reticularismo?* (Cajal, 1933). **(B)** Electron micrograph of a typical apical dendrite showing dendritic spines with different shapes (arrows). **(C)** high magnification of **A** to illustrate an axon terminal (*AX*) which establishes synaptic contacts (arrows) simultaneously with two dendritic spines. AP, spine apparatus. Scale bar: **(B)** 0,60 μm; **(C)** 0,15 μm. Taken from unpublished material (Alonso-Nanclares et al., 2008).

methylene blue procedure was modified by several authors, in particular Bethe (1895) who introduced fixation with ammonium molybdate to improve the preservation of the staining during the various steps of histological processing of the sections, and Dogiel (1896) who introduced some practical modifications allowing the application of the technique to thin, freshly-cut slices of central nervous tissue. Since dendritic spines were consistently stained with both the method of Golgi and with the variant of Cox, in specific regions of the neurons, Cajal interpreted this as clear evidence of their existence, and concluded that therefore dendritic spines must be key elements in the structure and function of neurons. Cajal (1896) noted:

> ...Dendritic spines are constantly present at the same regions of the [dendritic] arborizations, no matter what animal is studied, and are always lacking at certain sites, such as the [axon initial segment], cell body and origin of the thick [dendritic] processes.

However, due to the contradictory results of Meyer and the fact that Kölliker, who was much admired by Cajal, also denied the existence of dendritic spines, Cajal was prompted to re-examine this topic using the methylene blue method. Cajal used the same methodology as Meyer did and found that dendrites were stained so pale that their spines were not visible and therefore, the method applied by Meyer was inappropriate to show their existence. Cajal then modified the methylene blue procedure based on the procedures of Dogiel and Bethe, and found that dendritic spines were also stained with this method (Cajal, 1896; **Figure 6**). In addition, other authors confirmed the visualization of dendritic spines with the methylene blue method (e.g., Turner and Aber, 1900; Soukhanoff et al., 1904) and, therefore, it was concluded that they were not artifacts, but actual anatomical arrangements.

Interestingly, Golgi went on to publish an article (in 1901) where he drew dendritic spines (**Figure 7**). To my knowledge, it is the first time that he recognized the existence of these structures (Golgi, 1901). However, in the text he does not mention the dendritic spines. Therefore, it is clear that Golgi recognized the existence of dendritic spines, probably after the new evidence obtained with the methylene blue method used by Cajal and others scientists, but it seems that Golgi did not attribute any functional relevance to these structures.

OTHER INTERPRETATIONS OF THE DENDRITIC SPINES AND FINAL CONSIDERATIONS

Another interesting aspect of the early history of dendritic spines is that some authors confirmed their existence, but they proposed or interpreted their functions differently from Cajal. Among the most representative examples of these postulated functions

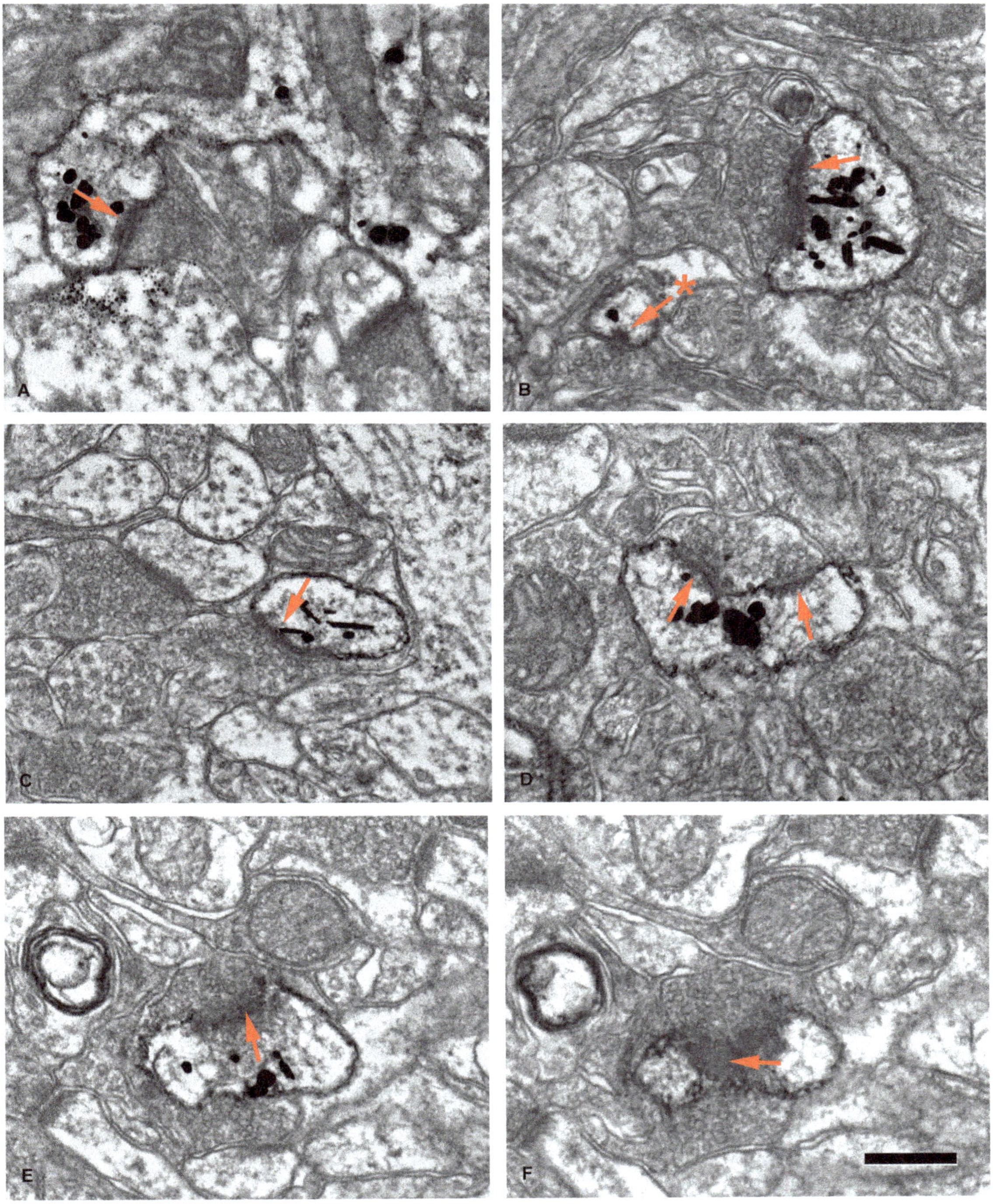

FIGURE 10 | Examples of dendritic spines forming synapses (A–F) in the adult mouse neocortex. The gold-particles allow the postsynaptic densities (PSDs; red arrows) to be clearly distinguished when present. Note the small size of the postsynaptic density (60 nm) in the head of a small spine in **(B)** (asterisk). **(E,F)** are consecutive sections of a spine head to illustrate a PSD cut tangentially. Scale bar: 560 nm in **(A)**; 350 nm in **(B,C)**; 300 nm in **(D)**; 280 nm in **(E,F)**. Taken from Arellano et al. (2007).

are those put forward by the distinguished neuroscientists Bethe and Held (**Figure 8**). Bethe (1903) drew dendritic spines as Cajal did, but he proposed that they were the initial points of an interstitial network of the gray matter that Nissl named *nervöse Grau* (**Figure 8A**). Held recognized the existence of dendritic spines but he proposed that they represented

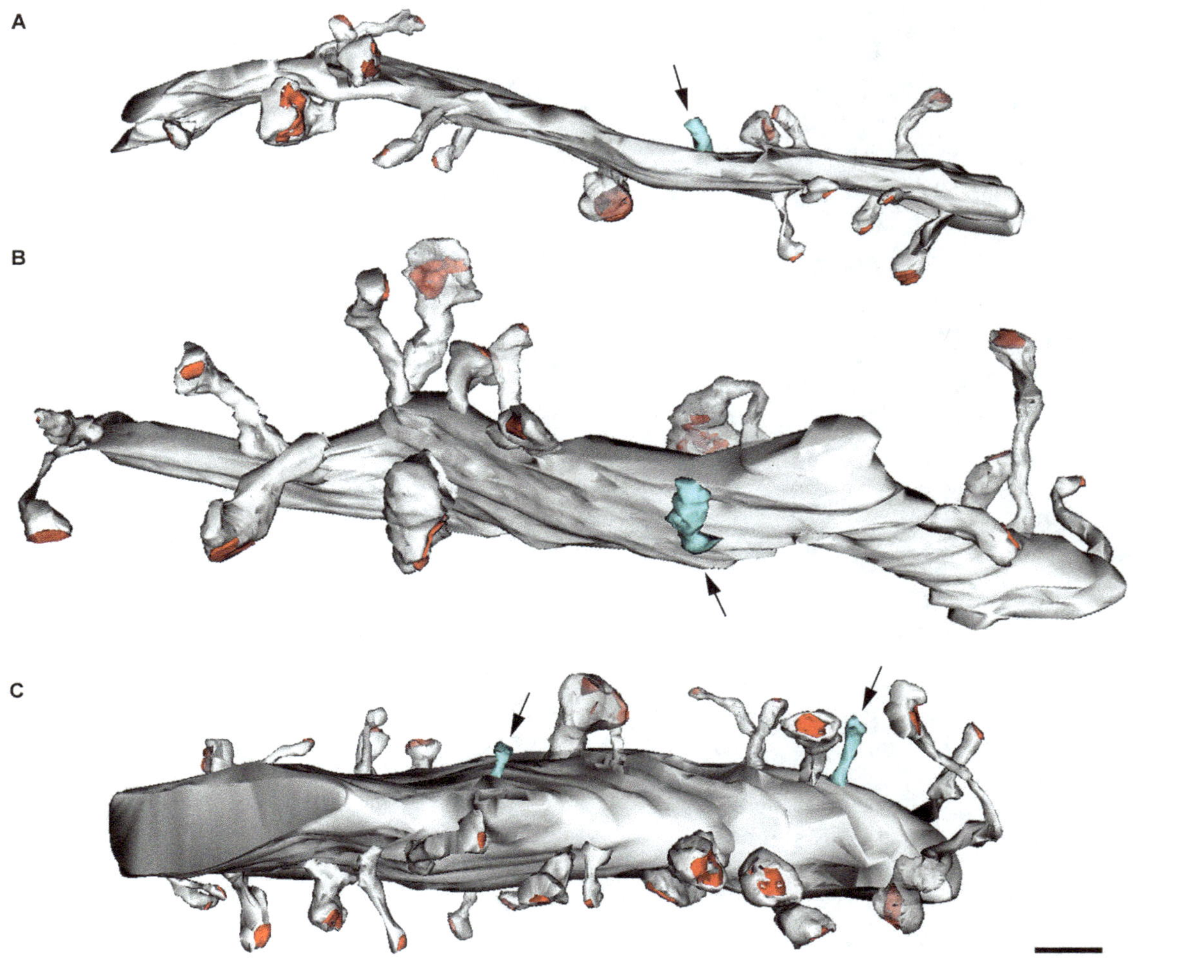

FIGURE 11 | Reconstructions from serial electron micrographs. Serial sections of dendritic segments in the adult mouse neocortex to illustrate the distribution of some non-synaptic spines (blue) indicated by arrows. The remaining spines establish synaptic contacts (red, PSD). **(A,B)** Basal dendrites; **(C)** apical dendrite. Scale bar: 2000 nm. Taken from Arellano et al. (2007).

the genuine end-feet (axons ended in distinct terminals) or *Endfüsse* that were incompletely stained or fragmented (**Figure 8B**). He thought that these axon terminals were fused with the dendrites, as occurred with the end-feet on the cell bodies (Held, 1897a,b, 1904, 1905, 1929). In addition, Held hypothesized the existence of an interstitial network that would allow communication between pyramidal cells thanks to the anastomoses between these "dendritic spines" and the nerve fibers (Held, 1929).

Cajal paid special attention to this publication and aimed to discredit it, driven by being at odds with the interpretation of Held, as well as by the fact that Held had wrongly attributed the discovery of dendritic spines to Golgi. Thus, in *¿Neuronismo o reticularismo?* (Cajal, 1933), Cajal presented a strong argument against the interpretation by Held basing his criticism on the fact that with the neurofibrillar methods the finest axon terminals are visualized, whereas the dendritic spines of pyramidal cells or Purkinje cells are never stained. To make this point clearer, in this article Cajal included an elegant schematic drawing (**Figure 9A**) in which the connections by contact of the collateral axonal branches of the pyramidal cells with dendritic spines were highlighted after analyzing the "extremely complex, diffuse nerve plexuses" of the cerebral cortex:

> I referred particularly to this intricate plexus when I lamented the insurmountable difficulties facing the analysis of the cortical synapses [...]. Note how these collaterals cross and enter into transversal or oblique contact with a great number of the dendritic shafts. It is probable that collaterals rest on the spines which cover the protoplasmic surfaces [dendrites] like down .... I have never seen anastomoses between the spines and the nerve fibers, despite having devoted particular attention to them since 1888.

Thus, after discovering dendritic spines, Cajal proposed that these elements established connections with axon terminals, and in his last articles he sometimes used the term "synapses" to refer to these connections (e.g., Cajal, 1933). Nevertheless, the advent and development of electron microscopy in the 1950s to study the nervous system (Robertson, 1953; Palade and Palay, 1954; De Robertis and Bennett, 1955; Palay, 1956; De Robertis, 1959) was necessary for the confirmation that they were really postsynaptic structures (**Figure 9**). The first electron microscope study of dendritic spines showing that they establish synaptic connections was published by Gray (1959), and these observations were confirmed and extended by several authors (e.g., Jones and Powell, 1969; Peters and Kaiserman-Abramof, 1969, 1970). Nevertheless, direct demonstration that the dendritic spines of Golgi-impregnated neurons established synapses came with the introduction of the combination of the Golgi method and electron microscopy, particularly the gold-toning technique of Fairén and colleagues (Fairén et al., 1977). This method involves de-impregnation of previously Golgi-impregnated neurons, followed by the study of their fine structure by electron microscope. The original impregnation deposit of silver chromate (which produces an intense, homogeneous intracellular labeling that masks postsynaptic densities) is replaced by a deposit of gold particles. At the electron microscope level, the deposit is visible as fine particles that mark the profiles of the de-impregnated neurons while allowing the visualization of the cytological details of the labeled neuron. Thus, this technique enables the accurate study of the ultrastructural characteristics and synaptic connections of Golgi-impregnated neurons, including dendritic spines, as the postsynaptic densities can be clearly distinguished (**Figure 10**). Further development of combinations of a variety of techniques (degeneration methods, immunocytochemistry, etc.,) for correlative light and electron microscopy soon followed. The application of these methods allowed the detailed examination of the afferent and efferent connections and chemical characteristics of Golgi-impregnated neurons (e.g., Frotscher and Léránth, 1986). Indeed, at present it is well established that almost all dendritic spines establish at least one excitatory glutamatergic synapse, as only a small portion of dendritic spines have been found to be non-synaptic (**Figure 11**; Arellano et al., 2007). Finally, the collective work of numerous authors have shown that dendritic spines are the major targets of excitatory connections in the cerebral cortex and that they seem to be key elements in learning, memory, and cognition (Yuste, 2010).

ACKNOWLEDGMENTS

This work was supported by grants from the following entities: Centro de Investigación en Red sobre Enfermedades Neurodegenerativas (CIBERNED, CB06/05/0066) and the Spanish Ministério de Economía y Competitividad (grant BFU2012-34963 and the Cajal Blue Brain Project, Spanish partner of the Blue Brain Project initiative from EPFL).

REFERENCES

Alonso-Nanclares, L., Gonzalez-Soriano, J., Rodriguez, J. R., and DeFelipe, J. (2008). Gender differences in human cortical synaptic density. *Proc. Natl. Acad. Sci. U S A* 105, 14615–14619. doi: 10.1073/pnas.0803652105

Andersen, P., Morris, R., Amaral, D., Bliss, T., O'Keefe, J. (eds) (2007). *The Hippocampus Book*. New York: Oxford University Press.

Arellano, J. I., Espinosa, A., Fairén, A., Yuste, R., and DeFelipe, J. (2007). Non-synaptic dendritic spines in neocortex. *Neuroscience* 145, 464–469. doi: 10.1016/j.neuroscience.2006.12.015

Bethe, A. (1895). Studien über das Centralnervensystem von Carcinus maenas nebst Angaben über ein neues verfahren der methylenblaufixation. *Arch. Mikrosk. Anat.* 44, 579–622. doi: 10.1007/bf02934031

Bethe, A. (1903). *Allgemeine Anatomie und Physiologie des Nervensystems*. Leipzig: Thieme.

Blazquez-Llorca, L., Garcia-Marin, V., Merino-Serrais, P., Ávila, J., and DeFelipe, J. (2011). Abnormal tau phosphorylation in the thorny excrescences of CA3 hippocampal neurons in patients with Alzheimer's. *J. Alzheimers Dis.* 26, 683–698. doi: 10.3233/JAD-2011-110659

Cajal, S. R. (1888). Estructura de los centros nerviosos de las aves. *Rev. Trim. Histol. Norm. Patol.* 1, 1–10.

Cajal, S. R. (1890). Textura de las circunvoluciones cerebrales de los mamíferos inferiores. Nota preventiva. *Gac. Méd. Catalana* 1, 22–31.

Cajal, S. R. (1892). Nuevo concepto de la histología de los centros nerviosos. *Rev. Cienc. Méd. Barc.* 18, 363–376; 457–476; 505–520; 529–540.

Cajal, S. R. (1893). Estructura del asta de Ammon y fascia dentate. *Anales Soc. Esp. Hist. Nat.* 22, 53–114.

Cajal, S. R. (1896). Las espinas colaterales de las células del cerebro teñidas por el azul de metileno. *Rev. Trim. Micrográf. Madrid* 1, 123–136.

Cajal, S. R. (1899). Estudios sobre la corteza cerebral humana. II. Estructura de la corteza motriz del hombre y mamíferos superiores. *Rev. Trim. Micrográf.* 4, 117–200.

Cajal, S. R. (1899–1904). *Textura del SistemaNervioso del Hombre y de Los Vertebrados*. Madrid: Imprenta y Librería de Nicolás Moya.

Cajal, S. R. (1909–1911). *Histologie du Système Nerveux de L'homme et des Vertébrés (Translated by L. Azoulay)*. Paris: Maloine

Cajal, S. R. (1917). *Recuerdos de mi Vida: Historia de mi Labor Científica*. Madrid: Imprenta y Librería de Nicolás Moya.

Cajal, S. R. (1933). ¿Neuronismo o Reticularismo? Las Pruebas Objetivas de la Unidad Anatómica de las Células Nerviosas. *Arch. Neurobiol.* 13, 217–291.

Cox, W. H. (1891). Imprägnation des centralen Nervensystems mit Quecksilbersalzen. *Arch. Mikrosk. Anat.* 37, 16–21.

DeFelipe, J. (2002). Sesquicentenary of the birthday of Santiago Ramón y Cajal, the father of modern neuroscience. *Trends Neurosci.* 25, 481–484. doi: 10.1016/s0166-2236(02)02214-2

DeFelipe, J. (2006). Brain plasticity and mental processes: Cajal again. *Nat. Rev. Neurosci.* 7, 811–817. doi: 10.1038/nrn2005

DeFelipe, J. (2010). *Cajal's Butterflies of the Soul: Science and Art*. New York: Oxford University Press.

DeFelipe, J. (2014). *El Jardín de la Neurología: Sobre lo Bello, el Arte y el Cerebro*. Madrid: Boletín Oficial del Estado y Consejo Superior de Investigaciones Científicas.

DeFelipe, J., and Jones, E. G. (1988). *Cajal on the Cerebral Cortex*. New York: Oxford University Press.

Demoor, J. (1896). La plasticité morphologique des neurones cérébraux. *Arch. Biol. Brux.* 14, 723–752.

De Robertis, E. (1959). Submicroscopy morphology of the synapse. *Int. Rev. Cytol.* 8, 61–96. doi: 10.1016/S0074-7696(08)62728-X

De Robertis, E. D., and Bennett, H. S. (1955). Some features of the submicroscopic morphology of synapses in frog and earthworm. *J. Biophys. Biochem. Cytol.* 1, 47–58. doi: 10.1083/jcb.1.1.47

Dogiel, A. S. (1896). Die nervenelemente in kleinhirne der Vögel und Säugethiere. *Arch. Mikrosk. Anat.* 47, 707–718. doi: 10.1007/bf02977417

Edinger, L. (1893). Vergleichend-entwickelungsgeschichtliche und anatomische studien im bereiche der hirnanatomie. *Anat. Anz.* 8, 305–321.

Ehrlich, P. (1881). Ueber das Methylenblau und seine klinisch-bakterioskopische Verwerthung. *Z. Klin. Med.* 2, 710–713.

Ehrlich, P. (1886). Ueber die Methyllenblau-reaction der lebenden nervensubstanz. *Dtsch. Med. Wochenschr.* 12, 49–52. doi: 10.1055/s-0028-113 c9684

Fairén, A., Peters, A., and Saldanha, J. (1977). A new procedure for examining Golgi impregnated neurons by light and electron microscopy. *J. Neurocytol.* 6, 311–337. doi: 10.1007/bf01175194

Fernandez, N., and Breathnach, C. S. (2001). Luis Simarro Lacabra [1851–1921]: from Golgi to Cajal through Simarro, via Ranvier? *J. His. Neurosci.* 10, 19–26. doi: 10.1076/jhin.10.1.19.5622

Foster, M., and Sherrington, C. S. (1897). *A Text-Book of Physiology. Part III: The Central Nervous System.* London: Macmillan.

Frotscher, M., and Léránth, C. (1986). The cholinergic innervation of the rat fascia dentata: identification of target structures on granule cells by combining choline acetyltransferase immunocytochemistry and Golgi impregnation. *J. Comp. Neurol.* 243, 58–70. doi: 10.1002/cne.902430106

Golgi, C. (1873). Sulla struttura della sostanza grigia del cervello (Comunicazione preventiva). *Gaz. Med. Ital. Lomb.* 33, 244–246.

Golgi, C. (1875). *Sulla Fina Struttura del Bulbi Olfattorii.* Reggio-Emilia: Printer Stefano Calderini.

Golgi, C. (1882–1883). "Sulla fina anatomia degli organi centrali del sistema nervoso. Rivista sperimentale di Freniatria, anni 1882–83," in *Opera Omnia, Vol. I. Istologia Normale (1870–1883)* (Milan: Ulrico Hoepli), 1903, 295–393.

Golgi, C. (1901). "Sulla fina anatomia degli organi centrali del sistema nervoso. *Lettera al Prof. Luigi Luciani* [La lettera fu pubblicata in parte nel Trattato di fisiologia dell'uomo del Professore Luigi Luciani ordinario di Fisiologia nell "Universita di Roma. (Societa editrice libraria. Milano 1901]," in *Opera Omnia. Vol. II. Istologia Normale (1883–1902)* (Milan: Ulrico Hoepli), 1903, 721–733.

Gray, E. G. (1959). Electron microscopy of synaptic contacts on dendrite spines of the cerebral cortex. *Nature* 183, 1592–1593. doi: 10.1038/1831592a0

Hatai, S. (1903). The finer structure of the neurones in the nervous system of the white rat. *Univ. Chicago. Dec. Publ.* 10, 170–190.

Held, H. (1897a). Beiträge zur structur der nervenzellen und ihrer Fortsätze. Zweite abhandlung. *Arch. Anat. Phys. Anat. Abt.* 204–294.

Held, H. (1897b). Beiträge zur structur der nervenzellen und ihrer Fortsätze. Dritte abhandlung. *Arch. Anat. Phys. Anat. Abt.* 273–312.

Held, H. (1904). Zur weiteren Kenntniss der Nervenendfüsse und zur Struktur der Sehzellen. *Abh. Math. Phys. Kl. Königl. Sächs. Ges Wiss.* 29, 143–185.

Held, H. (1905). Zur kenntniss einer neurofibrillären continuität im centralnervensystem der wirbelthiere. *Arch. Anat. Phys. Anat. Abt.* 55–78.

Held, H. (1929). "Die lehre von den neuronen und von neurencytium und ihr heutiger stand," in *Fortschritte der Naturwissenschftl. Forschung, N.F. Heft 8*, ed E. Abderhalden (Berlín: Urban und Schwarzenberg), 1–72.

Jones, E. G., and Powell, T. P. S. (1969). Morphological variations in the dendritic spines of the neocortex. *J. Cell Sci.* 5, 509–529.

Kölliker, A. (1896). *Handbuch der Gewebelehre des Menschen, 6th ed, Vol II. Nervensystem des Menschen und der Thiere.* Leipzig: Engelmann.

Mazzarello, P. (1999). *The Hidden Structure. A Scientific Biography of Camillo Golgi.* Oxford: Oxford University Press.

Meyer, S. (1895). Die subcutane Methylenblauinjection, ein mittel zur darstellung der elemente des Central-nervensystems Säugethieren. *Arch. Mikrosk. Anat.* 46, 282–290. doi: 10.1007/bf02906655

Meyer, S. (1896). Ueber eine verbindungsweise der neurone. Nebst mitteilungen über die technik und die erfolge der methode der subcutanen methylenblauinjection. *Arch. Mikrosk. Anat.* 47, 734–748. doi: 10.1007/bf02977419

Meyer, S. (1897). Ueber die funktion der Protoplasmafortsätze der nervenzellen. *Bericht. Math. Phys. Cl. Königl. Sächs. Gessells. Wiss. Leipzig* 49, 475–495.

Palade, G. E., and Palay, S. L. (1954). Electron microscope observations of interneuronal and neuromuscular synapses. *Anat. Rec.* 118, 335–336.

Palay, S. L. (1956). Synapses in the central nervous system. *J. Biophys. Biochem. Cytol.* 2, 193–202. doi: 10.1083/jcb.2.4.193

Peters, A., and Kaiserman-Abramof, I. R. (1969). The small pyramidal neuron of the rat cerebral cortex. the synapses upon dendritic spines. *Z. Zellforsch. Mikrosk. Anat.* 100, 487–506. doi: 10.1007/bf00344370

Peters, A., and Kaiserman-Abramof, I. R. (1970). The small pyramidal neuron of the rat cerebral cortex: the perikaryon, dendrites and spines. *Am. J. Anat.* 127, 321–355. doi: 10.1002/aja.1001270402

Retzius, G. (1891). Ueber den bau der oberflächeschicht der grosshirnrinde beim menschen und bei den Säugethieren. *Biologiska Foren. Förhandlingar* 3, 90–102.

Robertson, J. D. (1953). Ultrastructure of two invertebrate synapses. *Proc. Soc. Exp. Biol. Med.* 82, 219–223. doi: 10.3181/00379727-82-20071

Schaffer, K. (1892). Beitrag zur histologie der ammonshornformation. *Arch. Mikrosk. Anat.* 39, 611–632. doi: 10.1007/bf02961541

Sherrington, C. S. (1947). *The Integrative Action of the Nervous System.* Cambridge: University Press.

Soukhanoff, S., Geier, F., and Gourévitsch, M. (1904). Contribution á l'étude de l'aspect externe des prolongements protoplasmatiques des cellules nerveuses colorés par le bleu de méthilène. *Névraxe* 6, 117–122.

Stefanowska, M. (1897). Les appendices terminaux des dendrites cérébraux et leur différents états physiologiques. *Ann. Soc. Roy. Sc. Méd. Nat. Brux.* 6, 351–407.

Stefanowska, M. (1901). *Les Appendices Terminaux des Dendrites Cérébraux et leur Différents états Physiologiques.* Genève: Eggimann, 1–25 (Reprint of the article published in *Archives des Sciences Physiques et Naturelles* vol., 11).

Turner, J., and Aber, M. B. (1900). A note on the staining of brain in a mixture of methylene blue and peroxide of hydrogen—A *vital* reaction in *post-mortem* tissue. *Brain* 23, 524–529. doi: 10.1093/brain/23.3.524

von Gerlach, J. (1872). Über die struktur der grauen substanz des menschlichen grosshirns. *Zentralbl. Med. Wiss.* 10, 273–275.

Yuste, R. (2010). *Dendritic Spines.* Cambridge (MA): MIT Press.

18

The spine problem: finding a function for dendritic spines

Sarah Malanowski and Carl F. Craver *

Department of Philosophy, Washington University in St. Louis, St. Louis, MO, USA

Correspondence:
Carl F. Craver, Department of Philosophy, Washington University in St. Louis, Campus Box 1073, One Brookings Drive, St. Louis, MO 63130, USA
e-mail: ccraver@wustl.edu

Why do neurons have dendritic spines? This question—the heart of what Yuste calls "the spine problem"—presupposes that why-questions of this sort have scientific answers: that empirical findings can favor or count against claims about *why* neurons have spines. Here we show how such questions can receive empirical answers. We construe such why-questions as questions about how spines *make a difference to* the behavior of some mechanism that we take to be significant. Why-questions are driven fundamentally by the effort to understand how some item, such as the dendritic spine, is situated in the causal structure of the world (the *causal nexus*). They ask for a filter on that busy world that allows us to see a part's individual contribution to a mechanism, independent of everything else going on. So understood, answers to why-questions can be assessed by testing the claims these answers make about the causal structure of a mechanism. We distinguish four ways of making a difference to a mechanism (necessary, modulatory, component, background condition), and we sketch their evidential requirements. One consequence of our analysis is that there are many spine problems and that any given spine problem might have many acceptable answers.

Keywords: dendritic spines, function, functional attribution, causal-mechanical explanation, mechanisms

INTRODUCTION

Science, according to common wisdom, does not answer why questions. Science tells us only what and how things happen. Nowhere is this common wisdom more transparently false than in anatomy and physiology, where a central pre-occupation is to understand why organisms have the parts they do. These questions have been central to research on dendritic spines from the start. Cajal's pioneering judgment that spines are not merely artifacts of Golgi staining prompted the transparently teleological question: *why* do neurons have spines? Yuste (2011) refers to this as the "Spine Problem": "What exactly do spines contribute to the neuron?".

Cajal (1899) considered several answers to this question (García-López et al., 2007): that spines increase the "receptive surface" of the neuron, that they "absorb" nerve impulses, (Cajal, 1899, ibid. 119), and that they grow out to connect with distant axons. Theories of spine function have since proliferated. Shepherd, for example, reviews ten broad classes of theory, each of which can be specified in myriad ways (see Table 1, Shepherd, 1996, 2198). His list includes contributions spines might make to synaptic connectivity, development, synapse electrophysiology, synaptic plasticity, active processing of monosynaptic input, temporal processing of polysynaptic input, biochemical compartmentalization, and features of the membrane surface.

Here we explore the nature of these why-questions and the evidence required to test them. We show how these why-questions contribute to the search for neural mechanisms, distinguish several kinds of answers, and show how the mechanistic understanding of such why-questions and their answers connects those answers to empirical evidence about the causal structure of the world.

Our view of why-questions relies on the central idea that explanations in neuroscience describe mechanisms. Mechanisms consist of entities and activities organized in space and time so that they exhibit some behavior of the mechanism as a whole. Explanatory models of such mechanisms describe the spatial, temporal, and active organization of causally interacting parts. The effort to answer why-questions is a central part of the search for mechanisms that span multiple levels (Shepherd, 1983). Our focus is on these why-questions and, in particular, on what they contribute to our understanding of how the brain works, how it breaks, and how it might be improved. Why-questions, like how- and what- questions, are indispensable in the effort to understand hierarchically organized systems.

CAUSAL-MECHANICAL EXPLANATION

To answer a why-question about some item (such as dendritic spines) is to represent it as part of a causal-mechanical explanation for something else. Causal-mechanical explanations in general show how a phenomenon to be explained, the *explanandum phenomenon*, is situated in the causal nexus—how it was produced, how it acts, and how it interacts with other things in the world. One can situate the explanandum phenomenon in the causal nexus in three ways: etiologically, constitutively, and contextually.

Etiological explanations show *how* the phenomenon came to pass. They look back to reveal its antecedent causes. The tipped lantern, for example, is part of the etiological explanation for the fire. Likewise, spine loss may be part of the etiological explanation for several neuropsychological disorders (Penzes et al., 2011).

Constitutive explanations answer how questions by looking down to reveal the mechanisms that underlie or maintain the phenomenon. They look inside it and describe how parts, properties, and activities are organized together in space and time such that the phenomenon occurs. Constitutive explanations often span multiple levels: higher level mechanisms are explained by lower level mechanisms, which are in turn explained by mechanisms at a lower level still, and so on. The binding of neurotransmitters to receptors on dendritic spines is part of the constitutive explanation for many instances of excitatory synaptic transmission, which are themselves involved in most of the interesting things brains do. Looking down, synaptic transmission involves numerous chemical interactions and atomic processes well beneath the current grain of explanatory interest. Multilevel mechanisms in neuroscience thus typically require research in several different fields (cellular, cognitive, etc.), since different fields are better suited for studying different levels of mechanisms.

These two aspects of causal-mechanical explanation each relate the explanandum phenomenon to the causal structure of the world in a different way. Etiological explanations look back to the causal structures that brought it about. Constitutive explanations look down to the causal structures that make it work. Each, in its own way, tells us how the explanandum phenomenon comes about.

WHY-QUESTIONS AND CONTEXT: A THIRD ASPECT OF CAUSAL-MECHANICAL EXPLANATION

The third aspect of causal-mechanical explanation is contextual. Contextual explanations describe the *role* or *function* of spines. Like constitutive explanations, contextual explanation are interlevel, but rather than looking back or looking down, contextual explanations look up and around to situate the item in question within a higher-level mechanism (Cummins, 1983; Craver, 2001). They tell us *why* neurons have spines.

Recent reviews of dendritic spine function reflect this causal-mechanical understanding of why questions and their answers. Harris and Kater (1994) argue that to understand the function of dendritic spines one must consider them, "within the context of the overall synaptic complex" including not just the spine but "the post-synaptic density, the synaptic cleft, the presynaptic axonal bouton and its vesicles, and the neighboring astrocytic complexes" (Harris 348). Each theory in Shepherd's (1996) list situates dendritic spines within a more inclusive mechanism. Yuste (2011) focuses on one of Shepherd's contextual mechanisms: the construction and maintenance of a distributed network with independently modifiable synapses. In each case, the goal is to look up and see how dendritic spines make a difference to the behavior of some system of antecedently acknowledged significance.

More abstractly, the answer to a why-question for an item such as a dendritic spine involves attributing a function or role to the item. This attribution can be distilled into four components:

1. A mechanism displaying a behavior in salient conditions (e.g., forming a network of modifiable synapses).
2. The mechanism's behavior in these conditions is antecedently presumed to be important (e.g., because it affords flexible information processing).
3. Some item (part, property, or activity) is a spatio-temporal part of this system (e.g., spines, their morphology, or their growth).
4. The item makes a difference to the system behaving as it does in these conditions.

The mechanism and behavior described in (a) constitute the causal context in which the item functions. We place no constraints on the behaviors in (a) except that (b) they are antecedently presumed significant. Specifically, the behavior does not need to have contributed to the evolution (Neander, 1991) or development (Garson, 2011) of spines. Why-questions also arise in pathology and engineering: researchers study, for example, the role of spines in the etiological mechanisms of Down's syndrome (Kaufmann and Moser, 2000) and the role spines might play in the treatment of addiction (Robinson and Kolb, 1999).

Condition (c) distinguishes contextual or functional explanation from etiological and constitutive explanation by requiring that the functional item be part of (contained within) the mechanism. Condition (d) requires that the item must make a difference to how the system behaves. If a part can make no difference at all to how the mechanism behaves, the why-question has no answer.

Constitutive, etiological, and contextual explanations are separate aspects of the same, mechanistic explanatory objective: the what, the how, and the why combine to situate an item in the causal nexus (for more recent work on evidence-based discovery see Craver and Darden, 2013; Silva et al., 2013).

MANY ANSWERS TO THE SAME WHY QUESTION

Why-questions ask us to situate an item within the context of a higher-level mechanism. Clearly the same item can contribute to the behavior of many mechanisms at once—it can have many *functions*. This appears to be what Shepherd (1996) has in mind when he claims that dendritic spines are *multifunctional* units. Each theory in Shepherd's list of functions situates spines in a different causal context. This raises the reasonable prospect that there are many "spine problems" and many equally good solutions to each of them.

One reason to expect a multiplicity of functions is that distinct answers to the same why-question can be *hierarchically* related to one another. Harris and Kater (1994), for example, argue that spine shape *compartmentalizes* synaptic input, which *facilitates LTP induction* at single hippocampal synapses. Long-term potentiation, in turn, implements *weight adjustment* in computing networks that subserve *learning and memory*. These different functional attributions describe the same feature of spines in the context of different levels in one hierarchy of mechanisms (Craver, 2001, 2002; cf. Shepherd, 1983; Churchland and Sejnowski, 1992). The function attributed at one level (plasticity) requires or depends on the functions attributed in lower-level contexts (compartmentalization).

A second reason to expect that spines have multiple functions is that they make a difference to the behavior of many different systems. Spines have been hypothesized to stabilize dendrites

(Kasai et al., 2010; Koleske, 2013), to protect cells from calcium toxicity (Harris and Kater, 1994; Segal, 1995), and to prevent synaptic input from short-circuiting the dendritic membrane (Yuste, 2011). These hypotheses are not competitors—spines contribute to many higher-level phenomenon, and they do so in different ways.

The fact that an item might play different roles in different higher-level containing systems has important implications for extrapolating the results of experimental findings. Given that there are many different memory systems, in different brain regions, with different underlying mechanisms, dendritic spines might play different roles in different memory systems. The same item might also play a similar functional role when described with respect to some lower-level mechanism, but an altogether different functional role when described at higher levels. Similarities and differences at multiple levels of organization can influence the extent to which experimental findings extrapolate to other systems and other organisms.

WHAT QUESTIONS: ORGANIZATIONAL CONSTRAINTS ON FUNCTIONAL ATTRIBUTION

Many kinds of evidence can be used to argue for a particular theory concerning how an item is situated in a higher-level system. Some of this evidence is circumstantial in nature, concerning, e.g., spatial (size, shape, location, orientation) and temporal (order, rate, duration) findings about spines, their components, and their mechanistic context. Anatomical properties, such as spine locations, dimensions, morphologies, sub-structures, and organelles provide clues as to how spines might make a difference (Harris and Kater, 1994; Shepherd, 1996; García-López et al., 2007). Evidence about the time-course of intrinsic and activity-driven changes in spine morphology provides a dynamic, temporal perspective on the place of spines in the causal order of the brain (Kasai et al., 2010). Comparative evidence reveals correlations between spine density and specialization of certain brain areas (Elston et al., 2001). Such observations about *what* spines and their causal context are like can be combined with mathematical models to show how such properties would and would not influence the system's behavior (Koch and Zador, 1993; Yuste, 2013). Findings of this sort provide global constraints on what spines can do in any context and specific constraints on what they can contribute to a particular mechanism.

Yet such findings offer only indirect tests of the causal claims at the heart of functional attributions. Correlational studies provide clues to the causal structure of a system but are almost always compatible with multiple causal structures (Eberhardt and Scheines, 2007). Models are useful for exploring a space of possibilities, but models of dendritic spine function depend crucially on idealized assumptions about the relevant structures (Harris and Kater, 1994) and on the values of unmeasured parameters (Yuste, 2013). Evidence about the time-course of spine changes, by itself, does not tell us about the causal forces that drive the development of the system over time.

WAYS OF MAKING A DIFFERENCE

Functional attributions—answers to why-questions—can be tested more directly by evaluating experimentally the causal claims at their heart. Ideally, these causal claims are tested by intervening to change only the putative causal variable and observing whether this change makes a difference to the effect in question. Causal experiments test directly how an item can and does make a difference within a higher-level mechanism.

Four categories of functional attribution appear to be evidentially, explanatorily, and practically distinct. On one axis, an item might make a difference either by being *necessary* for a system's behavior or by *modulating* its behavior. Removing a necessary item prevents the behavior; removing a modulatory item merely changes it. On a second axis, an item might be either a *component* or a *background condition*. A component is a working part in the system; a background condition merely enables or assists the working parts. Combining the axes yields four kinds of functional role: necessary components, modulatory components, necessary background conditions, and modulatory background conditions.

Consider a specific example, which follows Stevens (1998) general framework. If changes in spine morphology are *necessary working components* in the mechanism of LTP, then the following causal claims should be true: (i) conditions that induce LTP should change spine morphology; (ii) preventing changes in spine morphology should prevent LTP; and (iii) inducing changes in spine morphology should be able to produce LTP in the right conditions. Condition (ii) expresses the idea of necessity in the relation; conditions (i) and (iii) combine to express the idea of componency—being a part that is sufficient in the circumstances to produce the mechanism's behavior (Mackie, 1980).

To put this causal analysis to work, consider the hypothesis that spine enlargement is a necessary component in the mechanism of LTP induction. Spines appear to enlarge following LTP induction in accordance with condition (i) (Matsuzaki et al., 2004). And if one blocks the polymerization of actin molecules thought to be required for spine enlargement, one can prevent late LTP (Ramachandran and Frey, 2009). This provides some evidence that actin-based remodeling of spines is necessary for LTP (Bosch et al., 2014).

The status of (iii) is more complicated. We know a lot about *what* potentiated synapses are like. The volume of the spine head is directly proportional to the size of the post-synaptic density, to the number of post-synaptic receptors, to the size of the pre-synaptic bouton, to the number of vesicles generally docked at the pre-synaptic bouton, and to the quantity of neurotransmitter available for release at the synapse (Nimchinsky et al., 2002; García-López et al., 2007). However, these correlations provide only circumstantial evidence that head size makes a difference to LTP. More direct causal experiments that induce LTP by changing spine morphology are required to establish (iii) directly. It thus remains to be seen whether spine enlargement *per se* makes a difference to LTP or whether it is merely a byproduct of processes that strengthen the synapse in other ways (Redondo and Morris, 2011).

A modulatory working component satisfies (i), but not (ii) or (iii). If spine enlargement modulates LTP, then preventing spine growth would alter LTP but not prevent it (contra ii). And changes in morphology would not, by themselves, produce LTP (contra iii). However, changes in morphology should make a difference to how LTP is induced or expressed. Whether a modulatory factor is considered a background condition or a working component depends on the relationship between the factor and the other components in the system: working components work together with other components to produce the phenomenon, while background conditions are less directly implicated in the phenomenon.

A necessary background condition satisfies (ii) but not (i) or (iii). Removing a necessary background condition prevents the system from functioning. Background conditions tend to be causally independent from the operating conditions of the system: changes induced in the background conditions are therefore considered to make no difference to the system's behavior in the relevant conditions.

This way of thinking about functional attributions and the evidence used to evaluate them can be extended to multiple levels of organization. It can be used as a framework to refine and evaluate causal evidence for distinct functional attributions. Focus on the role of dendritic spines in learning and memory. Experience-based changes in spine morphology have been proposed as a basis for long-term memory formation and retention (Bourne and Harris, 2007), but it is unclear just what this functional claim amounts to. The above framework can be used to more specifically describe how spine density changes make a difference in experience-based learning. The conditions that give rise to changes in experience also give rise to changes in spine formation (Sala and Segal, 2014), suggesting (i) is fulfilled. Other studies suggest that interfering with the formation of new spines impairs learning abilities (Soderling et al., 2007), but preventing spine formation may not eliminate learning entirely (contra ii). Studies showing that changes in spine density do not necessarily result in changes in learning and memory (Popov et al., 2007; Fester et al., 2012) suggest (iii) is not fulfilled. Spine formation thus appears to have a working modulatory role in some forms of learning and memory.

In short, this causal-mechanical analysis allows us to distinguish different kinds of functional hypotheses—different ways of making a difference to the behavior of a higher-level mechanism. Each situates an item differently within the causal context. Given that functional attributions are inherently multilevel, this analysis shows how functional attributions—answers to why-questions—integrate lower-level findings with findings about higher-level behaviors or mechanisms. Contextual explanation is inherently upward-looking and, in that sense, non-reductive.

CONCLUSION

Answering why-questions, like answering how and what questions, helps to reveal the causal structure of the world. When we ask why neurons have dendritic spines, we are asking how spines fit into the workings of this most spectacular machine. Seen in this light, to claim that dendritic spines have a function in the nervous system is, implicitly, to commit one's self to a set of causal claims about how that item makes a difference in a mechanistic context. Functional attributions gain their content from these causal claims and are evaluated most directly by testing whether those causal claims are true. Spines might play a role at many levels of organization in the nervous system and in many distinct causal systems, and might function as a necessary or modulatory component or background condition in each. Attention to the causal commitments of our functional claims helps to highlight and prioritize the diverse kinds of evidence required to evaluate them. So understood, Yuste's spine problem is likely not one problem but many, reflecting the many ways that spines might be situated in the complex causal nexus of the brain.

REFERENCES

Bosch, M., Castro, J., Saneyoshi, T., Matsuno, H., Sur, M., and Hayashi, Y. (2014). Structural and molecular remodeling of dendritic spine substructures during long-term potentiation. *Neuron* 82, 444–459. doi: 10.1016/j.neuron.2014.03.021

Bourne, J., and Harris, K. M. (2007). Do thin spines learn to be mushroom spines that remember? *Curr. Opin. Neurobiol.* 17, 381–386. doi: 10.1016/j.conb.2007.04.009

Cajal, S. R. (1899). *Reglas y Consejos Sobre Investigación Biológica.* Madrid: Imprenta de Fontanet.

Churchland, P. S., and Sejnowski, T. J. (1992). *The Computational Brain.* Cambridge, Massachusetts: The MIT Press.

Craver, C. F. (2001). Role functions, mechanisms and hierarchy. *Philos. Sci.* 68, 31–55. doi: 10.1086/392866

Craver, C. F. (2002). Interlevel experiments and multilevel mechanisms in the neuroscience of memory. *Philos. Sci. Supp.* 69, S83–S97. doi: 10.1086/341836

Craver, C. F., and Darden, L. (2013). *In Search of Biological Mechanisms: Discoveries Across the Life Sciences.* Chicago: University of Chicago Press.

Cummins, R. (1983). *The Nature of Psychological Explanation.* Cambridge: MIT Press.

Eberhardt, F., and Scheines, R. (2007). Interventions and causal inference. *Philos. Sci.* 74, 981–995. doi: 10.1086/525638

Elston, G. N., Benavides-Piccione, R., and DeFelipe, J. (2001). The pyramidal cell in cognition: a comparative study in human and monkey. *J. Neurosci.* 21, RC163–RC167.

Fester, L., Prange-Kiel, J., Zhou, L., Blittersdorf, B. V., Böhm, J., Jarry, H., et al. (2012). Estrogen-regulated synaptogenesis in the hippocampus: sexual dimorphism in vivo but not in vitro. *J. Steroid Biochem. Mol. Biol.* 131, 24–29. doi: 10.1016/j.jsbmb.2011.11.010

García-López, P., García-Marín, V., and Freire, M. (2007). The discovery of dendritic spines by Cajal in 1888 and its relevance in present-day neuroscience. *Prog. Neurobiol.* 83, 110–130. doi: 10.1016/j.pneurobio.2007.06.002

Garson, J. (2011). Selected effects functions and causal role functions in the brain: the case for an etiological approach to neuroscience. *Biol. Philos.* 26, 547–565. doi: 10.1007/s10539-011-9262-6

Harris, K. M., and Kater, S. B. (1994). Dendritic spines: cellular specializations imparting both stability and flexibility to synaptic function. *Annu. Rev. Neurosci.* 17, 341–371. doi: 10.1146/annurev.neuro.17.1.341

Kasai, H., Fukuda, M., Watanabe, S., Hayashi-Takagi, A., and Noguchi, J. (2010). Structural dynamics of dendritic spines in memory and cognition. *Trends Neurosci.* 33, 121–129. doi: 10.1016/j.tins.2010.01.001

Kaufmann, W. E., and Moser, H. W. (2000). Dendritic anomalies in disorders associated with mental retardation. *Cereb. Cortex* 10, 981–991. doi: 10.1093/cercor/10.10.981

Koch, C., and Zador, A. (1993). The function of dendritic spines: devices subserving biochemical rather than electrical compartmentalization. *J. Neurosci.* 13, 413–422.

Koleske, A. J. (2013). Molecular mechanisms of dendrite stability. *Nat. Rev. Neurosci.* 14, 536–550. doi: 10.1038/nrn3486

Mackie, J. L. (1980). *The Cement of the Universe: A Study of Causation.* Oxford: Clarendon Press.

Matsuzaki, M., Honkura, N., Ellis-Davies, G. C., and Kasai, H. (2004). Structural basis of long-term potentiation in single dendritic spines. *Nature* 429, 761–766. doi: 10.1038/nature02617

Neander, K. (1991). The teleological notion of function. *Australas. J. Philos.* 69, 454–468. doi: 10.1080/00048409112344881

Nimchinsky, E. A., Sabatini, B. L., and Svoboda, K. (2002). Structure and function of dendritic spines. *Annu. Rev. Physiol.* 64, 313–353. doi: 10.1146/annurev.physiol.64.081501.160008

Penzes, P., Cahill, M. E., Jones, K. A., VanLeeuwen, J. E., and Woolfrey, K. M. (2011). Dendritic spine pathology in neuropsychiatric disorders. *Nat. Neurosci.* 14, 285–293. doi: 10.1038/nn.2741

Popov, V. I., Medvedev, N. I., Patrushev, I. V., Ignat'ev, D. A., Morenkov, E. D., and Stewart, M. G. (2007). Reversible reduction in dendritic spines in CA1 of rat and ground squirrel subjected to hypothermia-normothermia in vivo: a three-dimensional electron microscope study. *Neuroscience* 149, 549–560. doi: 10.1016/j.neuroscience.2007.07.059

Ramachandran, B., and Frey, J. U. (2009). Interfering with the actin network and its effect on long-term potentiation and synaptic tagging in hippocampal CA1 neurons in slices *in vitro*. *J. Neurosci.* 29, 12167–12173. doi: 10.1523/JNEUROSCI.2045-09.2009

Redondo, R. L., and Morris, R. G. M. (2011). Making memories last: the synaptic tagging and capture hypothesis. *Nat. Rev. Neurosci.* 12, 17–30. doi: 10.1038/nrn2963

Robinson, T. E., and Kolb, B. (1999). Alterations in the morphology of dendrites and dendritic spines in the nucleus accumbens and prefrontal cortex following repeated treatment with amphetamine or cocaine. *Eur. J. Neurosci.* 11, 1598–1604. doi: 10.1046/j.1460-9568.1999.00576.x

Sala, C., and Segal, M. (2014). Dendritic spines: the locus of structural and functional plasticity. *Physiol. Rev.* 94, 141–188. doi: 10.1152/physrev.00012.2013

Segal, M. (1995). Dendritic spines for neuroprotection: a hypothesis. *Trends Neurosci.* 18, 468–471. doi: 10.1016/0166-2236(95)92765-i

Shepherd, G. M. (1983). *Neurobiology.* New York: Oxford University Press.

Shepherd, G. M. (1996). The dendritic spines: a multifunctional integrative unit. *J. Neurophysiol.* 75, 2197–2210.

Silva, A. J., Bickle, J., and Landreth, A. (2013). *Engineering the Next Revolution in Neuroscience: The New Science of Experiment Planning.* Oxford: Oxford University Press.

Soderling, S. H., Guire, E. S., Kaech, S., White, J., Zhang, F., Schutz, K., et al. (2007). A WAVE-1 and WRP signaling complex regulates spine density, synaptic plasticity and memory. *J. Neurosci.* 27, 355–365. doi: 10.1523/jneurosci.3209-06.2006

Stevens, C. F. (1998). A million dollar question: does LTP = memory? *Neuron* 20, 1–2. doi: 10.1016/s0896-6273(00)80426-2

Yuste, R. (2011). Dendritic spines and distributed circuits. *Neuron* 71, 772–781. doi: 10.1016/j.neuron.2011.07.024

Yuste, R. (2013). Electrical compartmentalization in dendritic spines. *Annu. Rev. Neurosci.* 36, 429–444. doi: 10.1146/annurev-neuro-062111-150455

Structural plasticity: mechanisms and contribution to developmental psychiatric disorders

Yann Bernardinelli, Irina Nikonenko and Dominique Muller *

Department of Basic Neurosciences, University of Geneva Medical School, Geneva, Switzerland

***Correspondence:**
Dominique Muller, Department of Basic Neurosciences, University of Geneva Medical School, 1, M. Servet, 1211 Geneva 4, Switzerland
e-mail: Dominique.Muller@unige.ch

Synaptic plasticity mechanisms are usually discussed in terms of changes in synaptic strength. The capacity of excitatory synapses to rapidly modify the membrane expression of glutamate receptors in an activity-dependent manner plays a critical role in learning and memory processes by re-distributing activity within neuronal networks. Recent work has however also shown that functional plasticity properties are associated with a rewiring of synaptic connections and a selective stabilization of activated synapses. These structural aspects of plasticity have the potential to continuously modify the organization of synaptic networks and thereby introduce specificity in the wiring diagram of cortical circuits. Recent work has started to unravel some of the molecular mechanisms that underlie these properties of structural plasticity, highlighting an important role of signaling pathways that are also major candidates for contributing to developmental psychiatric disorders. We review here some of these recent advances and discuss the hypothesis that alterations of structural plasticity could represent a common mechanism contributing to the cognitive and functional defects observed in diseases such as intellectual disability, autism spectrum disorders and schizophrenia.

Keywords: dendritic spines, excitatory synapses, plasticity, morphology, astrocyte

INTRODUCTION

Dendritic spines are the major site for excitatory transmission in the brain. They are usually contacted by en passant presynaptic terminals and most often surrounded by astrocytic processes, forming complex structures that dysplay a high degree of functional and structural plasticity. While most research attention has usually focused on the functional aspects of synaptic plasticity and their key contribution to learning and memory mechanisms, work in the last decade has clearly demonstrated the importance of the associated structural rearrangements. These consist of different types of morphological changes (enlargement, growth, pruning, stabilization), affecting different partners (spines, terminals, astrocytic processes) and taking place on different time scales (minutes to days), making them sometimes difficult to relate to the functional changes. These structural rearrangements are also tightly controlled by activity, they are usually NMDA receptor dependent, and have the potential to significantly affect the development and organization of local synaptic networks. Recent advances have started to unravel some of complex molecular mechanisms and signaling systems regulating these synaptic rearrangements, notably at the postsynaptic level. We will therefore mainly focus on these aspects in this review and highlight the multiplicity of mechanisms that may affect structural plasticity and the development of synaptic networks and thereby contribute to cognitive disorders.

MORPHOLOGICAL VARIABILITY OF EXCITATORY SYNAPSES

A particular characteristic of dendritic spines is the high variability of their morphological organization. They display major variations in volume, with large spines being several hundred times larger than small spines, but also in length, shape and content in organelles such as ribosomes, endosomal systems or spine apparatus. This high morphological variability is believed to reflect different functional properties of excitatory synapses linked to the size of the postsynaptic density, the number of postsynaptic receptors inserted in the postsynaptic density, the strength of the synapse, its developmental stage or even its stability over time. It is thus often considered that spine morphology correlates with functional parameters (Bourne and Harris, 2008). Large spines usually referred to as mushroom type of spines, or sometimes also as memory spines, are associated with mature, stable synapses that have been strengthened through a process of activity- or plasticity-mediated enlargement. In contrast, thin, elongated spines with small heads, sometimes called learning spines, are interpreted as representing young, newly formed synaptic structures that are more likely to be eliminated over time (Bourne and Harris, 2007). Several *in vitro* and *in vivo* studies have shown a high correlation between the size of the spine head, the size of the postsynaptic density, the size of glutamate-evoked responses and the stability of the spine (Kasai et al., 2003; Matsuzaki et al., 2004). In addition to thin spines, another type of protrusion often analyzed separately are filopodia, usually characterized by the absence of enlargement at the tip. Filopodia are believed to represent precursors of dendritic spines (Ziv and Smith, 1996; Petrak et al., 2005; Toni et al., 2007; Kayser et al., 2008) and they are mainly seen during early stages of development, where they can represent up to 20% of all protrusions. In adolescent and adult tissue however, they constitute only a few percent of all protrusions depending upon criteria used to identify them and their function remains largely unclear as a majority of filopodia just appear and disappear without transforming into spine synapses (Zuo et al., 2005; De Roo et al., 2008a). Overall, based on our current understanding of spine properties, it seems likely that the high morphological variability of dendritic spines reflects the different stages of maturation of excitatory synapses and their individual history. Accordingly, alterations of spine morphology or spine density, as seen in some developmental psychiatric disorders, are often interpreted as indicating defects in spine morphogenesis, stability or plasticity. A more in depth analysis of the dynamic properties of dendritic spines could however provide a better understanding of the underlying defects.

MECHANISM CONTRIBUTING TO STRUCTURAL PLASTICITY

A major breakthrough made possible by the development of *in vivo* confocal imaging approaches has been the demonstration that dendritic spines are highly plastic structures that not only continuously change in shape over time (Matus, 2000; Yasumatsu et al., 2008), but can also be formed and eliminated throughout life in an activity-dependent manner (Lendvai et al., 2000; Holtmaat et al., 2005; Caroni et al., 2012). These observations support the concept of a dynamic regulation of excitatory synaptic networks by activity and plasticity mechanisms. A striking aspect of this dynamic regulation of connectivity is its magnitude during periods of intense development such as critical periods and the fact that it then decreases with age (Zuo et al., 2005; Holtmaat and Svoboda, 2009). This is consistent with the notion that the control of spine dynamics by activity plays a central role in shaping the organization of local synaptic networks during development, whereas the reduced structural plasticity still present in older animals maintains possibilities of adaptation while minimizing the possible disruption of existing circuits.

These synaptic rearrangements involve multiple mechanisms to control the formation, maintenance and elimination of excitatory synapses. It is very likely that distinct molecular pathways regulate these different mechanisms independently, as specific manipulations can selectively affect formation, stabilization or elimination of protrusions (Mendez et al., 2010b; Koleske, 2013; Kehoe et al., 2014). Additionally there probably exists homeostatic regulations that coordinate these processes and can compensate for alterations of one or the other mechanism. For example, we have observed that transfection of pyramidal neurons with a dominant-negative mutant of N-cadherin, that strongly reduces spine stability, also leads to a compensatory increase in spine formation (Mendez et al., 2010a). Finally, these different mechanisms are finely tuned by activity and plasticity induction, adding another complexity to their regulation.

In the context of learning related paradigms (LTP), there appear to be two major structural types of changes that have been reported both in *in vitro* systems such as the hippocampal organotypic slice culture or under *in vivo* conditions in anesthetized mice (De Roo et al., 2008b; Hübener and Bonhoeffer, 2010). In slice cultures, induction of long-term potentiation results in two major changes: an increase in spine turnover, characterized by an increase in spine growth but also in spine elimination (Engert and Bonhoeffer, 1999; Nägerl et al., 2004; De Roo et al., 2008b), and a selective stabilization of activated synapses (De Roo et al., 2008b; Hill and Zito, 2013). In living mice, similar changes have also been observed in the visual or motor cortices (Keck et al., 2008; Xu et al., 2009). Notably, in mice trained for a dexterity motor task, spine turnover increases and correlates with the ability to learn the task, while there is also a specific stabilization of newly formed spines that correlates with the memory or retention of the task (Xu et al., 2009; Yang et al., 2009). Based on this type of results, one can thus propose that changes in spine turnover and changes in spine stability represent two key mechanisms associated with memory that could account for some of its antinomic properties: the capacity to learn, which requires adaptation of existing networks, and the capacity to retain information, which requires to maintain important functional circuits (Caroni et al., 2012; see **Figure 1**).

ACTIVITY-DEPENDENT CHANGES IN SPINE MORPHOLOGY AND STABILITY

Identification of stimulated synapses within a network has been and still is one of the important limitations for understanding how activity and plasticity regulate synapse properties. This has been overcome in only a few studies using either 2-photon uncaging of glutamate to achieve local stimulation of identified synapses or calcium imaging coupled to electrical stimulation to reveal functional synapses. Although previous electron microscopic (EM) analyses had already suggested that LTP could be associated with morphological changes (Fifková and Anderson, 1981; Geinisman, 1993; Buchs and Muller, 1996), the early, elegant studies by Kasai group (Matsuzaki et al., 2004) were the first to provide a direct demonstration that induction of plasticity was indeed associated with a rapid increase in size of stimulated synapses and an increased sensitivity to glutamate. Other experiments further showed that this enlargement can last several hours (Zito et al., 2009) and that it is correlated with a reorganization of the actin cytoskeleton (Honkura et al., 2008). These observations were thus perfectly in line with accumulating evidence suggesting an implication of the actin cytoskeleton and various actin-regulatory proteins in both LTP maintenance and spine morphology (Fukazawa et al., 2003; Lisman, 2003; Chen et al., 2007; Bramham, 2008). As previously mentioned and revelaed by the studies in hippocampal slice cultures, the structural changes affecting stimulated synapses are also correlated with a major increase in their long-term stability (De Roo et al., 2008b; Hill and Zito, 2013). Very few stimulated synapses disappeared within the days that followed their stimulation, while in contrast non stimulated synapses located on the same dendrite tended to be eliminated at a faster rate. Whether the change in spine stability is directly related to the activity-dependent enlargement remains however unclear. Spine size and spine stability show indeed a high degree of correlation. Repetitive imaging experiments indicate

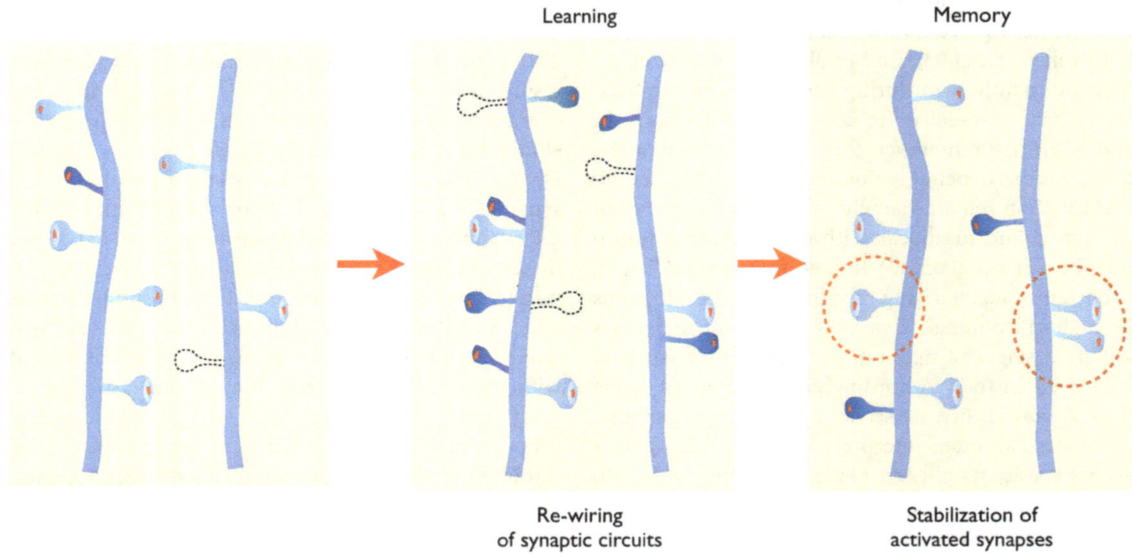

FIGURE 1 | Activity-mediated structural plasticity. Left panel: synaptic networks are characterized by a continuous process of growth (dark blue spine) and elimination (dotted line) of dendritic spines that is developmentally regulated. Middle panel: during learning or learning related activity, baseline turnover is significantly enhanced leading to an increased formation and elimination of synaptic contacts, thus allowing remodeling and adaptation of connectivity. New spines also tend to grow in the proximity of activated synapses favoring the formation of spine clusters. Right panel: newly formed and activated synapses are preferentially stabilized (dotted circles) allowing to maintain important functional connections.

that the size of spine heads continuously fluctuates over a time scale of days (Holtmaat et al., 2005; Yasumatsu et al., 2008). Furthermore, the fact that the activity-dependent spine enlargement seems to be only transient and to reverse within 24 h, while the improved stability can be measured over days suggests that they are regulated by different mechanisms (De Roo et al., 2008b).

The molecular nature of the mechanisms confering a high stability to activated spines remains also an open issue. Evidence from different studies suggest that the structural organization of the actin cytoskeleton within the spine head could contribute to modify spine stability (Fukazawa et al., 2003; Chen et al., 2007). Phosphorylation of the cytoskeleton-stabilizing protein beta-adducin appears to be required for spine stabilization (Bednarek and Caroni, 2011). Also, several molecules regulating actin polymerization and notably upstream and downstream regulators of Rho GTPases affect the capacity of spines to enlarge and their stability (Rex et al., 2009; Murakoshi et al., 2011; Dubos et al., 2012). Proteins that could also be important to confer stability are adhesion molecules expressed at excitatory synapses. Neuroligins, integrins, ephrins and N-cadherins have all been proposed to contribute to the persistence of spines (Wang et al., 2008; Matter et al., 2009; Bozdagi et al., 2010; McGeachie et al., 2011; Koleske, 2013), although a direct demonstration of their role in long-term activity-dependent spine stability is still often missing. In studies that we carried out to analyze the role of N-cadherin in structural plasticity, we found that an extracellular mutant of N-cadherin strongly affects the life time of dendritic spines and that it prevents activity-mediated spine stabilization (Mendez et al., 2010a). We also showed that N-cadherin is not expressed in all spines and that the spines in which it is expressed show an increased stability. Furthermore N-cadherin expression could be increased through activity patterns that induce LTP, and following stimulation we found that the adhesion molecule selectively accumulates in spines that had been activated. These results thus suggest that modifications in the adhesion profile of activated synapses contribute to regulate the stability and life time of spine synapses (Mendez et al., 2010a). It seems likely that this effect is mediated by increasing trans-synaptic interactions between pre- and postsynaptic structures as molecular complexes showing a periodic organization compatible with the existence of N-cadherin meshwork has been identified in the synaptic cleft of excitatory synapses (Zuber et al., 2005). Adhesion could also be reinforced between synaptic structures and the third partner of the tripartite synapse: the astroglial component. EM studies (Lushnikova et al., 2009) as well as work by Bernardinelli et al. (2014) suggest that synaptic activity and LTP induction can drive a reorganization of astrocytic processes around activated synapses. This glial structural remodeling is mediated by direct activation of glial metabotropic receptors by the released transmitter and calcium influx in the astrocytic process. This transient increase in motility of the astrocytic process leads to a better coverage of the synapse and an enhanced long-term stability of the synaptic contact. This effect has been observed both under *in vitro* and *in vivo* conditions in the somatosensory cortex and is summarized in **Figure 2**. These new results thus suggest a new role of astrocytic processes in the activity-dependent structural organization of the synapse and a contribution of the astrocyte to the generation of life-long, persistent synapses. In line

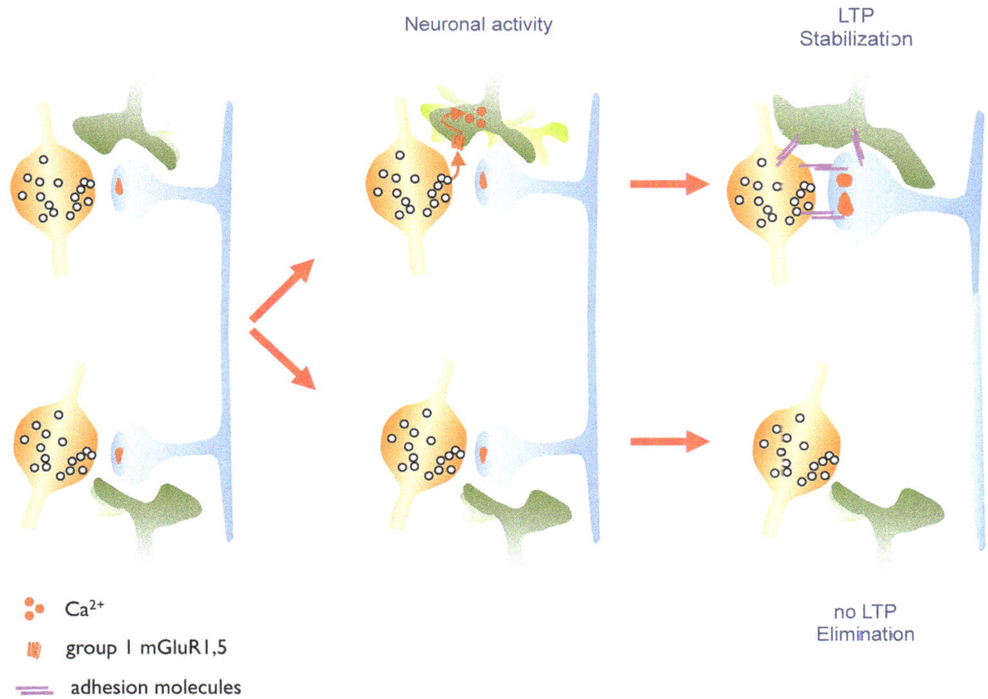

FIGURE 2 | Astrocytic structural plasticity contributes to the maintenance of activated synapses. Left panel: excitatory synapses are surrounded by astrocytic processes that show a high level of motility. Middle panel: this astrocytic motility is regulated by the released neurotransmitter, which activates glutamate metabotropic receptors on the astrocytic process leading to an increased calcium flux and motility of the astrocytic process. Right panel: when driven by learning related paradigms (LTP, upper synapse), this enhanced motility leads to an increased and more stable coverage of the synapse by the astrocytic process resulting in a long-lasting stabilization of the synapse. This mechanism might involve, among other possibilities, a contribution of adhesion molecules.

with these observations, recent work has also demonstrated a critical role of astrocytes in LTP mechanisms and long-term memory in mice (Suzuki et al., 2011). Conversely, there are multiple examples showing that molecular interference with the mechanisms of spine stabilization described above significantly affect cognitive functions (Allen et al., 1998; Sudhof, 2008; Redies et al., 2012; Vukojevic et al., 2012; Ba et al., 2013).

MECHANISMS OF ACTIVITY-DEPENDENT SPINE TURNOVER

The now classical experiments made by Engert and Bonhoeffer (1999) provided the first evidence that induction of plasticity could result in the growth of new dendritic spines. Further studies by several groups confirmed that these new spines display synapses with all the characteristics of morphologically mature and functional contacts (Toni et al., 1999; Nägerl et al., 2007). *In vivo* studies then showed that spine formation and elimination occurred continuously in a developmentally regulated manner and independently of activity (Lendvai et al., 2000; Holtmaat et al., 2005; Zuo et al., 2005). These mechanisms however are strongly enhanced by sensory or motor activity (Holtmaat et al., 2006; Xu et al., 2009). Consistently theta activity or induction of plasticity in hippocampal slices also strongly promotes spine turnover, enhancing both formation and elimination of dendritic spines, leading to a significant activity-dependent rewiring of the hippocampal circuit (De Roo et al., 2008b).

One interesting issue raised by these observations is whether mechanisms of spine growth and elimination are independently regulated. Although activity appears to stimulate both processes simultaneously, several recent results suggest that these two mechanisms are regulated independently of each other. For example, treatment with estrogens results in a significant increase in spine density both in *in vitro* and *in vivo* experiments (Yankova et al., 2001; Sakamoto et al., 2003; Mendez et al., 2010b). Turnover analyses revealed that this effect resulted from a significant increase in spine growth mechanisms, but without changes in spine elimination, thereby accounting for the changes in density. Similarly, specific effects on spine growth mechanisms without alterations of spine elimination have been observed following interference with P21 activated kinase (PAK3; Dubos et al., 2012), by direct activation of the cytoskeletal regulatory protein vasodilator-stimulated phosphoprotein (VASP; Lin et al., 2007; Nikonenko et al., 2013) and following application of BDNF or the phosphatase and tensin homolog (PTEN) inhibitor BpV (Tanaka et al., 2008; Boda et al., 2014). This suggests therefore that mechanisms that promote actin polymerization can directly stimulate spine growth and that signaling pathways implicated in the regulation of protein synthesis such as the PI3K-AKT-mTor pathway participate in the control of this growth process. Conversely, there are also mechanisms that selectively affect spine elimination without altering spine growth processes. This might be the case of long-term depression that has been shown in several recent studies to result in spine shrinkage and disappearance (Becker et al., 2008; Oh et al., 2013; Wiegert and Oertner, 2013). The molecular mechanisms implicated in this effect remain unclear but are likely to require activation of both NMDA and glutamate metabotropic receptors (Oh et al., 2013). Consistent with this interpretation, we recently identified a specific role of the inclusion of the GluN3A subunit in NMDA receptors in the regulation of spine pruning (Kehoe et al., 2013). The GluN3A subunit is highly expressed during critical periods of development and its expression is associated with a decrease in spine density (Roberts et al., 2009). By manipulating the expression of this subunit using gain or loss of function experiments, we found that a central mechanism accounting for these effects is a selective increase in spine pruning associated with expression of the GluN3A subunit (Kehoe et al., 2014). These results thus clearly indicate that spine density can be differentially regulated by interfering with either spine growth or elimination mechanisms.

Whether and how these mechanisms of spine turnover contribute to cognitive functions remains still unclear. However alterations of spine turnover have been reported for cases of intellectual disability or autism spectrum disorders (Cruz-Martín et al., 2010; Pan et al., 2010; Dubos et al., 2012) and mechanisms that regulate spine growth and turnover are also associated with cognitive defects and autism spectrum disorders (Sharma et al., 2010; Cao et al., 2013; Boda et al., 2014).

MECHANISMS UNDERLYING SPINE CLUSTERING

An interesting observation related to activity-dependent spine growth mechanisms is that the formation of the new spines occurs in a non-random fashion but is more readily observed in close proximity to activated synapses leading sometimes to the formation of spine clusters (De Roo et al., 2008b; Dubos et al., 2012). This phenomenon, initially detected in hippocampal slice cultures, was then also observed under *in vivo* conditions following a motor learning task (Fu et al., 2012). An intriguing question relates to the mechanism that could promote the growth of new spines in clusters or in regions of activity. Several hypotheses can be considered. First, there is evidence from *in vitro* work that application of glutamate or uncaging of glutamate on a dendrite can rapidly trigger the growth of a new spine (Richards et al., 2005; Kwon and Sabatini, 2011). The phenomenon was shown to depend upon the activity of protein kinases in the postsynaptic dendrite. One could thus consider that intense presynaptic activity and glutamate release could trigger the growth of new spines in small brain areas. One major difficulty with this interpretation is the timing of spine formation. Spine growth was observed to occur within minutes after glutamate uncaging, whereas activity-dependent spine growth is a much slower process that can only be visualized hours after stimulation, long after glutamate release has taken place (Engert and Bonhoeffer, 1999; De Roo et al., 2008b). Although this does not exclude a role for glutamate release, it certainly indicates that activity-induced spine growth is not equivalent to the effects of glutamate uncaging. Another interpretation has recently been proposed based on experiments analyzing the role of nitric oxide (NO) on synapse development (Nikonenko et al., 2013). Nitric oxide can be generated at excitatory synapses in response to NMDA receptor activation of NO synthase, which is closely associated with the postsynaptic density (Burette et al., 2002; Ishii et al., 2006; d'Anglemont de Tassigny et al., 2007). Interventions that blocked NO production or guanilate kinase, the main downstream effector of NO, strongly reduced spine growth mechanisms including the enhancement produced by induction of plasticity (Nikonenko et al., 2013). Conversely, application of cGMP enhanced spine formation, occluding the effects of synaptic activity. Interestingly, these effects could be traced to the phosphorylation of the actin regulatory protein VASP by cGMP kinase. Expression of VASP phospho-mutants that either mimicked or prevented phosphorylation by cGMP kinase reproduced or blocked the effects of activity on spine growth mechanisms (Nikonenko et al., 2013). Moreover in mice deficient in NO synthase, the development of spine synapses was considerably affected and exposure of these mice to an enriched environment failed to promote an increase in synapse density. Analysis of the distribution of spine synapses also revealed a lack of clustering of synapses, a phenomenon readily observed in wild type mice (Nikonenko et al., 2013). These findings thus suggest that one mechanism that may account for the activity-dependent clustering of spines around active sites could involve the production of NO by activated synapses, which in turn stimulates protrusion growth through the phosphorylation of the regulatory protein VASP, promoting in this way the formation of synapses in areas where active partners are found (summary in **Figure 3**).

While the functional importance of this clustering phenomenon remains still unclear, it is interesting that interference with NO production or signaling is associated with impaired cognitive performance and social dysfunction (Kirchner et al., 2004; Kelley et al., 2009; Tanda et al., 2009; Wass et al., 2009)

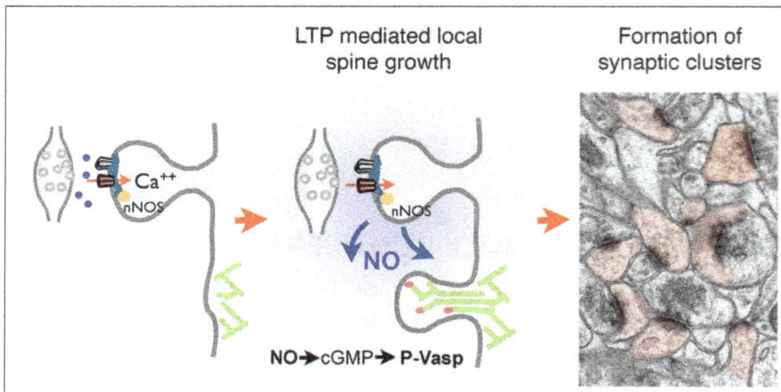

FIGURE 3 | Regulation of local spine growth by nitric oxide (NO). Left panel: neuronal NO synthase (nNOS), present in the postsynaptic density and tightly associated with PSD-95 and NMDA receptors, generates NO upon NMDA receptor activation and calcium influx. Middle panel: NO generated at activated synapses by LTP diffuses locally and triggers the activation of a cGMP-dependent cascade leading to the phosphorylation of the cytoskeleton regulatory protein VASP by cGMP-dependent kinase. This in turn promotes actin filament elongation and spine formation. Right panel: this mechanisms allows the formation of clusters of spine synapses around activated contacts, a phenomenon absent in nNOS deficient mice. The electron microscopy image illustrates clusters of dendritic spines (filled in rose) in the hippocampus of wild type mouse raised in an enriched environment.

and variants of the NO synthase 1 gene have been linked to schizophrenia (Shinkai et al., 2002; Bernstein et al., 2011).

SYNAPTIC DEFECTS IN DEVELOPMENTAL PSYCHIATRIC DISORDERS

All these data highlight the complexity of the mechanisms regulating the dynamics of excitatory synapses during development and strongly suggest that any interference with these structural plasticity properties may have a significant impact on the organization and functional properties of excitatory networks. Changes in spine stability or spine turnover can be expected to affect the number, but also the specificity of excitatory synapses resulting in the formation of synaptic circuits displaying various abnormal features such as hyper- or hypo-connectivity and hyper- or hypo-dynamic responses to activity (Mukai et al., 2008; Pan et al., 2010; Qiu et al., 2011). All these different alterations, by affecting the development and functional properties of synaptic networks, might decrease the reliability of information processing and lead to the formation of maladaptative brain circuits (Sigurdsson et al., 2010). Depending on the molecular mechanism involved, the alterations could affect differentially various brain areas or have a greater impact during different phases of development, thereby accounting for the variability in clinical or behavioral phenotypes. One would also anticipate that alterations of structural plasticity with a strong impact during critical periods of development might have more damaging consequences that could be difficult to reverse and would require very early interventions in order to compensate for the defects. Such early approaches are now tested in many situations related to autism spectrum disorders (Canitano, 2014).

Based on these observations, we propose that a possibly common feature of various developmental psychiatric disorders could be the existence of alterations in the dynamic properties of excitatory synapses. This would be consistent with the strong developmental component of these disorders and the multitude of synaptic proteins possibly implicated. This could also account for the fact that regions showing a high degree of plasticity, such as the prefrontal cortex and the hippocampus, are very often showing functional defects. Finally, in line with this hypothesis, signaling pathways that play an important role in regulating spine dynamics are major candidates for contributing to psychiatric disorders. Examples include Rho GTPases signaling and their regulation of the actin cytoskeleton and the signaling cascades implicated in the control of protein synthesis (Sawicka and Zukin, 2012; Ba et al., 2013). These two signaling systems are particularly important at excitatory synapses to control spine morphology and plasticity, and several genetic alterations associated with psychiatric disorders affect molecules implicated in these two pathways (Boda et al., 2010; Fromer et al., 2014).

The Rho GTPases signaling pathway comprises several molecules that have been associated with intellectual disability, autism spectrum disorders or schizophrenia. Examples include membrane receptors and adhesion molecules able to activate Rho GTPases (cadherins, ephrins), regulators of Rho GTPases (oligophrenin1, GDI1, ARHGEF6, EPAC2, CNK2 (connector enhancer of KSR-2), srGAP3, Disc1, SynGAP), effectors of Rho GTPases (PAK3), as well as cytoskeletal regulatory proteins (Endris et al., 2002; Govek et al., 2004; Nodé-Langlois et al., 2006; Woolfrey et al., 2009; Hayashi-Takagi et al., 2010; Clement et al., 2012; Lim et al., 2014). In many of these cases, alterations of synapse morphology or function have been reported, although analyses of spine dynamics are still often missing. There is one example that we have studied in more details and that concerns the intellectual disability protein PAK3. Several mutations of PAK3 are associated with intellectual disability in humans. Expression of the mutant PAK3 in hippocampal neurons or genetic and pharmacological suppression of PAK3 were all found to result in alterations of spine morphology and spine dynamics (Kreis et al., 2007; Dubos et al., 2012). The two main features observed following interference with PAK3 function were an increase in spontaneous spine growth mechanisms and a block of activity-dependent spine stabilization. Consequently, this resulted in an excessively dynamic synaptic network in which activity failed to selectively stabilize activated synapses (Dubos et al., 2012). This was also reflected by the presence of a high proportion of thin, immature spines and a reduced number of large mushroom type spines (Boda et al., 2004). It can be assumed therefore that these defects resulted in a failure to maintain important connections and to develop specificity in the wiring organization.

The second important pathway strongly implicated in psychiatric disorders involves a number of molecules regulating local protein synthesis. This includes membrane receptors (BDNF and TrkB, Insulin receptor, Ephrins) or adhesion and scaffold molecules (integrins, neuroligin/neurexin complex, shank, SynGAP), intracellular mediators implicated in mTOR signaling (PI3K, Akt, PTEN, TSC2) and regulators of protein synthesis (FMRP, CYFIP1) (Kumar et al., 2005; Lai and Ip, 2009; Mendez et al., 2010a; Sharma et al., 2010; Cuesto et al., 2011; Clement et al., 2012; Boda et al., 2014). This pathway is also critically implicated in the regulation of synaptic strength and in most cases alterations of spine morphology or density have been reported, suggesting impairments of structural plasticity. One of the most studied examples is certainly Fragile X syndrome, associated to multiple CGG repeats in the *fmr1* gene (Bhakar et al., 2012). Mice deficient in FMRP protein show alterations of spine morphology with an increased proportion of thin, elongated spines (Comery et al., 1997, but see also Wijetunge et al., 2014). Recent work using Fmr1 knocout mice provided evidence that these spines are hyper-dynamic, do not respond to sensory stimulation (Pan et al., 2010) and lack stability (Cruz-Martín et al., 2010). In slice culture experiments, we also found that spine turnover was excessively sensitive to activity and more specifically that induction of plasticity failed to induce a differential stabilization of activated spines. Interestingly, in these experiments, we were able to reverse this deficit through application of a PTEN inhibitor, which enhances the PI3K-Akt-mTOR signaling pathway (Boda et al., 2014), while interfering with metabotropic glutamate receptors was only partly effective (Cruz-Martín et al., 2010; Boda et al., 2014). This PTEN inhibitor also improved an associated deficit in LTP mechanisms and when injected in FMR1 deficient mice restored reversal learning in the Morris water maze task (Boda et al., 2014). While much remains to be understood regarding the mechanisms through which local protein synthesis could affect structural plasticity, these data suggest that this system may be an interesting target for modulating properties of spine dynamics and eventually counterbalance some of the deficits observed in the associated disorders.

CONCLUSION

Functional synaptic plasticity properties, by quickly changing synaptic strength, allow fast adaptations of network activity which are critical for information processing. However, on a longer time scale, structural plasticity properties may allow a more significant and stable rewiring of synaptic networks through both the formation of new connections and the stabilization of specific contacts. These properties of structural plasticity are particularly important during development where they contribute to shape the structural organization of brain circuits through activity. Molecular analyses of these structural properties started to identify key signaling pathways implicated in these synaptic reorganizations, which also appear to be strong candidates for contributing to cognitive and psychiatric disorders. Hence a common denominator of developmental disorders could involve alterations in spine dynamics that would affect the connectivity and specificity of brain circuits. More systematic analyses of these properties and their functional consequences should allow a better understanding of how they affect information processing and this could eventually lead to new possibilities of treatment of these disorders.

ACKNOWLEDGMENTS

This work was supported by the Swiss Science Foundation (grant 310030B_144080) and NCCR Synapsy.

REFERENCES

Allen, K. M., Gleeson, J. G., Bagrodia, S., Partington, M. W., MacMillan, J. C., Cerione, R. A., et al. (1998). PAK3 mutation in nonsyndromic X-linked mental retardation. *Nat. Genet.* 20, 25–30. doi: 10.1038/1675

Ba, W., van der Raadt, J., and Nadif Kasri, N. (2013). Rho GTPase signaling at the synapse: implications for intellectual disability. *Exp. Cell Res.* 319, 2368–2374. doi: 10.1016/j.yexcr.2013.05.033

Becker, N., Wierenga, C. J., Fonseca, R., Bonhoeffer, T., and Nägerl, U. V. (2008). LTD induction causes morphological changes of presynaptic boutons and reduces their contacts with spines. *Neuron* 60, 590–597. doi: 10.1016/j.neuron.2008.09.018

Bednarek, E., and Caroni, P. (2011). β-Adducin is required for stable assembly of new synapses and improved memory upon environmental enrichment. *Neuron* 69, 1132–1146. doi: 10.1016/j.neuron.2011.02.034

Bernardinelli, Y., Randall, J., Janett, E., Nikonenko, I., Konig, S., Jones, E. V., et al. (2014). Activity-dependent structural plasticity of perisynaptic astrocytic domains promotes excitatory synapse stability. *Curr. Biol.* 24, 1679–1688. doi: 10.1016/j.cub.2014.06.025

Bernstein, H. G., Keilhoff, G., Steiner, J., Dobrowolny, H., and Bogerts, B. (2011). Nitric oxide and schizophrenia: present knowledge and emerging concepts of therapy. *CNS Neurol. Disord. Drug Targets* 10, 792–807. doi: 10.2174/187152711798072392

Bhakar, A. L., Dölen, G., and Bear, M. F. (2012). The pathophysiology of fragile X (and what it teaches us about synapses). *Annu. Rev. Neurosci.* 35, 417–443. doi: 10.1146/annurev-neuro-060909-153138

Boda, B., Alberi, S., Nikonenko, I., Node-Langlois, R., Jourdain, P., Moosmayer, M., et al. (2004). The mental retardation protein PAK3 contributes to synapse formation and plasticity in hippocampus. *J. Neurosci.* 24, 10816–10825. doi: 10.1523/jneurosci.2931-04.2004

Boda, B., Dubos, A., and Muller, D. (2010). Signaling mechanisms regulating synapse formation and function in mental retardation. *Curr. Opin. Neurobiol.* 20, 519–527. doi: 10.1016/j.conb.2010.03.012

Boda, B., Mendez, P., Boury-Jamot, B., Magara, F., and Muller, D. (2014). Reversal of activity-mediated spine dynamics and learning impairment in a mouse model of Fragile X syndrome. *Eur. J. Neurosci.* 39, 1130–1137. doi: 10.1111/ejn.12488

Bourne, J., and Harris, K. M. (2007). Do thin spines learn to be mushroom spines that remember? *Curr. Opin. Neurobiol.* 17, 381–3886. doi: 10.1016/j.conb.2007.04.009

Bourne, J. N., and Harris, K. M. (2008). Balancing structure and function at hippocampal dendritic spines. *Annu. Rev. Neurosci.* 31, 47–67. doi: 10.1146/annurev.neuro.31.060407.125646

Bozdagi, O., Wang, X. B., Nikitczuk, J. S., Anderson, T. R., Bloss, E. B., Radice, G. L., et al. (2010). Persistence of coordinated long-term potentiation and dendritic spine enlargement at mature hippocampal CA1 synapses requires N-cadherin. *J. Neurosci.* 30, 9984–9989. doi: 10.1523/jneurosci.1223-10.2010

Bramham, C. R. (2008). Local protein synthesis, actin dynamics and LTP consolidation. *Curr. Opin. Neurobiol.* 18, 524–531. doi: 10.1016/j.conb.2008.09.013

Buchs, P. A., and Muller, D. (1996). Induction of long-term potentiation is associated with major ultrastructural changes of activated synapses. *Proc. Natl. Acad. Sci. U S A* 93, 8040–8045. doi: 10.1073/pnas.93.15.8040

Burette, A., Zabel, U., Weinberg, R. J., Schmidt, H. H., and Valtschanoff, J. G. (2002). Synaptic localization of nitric oxide synthase and soluble guanylyl cyclase in the hippocampus. *J. Neurosci.* 22, 8961–8970.

Canitano, R. (2014). New experimental treatments for core social domain in autism spectrum disorders. *Front. Pediatr.* 2:61. doi: 10.3389/fped.2014.00061

Cao, C., Rioult-Pedotti, M. S., Migani, P., Yu, C. J., Tiwari, R., Parang, K., et al. (2013). Impairment of TrkB-PSD-95 signaling in Angelman syndrome. *PLoS Biol.* 11:e1001478. doi: 10.1371/journal.pbio.1001848

Caroni, P., Donato, F., and Muller, D. (2012). Structural plasticity upon learning: regulation and functions. *Nat. Rev. Neurosci.* 13, 478–490. doi: 10.1038/nrn3258

Chen, L. Y., Rex, C. S., Casale, M. S., Gall, C. M., and Lynch, G. (2007). Changes in synaptic morphology accompany actin signaling during LTP. *J. Neurosci.* 27, 5363–5372. doi: 10.1523/jneurosci.0164-07.2007

Clement, J. P., Aceti, M., Creson, T. K., Ozkan, E. D., Shi, Y., Reish, N. J., et al. (2012). Pathogenic SYNGAP1 mutations impair cognitive development by disrupting maturation of dendritic spine synapses. *Cell* 151, 709–723. doi: 10.1016/j.cell.2012.08.045

Comery, T. A., Harris, J. B., Willems, P. J., Oostra, B. A., Irwin, S. A., Weiler, I. J., et al. (1997). Abnormal dendritic spines in fragile X knockout mice: maturation and pruning deficits. *Proc. Natl. Acad. Sci. U S A* 94, 5401–5404. doi: 10.1073/pnas.94.10.5401

Cruz-Martín, A., Crespo, M., and Portera-Cailliau, C. (2010). Delayed stabilization of dendritic spines in fragile X mice. *J. Neurosci.* 30, 7793–7803. doi: 10.1523/JNEUROSCI.0577-10.2010

Cuesto, G., Enriquez-Barreto, L., Caramés, C., Cantarero, M., Gasull, X., Sandi, C., et al. (2011). Phosphoinositide-3-kinase activation controls synaptogenesis and spinogenesis in hippocampal neurons. *J. Neurosci.* 31, 2721–2733. doi: 10.1523/JNEUROSCI.4477-10.2011

d'Anglemont de Tassigny, X., Campagne, C., Dehouck, B., Leroy, D., Holstein, G. R., Beauvillain, J. C., et al. (2007). Coupling of neuronal nitric oxide synthase to NMDA receptors via postsynaptic density-95 depends on estrogen and contributes to the central control of adult female reproduction. *J. Neurosci.* 27, 6103–6114. doi: 10.1523/jneurosci.5595-06.2007

De Roo, M., Klauser, P., Mendez, P., Poglia, L., and Muller, D. (2008a). Activity-dependent PSD formation and stabilization of newly formed spines in hippocampal slice cultures. *Cereb. Cortex* 18, 151–161. doi: 10.1093/cercor/bhm041

De Roo, M., Klauser, P., and Muller, D. (2008b). LTP promotes a selective long-term stabilization and clustering of dendritic spines. *PLoS Biol.* 6:e219. doi: 10.3410/f.1124276.581429

Dubos, A., Combeau, G., Bernardinelli, Y., Barnier, J. V., Hartley, O., Gaertner, H., et al. (2012). Alteration of synaptic network dynamics by the intellectual disability protein PAK3. *J. Neurosci.* 32, 519–527. doi: 10.1523/JNEUROSCI.3252-11.2012

Endris, V., Wogatzky, B., Leimer, U., Bartsch, D., Zatyka, M., Latif, F., et al. (2002). The novel Rho-GTPase activating gene MEGAP/ srGAP3 has a putative role in severe mental retardation. *Proc. Natl. Acad. Sci. U S A* 99, 11754–11759. doi: 10.1073/pnas.162241099

Engert, F., and Bonhoeffer, T. (1999). Dendritic spine changes associated with hippocampal long-term synaptic plasticity. *Nature* 399, 66–70. doi: 10.1038/19978

Fifková, E., and Anderson, C. L. (1981). Stimulation-induced changes in dimensions of stalks of dendritic spines in the dentate molecular layer. *Exp. Neurol.* 74, 621–627. doi: 10.1016/0014-4886(81)90197-7

Fromer, M., Pocklington, A. J., Kavanagh, D. H., Williams, H. J., Dwyer, S., Gormley, P., et al. (2014). De novo mutations in schizophrenia implicate synaptic networks. *Nature* 506, 179–184. doi: 10.1038/nature12929

Fu, M., Yu, X., Lu, J., and Zuo, Y. (2012). Repetitive motor learning induces coordinated formation of clustered dendritic spines in vivo. *Nature* 483, 92–95. doi: 10.1038/nature10844

Fukazawa, Y., Saitoh, Y., Ozawa, F., Ohta, Y., Mizuno, K., and Inokuchi, K. (2003). Hippocampal LTP is accompanied by enhanced F-actin content within the dendritic spine that is essential for late LTP maintenance in vivo. *Neuron* 38, 447–460. doi: 10.1016/s0896-6273(03)00206-x

Geinisman, Y. (1993). Perforated axospinous synapses with multiple, completely partitioned transmission zones: probable structural intermediates in synaptic plasticity. *Hippocampus* 3, 417–433. doi: 10.1002/hipo.450030404

Govek, E. E., Newey, S. E., Akerman, C. J., Cross, J. R., Van der Veken, L., and Van Aelst, L. (2004). The X-linked mental retardation protein oligophrenin-1 is required for dendritic spine morphogenesis. *Nat. Neurosci.* 7, 364–372. doi: 10.1038/nn1210

Hayashi-Takagi, A., Takaki, M., Graziane, N., Seshadri, S., Murdoch, H., Dunlop, A. J., et al. (2010). Disrupted-in-Schizophrenia 1 (DISC1) regulates spines of the glutamate synapse via Rac1. *Nat. Neurosci.* 13, 327–332. doi: 10.1038/nn.2487

Hill, T. C., and Zito, K. (2013). LTP-induced long-term stabilization of individual nascent dendritic spines. *J. Neurosci.* 33, 678–686. doi: 10.1523/JNEUROSCI.1404-12.2013

Holtmaat, A., and Svoboda, K. (2009). Experience-dependent structural synaptic plasticity in the mammalian brain. *Nat. Rev. Neurosci.* 10, 647–658. doi: 10.1038/nrn2699

Holtmaat, A. J., Trachtenberg, J. T., Wilbrecht, L., Shepherd, G. M., Zhang, X., Knott, G. W., et al. (2005). Transient and persistent dendritic spines in the neocortex in vivo. *Neuron* 45, 279–291. doi: 10.1016/j.neuron.2005.01.003

Holtmaat, A., Wilbrecht, L., Knott, G. W., Welker, E., and Svoboda, K. (2006). Experience-dependent and cell-type-specific spine growth in the neocortex. *Nature* 441, 979–983. doi: 10.1038/nature04783

Honkura, N., Matsuzaki, M., Noguchi, J., Ellis-Davies, G. C., and Kasai, H. (2008). The subspine organization of actin fibers regulates the structure and plasticity of dendritic spines. *Neuron* 57, 719–729. doi: 10.1016/j.neuron.2008.01.013

Hübener, M., and Bonhoeffer, T. (2010). Searching for engrams. *Neuron* 67, 363–371. doi: 10.1016/j.neuron.2010.06.033

Ishii, H., Shibuya, K., Ohta, Y., Mukai, H., Uchino, S., Takata, N., et al. (2006). Enhancement of nitric oxide production by association of nitric oxide synthase with N-methyl-D-aspartate receptors via postsynaptic density 95 in genetically engineered Chinese hamster ovary cells: real-time fluorescence imaging using nitric oxide sensitive dye. *J. Neurochem.* 96, 1531–1539. doi: 10.1111/j.1471-4159.2006.03656.x

Kasai, H., Matsuzaki, M., Noguchi, J., Yasumatsu, N., and Nakahara, H. (2003). Structure-stability-function relationships of dendritic spines. *Trends Neurosci.* 26, 360–368. doi: 10.1016/s0166-2236(03)00162-0

Kayser, M. S., Nolt, M. J., and Dalva, M. B. (2008). EphB receptors couple dendritic filopodia motility to synapse formation. *Neuron* 59, 56–69. doi: 10.1016/j.neuron.2008.05.007

Keck, T., Mrsic-Flogel, T. D., Vaz Afonso, M., Eysel, U. T., Bonhoeffer, T., and Hübener, M. (2008). Massive restructuring of neuronal circuits during functional reorganization of adult visual cortex. *Nat. Neurosci.* 11, 1162–1167. doi: 10.1038/nn.2181

Kehoe, L. A., Bellone, C., De Roo, M., Zandueta, A., Dey, P. N., Pérez-Otaño, I., et al. (2014). GluN3A promotes dendritic spine pruning and destabilization during postnatal development. *J. Neurosci.* 34, 9213–9221. doi: 10.1523/JNEUROSCI.5183-13.2014

Kehoe, L. A., Bernardinelli, Y., and Muller, D. (2013). GluN3A: an NMDA receptor subunit with exquisite properties and functions. *Neural Plast.* 2013:145387. doi: 10.1155/2013/145387

Kelley, J. B., Balda, M. A., Anderson, K. L., and Itzhak, Y. (2009). Impairments in fear conditioning in mice lacking the nNOS gene. *Learn. Mem.* 16, 371–378. doi: 10.1101/lm.1329209

Kirchner, L., Weitzdoerfer, R., Hoeger, H., Url, A., Schmidt, P., Engelmann, M., et al. (2004). Impaired cognitive performance in neuronal nitric oxide synthase knockout mice is associated with hippocampal protein derangements. *Nitric Oxide* 11, 316–330. doi: 10.1016/j.niox.2004.10.005

Koleske, A. J. (2013). Molecular mechanisms of dendrite stability. *Nat. Rev. Neurosci.* 14, 536–550. doi: 10.1038/nrn3486

Kreis, P., Thévenot, E., Rousseau, V., Boda, B., Muller, D., and Barnier, J. V. (2007). The p21-activated kinase 3 implicated in mental retardation regulates spine morphogenesis through a Cdc42-dependent pathway. *J. Biol. Chem.* 282, 21497–21506. doi: 10.1074/jbc.m703298200

Kumar, V., Zhang, M. X., Swank, M. W., Kunz, J., and Wu, G. Y. (2005). Regulation of dendritic morphogenesis by Ras-PI3K-Akt-mTOR and Ras-MAPK signaling pathways. *J. Neurosci.* 25, 11288–11299. doi: 10.1523/jneurosci.2284-05.2005

Kwon, H. B., and Sabatini, B. L. (2011). Glutamate induces de novo growth of functional spines in developing cortex. *Nature* 474, 100–104. doi: 10.1038/nature09986

Lai, K. O., and Ip, N. Y. (2009). Synapse development and plasticity: roles of ephrin/Eph receptor signaling. *Curr. Opin. Neurobiol.* 19, 275–283. doi: 10.1016/j.conb.2009.04.009

Lendvai, B., Stern, E. A., Chen, B., and Svoboda, K. (2000). Experience-dependent plasticity of dendritic spines in the developing rat barrel cortex in vivo. *Nature* 404, 876–881. doi: 10.1038/35009107

Lim, J., Ritt, D. A., Zhou, M., and Morrison, D. K. (2014). The CNK2 scaffold interacts with vilse and modulates Rac cycling during spine morphogenesis in hippocampal neurons. *Curr. Biol.* 24, 786–792. doi: 10.1016/j.cub.2014.02.036

Lin, Y. L., Lei, Y. T., Hong, C. J., and Hsueh, Y. P. (2007). Syndecan-2 induces filopodia and dendritic spine formation via the neurofibromin-PKA-Ena/VASP pathway. *J. Cell Biol.* 177, 829–841. doi: 10.1083/jcb.200608121

Lisman, J. (2003). Actin's actions in LTP-induced synapse growth. *Neuron* 38, 361–362. doi: 10.1016/s0896-6273(03)00257-5

Lushnikova, I., Skibo, G., Muller, D., and Nikonenko, I. (2009). Synaptic potentiation induces increased glial coverage of excitatory synapses in CA1 hippocampus. *Hippocampus* 19, 753–762. doi: 10.1002/hipo.20551

Matsuzaki, M., Honkura, N., Ellis-Davies, G. C., and Kasai, H. (2004). Structural basis of long-term potentiation in single dendritic spines. *Nature* 429, 761–766. doi: 10.1038/nature02617

Matter, C., Pribadi, M., Liu, X., and Trachtenberg, J. T. (2009). Delta-catenin is required for the maintenance of neural structure and function in mature cortex in vivo. *Neuron* 64, 320–327. doi: 10.1016/j.neuron.2009.09.026

Matus, A. (2000). Actin-based plasticity in dendritic spines. *Science* 290, 754–758. doi: 10.1126/science.290.5492.754

McGeachie, A. B., Cingolani, L. A., and Goda, Y. (2011). A stabilising influence: integrins in regulation of synaptic plasticity. *Neurosci. Res.* 70, 24–29. doi: 10.1016/j.neures.2011.02.006

Mendez, P., De Roo, M., Poglia, L., Klauser, P., and Muller, D. (2010a). N-cadherin mediates plasticity-induced long-term spine stabilization. *J. Cell Biol.* 189, 589–600. doi: 10.1083/jcb.201003007

Mendez, P., Garcia-Segura, L. M., and Muller, D. (2010b). Estradiol promotes spine growth and synapse formation without affecting pre-established networks. *Hippocampus* 21, 1263–1267. doi: 10.1002/hipo.20875

Mukai, J., Dhilla, A., Drew, L. J., Stark, K. L., Cao, L., MacDermott, A. B., et al. (2008). Palmitoylation-dependent neurodevelopmental deficits in a mouse model of 22q11 microdeletion. *Nat. Neurosci.* 11, 1302–1310. doi: 10.1038/nn.2204

Murakoshi, H., Wang, H., and Yasuda, R. (2011). Local, persistent activation of Rho GTPases during plasticity of single dendritic spines. *Nature* 472, 100–104. doi: 10.1038/nature09823

Nägerl, U. V., Eberhorn, N., Cambridge, S. B., and Bonhoeffer, T. (2004). Bidirectional activity-dependent morphological plasticity in hippocampal neurons. *Neuron* 44, 759–767. doi: 10.1016/j.neuron.2004.11.016

Nägerl, U. V., Köstinger, G., Anderson, J. C., Martin, K. A., and Bonhoeffer, T. (2007). Protracted synaptogenesis after activity-dependent spinogenesis in hippocampal neurons. *J. Neurosci.* 27, 8149–8156. doi: 10.1523/JNEUROSCI.0511-07.2007

Nikonenko, I., Nikonenko, A., Mendez, P., Michurina, T. V., Enikolopov, G., and Muller, D. (2013). Nitric oxide mediates local activity-dependent excitatory synapse development. *Proc. Natl. Acad. Sci. U S A* 110, E4142–E4151. doi: 10.1073/pnas.1311927110

Nodé-Langlois, R., Muller, D., and Boda, B. (2006). Sequential implication of the mental retardation proteins ARHGEF6 and PAK3 in spine morphogenesis. *J. Cell Sci.* 119, 4986–4993. doi: 10.1242/jcs.03273

Oh, W. C., Hill, T. C., and Zito, K. (2013). Synapse-specific and size-dependent mechanisms of spine structural plasticity accompanying synaptic weakening. *Proc. Natl. Acad. Sci. U S A* 110, E305–E312. doi: 10.1073/pnas.1214705110

Pan, F., Aldridge, G. M., Greenough, W. T., and Gan, W. B. (2010). Dendritic spine instability and insensitivity to modulation by sensory experience in a mouse model of fragile X syndrome. *Proc. Natl. Acad. Sci. U S A* 107, 17768–17773. doi: 10.1073/pnas.1012496107

Petrak, L. J., Harris, K. M., and Kirov, S. A. (2005). Synaptogenesis on mature hippocampal dendrites occurs via filopodia and immature spines during blocked synaptic transmission. *J. Comp. Neurol.* 484, 183–190. doi: 10.1002/cne.20468

Qiu, S., Anderson, C. T., Levitt, P., and Shepherd, G. M. (2011). Circuit-specific intracortical hyperconnectivity in mice with deletion of the autism-associated Met receptor tyrosine kinase. *J. Neurosci.* 31, 5855–5864. doi: 10.1523/JNEUROSCI.6569-10.2011

Redies, C., Hertel, N., and Hübner, C. A. (2012). Cadherins and neuropsychiatric disorders. *Brain Res.* 1470, 130–144. doi: 10.1016/j.brainres.2012.06.020

Rex, C. S., Chen, L. Y., Sharma, A., Liu, J., Babayan, A. H., Gall, C. M., et al. (2009). Different Rho GTPase-dependent signaling pathways initiate sequential steps in the consolidation of long-term potentiation. *J. Cell Biol.* 186, 85–97. doi: 10.1083/jcb.200901084

Richards, D. A., Mateos, J. M., Hugel, S., de Paola, V., Caroni, P., Gahwiler, B. H., et al. (2005). Glutamate induces the rapid formation of spine head protrusions in hippocampal slice cultures. *Proc. Natl. Acad. Sci. U S A* 102, 6166–6171. doi: 10.1073/pnas.0501881102

Roberts, A. C., Díez-García, J., Rodriguiz, R. M., López, I. P., Luján, R., Martínez-Turrillas, R., et al. (2009). Downregulation of NR3A-containing NMDARs is required for synapse maturation and memory consolidation. *Neuron* 63, 342–356. doi: 10.1016/j.neuron.2009.06.016

Sakamoto, H., Mezaki, Y., Shikimi, H., Ukena, K., and Tsutsui, K. (2003). Dendritic growth and spine formation in response to estrogen in the developing Purkinje cell. *Endocrinology* 144, 4466–4477. doi: 10.1210/en.2003-0307

Sawicka, K., and Zukin, R. S. (2012). Dysregulation of mTOR signaling in neuropsychiatric disorders: therapeutic implications. *Neuropsychopharmacology* 37, 305–306. doi: 10.1038/npp.2011.210

Sharma, A., Hoeffer, C. A., Takayasu, Y., Miyawaki, T., McBride, S. M., Klann, E., et al. (2010). Dysregulation of mTOR signaling in fragile X syndrome. *J. Neurosci.* 30, 694–702. doi: 10.1523/jneurosci.3696-09.2010

Shinkai, T., Ohmori, O., Hori, H., and Nakamura, J. (2002). Allelic association of the neuronal nitric oxide synthase (NOS1) gene with schizophrenia. *Mol. Psychiatry* 7, 560–563. doi: 10.1038/sj.mp.4001041

Sigurdsson, T., Stark, K. L., Karayiorgou, M., Gogos, J. A., and Gordon, J. A. (2010). Impaired hippocampal-prefrontal synchrony in a genetic mouse model of schizophrenia. *Nature* 464, 763–767. doi: 10.1038/nature08855

Sudhof, T. C. (2008). Neuroligins and neurexins link synaptic function to cognitive disease. *Nature* 455, 903–911. doi: 10.1038/nature07456

Suzuki, A., Stern, S. A., Bozdagi, O., Huntley, G. W., Walker, R. H., Magistretti, P. J., et al. (2011). Astrocyte-neuron lactate transport is required for long-term memory formation. *Cell* 144, 810–823. doi: 10.1016/j.cell.2011.02.018

Tanaka, J., Horiike, Y., Matsuzaki, M., Miyazaki, T., Ellis-Davies, G. C., and Kasai, H. (2008). Protein synthesis and neurotrophin-dependent structural plasticity of single dendritic spines. *Science* 319, 1683–1687. doi: 10.1126/science.1152864

Tanda, K., Nishi, A., Matsuo, N., Nakanishi, K., Yamasaki, N., Sugimoto, T., et al. (2009). Abnormal social behavior, hyperactivity, impaired remote spatial memory and increased D1-mediated dopaminergic signaling in neuronal nitric oxide synthase knockout mice. *Mol. Brain* 2:19. doi: 10.1186/1756-6606-2-19

Toni, N., Buchs, P. A., Nikonenko, I., Bron, C. R., and Muller, D. (1999). LTP promotes formation of multiple spine synapses between a single axon terminal and a dendrite. *Nature* 402, 421–425. doi: 10.1038/46574

Toni, N., Teng, E. M., Bushong, E. A., Aimone, J. B., Zhao, C., Consiglio, A., et al. (2007). Synapse formation on neurons born in the adult hippocampus. *Nat. Neurosci.* 10, 727–734. doi: 10.1038/nn1908

Vukojevic, V., Gschwind, L., Vogler, C., Demougin, P., de Quervain, D. J., Papassotiropoulos, A., et al. (2012). A role for alpha-adducin (ADD-1) in nematode and human memory. *EMBO J.* 31, 1453–1466. doi: 10.1038/emboj.2012.14

Wang, X. B., Bozdagi, O., Nikitczuk, J. S., Zhai, Z. W., Zhou, Q., and Huntley, G. W. (2008). Extracellular proteolysis by matrix metalloproteinase-9 drives dendritic spine enlargement and long-term potentiation coordinately. *Proc. Natl. Acad. Sci. U S A* 105, 19520–19525. doi: 10.1073/pnas.0807248105

Wass, C., Klamer, D., Fejgin, K., and Palsson, E. (2009). The importance of nitric oxide in social dysfunction. *Behav. Brain Res.* 200, 113–116. doi: 10.1016/j.bbr.2009.01.002

Wiegert, J. S., and Oertner, T. G. (2013). Long-term depression triggers the selective elimination of weakly integrated synapses. *Proc. Natl. Acad. Sci. U S A* 110, E4510–E4519. doi: 10.1073/pnas.1315926110

Wijetunge, L. S., Angibaud, J., Frick, A., Kind, P. C., and Nägerl, U. V. (2014). Stimulated emission depletion (STED) microscopy reveals nanoscale defects in the developmental trajectory of dendritic spine morphogenesis in a mouse model of fragile X syndrome. *J. Neurosci.* 34, 6405–6412. doi: 10.1523/jneurosci.2974-14.2014

Woolfrey, K. M., Srivastava, D. P., Photowala, H., Yamashita, M., Barbolina, M. V., Cahill, M. E., et al. (2009). Epac2 induces synapse remodeling and depression and its disease-associated forms alter spines. *Nat. Neurosci.* 12, 1275–1284. doi: 10.1038/nn.2386

Xu, T., Yu, X., Perlik, A. J., Tobin, W. F., Zweig, J. A., Tennant, K., et al. (2009). Rapid formation and selective stabilization of synapses for enduring motor memories. *Nature* 462, 915–919. doi: 10.1038/nature08389

Yang, G., Pan, F., and Gan, W. B. (2009). Stably maintained dendritic spines are associated with lifelong memories. *Nature* 462, 920–924. doi: 10.1038/nature08577

Yankova, M., Hart, S. A., and Woolley, C. S. (2001). Estrogen increases synaptic connectivity between single presynaptic inputs and multiple postsynaptic CA1 pyramidal cells: a serial electron-microscopic study. *Proc. Natl. Acad. Sci. U S A* 98, 3525–3530. doi: 10.1073/pnas.051624598

Yasumatsu, N., Matsuzaki, M., Miyazaki, T., Noguchi, J., and Kasai, H. (2008). Principles of long-term dynamics of dendritic spines. *J. Neurosci.* 28, 13592–13608. doi: 10.1523/jneurosci.0603-08.2008

Zito, K., Scheuss, V., Knott, G., Hill, T., and Svoboda, K. (2009). Rapid functional maturation of nascent dendritic spines. *Neuron* 61, 247–258. doi: 10.1016/j.neuron.2008.10.054

Ziv, N. E., and Smith, S. J. (1996). Evidence for a role of dendritic filopodia in synaptogenesis and spine formation. *Neuron* 17, 91–102. doi: 10.1016/s0896-6273(00)80283-4

Zuber, B., Nikonenko, I., Klauser, P., Muller, D., and Dubochet, J. (2005). The mammalian central nervous synaptic cleft contains a high density of periodically organized complexes. *Proc. Natl. Acad. Sci. U S A* 102, 19192–19197. doi: 10.1073/pnas.0509527102

Zuo, Y., Lin, A., Chang, P., and Gan, W. B. (2005). Development of long-term dendritic spine stability in diverse regions of cerebral cortex. *Neuron* 46, 181–189. doi: 10.1016/j.neuron.2005.04.001

20

The BDNF effects on dendritic spines of mature hippocampal neurons depend on neuronal activity

Yves Kellner, Nina Gödecke, Tobias Dierkes, Nils Thieme, Marta Zagrebelsky *† and Martin Korte *†

Division of Cellular Neurobiology, Zoological Institute, TU Braunschweig, Braunschweig, Germany

Correspondence:
Marta Zagrebelsky and Martin Korte, Division of Cellular Neurobiology, Zoological Institute, TU Braunschweig, Germany, Spielmannstr 7, 38106 Braunschweig, Germany
e-mail: m.korte@tu-bs.de; m.zagrebelsky@tu-bs.de

† These authors have contributed equally to this work.

The fine tuning of neural networks during development and learning relies upon both functional and structural plastic processes. Changes in the number as well as in the size and shape of dendritic spines are associated to long-term activity-dependent synaptic plasticity. However, the molecular mechanisms translating functional into structural changes are still largely unknown. In this context, neurotrophins, like Brain-Derived Neurotrophic Factor (BDNF), are among promising candidates. Specifically BDNF-TrkB receptor signaling is crucial for activity-dependent strengthening of synapses in different brain regions. BDNF application has been shown to positively modulate dendritic and spine architecture in cortical and hippocampal neurons as well as structural plasticity *in vitro*. However, a global BDNF deprivation throughout the central nervous system (CNS) resulted in very mild structural alterations of dendritic spines, questioning the relevance of the endogenous BDNF signaling in modulating the development and the mature structure of neurons *in vivo*. Here we show that a loss-of-function approach, blocking BDNF results in a significant reduction in dendritic spine density, associated with an increase in spine length and a decrease in head width. These changes are associated with a decrease in F-actin levels within spine heads. On the other hand, a gain-of-function approach, applying exogenous BDNF, could not reproduce the increase in spine density or the changes in spine morphology previously described. Taken together, we show here that the effects exerted by BDNF on the dendritic architecture of hippocampal neurons are dependent on the neuron's maturation stage. Indeed, in mature hippocampal neurons *in vitro* as shown *in vivo* BDNF is specifically required for the activity-dependent maintenance of the mature spine phenotype.

Keywords: dendrites, spines, structural plasticity, hippocampus, neurotrophins

INTRODUCTION

Neurotrophins are essential for multiple aspects of neuronal development and function. Especially Brain-derived Neurotrophic Factor (BDNF) has been shown to play an important role in neuronal survival and in the maintenance of several neuronal systems. In addition, BDNF has been implicated in numerous processes of functional and structural synaptic plasticity (Gottmann et al., 2009; Park and Poo, 2012; Zagrebelsky and Korte, 2013). The role of BDNF has been extensively analyzed *in vitro* upon the application of exogenous BDNF. The data obtained support the notion that during development BDNF is involved in regulating the fine-tuning of the cortical network by selectively enhancing dendritic growth in an activity-dependent manner (Mcallister et al., 1995, 1996; Horch et al., 1999). Application of exogenous BDNF to developing primary hippocampal neurons has been shown to result in a significant increase in the number of primary neurites as well as an increase in neurite complexity and length (Ji et al., 2005; Kwon and Sabatini, 2011). Furthermore, dendritic spine density and morphology of mature primary hippocampal neurons are significantly influences by a BDNF application (Ji et al., 2005, 2010). Similarly, mature organotypic hippocampal neurons treated with BDNF show a significant increase in dendritic spine density and in the number of synapses (Tyler and Pozzo-Miller, 2001, 2003). Taken together, the *in vitro* studies described above strongly support the notion that, in the hippocampus exogenous BDNF promotes dendritic formation and growth during development and regulates dendritic spine density and morphology in mature neurons. But as strong as the evidence for a role of BDNF in modulating dendritic architecture might appear, the preparation techniques (Danzer et al., 2004) and the culture conditions (Chapleau et al., 2008) have been shown to influence the expression levels as well as the cellular response to BDNF, possibly confounding the analysis under these conditions. Suggestive for a role of BDNF *in vivo* is the correlation between the physiological variability in BDNF expression levels in the mouse dentate gyrus and the dendritic spine density in granule cells (Stranahan, 2011). Moreover, a reduction in BDNF serum levels is associated to a reduction in hippocampus volume in aging humans (Erickson et al., 2011) as well as in dendritic complexity and spine density in senescent rats (Von Bohlen Und Halbach, 2010). The *in vivo* role of BDNF has been very difficult to evaluate in the post-natal brain as $bdnf^{-/-}$ mouse mutants die too early for the role of BDNF to be assessed after its increased post-natal expression caused by neuronal activity (Zafra et al., 1990; Hong et al., 2008). The analysis of $bdnf^{+/-}$ mouse mutants, showing reduced BDNF levels provided evidence that, *in vivo* BDNF plays an important role in the induction of LTP in the hippocampus (Korte et al., 1995), the acquisition of extinction learning (Psotta et al., 2013) and in the structural rearrangement of adult cortical circuitry upon increased sensory input (Genoud et al., 2004). On the other hand, in *bdnf*$^{+/-}$ mice synapse density and spine morphology are indistinguishable from those in WT mice (Korte et al., 1995; Genoud et al., 2004) and a compensatory increase in TrkB receptor expression occurs (Carreton et al., 2012), leaving open the question of whether BDNF modulates dendritic architecture *in vivo*. Thus, a number of studies have been performed using different conditional gene targeted mouse lines and Cre-loxP-mediated excision of *bdnf* (Rios et al., 2001; Gorski et al., 2003; Baquet et al., 2004; He et al., 2004; Chan et al., 2006, 2008; Monteggia et al., 2007; Unger et al., 2007; Rauskolb et al., 2010). Surprisingly, the effect on excitatory neurons in the hippocampus and cortex of a global BDNF deprivation throughout the central nervous system (CNS) is extremely mild when compared to the effects observed upon a BDNF application *in vitro*. Rauskolb et al. (2010) showed that in a Tau-BDNF^{KO} mouse the volume of the cortex is only slightly reduced and the one of the hippocampus unchanged. Accordingly, dendritic complexity of CA1 pyramidal cells is only mildly reduced and while no changes could be observed in dendritic spine density the spine type distribution in Tau-BDNF^{KO} neurons is significantly shifted toward a more immature phenotype, pointing to a specific role of BDNF in the maintenance of mature dendritic spines in the mature hippocampus. These results are consistent with the observation that a conditional deletion of TrkB in the hippocampus does not affect the gross dendritic morphology of CA1 pyramidal neurons (Minichiello et al., 1999; Luikart et al., 2005).

So overall it is noteworthy that while most of the published data supporting a role for BDNF in modulating dendrite and dendritic spine morphology derive from *in vitro* experiments applying exogenous BDNF, a role for endogenous BDNF in this context is still unclear. Moreover, *in vivo* the effects of endogenous BDNF in modulating the structure of neurons seem to be extremely specific, depending on the developmental stage, the brain area as well as the cell-type. Therefore, in this study we set out to address the discrepancies in the role of BDNF in modulating the architecture of mature hippocampal neurons. In order to contribute to a better understanding of the BDNF activity, we analyzed the effects of several manipulations of its signaling on dendrites and dendritic spines at different developmental stages and under different levels of neuronal activity in primary neuronal cultures. The results we obtained in our culture system confirm the observations previously obtained *in vivo* and show that BDNF exerts a highly precise role on different aspects of neuronal architecture in an age-dependent manner. In mature hippocampal neurons *in vitro*, as shown *in vivo* endogenous BDNF is specifically required for the activity-dependent maintenance of the mature spine phenotype.

MATERIALS AND METHODS

PREPARATION OF PRIMARY HIPPOCAMPAL CULTURES

Primary hippocampal cultures were prepared from C57BL/6 mice at embryonic day 18. All procedures were approved by guidelines from the Animal Committee on Ethics in the Care and Use of Laboratory Animals of TU Braunschweig. Embryos were decapitated and the brains were kept in ice-cold Gey's balanced salt solution (GBSS) containing of 1% kynurenic acid, 1% glucose and adjusted to pH 7.2. The dissected hippocampi were incubated for 30 min in trypsin/EDTA at 37°C and then mechanically dissociated. Cells were plated at high density (10^5/well) on poly-L-lysine-coated coverslips (13 mm) and kept in Neurobasal medium (Invitrogen) supplemented with 2% B27 (Invitrogen) and 0.5 mM Glutamax at 37°C, 5% CO_2, and 99% humidity. For analysis of neurite growth in 3–6 days *in vitro* to the cells were plated at a density of 10^4 cells per well. For the experiments performed in high Magnesium (Mg^{2+}) containing medium, the cells were plated at a density of 70,000 cells per well and kept in Neurobasal medium (Gibco) supplemented with 2% BSA (Gibco), 200 μM L-Glutamin and 1% 100 × N2 (Invitrogen) at 37°C, 5% CO_2, and 99% humidity.

TRANSFECTION OF PRIMARY HIPPOCAMPAL NEURONS

Hippocampal neurons were transfected at various time points with a farnesylated form of the enhanced green fluorescent protein (fEGFP) using Lipofectamine 2000 according to the manufacturer's protocol. To specifically label F-actin without adverse effects on actin dynamics the cells were co-transfected with fEGFP and an expression plasmid for the Lifeact peptide fused to a red fluorescent protein (RFP-LA) (Riedl et al., 2008, 2010). Briefly, 0.8 μg DNA or, for a co-transfection 0.4 μg pfEGFP and 0.6 μg pRFP-LA and 2 μl Lipofectamine 2000 per well were mixed in 100 μl Neurobasal medium, and added to the cultures dropwise. After 50 min of incubation the transfection medium was exchanged for the original Neurobasal medium. The cultures were kept for 24 h at 37°C, 5% CO_2, and 99% humidity before the treatment.

TREATMENT OF PRIMARY HIPPOCAMPAL NEURONS

Twenty-four hours after transfection, 1/3 of the culture medium was exchanged for a medium containing 0.1% Bovine Serum Albumine (BSA, Sigma; 0.1% BSA/PBS) as a control treatment or 0.1% BSA combined with BDNF (Recombinant Human BDNF, 40 ng/ml, R&D Systems), BDNF blocking antibodies (BDNF-Abs, 1:500, M. Sendtner, Wuerzburg Germany) or TrkB receptor bodies (TrkB-Fc, Recombinant Human TrkB-Fc, 500 ng/ml, R&D Systems). The BSA was added to the medium to prevent BDNF or the antibodies from sticking to the plastic (Chen et al., 1999). In a second set of control experiments the cultures were kept in Neurobasal medium without addition of BSA. As no significant difference between the two control conditions could be observed only the BSA control was used in the result part. The cultures were fixed 24 h after the treatment in 4% paraformaldehyde (PFA) in 0.1 M phosphate buffer (PBS), washed and mounted with an anti-fading aqueous mounting medium (Fluoro-Gel Emsdiasum).

In a second set of experiments neuronal activity was reduced in primary hippocampal cultures by increasing the Mg^{2+}concentration in the medium. Indeed, Mg^{2+} decreases the activation of voltage-gated channels thereby reducing neuronal excitability (Mayer and Westbrook, 1987; Dribben et al., 2010). To avoid effects on the early developmental stages Mg^{2+} concentration in the medium was increased starting at 7 DIV from 1.5

to 3.5 mM by adding $MgCl_2$, for 2 weeks and fresh medium was added once a week. The treatment with BDNF or TrkB receptor bodies was performed for 24 h either in low (1.5 mM) or high (3.5 mM) Mg^{2+} containing medium.

IMMUNOCYTOCHEMISTRY

Primary hippocampal cultures (6 or 23 DIV) were fixed with 4% PFA, permeabilized and blocked with a solution containing 0.2% Triton X-100, 10% goat serum, and 0.1% BSA in PBS. A rabbit polyclonal antibody anti-c-fos (Santa Cruz Biotechnology, Inc., sc-52; dilution 1:500), a mouse monoclonal antibody anti-CaMKII (Invitrogen, dilution 1:500), a rabbit polyclonal anti-MAP2 (Abcam, dilution 1:500) or a primary rabbit monoclonal anti-phospho-TrkA (Tyr674/675)/TrkB (Tyr706/707) antibody (Cell Signaling Technology; dilution 1:200) were diluted in blocking solution (10% goat serum and 0.1% BSA in PBS) and incubated at 4°C overnight. Secondary anti-rabbit or anti-mouse antibodies conjugated with Cy2, Cy3, or Cy5 (Jackson Immuno Research) were diluted 1:500 in PBS and incubated for 2 h at room temperature. Alexa Fluor 350 phalloidin (Lifetechnologies) was diluted 1:50 in PBS and incubated for 3 h at room temperature to selectively stain F-actin. Finally, cultures were counterstained with DAPI (4′,6-diamidino-2-phenylindole) (Biotium) diluted 1:1000 in PBS for 5 min, washed and mounted using an anti-fading aquous mounting medium (Fluoro-Gel Emsdiasum).

NEURON SELECTION

The transfection of the fEGFP expression plasmid under the control of the CMV promoter resulted in the intense labeling of the entire dendritic arbor as well as of all dendritic spines of individual pyramidal neurons. A small number of individual pyramidal neurons were transfected in each culture allowing to following the complete dendritic processes of each labeled neuron. Only non-overlapping labeled neurons were selected for our analysis allowing for an unambiguous reconstruction of the entire dendritic tree as well as the analysis for the spine density. Degenerating neurons were identified according to the presence of retraction bulbs and fragmentation of the dendritic processes and excluded from the analysis. Due to a recent report showing that Mg^{2+} (5 to 10 mM) increases neuronal apoptosis in primary hippocampal neurons (Dribben et al., 2010), special care was used in selecting neurons kept in high magnesium medium (3.5 mM). Indeed, all neurons selected for the analysis showed a healthy cell body and dendritic tree with no signs of apoptosis.

NEURONAL IMAGING AND ANALYSIS

The neurons selected for analysis were imaged using an Axioplan 2 microscope equipped with an ApoTome module (Zeiss). Each neuron was first imaged using a 20× objective [1.25 numerical aperture (NA)] and the images were used to analyze dendritic complexity and length using a Sholl analysis (Sholl, 1953). The neurons were traced using the Neurolucida software (MicroBrightField), and the Sholl analysis was obtained with Neuroexplorer software (MicroBrightField), calculating the cumulative number of dendritic intersections at 10 µm interval distance points starting from the cell body. The total number of crossings for each cell was used as an index for total dendritic complexity. The total neurite length, number of primary neurites and number of branching points of 6 DIV neurons were analyzed by tracing MAP2 labeled neurites using the NeuronJ (Meijering et al., 2004) plugin for ImageJ (NIH) Software. Spine density was measured separately for portions of selected second or third order dendrite branches and imaged using a 63× objective (1.32 NA) acquiring three-dimensional stacks z-sectioned at 0.5 µm. The number of spines and the dendritic length were measured using the ImageJ software. The number of spines was normalized per micrometer of dendritic length and a minimal length of 250 µm of dendrite per cell was analyzed. The maximal spine head diameter and maximal spine length (from the dendritic shaft to the spine head tip) were measured on three-dimensional stacks using the ImageJ (NIH) software. To examine the actin content in dendritic spine heads the mean fluorescent intensity of RFP-lifeact was measured with the area selection tool of ImageJ and normalized to the mean fluorescent intensity of the dendritic shaft (for normalization of the RFP overexpression, **Figure 3B**, indicated with the arrow heads). RFP-Lifeact and the immunocytochemistry for c-fos and phosphorylated TrkB were imaged keeping a constant exposure time. The mean fluorescent intensity values for the immunocytochemistry of c-fos and phosphorylated TrkB were measured with ImageJ (NIH) and normalized to the control condition. The analysis was performed blindly.

CALCIUM IMAGING

Primary hippocampal cultures 16 and 23 DIV were loaded with calcium indicator by incubating them for 15 min with the indicator solution (50 µg Oregon Green 488 BAPTA-1 AM (Invitrogen), dissolved in 50 µl DMSO and 2.5% Pluronic acid) at 37°C, 5% CO_2, and 99% humidity. The cells were then transferred to HBSS (Hanks balanced salt solution) and kept 45 min at 37°C, 5% CO_2, and 99% humidity. The coverslips were thentransferred to the recording chamber, continuously perfused with HBSS and kept at 32°C. The live imaging was performed using an Olympus BX61WI microscope system (Cell^M software) and a CCD camera (VisiCam QE, Visitron Systems). Images were recorded at 6 Hz for 75 sec with an Olympus 20× water immersion objective (0.95 NA XLUMPLAN FL, Olympus), whereby a pixel resolution of 0.77 µm/pixel was achieved. A frame rate of 150 ms and an exposure time of 61 ms were used. Primary hippocampal cultures were treated with BSA (serial 0.1% BSA/1× PBS) or BDNF (Recombinant Human BDNF, 40 ng/ml, R&D Systems) by a 5 min bath-application.

The analysis of calcium transients was performed using ImageJ (NIH) and calculating the fluorescence changes as average of all pixels within regions of interests (ROIs). The ROIs were set around the cell bodies of the neurons. For the background subtraction the ROI was drawn on a neighboring area containing neuropil. The resulting changes in the intracellular calcium concentration are represented as $\Delta F/F_0$ in percent, where F_0 is the fluorescence at resting conditions $[\Delta F/F_0 = (F - F_0)/F_0]$ taken before the application of BDNF (Lang et al., 2006). In addition to it we generated using the plugin "reslice" of the ImageJ Software a pseudo-line scan to visualize changes in the fluorescence intensity for the whole ΔF-stack. In the pseudo-line scan the y-axis corresponds to the respective line drawn on the stack whereas the x-axis corresponds to time.

STATISTICAL ANALYSIS

The statistical analysis was performed using Microsoft Excel or GraphPad Prism. The data obtained were compared between two different experimental conditions using an unpaired two-tailed Student's *t*-test. Data including more than 2 different groups were analyzed using a One-Way ANOVA followed by a *post-hoc* Tukey's Multiple Comparison Test. Values of $p = 0.05$ were considered significant and plotted as follows $^{*}p < 0.05$; $^{**}p < 0.01$; $^{***}p < 0.001$. All data are indicated as mean ± s.e.m.

RESULTS

ENDOGENOUS BDNF REGULATES DENDRITIC SPINE DENSITY AND MORPHOLOGY IN MATURE PRIMARY HIPPOCAMPAL NEURONS

In view of the discrepancy existing between a described action of exogenous BDNF in modulating the dendritic architecture of hippocampal neurons *in vitro* (Tyler and Pozzo-Miller, 2001; Ji et al., 2005, 2010) and previous data showing that a global deprivation of BDNF throughout the CNS *in vivo* results in only minimal morphological alterations of mature hippocampal neurons (Minichiello et al., 1999; Zakharenko et al., 2003; Rauskolb et al., 2010, for a review see Zagrebelsky and Korte, 2013), we analyzed the role of BDNF in modulating dendritic spine number and spine morphology as well as dendritic architecture of primary hippocampal neurons. The dendrite and dendritic spine architecture of mature 3-week-old (22 DIV) primary hippocampal neurons (Papa et al., 1995), expressing a membrane targeted farnesylated EGFP (fEGFP; **Figure 1B**) and identified as excitatory by their pyramidal like morphology (**Figure 1B**) and by the expression of the Ca^{2+}/calmodulin-dependent protein kinase (CaMKII; **Figure 1B** inserts) were analyzed upon the application of either a gain- or loss-of-function approach for BDNF (**Figure 1A**). While 22 DIV fEGFP-expressing neurons treated for 24 h with exogenous BDNF showed no obvious alterations in dendritic spine density when compared to control neurons, (**Figure 1B′**), treating the neurons with BDNF function blocking antibodies (BDNF-Abs) led to a strong reduction in dendritic spine density (**Figure 1B′**). This observation was confirmed by the quantification of dendritic spine density showing no significant difference between BDNF and control treated cells (**Figure 1C**, Table S1). On the other hand, a significant reduction in dendritic spine density was observed for neurons treated with BDNF blocking antibodies (**Figure 1C**, Table S1; control vs. BDNF-Abs, $p < 0.001$; BDNF vs. BDNF-Abs $p < 0.001$). These observations suggest that while the endogenous BDNF may be crucial for the maintenance of dendritic spines in mature primary hippocampal neurons, exogenous BDNF does not play a role in this context. We next assessed whether BDNF regulates spine morphology in mature hippocampal neurons by analyzing the effects of adding or blocking BDNF on dendritic spine head width and length. When compared spine head width as well as spine length (**Figure 1B′**) did not show any major difference after a 24 h treatment with BDNF in comparison to the control condition. On the other hand neurons treated with BDNF blocking antibodies showed clearly elongated and thinner spines than control neurons (**Figure 1B′**). Indeed, quantification of spine morphology upon BDNF antibody treatment showed a significant decrease in spine head width (**Figure 1D**, Table S1; control vs. BDNF-Abs and BDNF vs. BDNF-Abs, $p < 0.05$) associated to a significant increase in dendritic spine length (**Figure 1E**, Table S1; control *vs.* BDNF-Abs $p < 0.01$, BDNF vs. BDNF-Abs $p < 0.001$). Treatment with exogenous BDNF did not result in any significant change in dendritic spine head width (**Figure 1D**, Table S1). Under these conditions dendritic spine length was only slightly reduced when compared to controls but significantly lower than in neurons treated with BDNF blocking antibodies (**Figure 1E**, Table S1; BDNF vs. BDNF-Abs, $p < 0.001$). Next dendritic spines were separated according on their stage of maturation into four categories based on their head width. Comparing the effect of the different treatments within each spine head category showed a significant increase in spines with a small head ($<0.3\,\mu m$; control vs. BDNF-Abs $p < 0.001$, BDNF vs. BDNF-Abs $p < 0.01$) accompanied by a significant decrease in larger spine heads ($\geq 0.5\,\mu m$ $<1\,\mu m$; control vs. BDNF-Abs $p < 0.01$, BDNF vs. BDNF-Abs $p < 0.001$) when a treatment with BDNF blocking antibodies was compared to a control treatment or to a treatment with exogenous BDNF (**Figure 1F**). Application of BDNF (gain-of-function experiment) did not result in any significant alteration in spine head size when compared to the control conditions (**Figure 1F**). Binning the spines according to their length did not show any difference for BDNF treated neurons but resulted in a significant alteration in spine length distribution upon BDNF antibody treatment (loss-of-function) (**Figure 1G**). While under these conditions spines shorter than $1.5\,\mu m$ were significantly decreased (**Figure 1G**; $\geq 0.5\,\mu m$ $<1\,\mu m$ $p < 0.01$ to the BDNF treatment; $\geq 1\,\mu m$ $<1.5\,\mu m$ $p < 0.05$ to the control), those longer that $1.5\,\mu m$ were significantly increased when compared to the control conditions or the BDNF treatment (**Figure 1G**; $p < 0.01$ to the control, $p < 0.001$ to BDNF treatment). Finally, the effects of either a gain- or a loss-of-function for BDNF on dendritic architecture were analyzed using a Sholl analysis to compare dendritic complexity. No significant differences in dendritic complexity could be observed between the three different treatments (**Figure 1H**; control, BDNF, BDNF-Abs). Accordingly, also total dendritic complexity was not significantly different in BDNF or BDNF- antibody-treated cells vs. control cells (**Figure 1H′**, Table S1).

Taken together, these results demonstrate that the exogenous application of BDNF, in mature primary hippocampal neurons, does not influence dendritic spine density, morphology and dendrite complexity. On the other hand, the loss-of-function experiments show that the endogenous BDNF is essential for maintaining spine density and the mature morphology of dendritic spines in primary hippocampal neurons.

ENDOGENOUS BDNF REGULATES DENDRITIC SPINE DENSITY AND MORPHOLOGY IN DEVELOPING PRIMARY HIPPOCAMPAL NEURONS

In the next series of experiments we tested whether the different effects of exogenous vs. endogenous BDNF on neuronal structure might depend on the age of the treated primary hippocampal neurons. To this aim we analyzed whether a gain- or a loss-of-function approach for BDNF regulates the dendritic

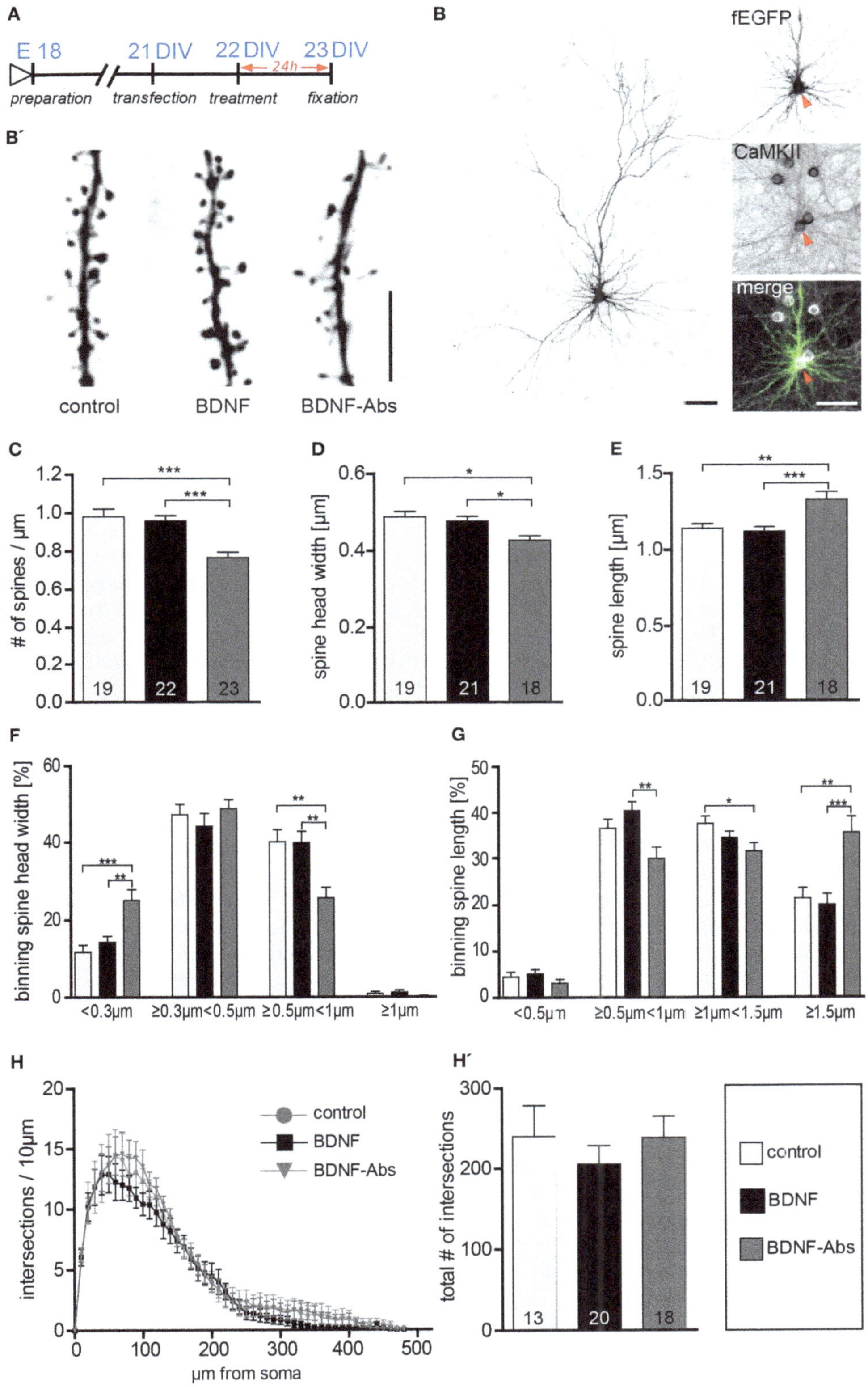

FIGURE 1 | (A) Experimental timeline. DIV23 hippocampal neurons were treated for 24 h before fixation. **(B)** Representative image of a typical DIV23 fEGFP expressing hippocampal neuron used in the experiments; the inserts on the right show a close up of the cell body labeled with fEGFP (above) or with an immunohistochemistry against CaMKII (middle) merged to show colocalization (below): scale bars are 50 µm. **(B′)** High-magnification image of typical dendritic stretches from control (left), BDNF (middle) and BDNF

(Continued)

FIGURE 1 | Continued
antibodies (right) treated neurons. Scale bar, 5 μm. **(C)** Graphs comparing dendritic spine density between BSA (control), BDNF and BDNF antibodies (BDNF-Abs) treated DIV22 hippocampal neurons. **(D)** Histogram comparing the spine head width between hippocampal neurons upon BSA (control), BDNF or BDNF antibodies (BDNF-Abs) treatment. **(E)** Histogram of the dendritic spine length in control, BDNF or BDNF antibodies (BDNF-Abs) treated neurons. **(F)** Graph showing the binning of spines according to their spine head width and comparing the proportion of spines within each category in response to a BSA (control), BDNF or BDNF antibodies (BDNF-Abs) treatment. **(G)** Graph showing the binning of spines according to their spine length and comparing the proportion of spines within each category in response to a BSA (control), BDNF or BDNF antibodies (BDNF-Abs) treatment. **(H)** Graph plotting dendritic complexity in relation to the distance to the cell body of hippocampal neurons under control conditions or treated with BDNF or BDNF antibodies (BDNF-Abs). **(H′)** Histogram of the total number of intersections for BSA (control), BDNF and BDNF antibodies (BDNF-Abs) treated neurons. The number in the columns represents the number of cells analyzed. Significance is indicated as follows: $^{*}p < 0.05$; $^{**}p < 0.01$; $^{***}p < 0.001$. Error bars indicate s.e.m. ANOVA, *post-hoc* Tukey's Multiple Comparison Test.

architecture or spine number and morphology in 2 weeks-old primary hippocampal neurons (15 DIV; **Figure 2A**). When 15 DIV fEGFP-expressing neurons treated for 24 hours with BDNF were compared to control neurons, no obvious difference in dendritic spine density or morphology could be observed. Accordingly, the quantification of spine density did not result in any significant difference between BDNF treated and control neurons (**Figure 2B**, Table S1). However, as for mature hippocampal neurons, also here the application of BDNF blocking antibodies led to a highly significant reduction in dendritic spine density (**Figure 2B**, Table S1; control vs. BDNF-Abs and BDNF vs. BDNF-Abs $p < 0.001$). We then assessed whether BDNF regulates spine morphology comparing the maximal spine head width and spines length between different treatments. Application of exogenous BDNF for 24 h did not result in any significant alteration of the spine head width (**Figure 2C**, Table S1) and length (**Figure 2D**, Table S1) in comparison to the control condition. Interestingly, while the loss-of-function experiments did not result in any significant change in spine head width (**Figure 2C**, Table S1) a significant increase in dendritic spine length could be observed after application of BDNF blocking antibodies in comparison to both the control and the BDNF treatment (**Figure 2D**, Table S1; control vs. BDNF-Abs and BDNF vs. BDNF-Abs $p < 0.001$). Binning the spines according to their head width and comparing the different treatments within each spine head category resulted in a significant increase in the proportion of spines with a small head for the BDNF blocking antibody treatment only when compared to the BDNF treatment (**Figure 2E**; BDNF vs. BDNF-Abs $p < 0.05$). No significant changes could be observed for the spine head width distribution upon BDNF application (**Figure 2E**) when compared to the control condition. Binning the spines according to their length showed for neurons treated with BDNF blocking antibodies a significant decrease in the shorter spine category (**Figure 2F**; <0.5 μm, control vs. BDNF-Abs $p < 0.01$, BDNF vs. BDNF-Abs $p < 0.001$; and ≥0.5 μm <1 μm, control vs. BDNF-Abs $p < 0.01$, BDNF vs. BNF-Abs $p < 0.001$) accompanied by a significant increase in longer spines (**Figure 2F**; >1.5 μm, control vs. BDNF-Abs $p < 0.01$, BDNF vs. BDNF-Abs $p < 0.001$). Finally, we also analyzed whether the effect of BDNF on dendrite architecture might be age dependent. However, also for 15 DIV hippocampal neurons when either a BDNF or a BDNF antibody treatment was compared to the controls, no significant alteration in dendritic complexity could be observed for the Sholl analysis (**Figure 2G**). Accordingly, we did not observe any significant differences in total complexity between the different treatments (**Figure 2G′**, Table S1).

All in all the results described above indicate that endogenous BDNF is necessary for dendritic spine growth and to regulate spine length in developing primary hippocampal neurons. Interestingly, the spine head width in younger hippocampal neurons is not dependent on endogenous BDNF signaling.

ENDOGENOUS BDNF REGULATES ACTIN CONCENTRATION WITHIN DENDRITIC SPINE

Because the actin cytoskeleton is involved in regulating cell mobility and morphology and actin is highly enriched within the dendritic spine head—for a review see (Cingolani and Goda, 2008)—we hypothesized that BDNF may regulate actin in dendritic spines in order to shape and change spine morphology. To test this hypothesis we used RFP-Lifeact (Riedl et al., 2008 and 2010) to detect possible changes in the F-actin content in dendritic spines upon changes in BDNF signaling. The RFP-Lifeact expression plasmid was co-transfected with fEGFP and resulted in 99.7% colocalization of RFP-Lifeact within spines (**Figures 3A/B**) as well as with F-actin labeled using Alexa Fluor 350 Phalloidin (**Figure 3B**). In line with our observations the exogenous application of BDNF for 24 hours to 22 or 15 DIV primary hippocampal neurons did not result in any change in the normalized mean fluorescent intensity for RFP-Lifeact in comparison to control (**Figures 3C,D**, Table S1). However, in the loss-of-function experiments the treatment with BDNF blocking antibodies resulted in a highly significant decrease in the F-actin content within the head of dendritic spines both in 16 DIV (**Figure 3D**, Table S1; control vs. BDNF-Abs $p < 0.001$, BDNF vs. BDNF-Abs $p < 0.001$) and 23 DIV primary hippocampal neurons (**Figure 3D**, Table S1; control vs. BDNF-Abs $p < 0.01$, BDNF vs. BDNF-Abs $p < 0.001$).

Taken together our results show that endogenous BDNF modulates the actin cytoskeleton within dendritic spines as well as their morphology.

MATURE PRIMARY HIPPOCAMPAL NEURONS ARE RESPONSIVE TO AN ACUTE TREATMENT WITH EXOGENOUS BDNF

Our results so far clearly support a role for endogenous BDNF in the hippocampus by completely reproducing *in vitro* the mild alterations observed in the morphology of hippocampal neurons *in vivo* upon a global BDNF deprivation (Rauskolb et al., 2010). On the other hand our data fail to replicate previous work showing an effect of BDNF application in regulating dendrite and spine architecture (Tyler and Pozzo-Miller, 2001; Ji et al., 2005). To address this discrepancy we first confirmed that the BDNF used in this study is indeed active and that it is able

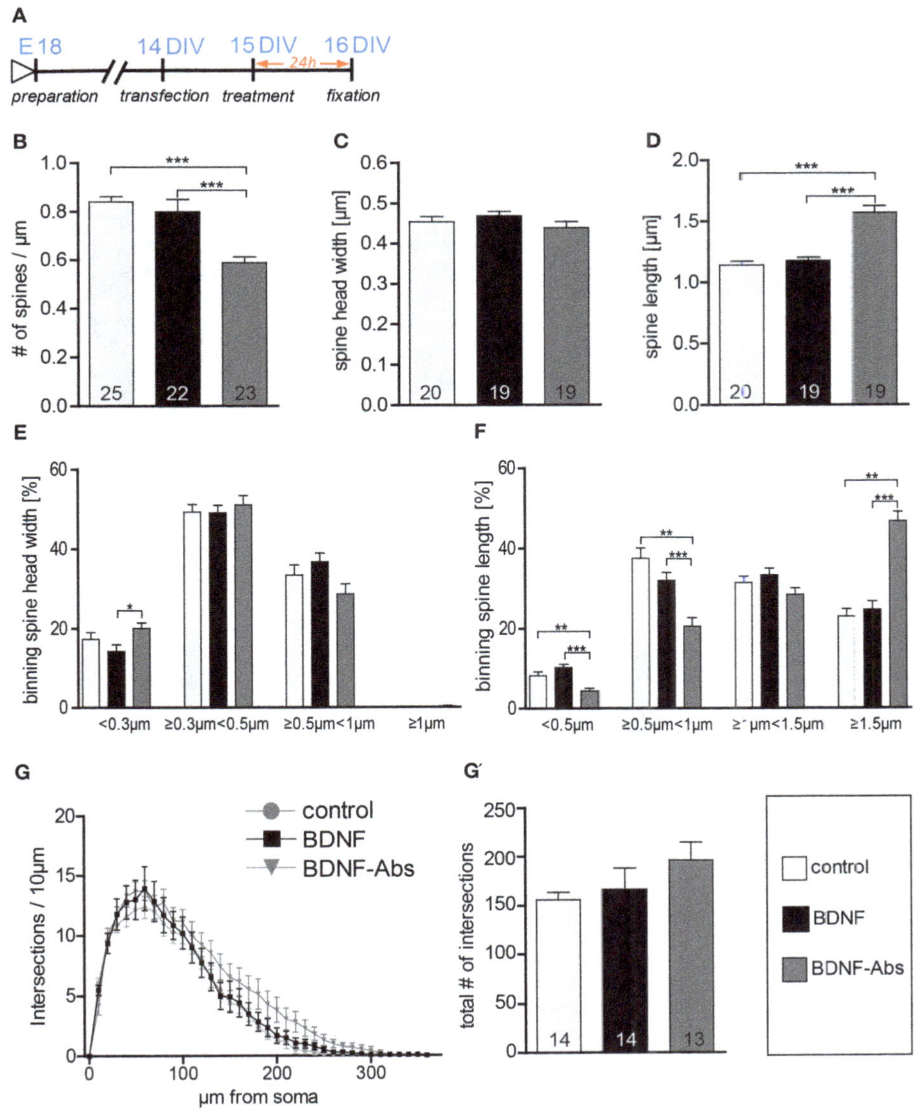

FIGURE 2 | (A) Experimental timeline. DIV16 hippocampal neurons were treated for 24 h before fixation **(B)** Graphs comparing dendritic spine density between control, BDNF and BDNF-antibodies (BDNF-Abs) treated DIV16 hippocampal neurons. **(C)** Histogram comparing the spine head width between hippocampal neurons upon BSA (control), BDNF or BDNF antibodies treatment. **(D)** Histogram of the dendritic spine length in BSA (control), BDNF or BDNF antibodies (BDNF-Abs) treated neurons. **(E)** Graph showing the binning of spines according to their spine head width and comparing the proportion of spines within each category in response to a BSA (control), BDNF or BDNF antibodies (BDNF-Abs) treatment. **(F)** Graph showing the binning of spines according to their spine length and comparing the proportion of spines within each category in response to a BSA (control), BDNF or BDNF antibodies (BDNF-Abs) treatment. **(G)** Graph plotting dendritic complexity in relation to the distance to the cell body of hippocampal neurons under control conditions or treated with BDNF or BDNF antibodies (BDNF-Abs). **(G′)** Histogram of the total number of intersections for BSA (control), BDNF and BDNF antibodies (BDNF-Abs) treated neurons. The number in the columns represents the number of cells analyzed. Significance is indicated as follows: $^{*}p < 0.05$; $^{**}p < 0.01$; $^{***}p < 0.001$. Error bars indicate s.e.m. ANOVA, *post-hoc* Tukey's Multiple Comparison Test.

to elicit clear neuronal responses in primary hippocampal neuronal cultures. To this aim we tested three critical events known to occur upon a BDNF application: (a) activation of the TrkB receptor was tested by analyzing its phosphorylation levels (Ji et al., 2010); (b) calcium imaging was used to test the ability of BDNF to induce local calcium transients in hippocampal neurons (Berninger et al., 1993) and (c) immunohistochemistry was used to visualize the activation of the immediate early gene (IEG) *c-fos* (Marty et al., 1996). An immunohistochemistry against phosphorylated TrkB receptor performed 15 min after BDNF application (**Figure 4A**) showed an obvious increase in the levels of TrkB receptor phosphorylation when compared to control treated neurons (**Figure 4B**). This observation was confirmed by a significant increase in the normalized intensity for the phospho-TrkB

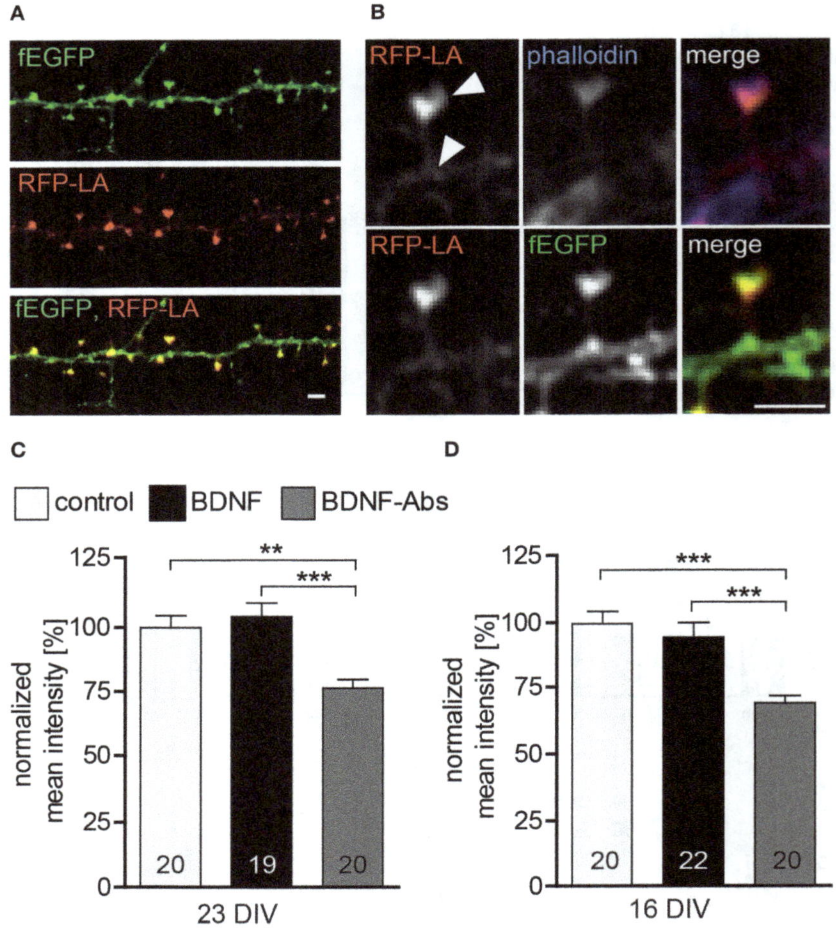

FIGURE 3 | (A) Maximal intensity projection of a representative dendrite of hippocampal neurons expressing fEGFP (above) and RFP-Lifeact (middle) merged to show colocalization (below). Scale bar, 2 μm. **(B)** High magnification images showing a single dendritic spine expressing fEGFP (above) and RFP-Lifeact (middle) and merged to show their colocalization in the spine head (below) Scale bar, 2 μm. **(C)** Histogram plotting the normalized mean fluorescent intensity for RFP-Lifeact within the spine head of DIV23 BSA (control), BDNF and BDNF antibodies (BDNF-Abs) treated neurons. **(D)** Histogram showing the normalized mean intensity for RFP-Lifeact within the spine head of DIV16 hippocampal neurons. The number in the columns represents the number of cells analyzed. Significance is indicated as follows: $^{**}p < 0.01$; $^{***}p < 0.001$. Error bars indicate s.e.m. ANOVA, *post-hoc* Tukey's Multiple Comparison Test.

immunohistochemistry (**Figure 4C**, Table S2; $p < 0.001$) as well as by a clear shift in the proportion of positive vs. negative cells for phospho-TrkB. Indeed, upon BDNF treatment significantly more neurons resulted to be positive for phospho-TrkB immunohistochemistry and significantly less to be negative for it (**Figure 4D**, Table S2; $p < 0.01$). The activation of the PLCγ signaling pathway upon BDNF binding to the TrkB receptor leads to an increase in the intracellular calcium levels (Segal and Greenberg, 1996; Blum and Konnerth, 2005; Minichiello, 2009) and was specifically shown for hippocampal cultures (Berninger et al., 1993; Canossa et al., 1997; Finkbeiner et al., 1997). Here we analyzed the frequency of global calcium transients as readout for a neuronal response to an acute BDNF application (**Figure 4E**; Lang et al., 2007; Lohmann, 2009). A clear increase in the frequency of calcium transients in DIV22 primary hippocampal neurons could be observed upon the acute application of BDNF (**Figure 4F**). Indeed, at a quantitative analysis calcium transient frequency resulted to be significantly increased after BDNF treatment in comparison to a control treatment (**Figure 4G**, Table S2; BDNF vs. control $p < 0.05$). The increase in the frequency in calcium transients upon BDNF application was transient as 10 min after BDNF washout the frequency was back to the pre-treatment levels (**Figure 4G**, Table S2). Finally, to verify that the application of BDNF leads to the expression of immediate early genes (IEGs) we used an immunohistochemistry for c-fos known to be activated upon an acute treatment with BDNF (**Figure 4H**; Marty et al., 1996; Gascon et al., 2005). An immunohistochemistry for c-fos showed a clear colocalization between c-fos and the nucleus of neurons (**Figure 4E**). Quantitative analysis performed 3 h after the stimulation with BDNF (**Figure 4H**) showed significantly higher intensity values for the c-fos immunohistochemistry (**Figure 4J**, Table S2; $p < 0.01$) and a significant increase in the number of c-fos positive cells in comparison to control (**Figure 4K**, Table S2; $p < 0.001$).

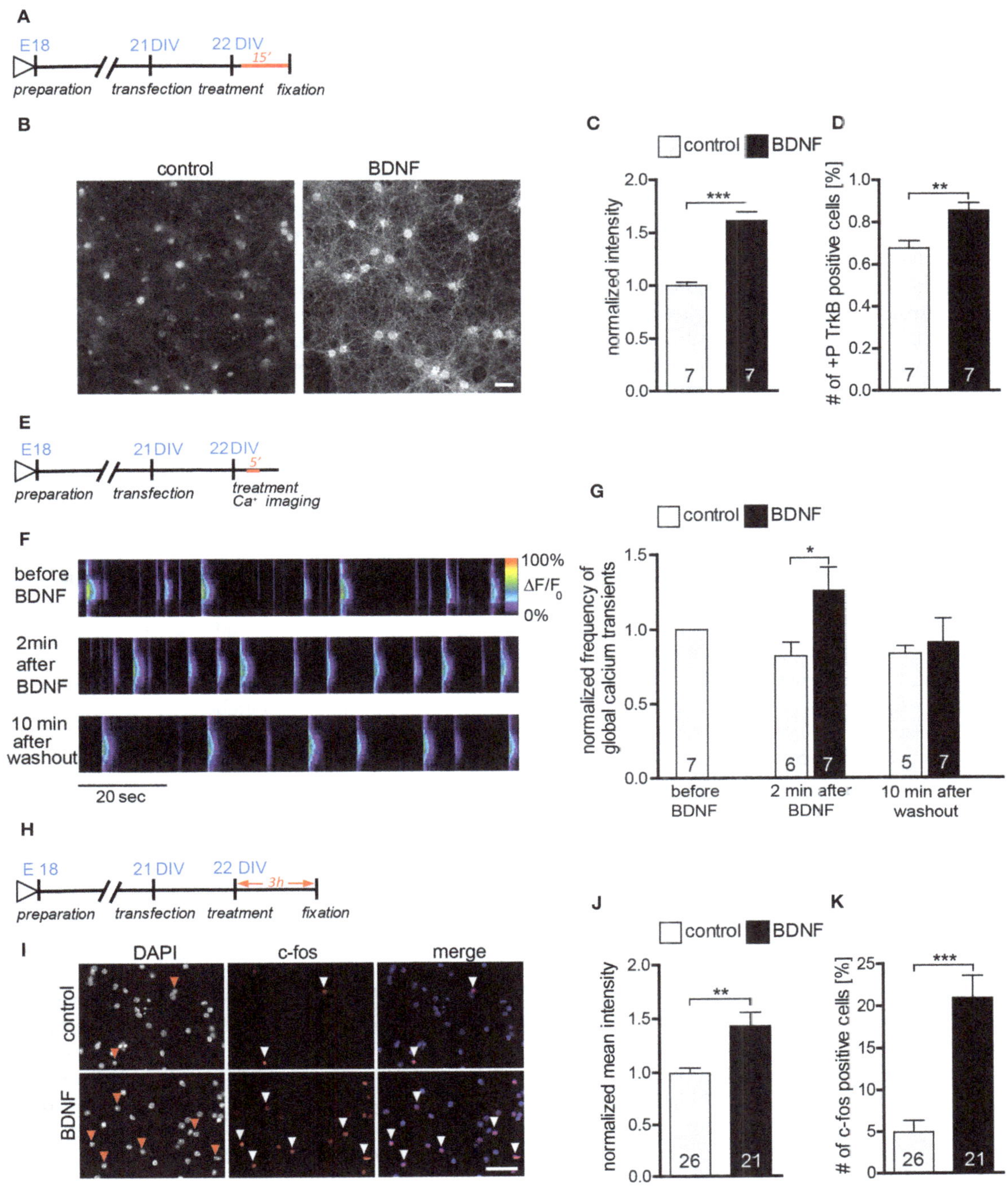

FIGURE 4 | (A) Experimental timeline. DIV22 primary hippocampal neurons were treated 15 min with BDNF before fixation. **(B)** Images of primary hippocampal cultures (22 DIV) treated with either BSA (control) (left) or BDNF (right) and stained with an anti-phospho-TrkB receptor antibodies. Scale bar, 40 μm. **(C)** Histogram showing the normalized fluorescence intensity for the phospho-TrkB receptor under control conditions or treated with BDNF. **(D)** Graph showing the number of phospho-TrkB positive hippocampal neurons in control and BDNF treated hippocampal primary cultures. **(E)** Experimental timeline. DIV22 primary hippocampal neurons were treated 5 min with BDNF during calcium imaging. **(F)** Pseudo line-scan showing the global calcium transients occurring in hippocampal primary cultures before, during and after BDNF applications. **(G)** Graph showing the frequency of calcium transients in hippocampal primary neurons before, during and after BDNF application. **(H)** Experimental timeline. DIV22 primary hippocampal neurons were treated for 3 h with BDNF before fixation. **(I)** Images of primary hippocampal cultures (22 DIV) treated with either BSA (control) (above) or BDNF (below) and stained with an anti-c-fos antibody. Scale bar, 20 μm. **(J)** Graph comparing the normalized mean intensity for the immunohistochemistry against c-fos in control or BDNF treated hippocampal primary neurons. **(K)** Histogram of the number of c-fos positive neurons in control and BDNF treated hippocampal cultures. The number in the columns represents the number of analyzed experiments. Significance is indicated as follows: $*p < 0.05$; $**p < 0.01$; $***p < 0.001$. Error bars indicate s.e.m. Unpaired two-tailed Student Test.

In summary we could show that the BDNF used in these experiments is active and clearly leads to an activation of the TrkB-receptor, an increase in the frequency of calcium transients and an activation of transcription (up regulation of the immediate early gene *c-fos*) in mature primary hippocampal neurons.

EXOGENOUS BDNF REGULATES NEURITE OUTGROWTH AND COMPLEXITY IN YOUNG PRIMARY HIPPOCAMPAL NEURONS

Previous studies have shown BDNF to promote neurite outgrouth and dendritic complexity (Mcallister et al., 1995; Shimada et al., 1998). In view of the lack of effects on dendritic architecture observed in this study upon BDNF application to either DIV15 or DIV22 hippocampal primary neurons, we tested whether the effect of BDNF on dendrites might be age-dependent. Indeed, BDNF has been shown to regulate neurite outgrowth in development hippocampal neurons (Ji et al., 2005, 2010). Therefore, we treated young hippocampal neurons 3 DIV with either a gain- or a loss-of-function approach for BDNF. After 3 days of treatment (**Figure 5A**) an immunohistochemistry for Microtubule-associated protein 2 (MAP2) was used to visualize the developing neurites (**Figure 5B**; up control, middle BDNF, lower TrkB-Fc). Morphometric analysis for neurite growth was performed by quantifying three parameters: total neurite length, number of primary neurites and number of branching points (**Figures 5C–E**, Table S3). The total neurite length was higher after BDNF application than in control treated neurons (**Figure 5C**, Table S3; BDNF vs. control, $p < 0.001$). Interestingly the loss-of-function experiments with either a BDNF-Abs or TrkB-Fc did not show any significant difference in neurite length when compared to the control conditions (**Figure 5C**, Table S3). The specificity of the TrkB-Fc in neutralizing BDNF was determined by a co-application of BDNF and TrkB-Fc. Quantitative analysis revealed that application of TrkB-Fc completely prevented the positive effect of a BDNF treatment on the total neurite length (**Figure 5C**, Table S3). The number of primary neurites after BDNF application showed a slight increase when compared to the control (**Figure 5D**, Table S3; BDNF vs. control, $p < 0.01$), whereas the treatment with BDNF-Abs or TrkB-Fc did not alter neurite number (**Figure 5D**, Table S3). The significant increase in primary neurites observed after BDNF treatment could be prevented by a co-treatment with TrkB-Fc (**Figure 5D**, Table S3). Next we determined whether a BDNF application might affect neurite complexity by analyzing the number of branching points of MAP2 labeled processes. Indeed, a BDNF treatment resulted in a 2-fold increase in complexity in comparison to control (**Figure 5E**, Table S3; BDNF vs. control, $p < 0.001$). On the contrary, treatment with BDNF-Abs or TrkB-Fc did not influence the number of branching points when compared to the control (**Figure 5E**, Table S3). Additionally, the positive effect of BDNF on neurite complexity was prevented by a co-treatment with BDNF and TrkB-Fc (**Figure 5E**, Table S3).

Our results suggest that the application of BDNF promotes neurite outgrowth by increasing both neurite elongation and branching in developing DIV3 hippocampal primary neurons. Interestingly, two loss-of-function approaches for BDNF did not affect the neurite architecture of primary hippocampal neurons (3–6 DIV) during their early development.

ROLE OF NEURONAL ACTIVITY IN REGULATING THE SENSITIVITY OF MATURE HIPPOCAMPAL NEURONS UPON EXOGENOUS BDNF APPLICATION

BDNF synthesis and release have been shown to occur in an activity-dependent way (Thoenen, 1991; Gärtner and Staiger, 2002). Therefore, one possible explanation for the discrepancies in the effect of BDNF application on neuronal morphology *in vitro* (Ji et al., 2005, 2010; Rauskolb et al., 2010) may lie in the different levels of neuronal activity in the primary cultures. Indeed, in cultures with a higher neuronal activity the levels of endogenous BDNF may be already high and might mask the effects of BDNF application. To test this hypothesis primary hippocampal neurons were kept for 2 weeks in a medium containing a higher concentration of Magnesium (3.5 mM Mg^{2+}; **Figure 6A**) and the effects of a 24 h treatment with BDNF (in NB medium with low, 1.5 mM Mg^{2+}) on the number and structure of dendritic spines were analyzed. Calcium imaging was used to compare the levels of neuronal activity in hippocampal neurons grown under high Mg^{2+} to those of neurons grown under control (low Mg^{2+}) conditions. While no significant difference could be detected regarding the amplitude of global calcium transients between the two groups (**Figure 6C**, Table S4), their frequency was significantly decreased in neurons kept in high Mg^{2+} when compared to control neurons (**Figure 6B**, Table S4; $p < 0.001$) suggesting a long-term reduction in neuronal activity. Accordingly, while dendritic complexity was unchanged (**Figure 6D**, Table S4), a significantly lower dendritic spine density could be observed when comparing control neurons kept in high Mg^{2+} with control neurons kept in low Mg^{2+} medium (**Figure 6E**, Table S4; $p < 0.001$). On the other hand, no significant differences in spine density could be detected upon a BDNF or a TrkB-Fc treatment for neurons grown under high Mg^{2+} conditions when compared to the control high Mg^{2+} conditions (**Figure 6E**, Table S4). Next, a possible effect of BDNF on dendritic spine morphology was analyzed. Interestingly, compared to control treated neurons BDNF treatment in cultures kept in high Mg^{2+} resulted in a slight increase in dendritic spine width (**Figure 6F**, Table S4) and a slight decrease in spine length (**Figure 6G**, Table S4), but the difference did not reach significance. No significant differences were observed both for the head width and for the length when TrkB-Fc treated cells in high Mg^{2+} were compared to high Mg^{2+} controls (**Figures 6F,G**, Table S4). To better clarify the mild spine head increase observed in neurons kept in high Mg^{2+} medium upon BDNF treatment spines were binned into four categories according to their head width. Comparing spine head width within each category showed a significant increase upon BDNF treatment in the proportion of spines with larger heads (**Figure 6H**; $\geq 0.5\,\mu m$ $< 1\,\mu m$; $p < 0.05$) with a comparable significant decrease in the proportion of spine with small heads (**Figure 6H**; $< 0.3\,\mu m$; $p < 0.05$) when compared to control neurons cultivated in high Mg^{2+}. No significant difference was observed between the control and TrkB-Fc treatments in any of the spine head width categories under the same conditions (**Figure 6H**). Comparing the effect of a control, a BDNF or a TrkB-Fc treatment within different categories of dendritic spine binned according to their length did not show any significant

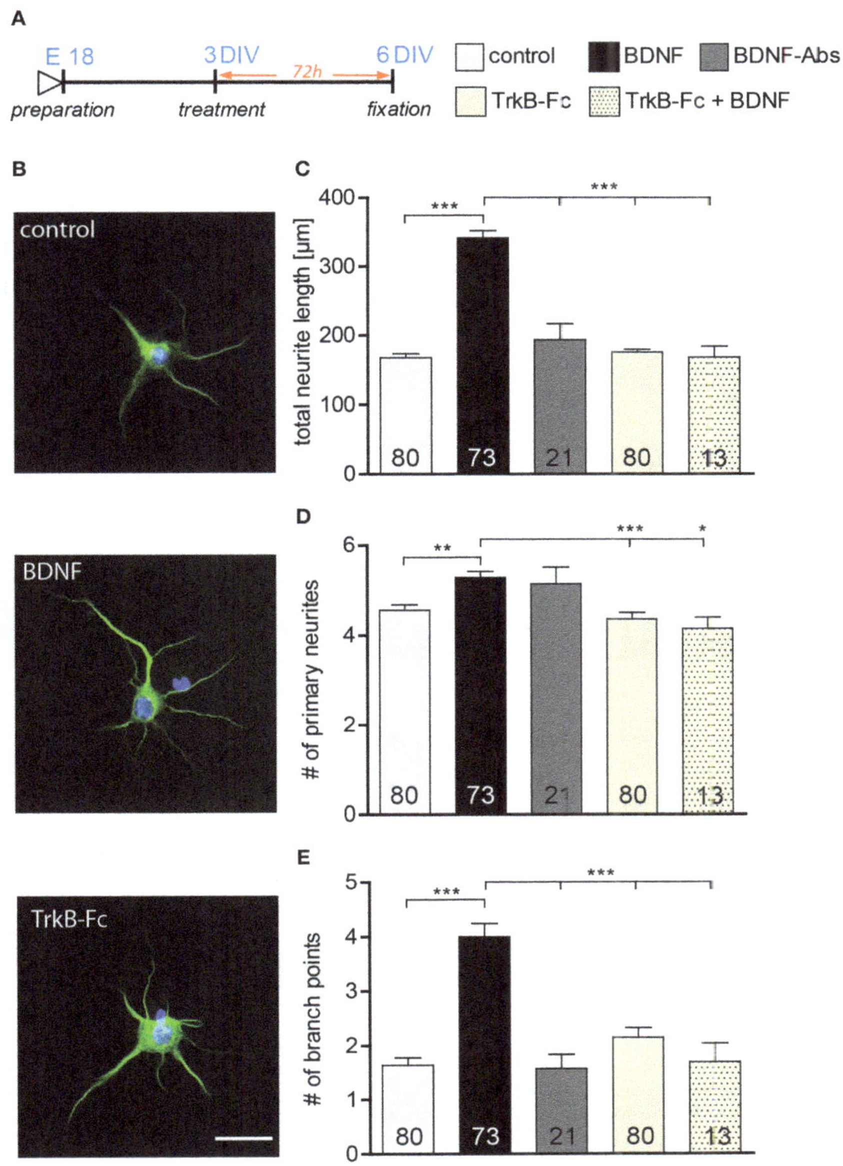

FIGURE 5 | (A) Experimental timeline. BSA, BDNF, BDNF antibodies (BDNF-Abs) or TrkB receptor bodies (TrkB-Fc) were applied on DIV3 hippocampal neurons for 72 h. **(B)** Micrographs showing MAP2 positive BSA (control) (above), BDNF (middle) or BDNF antibodies (BDNF-Abs; below) treated primary hippocampal neurons. Scale bar, 25 µm. **(C)** Histogram comparing neurite length of DIV6 hippocampal neurons after application of BSA (control), BDNF, BDNF antibodies (BDNF-Abs), TrkB receptor bodies (TrkB-Fc) or combined BDNF and TrkB receptor bodies (TrkB-Fc). **(D)** Histogram comparing the number of primary neurites of DIV6 hippocampal neurons after application of BSA (control), BDNF, BDNF antibodies (BDNF-Abs), TrkB receptor bodies (TrkB-Fc) or combined BDNF and TrkB receptor bodies (TrkB-Fc). **(E)** Histogram comparing the number of branching points for the dendrites of DIV6 hippocampal neurons after application of BSA (control), BDNF, BDNF antibodies (BDNF-Abs), TrkB receptor bodies (TrkB-Fc) or combined BDNF and TrkB receptor bodies (TrkB-Fc). The number in the columns represents the number of cells analyzed. Significance is indicated as follows: $*p < 0.05$; $**p < 0.01$; $***p < 0.001$. Error bars indicate s.e.m. ANOVA, *post-hoc* Tukey's Multiple Comparison Test.

difference (**Figure 6I**). The data described above suggest that indeed a chronic reduction in neuronal activity during the cultivation time might reduce the endogenous BDNF levels in hippocampal primary neurons and thereby increase their sensitivity to an exogenous BDNF application to modulate dendritic spine morphology.

THE ACTION OF EXOGENOUS BDNF IN MODULATING DENDRITIC SPINE MORPHOLOGY DEPEND ON NEURONAL ACTIVITY

BDNF has been shown to modulate dendritic spine morphology upon activity-dependent synaptic plasticity Tanaka (Tanaka et al., 2008). To assess whether under our culture condition neuronal activity governs the BDNF effect on dendritic spine

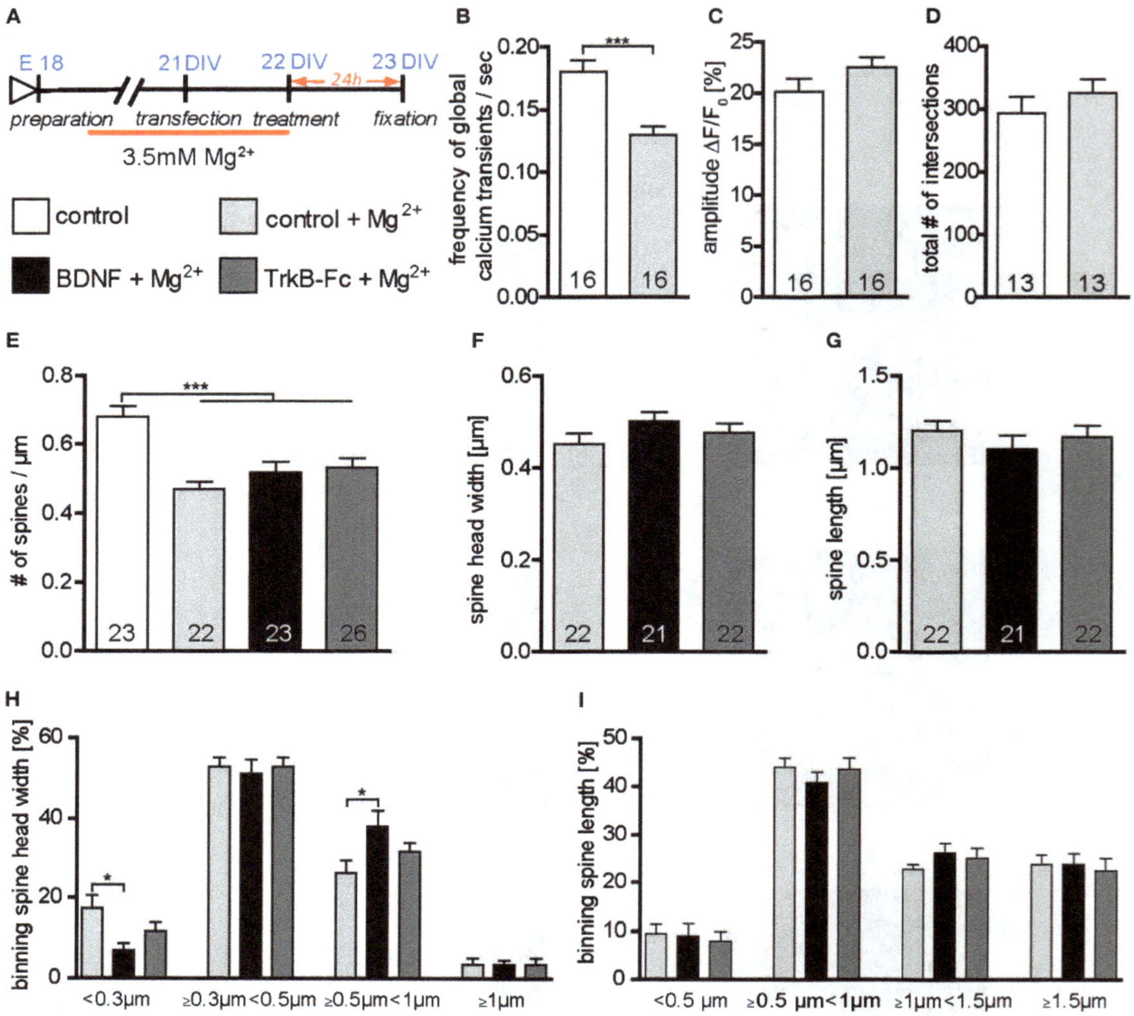

FIGURE 6 | (A) Experimental timeline. Primary neurons were cultivated for 2 weeks in high (3.5 mM) Mg^{2+} medium and treated with BSA (control), BDNF or TrkB-Fc in low (1.5 mM) Mg^{2+}. **(B)** Graph comparing the frequency of calcium transients in hippocampal primary neurons cultivated in high or low Mg^{2+} containing medium. **(C)** Graph comparing the amplitude of calcium transients in hippocampal primary neurons cultivated in high or low Mg^{2+} containing medium. **(D)** Histogram of the total number of intersections in hippocampal primary neurons cultivated in high or low Mg^{2+} containing medium. **(E)** Graphs comparing dendritic spine density between neurons cultivated in low or high Mg^{2+} and treated with BSA (control), BDNF and TrkB receptor bodies (TrkB-Fc). **(F)** Histogram comparing the spine head width between primary hippocampal neurons cultivated in high Mg^{2+} and treated with BSA (control), BDNF and TrkB receptor bodies (TrkB-Fc). **(G)** Histogram of the dendritic spine length between primary hippocampal neurons cultivated in high Mg^{2+} and treated with BSA (control), BDNF and TrkB receptor bodies (TrkB-Fc). **(H)** Graph showing the binning of spines according to their spine head width and comparing the proportion of spines within each category in response to a BSA (control), BDNF or BDNF antibodies (BDNF-Abs) treatment. **(I)** Graph showing the binning of spines according to their spine length and comparing the proportion of spines within each category in response to a control, BDNF or TrkB receptor bodies (TrkB-Fc) treatment. The number in the columns represents the number of cells analyzed. Significance is indicated as follows: $^{*}p < 0.05$; $^{***}p < 0.001$. Error bars indicate s.e.m. Unpaired two-tailed Student Test and ANOVA, *post-hoc* Tukey's Multiple Comparison Test.

morphology, hippocampal primary neurons were kept for 2 weeks and treated with BDNF in a high Mg^{2+} (3.5 mM) medium (**Figure 7A**) in order to reduce neuronal activity. Under these conditions a significantly lower dendritic spine density could be observed when comparing control neurons kept in high Mg^{2+} to control neurons in low Mg^{2+} medium (**Figure 7B**, Table S4; $p < 0.05$). Moreover, dendritic spine density of neurons treated either with BDNF or with TrkB-Fc in high Mg^{2+} was significantly lower than in controls (low Mg^{2+}) neurons (**Figure 7B**, Table S4; BDNF vs. low Mg^{2+} control $p < 0.05$; TrkB-Fc *vs.* low Mg^{2+} control $p < 0.001$). Interestingly, both a BDNF treatment as well as a treatment with TrkB-Fc performed in high Mg^{2+} did not affect either spine head width (**Figure 7C**, Table S4) or spine length (**Figure 7D**, Table S4) when compared to a control treatment in high Mg^{2+}. Also binning the spines according to their head width (**Figure 7E**) or to their length (**Figure 7F**) did not show any alteration in the spine size distributions both for a BDNF and a TrkB-Fc

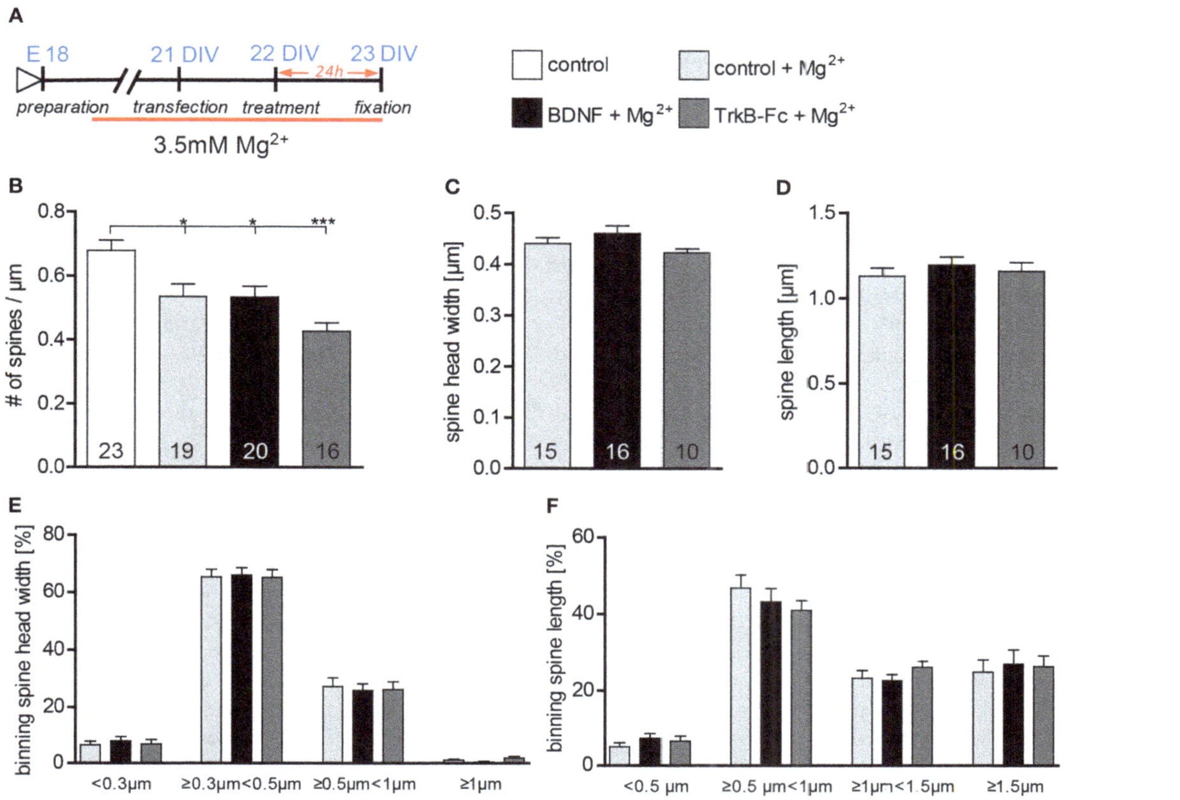

FIGURE 7 | (A) Experimental timeline. Primary neurons were cultivated for 2 weeks in high Mg^{2+} medium and treated with BSA (control), BDNF or TrkB-Fc in high Mg^{2+}. **(B)** Graphs comparing dendritic spine density between neurons cultivated in low or high Mg^{2+} and treated with BSA (control), BDNF and TrkB receptor bodies (TrkB-Fc) in high Mg^{2+}. **(C)** Histogram comparing the spine head width between primary hippocampal neurons cultivated and treated in high Mg^{2+} with BSA (control), BDNF and TrkB receptor bodies (TrkB-Fc). **(D)** Histogram of the dendritic spine length between primary hippocampal neurons cultivated and treated in high Mg^{2+} with BSA (control), BDNF and TrkB receptor bodies (TrkB-Fc). **(E)** Graph showing the binning of spines according to their spine head width and comparing the proportion of spines within each category in response to a BSA (control), BDNF or BDNF antibodies (BDNF-Abs) treatment in high Mg^{2+}. **(F)** Graph showing the binning of spines according to their spine length and comparing the proportion of spines within each category in response to a BSA (control), BDNF or TrkB receptor bodies (TrkB-Fc) treatment in high Mg^{2+}. The number in the columns represents the number of cells analyzed. Significance is indicated as follows: $^*p < 0.05$; $^{***}p < 0.001$. Error bars indicate s.e.m. Unpaired two-tailed Student Test and ANOVA, *post-hoc* Tukey's Multiple Comparison Test.

applications compared to a control treatment performed in high Mg^{2+}.

The results above indicate that BDNF application indeed modulates dendritic spine architecture in an activity-dependent manner.

DISCUSSION

The main findings in this study are that the effects exerted by BDNF on the dendritic architecture of hippocampal neurons are dependent on the neuron's maturation stage and that BDNF is specifically required for the activity-dependent maintenance of the mature spine phenotype in mature excitatory hippocampal neurons *in vitro*. Indeed, our current results reproduce previous results obtained *in vivo* (Rauskolb et al., 2010). These observations further support the notion, that BDNF is a precise mediator of specific effects on neurons rather than a pleiotropic molecule unspecifically promoting cell health and survival. Indeed, besides its role in promoting neurite outgrowth (Ji et al., 2005, 2010), which we can confirm in the data presented here, BDNF is required for the activity-dependent maturation and stabilization of dendritic spines.

Our results are in line with previous work showing a surprising selectivity in the brain areas requiring BDNF-signaling for normal post-natal development (Minichiello et al., 1999; Zakharenko et al., 2003; Rauskolb et al., 2010; Zagrebelsky and Korte, 2013). Indeed, while a global BDNF deprivation throughout the CNS impairs the proper post-natal growth of striatal medium spiny neurons, BDNF deprivation fails to cause major alterations in the fine structure of mature CA1 pyramidal neurons (Rauskolb et al., 2010). These observations suggest a crucial but rather limited and specific effect of BDNF in maintaining the mature phenotype of dendritic spines without affecting the general architecture of hippocampal neurons. Our results *in vitro* show a very similar effect upon the application of two loss-of-function approaches for BDNF (function blocking BDNF antibodies, TrkB receptor bodies) confirming a physiological role of the endogenous BDNF in this context. On the other hand, our experiments fail to reproduce previously published data showing a highly significant increase in dendritic spine density and alterations in spine morphology upon the application of exogenous BDNF to mature hippocampal primary neurons (Ji et al., 2005, 2010) or to hippocampal slice cultures (Tyler and Pozzo-Miller, 2001). The discrepancy between the data presented here and other previously published data regarding the role of exogenous BDNF in regulating the architecture of mature hippocampal neurons may have different reasons. One possible explanation is the different animal species used for the experiments. While studies showing an effect of a BDNF loss-of-function either *in vivo* (Rauskolb et al., 2010) or *in vitro* (our current study) were mostly performed in mouse derived cultures, most of the previous *in vitro* work describing an effect for a BDNF gain-of-function was done in rat hippocampal neurons (Tyler and Pozzo-Miller, 2001; Ji et al., 2005, 2010) suggesting a possible difference in the sensitivity to BDNF signaling in the two different species—or simply a different level of BDNF release from neurons into the medium. Moreover, culture conditions have been shown to possibly influence the expression levels as well as the cellular response to BDNF (Chapleau et al., 2008). Indeed, here we show that the levels of neuronal activity in the cultures determine the responsiveness to the exogenous or the endogenous BDNF (**Figures 6**, **7**). Low levels of neuronal activity during the cultivation period result in lower spine density values and an increased responsiveness of the hippocampal neurons to the applications of exogenous BDNF. Indeed, the synthesis and secretion of BDNF have been shown to be directly controlled by neuronal activity (reviewed in Thoenen, 1991; see also Gärtner and Staiger, 2002). Accordingly, control neurons in previous publications showing a strong effect upon a BDNF application (Ji et al., 2005, 2010) had a spine density which is about 10 times smaller than the one measured in the current study or described *in vivo* (De Simoni et al., 2003) and 5 times smaller than the one described for a more complex *in vitro* system (De Simoni et al., 2003; Rauskolb et al., 2010). It should also be noted that in our culture system the levels of neuronal activity as well as the cellular responsiveness to BDNF were tested in different ways (**Figures 4A–K**). Application of exogenous BDNF has been shown to trigger a direct response of the neuronal network via a transient elevation of the intracellular calcium concentration (Berninger et al., 1993; Lang et al., 2007). In contrast, blocking intrinsic BDNF signaling was shown to reduce the frequency of spontaneously occurring calcium rises in developing rat hippocampal neurons (Lang et al., 2007). In our study calcium imaging was used first to test the responsiveness of the hippocampal neurons to BDNF and also to test the effects on neuronal activity of manipulating the Mg^{2+} concentration in the culture medium. Thereby we could confirm that increasing Mg^{2+} concentration in the medium results in a long lasting reduction in neuronal excitability and network activity of primary hippocampal cultures (Dribben et al., 2010). While this reduction in neuronal activity does not influence dendritic morphology and complexity, it's accompanied by a significant decrease in dendritic spine density as well as by an increased cellular sensitivity to the application of exogenous BDNF. The cellular responsiveness to BDNF was tested also quantifying the changes in TrkB phosphorylation as well as the activation of the IEG c-fos, two critical events known to occur upon the acute activation of BDNF signaling (Marty et al., 1996; Ji et al., 2005, 2010). Our results indicate that in spite of the lack of morphological effects of an application of BDNF, mature excitatory, hippocampal neurons under the culture conditions used in this work are responsive to BDNF. In addition, their responsiveness is increased under low neuronal activity conditions. Whether the increase neuronal responsiveness to BDNF is due to an activity-dependent decrease in BDNF release from neurons or, as recently described from microglia (Parkhurst et al., 2013) will be very interesting to address. Indeed, changes in magnesium concentration have been shown to possibly influence ATP release (Li et al., 1997) and could thereby indirectly influence BDNF release from microglia (Trang et al., 2009; Parkhurst et al., 2013). Moreover, it will be crucial to explore the possibility that different amounts of microglia may influence the BDNF levels in the primary hippocampal cultures and thereby their responsiveness to a BDNF exogenous application.

Our results show a requirement for neuronal-activity during the application for BDNF to exert its effect on dendritic spines. This observation is in line with previous work showing that during the early development of cortical pyramidal neurons in ferrets BDNF regulates dendritic architecture in an activity-dependent manner (Mcallister et al., 1996). Moreover, in cultures of cerebellar neurons, BDNF increases the spine density of Purkinje cells only in the presence of granule cells suggesting a crucial role of neuronal activity in mediating this BDNF effect (Shimada et al., 1998). In line with this observation is the role of BDNF in regulating structural changes at dendritic spines upon activity-dependent synaptic plasticity in mature hippocampal neurons (Tanaka et al., 2008).

One important open question concerns the functional consequences of the observed structural changes at spines regulated by BDNF signaling. Our results upon a BDNF loss-of-function confirm the structural alterations at spine observed already *in vivo* (Rauskolb et al., 2010). Specifically, a BDNF deprivation results in a decrease in dendritic spine density accompanied by a decrease in spine head width and an increase in spine length suggesting a loss of the mature phenotype of spines possibly resulting in a decrease and a weakening of synaptic connections under these conditions. Indeed, spine head width is correlated with the size of the post-synaptic density and the number of AMPA receptors (Holtmaat and Svoboda, 2009) and a shrinking of the spine head width has been correlated to the synaptic weakening occurring upon long term depression induction (Zhou et al., 2004). Moreover, the spine neck has been suggested to act as a diffusion barrier regulating the biochemical compartmentalization in the spine head (Sjostrom et al., 2008; Holthoff et al., 2010). Indeed, spines with long necks have been shown to be electrically silent at the soma, although their heads are activated by an uncaging event (Araya et al., 2006) and a BDNF-dependent shortening of the spine neck was observed upon inducing long term potentiation at single spines (Tanaka et al., 2008). It has been show that upon maturation the proportion of mushroom spines increases while the one of thin long spines decreases (De Simoni et al., 2003). Taken together these data suggest that BDNF signaling plays a crucial role in maintaining the mature architecture of dendritic spines.

Finally, we show in our experiments that endogenous BDNF modulates the actin cytoskeleton within dendritic spines as well as their morphology. This is of interest with respect to the fact that activity-dependent as well as spontaneous structural changes of dendritic spines are dependent on the modulation of actin dynamics within spines (Krucker et al., 2000; Fukazawa et al., 2003; Kramar et al., 2004). Noteworthy in this context is the observation that BDNF modulates actin regulatory binding proteins which control the turnover of the actin cytoskeleton as well as cytoskeleton-associated proteins like Arc/Arg3.1 (Ying et al., 2002; Messaoudi et al., 2007; Rex et al., 2007; Bramham, 2008). Interestingly, while a gain-of-function approach performed in this study did not affect the F-actin content within dendritic spines, a loss-of-function experiment resulted in a significant decrease in polymerized actin (see **Figure 3**). This is in line with the results of Rex et al. (2007) which show that exogenous application of BDNF to rat hippocampal slices increased the number of F-actin labeled spines only when theta burst stimulation was applied (Rex et al., 2007). Moreover, the effect of theta burst stimulation on F-actin was completely abolished by a BDNF scavenger (TrkB-Fc; Rex et al., 2007) suggesting a role for the TrkB receptor in this context. On the other hand, BDNF might also modulate actin dynamics via the p75 Neurotrophin Receptor ($p75^{NTR}$). In a series of gain- and loss-of-function experiments we previously showed that the $p75^{NTR}$ negatively modulates dendritic spine density and morphology (Zagrebelsky et al., 2005), in addition to its effect on long-term depression (Rösch et al., 2005; Woo et al., 2005). It has been shown that signaling via the $p75^{NTR}$ controls the activity of the small GTPase RhoA, thereby regulating the actin cytoskeleton (Yamashita et al., 1999; Yamashita and Tohyama, 2003; Gehler et al., 2004) and possibly preparing it for processes of negative synaptic plasticity.

In summary our study reports highly specific effects of BDNF on the maintenance of mature spines in excitatory hippocampal neurons and it also shed some light on why published *in vivo* and *in vitro* results concerning morphological effects of BDNF are often contradictory.

ACKNOWLEDGMENTS

We are grateful for the excellent technical assistance of Diane Mundil. This work was supported by the DFG (Martin Korte and Marta Zagrebelsky).

REFERENCES

Araya, R., Jiang, J., Eisenthal, K. B., and Yuste, R. (2006). The spine neck filters membrane potentials. *Proc. Natl. Acad. Sci. U.S.A.* 103, 17961–17966. doi: 10.1073/pnas.0608755103

Baquet, Z. C., Gorski, J. A., and Jones, K. R. (2004). Early striatal dendrite deficits followed by neuron loss with advanced age in the absence of anterograde cortical brain-derived neurotrophic factor. *J. Neurosci.* 24, 4250–4258. doi: 10.1523/JNEUROSCI.3920-03.2004

Berninger, B., Garcia, D. E., Inagaki, N., Hahnel, C., and Lindholm, D. (1993). BDNF and NT-3 induce intracellular Ca2+ elevation in hippocampal neurones. *Neuroreport* 4, 1303–1306. doi: 10.1097/00001756-199309150-00004

Blum, R., and Konnerth, A. (2005). Neurotrophin-mediated rapid signaling in the central nervous system: mechanisms and functions. *Physiology. (Bethesda)* 20, 70–78. doi: 10.1152/physiol.00042.2004

Bramham, C. R. (2008). Local protein synthesis, actin dynamics, and LTP consolidation. *Curr. Opin. Neurobiol* 18, 524–531. doi: 10.1016/j.conb.2008.09.013

Canossa, M., Griesbeck, O., Berninger, B., Campana, G., Kolbeck, R., and Thoenen, H. (1997). Neurotrophin release by neurotrophins: implications for activity-dependent neuronal plasticity. *Proc. Natl. Acad. Sci. U.S.A.* 94, 13279–13286. doi: 10.1073/pnas.94.24.13279

Carreton, O., Giralt, A., Torres-Peraza, J. F., Brito, V., Lucas, J. J., Gines, S., et al. (2012). Age-dependent decline of motor neocortex but not hippocampal performance in heterozygous BDNF mice correlates with a decrease of cortical PSD-95 but an increase of hippocampal TrkB levels. *Exp. Neurol.* 237, 335–345. doi: 10.1016/j.expneurol.2012.06.033

Chan, J. P., Cordeira, J., Calderon, G. A., Iyer, L. K., and Rios, M. (2008). Depletion of central BDNF in mice impedes terminal differentiation of new granule neurons in the adult hippocampus. *Mol. Cell. Neurosci.* 39, 372–383. doi: 10.1016/j.mcn.2008.07.017

Chan, J. R., Jolicoeur, C., Yamauchi, J., Elliott, J., Fawcett, J. P., Ng, B. K., et al. (2006). The polarity protein Par-3 directly interacts with p75NTR to regulate myelination. *Science* 314, 832–836. doi: 10.1126/science.1134069

Chapleau, C. A., Carlo, M. E., Larimore, J. L., and Pozzo-Miller, L. (2008). The actions of BDNF on dendritic spine density and morphology in organotypic slice cultures depend on the presence of serum in culture media. *J. Neurosci. Methods* 169, 182–190. doi: 10.1016/j.jneumeth.2007.12.006

Chen, G., Kolbeck, R., Barde, Y. A., Bonhoeffer, T., and Kossel, A. H. (1999). Relative contribution of endogenous neurotrophins in hippocampal long-term potentiation. *J. Neurosci.* 19, 7983–7990.

Cingolani, L. A., and Goda, Y. (2008). Actin in action: the interplay between the actin cytoskeleton and synaptic efficacy. *Nat. Rev. Neurosci.* 9, 344–356. doi: 10.1038/nrn2373

Danzer, S. C., Pan, E., Nef, S., Parada, L. F., and Mcnamara, J. O. (2004). Altered regulation of brain-derived neurotrophic factor protein in hippocampus following slice preparation. *Neuroscience* 126, 859–869. doi: 10.1016/j.neuroscience.2004.03.025

De Simoni, A., Griesinger, C. B., and Edwards, F. A. (2003). Development of rat CA1 neurones in acute versus organotypic slices: role of experience in synaptic morphology and activity. *J. Physiol.* 550, 135–147. doi: 10.1113/jphysiol.2003.039099

Dribben, W. H., Eisenman, L. N., and Mennerick, S. (2010). Magnesium induces neuronal apoptosis by suppressing excitability. *Cell Death Dis.* 1:e63. doi: 10.1038/cddis.2010.39

Erickson, K. I., Voss, M. W., Prakash, R. S., Basak, C., Szabo, A., Chaddock, L., et al. (2011). Exercise training increases size of hippocampus and improves memory. *Proc. Natl. Acad. Sci. U.S.A.* 108, 3017–3022. doi: 10.1073/pnas.1015950108

Finkbeiner, S., Tavazoie, S. F., Maloratsky, A., Jacobs, K. M., Harris, K. M., and Greenberg, M. E. (1997). CREB: a major mediator of neuronal neurotrophin responses. *Neuron* 19, 1031–1047. doi: 10.1016/S0896-6273(00)80395-5

Fukazawa, Y., Saitoh, Y., Ozawa, F., Ohta, Y., Mizuno, K., and Inokuchi, K. (2003). Hippocampal LTP is accompanied by enhanced F-actin content within the dendritic spine that is essential for late LTP maintenance *in vivo*. *Neuron* 38, 447–460. doi: 10.1016/S0896-6273(03)00206-X

Gärtner, A., and Staiger, V. (2002). Neurotrophin secretion from hippocampal neurons evoked by long-term-potentiation-inducing electrical stimulation patterns. *Proc. Natl. Acad. Sci. U.S.A.* 99, 6386–6391. doi: 10.1073/pnas.092129699

Gascon, E., Vutskits, L., Zhang, H., Barral-Moran, M. J., Kiss, P. J., Mas, C., et al. (2005). Sequential activation of p75 and TrkB is involved in dendritic development of subventricular zone-derived neuronal progenitors *in vitro*. *Eur. J. Neurosci.* 21, 69–80. doi: 10.1111/j.1460-9568.2004.03849.x

Gehler, S., Gallo, G., Veien, E., and Letourneau, P. C. (2004). p75 neurotrophin receptor signaling regulates growth cone filopodial dynamics through modulating RhoA activity. *J. Neurosci.* 24, 4363–4372. doi: 10.1523/JNEUROSCI.0404-04.2004

Genoud, C., Knott, G. W., Sakata, K., Lu, B., and Welker, E. (2004). Altered synapse formation in the adult somatosensory cortex of brain-derived neurotrophic factor heterozygote mice. *J. Neurosci.* 24, 2394–2400. doi: 10.1523/JNEUROSCI.4040-03.2004

Gorski, J. A., Zeiler, S. R., Tamowski, S., and Jones, K. R. (2003). Brain-derived neurotrophic factor is required for the maintenance of cortical dendrites. *J. Neurosci.* 23, 6856–6865.

Gottmann, K., Mittmann, T., and Lessmann, V. (2009). BDNF signaling in the formation, maturation and plasticity of glutamatergic and GABAergic synapses. *Exp. Brain Res.* 199, 203–234. doi: 10.1007/s00221-009-1994-z

He, X. P., Kotloski, R., Nef, S., Luikart, B. W., Parada, L. F., and Mcnamara, J. O. (2004). Conditional deletion of TrkB but not BDNF prevents epileptogenesis in the kindling model. *Neuron* 43, 31–42. doi: 10.1016/j.neuron.2004.06.019

Holthoff, K., Zecevic, D., and Konnerth, A. (2010). Rapid time course of action potentials in spines and remote dendrites of mouse visual cortex neurons. *J. Physiol.* 588, 1085–1096. doi: 10.1113/jphysiol.2009.184960

Holtmaat, A., and Svoboda, K. (2009). Experience-dependent structural synaptic plasticity in the mammalian brain. *Nat. Rev. Neurosci.* 10, 647–658. doi: 10.1038/nrn2699

Hong, E. J., Mccord, A. E., and Greenberg, M. E. (2008). A biological function for the neuronal activity-dependent component of Bdnf transcription in the development of cortical inhibition. *Neuron* 60, 610–624. doi: 10.1016/j.neuron.2008.09.024

Horch, H. W., Krüttgen, A., Portbury, S. D., and Katz, L. C. (1999). Destabilization of cortical dendrites and spines by BDNF. *Neuron* 23, 353–364. doi: 10.1016/S0896-6273(00)80785-0

Ji, Y., Lu, Y., Yang, F., Shen, W., Tang, T. T., Feng, L., et al. (2010). Acute and gradual increases in BDNF concentration elicit distinct signaling and functions in neurons. *Nat. Neurosci.* 13, 302–309. doi: 10.1038/nn.2505

Ji, Y., Pang, P. T., Feng, L., and Lu, B. (2005). Cyclic AMP controls BDNF-induced TrkB phosphorylation and dendritic spine formation in mature hippocampal neurons. *Nat. Neurosci.* 8, 164–172. doi: 10.1038/nn1381

Korte, M., Carroll, P., Wolf, E., Brem, G., Thoenen, H., and Bonhoeffer, T. (1995). Hippocampal long-term potentiation is impaired in mice lacking brain-derived neurotrophic factor. *Proc. Natl. Acad. Sci. U.S.A.* 92, 8856–8860. doi: 10.1073/pnas.92.19.8856

Kramar, E. A., Lin, B., Lin, C. Y., Arai, A. C., Gall, C. M., and Lynch, G. (2004). A novel mechanism for the facilitation of theta-induced long-term potentiation by brain-derived neurotrophic factor. *J. Neurosci.* 24, 5151–5161. doi: 10.1523/JNEUROSCI.0800-04.2004

Krucker, T., Siggins, G. R., and Halpain, S. (2000). Dynamic actin filaments are required for stable long-term potentiation (LTP) in area CA1 of the hippocampus. *Proc. Natl. Acad. Sci. U.S.A.* 97, 6856–6861. doi: 10.1073/pnas.100139797

Kwon, H. B., and Sabatini, B. L. (2011). Glutamate induces de novo growth of functional spines in developing cortex. *Nature* 474, 100–104. doi: 10.1038/nature09986

Lang, S. B., Bonhoeffer, T., and Lohmann, C. (2006). Simultaneous imaging of morphological plasticity and calcium dynamics in dendrites. *Nat. Protoc.* 1, 1859–1864. doi: 10.1038/nprot.2006.267

Lang, S. B., Stein, V., Bonhoeffer, T., and Lohmann, C. (2007). Endogenous brain-derived neurotrophic factor triggers fast calcium transients at synapses in developing dendrites. *J. Neurosci.* 27, 1097–1105. doi: 10.1523/JNEUROSCI.3590-06.2007

Li, C., Peoples, R. W., and Weight, F. F. (1997). Mg^{2+} inhibition of ATP-activated current in rat nodose ganglion neurons: evidence that Mg^{2+} decreases the agonist affinity of the receptor. *J. Neurophysiol.* 77, 3391–3395.

Lohmann, C. (2009). Calcium signaling and the development of specific neuronal connections. *Prog. Brain Res.* 175, 443–452. doi: 10.1016/S0079-6123(09)17529-5

Luikart, B. W., Nef, S., Virmani, T., Lush, M. E., Liu, Y., Kavalali, E. T., et al. (2005). TrkB has a cell-autonomous role in the establishment of hippocampal Schaffer collateral synapses. *J. Neurosci.* 25, 3774–3786. doi: 10.1523/JNEUROSCI.0041-05.2005

Marty, S., Berninger, B., Carroll, P., and Thoenen, H. (1996). GABAergic stimulation regulates the phenotype of hippocampal interneurons through the regulation of brain-derived neurotrophic factor. *Neuron* 16, 565–570. doi: 10.1016/S0896-6273(00)80075-6

Mayer, M. L., and Westbrook, G. L. (1987). Permeation and block of N-methyl-D-aspartic acid receptor channels by divalent cations in mouse cultured central neurones. *J. Physiol.* 394, 501–527.

Mcallister, A. K., Katz, L. C., and Lo, D. C. (1996). Neurotrophin regulation of cortical dendritic growth requires activity. *Neuron* 17, 1057–1064. doi: 10.1016/S0896-6273(00)80239-1

Mcallister, A. K., Lo, D. C., and Katz, L. C. (1995). Neurotrophins regulate dendritic growth in developing visual cortex. *Neuron* 15, 791–803. doi: 10.1016/0896-6273(95)90171-X

Meijering, E., Jacob, M., Sarria, J. C., Steiner, P., Hirling, H., and Unser, M. (2004). Design and validation of a tool for neurite tracing and analysis in fluorescence microscopy images. *Cytometry A* 58, 167–176. doi: 10.1002/cyto.a.20022

Messaoudi, E., Kanhema, T., Soule, J., Tiron, A., Dagyte, G., Da, S. B., et al. (2007). Sustained Arc/Arg3.1 synthesis controls long-term potentiation consolidation through regulation of local actin polymerization in the dentate gyrus *in vivo*. *J. Neurosci.* 27, 10445–10455. doi: 10.1523/JNEUROSCI.2883-07.2007

Minichiello, L. (2009). TrkB signalling pathways in LTP and learning. *Nat. Rev. Neurosci.* 10, 850–860. doi: 10.1038/nrn2738

Minichiello, L., Korte, M., Wolfer, D., Kuhn, R., Unsicker, K., Cestari, V., et al. (1999). Essential role for TrkB receptors in hippocampus-mediated learning. *Neuron* 24, 401–414. doi: 10.1016/S0896-6273(00)80853-3

Monteggia, L. M., Luikart, B., Barrot, M., Theobold, D., Malkovska, I., Nef, S., et al. (2007). Brain-derived neurotrophic factor conditional knockouts show gender differences in depression-related behaviors. *Biol. Psychiatry* 61, 187–197. doi: 10.1016/j.biopsych.2006.03.021

Papa, M., Bundman, M. C., Greenberger, V., and Segal, M. M. (1995). Morphological analysis of dendritic spine development in primary cultures of hippocampal neurons. *J. Neurosci.* 15, 1–11.

Park, H., and Poo, M. M. (2012). Neurotrophin regulation of neural circuit development and function. *Nat. Rev. Neurosci.* 14, 7–23. doi: 10.1038/nrn3379

Parkhurst, C. N., Yang, G., Ninan, I., Savas, J. N., Yates, J. R. 3rd., Lafaille, J. J., et al. (2013). Microglia promote learning-dependent synapse formation through brain-derived neurotrophic factor. *Cell* 155, 1596–1609. doi: 10.1016/j.cell.2013.11.030

Psotta, L., Lessmann, V., and Endres, T. (2013). Impaired fear extinction learning in adult heterozygous BDNF knock-out mice. *Neurobiol. Learn. Mem.* 103, 34–38. doi: 10.1016/j.nlm.2013.03.003

Rauskolb, S., Zagrebelsky, M., Dreznjak, A., Deogracias, R., Matsumoto, T., Wiese, S., et al. (2010). Global deprivation of brain-derived neurotrophic factor in the CNS reveals an area-specific requirement for dendritic growth. *J. Neurosci.* 30, 1739–1749. doi: 10.1523/JNEUROSCI.5100-09.2010

Rex, C. S., Lin, C. Y., Kramar, E. A., Chen, L. Y., Gall, C. M., and Lynch, G. (2007). Brain-derived neurotrophic factor promotes long-term potentiation-related cytoskeletal changes in adult hippocampus. *J. Neurosci.* 27, 3017–3029. doi: 10.1523/JNEUROSCI.4037-06.2007

Riedl, J., Crevenna, A. H., Kessenbrock, K., Yu, J. H., Neukirchen, D., Bista, M., et al. (2008). Lifeact: a versatile marker to visualize F-actin. *Nat. Methods* 5, 605–607. doi: 10.1038/nmeth.1220

Riedl, J., Flynn, K. C., Raducanu, A., Gartner, F., Beck, G., Bosl, M., et al. (2010). Lifeact mice for studying F-actin dynamics. *Nat. Methods* 7, 168–169. doi: 10.1038/nmeth0310-168

Rios, M., Fan, G., Fekete, C., Kelly, J., Bates, B., Kuehn, R., et al. (2001). Conditional deletion of brain-derived neurotrophic factor in the postnatal brain leads to obesity and hyperactivity. *Mol. Endocrinol.* 15, 1748–1757. doi: 10.1210/mend.15.10.0706

Rösch, H., Schweigreiter, R., Barde, Y. A., Bonhoeffer, T., and Korte, M. (2005). The neurotrophin receptor p75NTR modulates long-term depression and regulates the expression of AMPA receptor subunits in the hippocampus. *Proc. Natl. Acad. Sci. U.S.A.* 102, 7362–7367. doi: 10.1073/pnas.0502460102

Segal, R. A., and Greenberg, M. E. (1996). Intracellular signaling pathways activated by neurotrophic factors. *Annu. Rev. Neurosci.* 19, 463–489. doi: 10.1146/annurev.ne.19.030196.002335

Shimada, A., Mason, C. A., and Morrison, M. E. (1998). TrkB signaling modulates spine density and morphology independent of dendrite structure in cultured neonatal purkinje cells [Review]. *J. Neurosci.* 18, 8559–8570.

Sholl, D. A. (1953). Dendritic organization in the neurons of the visual and motor cortices of the cat. *J. Anat.* 87, 387–406.

Sjostrom, P. J., Rancz, E. A., Roth, A., and Hausser, M. (2008). Dendritic excitability and synaptic plasticity. *Physiol. Rev.* 88, 769–840. doi: 10.1152/physrev.00016.2007

Stranahan, A. M. (2011). Physiological variability in brain-derived neurotrophic factor expression predicts dendritic spine density in the mouse dentate gyrus. *Neurosci. Lett.* 495, 60–62. doi: 10.1016/j.neulet.2011.03.037

Tanaka, J., Horiike, Y., Matsuzaki, M., Miyazaki, T., Ellis-Davies, G. C., and Kasai, H. (2008). Protein synthesis and neurotrophin-dependent structural plasticity of single dendritic spines. *Science* 319, 1683–1687. doi: 10.1126/science.1152864

Thoenen, H. (1991). The changing scene of neurotrophic factors. *Trends Neurosci.* 14, 165–170. doi: 10.1016/0166-2236(91)90097-E

Trang, T., Beggs, S., Wan, X., and Salter, M. W. (2009). P2X4-receptor-mediated synthesis and release of brain-derived neurotrophic factor in microglia is dependent on calcium and p38-mitogen-activated protein kinase activation. *J. Neurosci.* 29, 3518–3528. doi: 10.1523/JNEUROSCI.5714-08.2009

Tyler, W. J., and Pozzo-Miller, L. (2003). Miniature synaptic transmission and BDNF modulate dendritic spine growth and form in rat CA1 neurones. *J. Physiol.* 553, 497–509. doi: 10.1113/jphysiol.2003.052639

Tyler, W. J., and Pozzo-Miller, L. D. (2001). BDNF enhances quantal neurotransmitter release and increases the number of docked vesicles at the active zones of hippocampal excitatory synapses. *J. Neurosci.* 21, 4249–4258.

Unger, T. J., Calderon, G. A., Bradley, L. C., Sena-Esteves, M., and Rios, M. (2007). Selective deletion of Bdnf in the ventromedial and dorsomedial hypothalamus of adult mice results in hyperphagic behavior and obesity. *J. Neurosci.* 27, 14265–14274. doi: 10.1523/JNEUROSCI.3308-07.2007

Von Bohlen Und Halbach, O. (2010). Involvement of BDNF in age-dependent alterations in the hippocampus. *Front. Aging Neurosci.* 2:36. doi: 10.3389/fnagi.2010.00036

Woo, N. H., Teng, H. K., Siao, C. J., Chiaruttini, C., Pang, P. T., Milner, T. A., et al. (2005). Activation of p75(NTR) by proBDNF facilitates hippocampal long-term depression. *Nat. Neurosci.* 8, 1069–1077. doi: 10.1038/nn1510

Yamashita, T., and Tohyama, M. (2003). The p75 receptor acts as a displacement factor that releases Rho from Rho-GDI. *Nat. Neurosci.* 6, 461–467. doi: 10.1038/nn1045

Yamashita, T., Tucker, K. L., and Barde, Y. A. (1999). Neurotrophin binding to the p75 receptor modulates Rho activity and axonal outgrowth. *Neuron* 24, 585–593. doi: 10.1016/S0896-6273(00)81114-9

Ying, S. W., Futter, M., Rosenblum, K., Webber, M. J., Hunt, S. P., Bliss, T. V., et al. (2002). Brain-derived neurotrophic factor induces long-term potentiation in intact adult hippocampus: requirement for ERK activation coupled to CREB and upregulation of Arc synthesis. *J. Neurosci.* 22, 1532–1540.

Zafra, F., Hengerer, B., Leibrock, J., Thoenen, H., and Lindholm, D. (1990). Activity dependent regulation of BDNF and NGF mRNAs in the rat hippocampus is mediated by non-NMDA glutamate receptors. *EMBO J.* 9, 3545–3550.

Zagrebelsky, M., Holz, A., Dechant, G., Barde, Y. A., Bonhoeffer, T., and Korte, M. (2005). The p75 neurotrophin receptor negatively modulates dendrite complexity and spine density in hippocampal neurons. *J. Neurosci.* 25, 9989–9999. doi: 10.1523/JNEUROSCI.2492-05.2005

Zagrebelsky, M., and Korte, M. (2013). Form follows function: BDNF and its involvement in sculpting the function and structure of synapses. *Neuropharmacology* 76, 628–638. doi: 10.1016/j.neuropharm.2013.05.029

Zakharenko, S. S., Patterson, S. L., Dragatsis, I., Zeitlin, S. O., Siegelbaum, S. A., Kandel, E. R., et al. (2003). Presynaptic BDNF required for a presynaptic but not postsynaptic component of LTP at hippocampal CA1-CA3 synapses. *Neuron* 39, 975–990. doi: 10.1016/S0896-6273(03)00543-9

Zhou, Q., Homma, K. J., and Poo, M. M. (2004). Shrinkage of dendritic spines associated with long-term depression of hippocampal synapses. *Neuron* 44, 749–757. doi: 10.1016/j.neuron.2004.11.011

Permissions

All chapters in this book were first published by Frontiers; hereby published with permission under the Creative Commons Attribution License or equivalent. Every chapter published in this book has been scrutinized by our experts. Their significance has been extensively debated. The topics covered herein carry significant findings which will fuel the growth of the discipline. They may even be implemented as practical applications or may be referred to as a beginning point for another development.

The contributors of this book come from diverse backgrounds, making this book a truly international effort. This book will bring forth new frontiers with its revolutionizing research information and detailed analysis of the nascent developments around the world.

We would like to thank all the contributing authors for lending their expertise to make the book truly unique. They have played a crucial role in the development of this book. Without their invaluable contributions this book wouldn't have been possible. They have made vital efforts to compile up to date information on the varied aspects of this subject to make this book a valuable addition to the collection of many professionals and students.

This book was conceptualized with the vision of imparting up-to-date information and advanced data in this field. To ensure the same, a matchless editorial board was set up. Every individual on the board went through rigorous rounds of assessment to prove their worth. After which they invested a large part of their time researching and compiling the most relevant data for our readers.

The editorial board has been involved in producing this book since its inception. They have spent rigorous hours researching and exploring the diverse topics which have resulted in the successful publishing of this book. They have passed on their knowledge of decades through this book. To expedite this challenging task, the publisher supported the team at every step. A small team of assistant editors was also appointed to further simplify the editing procedure and attain best results for the readers.

Apart from the editorial board, the designing team has also invested a significant amount of their time in understanding the subject and creating the most relevant covers. They scrutinized every image to scout for the most suitable representation of the subject and create an appropriate cover for the book.

The publishing team has been an ardent support to the editorial, designing and production team. Their endless efforts to recruit the best for this project, has resulted in the accomplishment of this book. They are a veteran in the field of academics and their pool of knowledge is as vast as their experience in printing. Their expertise and guidance has proved useful at every step. Their uncompromising quality standards have made this book an exceptional effort. Their encouragement from time to time has been an inspiration for everyone.

The publisher and the editorial board hope that this book will prove to be a valuable piece of knowledge for researchers, students, practitioners and scholars across the globe.

List of Contributors

Menahem Segal and Eduard Korkotian
Department of Neurobiology, The Weizman Institute, Rehovot, Israel

Michal Stawarski and Jakub Wlodarczyk
Laboratory of Cell Biophysics, Department of Molecular and Cellular Neurobiology, Nencki Institute of Experimental Biology, Warsaw, Mazowieckie, Poland

Marzena Stefaniuk
Laboratory of Neurobiology, Department of Molecular and Cellular Neurobiology, Nencki Institute of Experimental Biology, Warsaw, Mzowieckie, Poland

Guy N. Elston
Centre for Cognitive Neuroscience, Sunshine Coast, QLD, Australia

Ichiro Fujita
Graduate School of Frontier Biosciences and Center for Information and Neural Networks, Osaka University and National Institute of Communication Technology, Suita, Japan

Saturnino Spiga
Department of Animal Biology and Ecology, University of Cagliari, Cagliari, Italy

Giovanna Mulas
Department of Animal Biology and Ecology, University of Cagliari, Cagliari, Italy
"G.Minardi" Laboratory of Cognitive Neuroscience, Department of Chemistry and Pharmacy, University of Sassari, Sassari, Italy

Francesca Piras
Department of Animal Biology and Ecology, University of Cagliari, Cagliari, Italy
Department of Natural Science and the Territory, University of Sassari, Sassari, Italy

Marco Diana
"G.Minardi" Laboratory of Cognitive Neuroscience, Department of Chemistry and Pharmacy, University of Sassari, Sassari, Italy

Carlos Gerardo Dotti, Jose Antonio Esteban and María Dolores Ledesma
Centro Biología Molecular Severo Ochoa, CSIC-UAM, Madrid, Spain

Daniel Studer and Werner Graber
Institute of Anatomy, University of Bern, Bern, Switzerland

Xin Xu, Eric C. Miller and Lucas Pozzo-Miller
Department of Neurobiology, Civitan International Research Center, The University of Alabama at Birmingham, Birmingham, AL, USA

Emily A. Kelly and Ania K. Majewska
Department of Neurobiology and Anatomy, Center for Visual Science, School of Medicine and Dentistry, University of Rochester, Rochester, NY, USA

Lisa A. Opanashuk
Department of Environmental Medicine, University of Rochester, Rochester, NY, USA

Kevin Takasaki and Bernardo L. Sabatini
Department of Neurobiology, Harvard Medical School, Howard Hughes Medical Institute, Boston, MA, USA

Michael Frotscher, Xuejun Chai and Shanting Zhao
Institute for Structural Neurobiology, Center for Molecular Neurobiology Hamburg, University Medical Center Hamburg-Eppendorf, Hamburg, Germany

Sigrun Nestel
Institute of Anatomy and Cell Biology, University of Freiburg, Freiburg, Germany

Connie Cheng, Olivia Trzcinski and Laurie C. Doering
Department of Pathology and Molecular Medicine, McMaster University, Hamilton, ON, Canada

James J. Mancuso, Jie Cheng, Zheng Yin, Jared C. Gilliam, Xiaofeng Xia, Xuping Li and Stephen T. C. Wong
Department of Systems Medicine and Bioengineering, Houston Methodist Research Institute, Houston, TX, USA
TT and WF Chao Center for Bioinformatics Research and Imaging for Neurosciences, Houston Methodist Research Institute, Houston, TX, USA

Aaron D. Levy and Mitchell H. Omar
Interdepartmental Neuroscience Program, Yale University, New Haven, CT, USA
Department of Molecular Biophysics and Biochemistry, Yale University, New Haven, CT, USA

Max Adrian, Corette J. Wierenga, Casper C. Hoogenraad and Lukas C. Kapitein
Cell Biology, Department of Biology, Faculty of Science, Utrecht University, Utrecht, Netherlands

Anthony J. Koleske
Interdepartmental Neuroscience Program, Yale University, New Haven, CT, USA
Department of Molecular Biophysics and Biochemistry, Yale University, New Haven, CT, USA
Department of Neurobiology, Yale University, New Haven, CT, USA

Remy Kusters
Department of Applied Physics, Eindhoven University of Technology, Eindhoven, Netherlands

Cornelis Storm
Department of Applied Physics, Eindhoven University of Technology, Eindhoven, Netherlands
Institute for Complex Molecular Systems, Eindhoven University of Technology, Eindhoven, Netherlands

Chia-Chien Chen and Yi Zuo
Department of Molecular, Cell and Developmental Biology, University of California at Santa Cruz, Santa Cruz, CA, USA

Ju Lu
Department of Biological Sciences and James H. Clark Center, Stanford University, Stanford, CA, USA

Roberto Araya
Department of Neurosciences, Faculty of Medicine, University of Montreal, Montreal, QC, Canada

Mikko Koskinen and Pirta Hotulainen
Neuroscience Center, University of Helsinki, Helsinki, Finland

Javier DeFelipe
Instituto Cajal (CSIC), Madrid, Spain
Laboratorio Cajal de Circuitos Corticales (Centro de Tecnología Biomédica: UPM), and CIBERNED, Madrid, Spain

Sarah Malanowski and Carl F. Craver
Department of Philosophy, Washington University in St. Louis, St. Louis, MO, USA

Yann Bernardinelli, Irina Nikonenko and Dominique Muller
Department of Basic Neurosciences, University of Geneva Medical School, Geneva, Switzerland

Yves Kellner, Nina Gödecke, Tobias Dierkes, Nils Thieme, Marta Zagrebelsky and Martin Korte
Division of Cellular Neurobiology, Zoological Institute, TU Braunschweig, Braunschweig, Germany

Index